THE NETTER COLLECTION

OF MEDICAL ILLUSTRATIONS

Nervous System

Part I—Brain

3rd Edition

VOLUME 7

A compilation of paintings prepared by **FRANK H. NETTER, MD**

Edited by

Michael J. Aminoff, MD, DSc, FRCP
Distinguished Professor Emeritus
Department of Neurology
School of Medicine
University of California
San Francisco, California

Scott L. Pomeroy, MD, PhD
Bronson Crothers Professor of Neurology
Harvard Medical School
Chair, Department of Neurology
Neurologist-in-Chief
Boston Children's Hospital
Boston, Massachusetts

Kerry H. Levin, MD
Professor of Neurology
Cleveland Clinic Lerner College of Medicine of Case Western
Reserve University
Chairman, Department of Neurology
Director, Neuromuscular Center
Cleveland Clinic
Cleveland, Ohio

Additional Illustrations by

Carlos A.G. Machado, MD

CONTRIBUTING ILLUSTRATORS
John A. Craig, MD
Tiffany S. DaVanzo, MA, CMI
DragonFly Media
Anita Impagliazzo, MA, CMI
Paul Kim, MS
Kristen W. Marzejon, CMI
James A. Perkins, MS, MFA

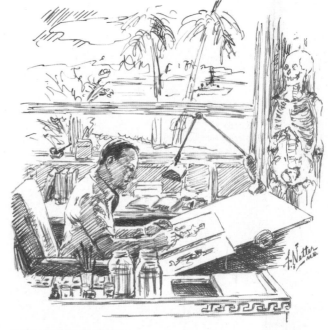

Self portrait by Dr. Netter

ELSEVIER

Elsevier
1600 John F. Kennedy Blvd.
Suite 1600
Philadelphia, Pennsylvania

THE NETTER COLLECTION OF MEDICAL ILLUSTRATIONS:
NERVOUS SYSTEM, PART I: BRAIN, VOLUME 7, THIRD EDITION   ISBN: 978-0-323-88084-8

Notices

Publisher: Elyse O'Grady
Senior Content Strategist: Marybeth Thiel
Publishing Services Manager: Catherine Jackson
Senior Project Manager/Specialist: Carrie Stetz
Book Design: Patrick Ferguson

Printed in India

Last digit is the print number: 9 8 7 6 5 4 3 2 1

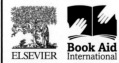

Working together
to grow libraries in
developing countries

www.elsevier.com • www.bookaid.org

"Clarification is the goal. No matter how beautifully it is painted, a medical illustration has little value if it does not make clear a medical point."
—Frank H. Netter, MD

Dr. Frank Netter created an illustrated legacy unifying his perspectives as physician, artist, and teacher. Both his greatest challenge and greatest success was charting a middle course between artistic clarity and instructional complexity. That success is captured in *The Netter Collection,* beginning in 1948 when the first comprehensive book of Netter's work was published by CIBA Pharmaceuticals. It met with such success that over the following 40 years the collection was expanded into an 8-volume series—with each title devoted to a single body system. Between 2011 and 2016, these books were updated and rereleased. Now, after another decade of innovation in medical imaging, renewed focus on patient-centered care, conscious efforts to improve inequities in healthcare and medical education, and a growing understanding of many clinical conditions, including multisystem effects of COVID-19, we are happy to make available a third edition of Netter's timeless work enhanced and informed by modern medical knowledge and context.

Inside the classic green covers, students and practitioners will find hundreds of original works of art. This is a collection of the human body in pictures— Dr. Netter called them *pictures,* never paintings. The latest expert medical knowledge is anchored by the sublime style of Frank Netter that has guided physicians' hands and nurtured their imaginations for more than half a century.

Noted artist-physician Carlos Machado, MD, the primary successor responsible for continuing the Netter tradition, has particular appreciation for the Green Book series. "*The Reproductive System* is of special significance for those who, like me, deeply admire Dr. Netter's work. In this volume, he masters the representation of textures of different surfaces, which I like to call 'the rhythm of the brush,' since it is the dimension, the direction of the strokes, and the interval separating them that create the illusion of given textures: organs have their external surfaces, the surfaces of their cavities, and texture of their parenchymas realistically represented. It set the style for the subsequent volumes of *The Netter Collection*—each an amazing combination of painting masterpieces and precise scientific information."

This third edition could not exist without the dedication of all those who edited, authored, or in other ways contributed to the second edition or the original books, nor, of course, without the excellence of Dr. Netter. For this third edition, we also owe our gratitude to the authors, editors, and artists whose relentless efforts were instrumental in adapting these classic works into reliable references for today's clinicians in training and in practice. From all of us with the Netter Publishing Team at Elsevier, thank you.

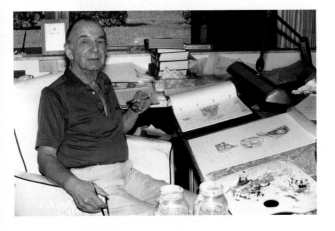

Dr. Frank Netter at work.

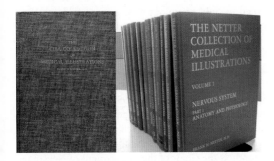

The single-volume "Blue Book" that preceded the multivolume *Netter Collection of Medical Illustrations* series, affectionately known as the "Green Books."

**The
Netter Collection**
OF MEDICAL ILLUSTRATIONS
3rd Edition

Volume 1 **Reproductive System**
Volume 2 **Endocrine System**
Volume 3 **Respiratory System**
Volume 4 **Integumentary System**
Volume 5 **Urinary System**
Volume 6 **Musculoskeletal System**
Volume 7 **Nervous System**
Volume 8 **Cardiovascular System**
Volume 9 **Digestive System**

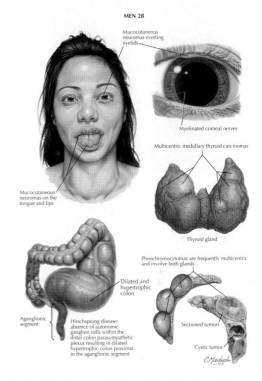

An illustrated plate painted by Carlos Machado, MD.

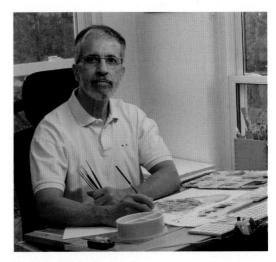

Dr. Carlos Machado at work.

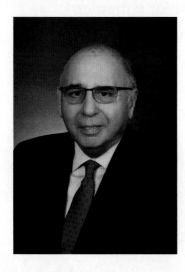

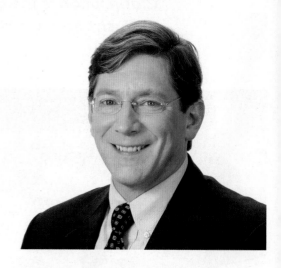

Michael J. Aminoff, MD, DSc, was born and educated in England, graduating from University College London in 1962 and from University College Hospital Medical School as a physician in 1965. He subsequently trained in neurology and clinical neurophysiology at The National Hospital for Neurology and Neurosurgery (Queen Square) in London and also undertook basic research on spinal physiology at its affiliated Institute of Neurology, which led to the award of an MD degree (which, in England, is an advanced medical degree based on research) on completion of his thesis. In 1974 he moved from England to the University of California San Francisco (UCSF) School of Medicine, where he became Professor of Neurology in 1982 and Distinguished Professor of Neurology in 2010 and is now Distinguished Professor Emeritus. He directed the Clinical Neurophysiology Laboratories at UCSF until July 2004 and then served as Executive Vice Chair of the Department of Neurology (2004–2017).

Dr. Aminoff is the author of over 240 original medical and scientific articles, more than 200 book chapters on neurologic topics, and the author or editor of numerous books, many of which have gone into several editions. His published scientific contributions led to the award of a Doctorate in Science (an advanced doctorate in the Faculty of Science) in 2000 by the University of London. He is the one of the two editors-in-chief of the four-volume *Encyclopedia of the Neurological Sciences*

published by Academic Press in 2003 (2nd edition, 2014). He is also one of the series editors of the prestigious multivolume *Handbook of Clinical Neurology* (Elsevier). He was Editor-in Chief of the journal *Muscle and Nerve* from 1998 to 2007 and also serves on numerous other editorial boards of medical and scientific journals. His other interests include medical history, and he has written biographies of Brown-Séquard (Raven Press, 1993; Oxford University Press, 2011), Sir Charles Bell (Oxford University Press, 2016), and Victor Horsley (Cambridge University Press, 2022).

The awards that he has received include the Lifetime Achievement Award of the American Association of Neuromuscular and Electrodiagnostic Medicine in 2006, the A.B. Baker Award of the American Academy of Neurology in 2007 for lifetime achievements and contributions to medical education, and the Robert S. Schwab Award for outstanding contributions to research in peripheral clinical neurophysiology from the American Clinical Neurophysiology Society in 2019. An endowed chair is to be named after him at UCSF, and a lectureship has been named for him within the Division of Neurology at Miami Neuroscience Institute, South Florida.

He served for 8 years as a director of the American Board of Psychiatry and Neurology, serving as chairman of the board in 2011. He is married, lives in San Francisco, and has a daughter who is a pediatrician and two sons who are attorneys.

Scott L. Pomeroy, MD, PhD, was born and educated in Southwest Ohio, graduating from Miami University in 1975 and the MD/PhD program of the University of Cincinnati in 1982. His doctoral research focused on brainstem neurophysiology and pain inhibition. After a pediatric residency at Boston Children's Hospital, he trained in child neurology at St. Louis Children's Hospital and studied nervous system development as a postdoctoral fellow of Dale Purves at Washington University in St. Louis, work for which he won the Child Neurology Society Young Investigator Award in 1989. After returning to Boston Children's Hospital and Harvard Medical School in 1991, he cofounded the neuro-oncology service and conducts basic research to understand how normal development of brain cells becomes derailed to cause childhood brain tumors. He currently is the Chair of the Department of Neurology and Neurologist-in-Chief of Boston Children's Hospital, the Bronson Crothers Professor of Neurology at Harvard Medical School, and Co-director of the Eunice K. Shriver National Institutes of Child Health and Human Development–funded Intellectual and Developmental Disabilities Research Center of Boston Children's Hospital and Harvard Medical School.

Dr. Pomeroy served as an editor of the second edition of this atlas and is one of four editors of the widely read textbook *Bradley and Daroff's Neurology in Clinical Practice* (Elsevier). He served as Associate Editor of *Annals of Neurology* from 2013 to 2021 and has served on the editorial boards of several other journals in the fields of neurology and neuro-oncology. He has contributed more than 200 peer-reviewed papers and book chapters.

Dr. Pomeroy has won numerous awards for his research and clinical care of children with brain tumors, including the Sidney Carter Award of the American Academy of Neurology, the Daniel Drake Medal of the University of Cincinnati College of Medicine, the Compassionate Caregiver Award of the Schwartz Center for Compassionate Healthcare, and the Bernard Sachs Award of the Child Neurology Society. He was elected as a member of the National Academy of Medicine in 2017. Dr. Pomeroy and his wife, Marie, live in Boston and spend much of their time devoted to their children and seven grandchildren, who live in Maryland and Colorado.

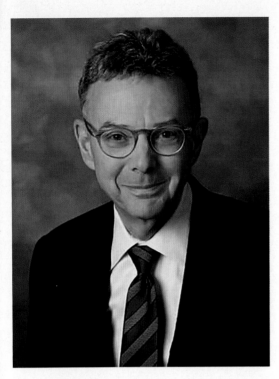

Kerry Levin, MD, graduated from the Johns Hopkins University School of Arts and Sciences in 1973 and the Johns Hopkins University School of Medicine in 1977. After an internal medicine residency at the Case Western Reserve University Hospitals of Cleveland, he completed a neurology residency at the Hospital of the University of Chicago and an EMG/Neuromuscular Fellowship at Mayo Clinic, Rochester, Minnesota.

Dr. Levin has practiced neurology and neuromuscular medicine at Cleveland Clinic since 1984. He has served as Director of the Neurology Residency Program and the Clinical Neurophysiology and Neuromuscular Medicine Fellowship programs. At Cleveland Clinic he has been Chair of the Department of Neurology since 2008 and Director of the Neuromuscular Center since 2006. He has authored and edited numerous publications and texts, including two clinical neurophysiology volumes of the *Handbook of Clinical Neurology* (Elsevier). He formerly served on the editorial board of *Continuum*, a publication of the American Academy of Neurology. Dr. Levin was a director of the American Board of Psychiatry and Neurology for 8 years and served as its chairman in 2017. In 2021 he received the Distinguished Physician Award of the American Association of Neuromuscular and Electrodiagnostic Medicine. He has one daughter and lives with his wife in Cleveland.

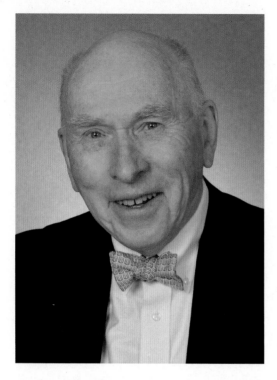

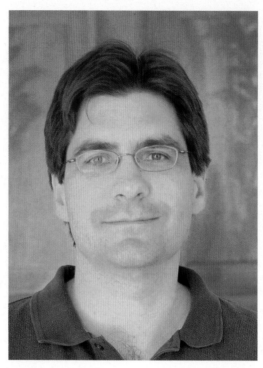

H. Royden Jones Jr, MD, died in June 2013, shortly after the previous edition of this book was published. He had been instrumental in its development, assembling us as an editorial team to see it to fruition, and was particularly proud of it, for he had known Frank Netter personally. He was greatly missed as we worked on this new (third) edition.

Dr. Jones received his medical degree in 1962 from Northwestern University Medical School and trained in neurology and clinical neurophysiology at the Mayo Clinic. He joined the Lahey Clinic in 1972 and was appointed the Jaime Ortiz-Patiño Chair in Neurology in 1996. He was an outstanding physician and teacher who specialized in neuromuscular disorders and a clinical electromyographer who founded the EMG Laboratory at the Lahey Clinic; he also directed the laboratory at Boston Children's Hospital. He was a Director of the American Board of Psychiatry and Neurology (1997–2004) and in 2007 received the Distinguished Physician Award from the American Association of Neuromuscular and Electrodiagnostic Medicine, a well-deserved tribute. Dr. Jones taught each of us and touched our lives in many other ways. He is missed by all who knew him.

Ted M. Burns, MD, died in June 2022. He was one of the editors of the second edition of this book, and his contributions to its structure and content live on in this new edition. A leader in American neurology, he has left a legacy of excellence in clinical care, scholarship, and service to his own institution and many professional societies. Although his chosen area of interest was neuromuscular disorders, his goal was to advance neurologic knowledge and its access to practicing neurologists nationally and internationally. In his honor, the American Brain Foundation and American Academy of Neurology established the annual Ted M. Burns Humanism in Neurology Award in 2020. At the time of his death, Ted was the Vice Chair of Clinical Affairs in the Department of Neurology at the University of Virginia and held an Endowed Chair as the Harrison Distinguished Teaching Professor. He was head of the Neuromuscular Disorders Division and Director of the Electromyography Laboratory. We miss him.

PREFACE, ACKNOWLEDGMENTS, AND DEDICATION

PREFACE

Ten years have passed since the last edition of this volume was published. They have been exciting years in the neurosciences and in clinical neurology. Advances in molecular biology have led to a greater understanding of many disease processes. Disease prediction, prognostication, and treatment are becoming tailored more completely to individual patients, as exemplified by the management of brain tumors. With advances in genomics and other factors, personalized medicine is becoming an increasing reality, something quite unimaginable just a few years ago.

Recent advances, expanding knowledge, and increasing specialization within all branches of clinical medicine have made it difficult for trainees and non-neurologists to grasp the essentials of clinical neurology and for established neurologists to remain abreast of developments in subspecialities other than their own. These factors have prompted the development of this new edition of *The Netter Collection of Medical Illustrations: Nervous System*.

Frank Netter's initial atlas of neurologic structure and function, first published in 1957, provided a very concise introduction to the nervous system for generations of students. He was able to simplify complicated anatomic components and physiologic processes and to illustrate them memorably in paintings that were both arresting and pleasing. The initial single-part publication provided a stimulating introduction to many intriguing and important clinical aspects of neurologic medicine. Although the scope was somewhat limited in its clinical depth, the vivid and intriguing plates that accompanied each topic provided a means of learning about the neurosciences that was both exciting and satisfying. To widen the content of the work, a second volume was published in 1986, and these two parts are generally referred to as the first edition of *Netter's Collection of Medical Illustrations of the Nervous System*.

When we developed the second edition, published in 2013, we expanded the scope of the volumes to bring them up to date and make them more comprehensive, helped by a superb group of medical artists who were able to follow Frank Netter's original style. We discussed many neurologic disorders from both basic science and clinical perspectives, supplementing the system-based approach now used in many medical schools. Encompassing the many advances in genetics, immunology, and imaging that had occurred was challenging, especially because the size of the volume had to be limited if it was to retain its utility.

Such is the pace of medical advance that now—just 10 years later—we have felt the need to prepare this new edition. We hope that today's medical students will find it an exciting introduction to the study of the nervous system in health and disease and will derive as much pleasure from the illustrations as we have been fortunate enough to enjoy.

ACKNOWLEDGMENTS

The editors thank their many neuroscience colleagues who contributed to this text, as well as our many patients through whom we learned the art and science of neurology. We also express our admiration and thanks to our artist colleagues Carlos A.G. Machado, MD, Kristen W. Marzejon, MS, MFA, Tiffany S. DaVanzo, MA, CMI, Paul Kim, MS, and James A. Perkins, MS, MFA, who have so carefully upheld Frank Netter's approach to medical illustration. These dedicated artists have expertly created a number of outstanding new plates for these volumes. Finally, the entire Elsevier editorial team, particularly Marybeth Thiel, Elyse O'Grady, and Carrie Stetz, have been gracious and cooperative in supporting our goals. It has been a distinct pleasure having such professional and dedicated colleagues.

DEDICATION

These two volumes are dedicated to our wives, children, and grandchildren, whose love and support gave us the time to work on this project; to our students, residents, and fellows, who challenged us to be fine teachers; and to our many and dear patients for whom we have been honored to care.

Michael J. Aminoff
Scott L. Pomeroy
Kerry H. Levin

FOREWORD TO THE SECOND EDITION

Combining Dr. Frank Netter's classic medical illustrations with a first-rate, current text is a brilliant idea. The choice of authors could not be better; as a group they are well-regarded clinicians whose experience as teachers, having national and sometimes international reputations, is well illustrated by the clarity of their writing. Very clearly there has been great attention to achieving a supple, readable style. The added images, such as the MRIs and other visual tools, are very well chosen. Their clarity for teaching purposes matches the text in quality, and these are nicely integrated with Netter's classic imagery. The most impressive thing about this effort is the marvelous embedding of Netter's illustrations into the text with preservation of coherence.

The original publication of these illustrations in the first Netter atlas was a regular, albeit unofficial, part of medical school neurologic learning early in my career during the 1960s. Concomitantly, Netter's corollary bimonthly white-covered slim paperback *Clinical Symposia* was always welcome with the new mail...more than one issue was frequently strewn on my desk. These were essentially mini atlases always centered by a striking illustration immediately telling you what the dedicated subject would be. Each new edition was always accompanied by 15 to 20 new and now classic Netter illustrations. It was not clear how Ciba Pharmaceutical wanted to specifically influence us in trade for their marvelous free teaching aids. Now I wish I had saved many of them.

Dr. Netter's style is absolutely distinctive. It has the look of mid-20th-century illustration art, somewhat like Norman Rockwell's. Not unlike a Rockwell, one can recognize a Netter illustration across the room. He is consistent no matter what his subject; his work, including its vivid coloration, is always particularly serious despite its sometimes cartoonish appearance. Netter is distinctive the way all truly great artists' work invariably is, no matter what the level of sophistication. Think of Mondrian. Think of Francis Bacon. Totally different than Netter, they are good examples of great "high" art that are similarly distinctive and consistent. And such consistency, regardless of the subject, is surely part of what makes for genius with subsequent fame and greatness. Accompanied by their new text in two detailed parts covering the brain as well as the spinal cord and its related peripheral motor sensory units, Frank Netter's art has been beautifully resurrected once again. These will surely provide learning with pleasure to yet another generation of medical students during their neurologic studies.

Nicholas A. Vick, MD
Clinical Professor of Neurology
Pritzker School of Medicine
University of Chicago
Chicago, Illinois
Department of Neurology
NorthShore University Health System
Evanston, Illinois

While attending a major medical meeting more than 2 decades after using the first Netter *Nervous System,* published in 1957, I met a representative of the Ciba Pharmaceutical Medical Education division—the corporation that sponsored Dr. Frank Netter's medical artistic career for more than 40 years—and inquired about the possibility of having him create paintings relevant to the peripheral motor and sensory unit and, particularly, the major peripheral nerves. Within a few months, I was surprised to receive a handwritten letter from Dr. Netter, asking for more detailed suggestions. This led to an invitation to meet with him at his Florida beachfront home and to advise him in reference to his current orthopedic disorders project.

Frank was a humble and engaging person entirely dedicated to his goal of illustrating all human anatomy and related clinical disorders. A day in his studio might be dedicated to interviewing physicians to discuss their area of expertise, who would provide him with a full appreciation of the subject before he started on his drawings. Sometimes after lunch he took a break from his ever-present cigars and his studio to play two or three holes of golf before returning to his various challenges. Most other days were dedicated to conceptualization, drawing, or painting sessions. Dr. Netter had an unbridled passion for his work. His artistic abilities were truly amazing—he was under contract to provide 93 new illustrations annually, which amounts to one every 4 days. He worked with vigor every day of the week until his death at age 85.

Unknown to me when we initially met, Frank previously had commenced his work on a new edition of his *Neuroscience Atlas,* having recognized the relatively limited scope of his initial volume. After we worked together for awhile, he showed this project to me, noting that it had remained dormant for a few years; subsequently, he asked me to become its clinical editor. There were to be two parts. *Part I,* dedicated to traditional basic neuroanatomy and neurophysiology, was essentially completed. The clinical portion of his revised atlas, *Part II, Neurologic and Neuromuscular Disorders,* required extensive new artwork and text and was first published in 1986. However, production costs and time restraints limited its clinical breadth and depth. Therefore Frank and I envisioned production of a more complete set of texts within 5 to 10 years to add further to these volumes. Although long overdue, thanks to the foresight of Elsevier, these volumes are now completed. There is no doubt that Dr. Netter would be extremely pleased with these results subsequent to the dedication of so many expert neurologic physicians. The new two-part volume supports his dream of very comprehensive, relevant, and totally up-to-date neuroscience atlases.

H. Royden Jones, MD

The Ciba Collection of Medical Illustrations was originally conceived as a series of atlases picturing the anatomy, embryology, physiology, pathology, and diseases of mankind, system by system. The creation of these atlases has been for me a labor of love to which I have devoted most of my working career. The first volume of this series was *Nervous System.* That volume was very well received and acclaimed by students, physicians, and members of allied professions throughout the world. It has been reprinted many times and published in a number of languages. The multitude of letters of appreciation I have received in the more than 30 years since its first publication have been a great source of satisfaction to me, even as I progressed with other volumes in the series.

From the beginning, however, certain deficiencies in the *Nervous System* volume became evident. It contained, for example, practically no coverage of the peripheral nervous system, of embryology, of basic neurophysiology—that is, nerve impulse transmissions and synapse—and the presentation of the neurologic and neuromuscular diseases was far too skimpy and incomplete. Furthermore, as time progressed and our knowledge advanced, the deficiencies became more significant. Advances in neuroradiology and neurosurgery made it important to update the illustrations of the blood vessels of the brain and spinal cord. The advent of the CT scan as a valuable diagnostic tool necessitated its inclusion as a specific procedure. Our improved understanding of the neuromuscular diseases and increased application of electromyography, electroencephalography, and nerve conduction studies called for a better presentation of basic neurophysiology and nerve-muscle relationships. The great progress in the study of neurologic disorders such as poliomyelitis, parkinsonism, myasthenia gravis, stroke, trauma, Alzheimer disease, and many others demanded amplification of the section on specific diseases of the nervous system. Finally, the better definition of the congenital and developmental disorders not only prompted presentation of those disorders but emphasized the importance of including a section on neuroembryology.

Accordingly, it has for many years been my desire to revise and expand this atlas in a new edition. I was, however, so busy with preparing other volumes of the *Ciba Collection* that it took me a long time to accomplish it. This was, to a certain extent, fortuitous, for it allowed me to include newer material that would not have been available for an earlier revision. But the volume of illustrations and accompanying texts grew to such an extent that they could not all be included in a single book. It was therefore decided to issue the atlas in two parts: Part I to include anatomy, embryology, physiology, and functional neuroanatomy and Part II, shortly forthcoming, to include all neurologic and neuromuscular diseases.

At the same time that I was working on this revision I was also occupied with preparing an atlas on the musculoskeletal system, and the great overlap between the fields of orthopedics—that is, musculoskeletal disorders and neurologic or neurosurgical disorders—became apparent. Indeed, many of the disorders to be covered lay in the realm of both specialties. Thus the two-part presentation of this atlas is advantageous because Part II bridges the gap between the two fields, and I believe this will be pertinent to both neurology-neurosurgery and orthopedics, as well as to the fields of general practice and internal medicine. Part I, on the other hand, will serve as a reference for basic understanding of much of the material in Part II and will be very useful for the student and for those in allied professions such as physical therapy, speech therapy, and psychology. All in all, I believe that in this revised edition of *Nervous System* I have corrected the deficiencies referred to above, as well as many others, and I hope it will prove as useful and helpful to all those who refer to it as the original edition apparently was in its day.

I take this opportunity to express my appreciation to all the collaborators and consultants who helped me with preparing this volume. They are all credited separately herein. I admire their erudition and I thank them for the time they gave me and the knowledge they imparted to me. It was a great pleasure for me to learn from them, and I cherish the friendships we established during our collaboration. The creation of this volume would have been impossible without their help. I also thank the Ciba-Geigy Corporation and its executives for the free hand they have given me in this project and the members of the editorial staff for their very helpful and dedicated cooperation.

Since the foundation for this volume was laid in its earlier edition, I reiterate here, with much nostalgia, my appreciation for the great men who guided me through that original endeavor. They were Dr. Abraham Kaplan, neurosurgeon and gifted student of Dr. Harvey Cushing; Dr. Albert Kuntz, pioneer in unraveling the mysteries of the autonomic nervous system; Dr. Gerhardt von Bonin, brilliant neurophysiologist; and Dr. W. R. Ingram, professor of anatomy at the University of Iowa, who devoted much of his career to study the hypothalamus. In regard to the editor of that original edition, I quote herewith the last paragraph from my introduction to that volume:

Every artist thrives on appreciation, understanding, and encouragement. In this respect I have been double fortunate. First, the warm reception which the medical profession as accorded my pictures has been a wonderful source of satisfaction to me. Second, more personal and close at hand, has been the inspiring personality of Dr. Ernst Oppenheimer. His understanding of the things I was trying to do, his appreciation of what I had done, and his encouragement to do more were a constant assurance that I was not alone. In addition, his vision of the scope and value of this atlas and his many coordinating activities in its behalf have been vital factors in the project.

Frank H. Netter, 1983

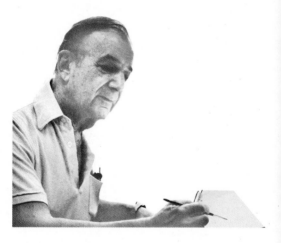

EDITORS-IN-CHIEF

Michael J. Aminoff, MD, DSc, FRCP
Distinguished Professor Emeritus
Department of Neurology
UCSF School of Medicine
University of California
San Francisco, California
EDITOR: PART I: SECTIONS 6, 7, 11, 14;
  PART II: SECTIONS 1, 2, 3, 7, 9
AUTHOR: PART I: PLATE 7.18; PART II: PLATES 2.1–2.29

Scott L. Pomeroy, MD, PhD
Bronson Crothers Professor of Neurology
Harvard Medical School
Chair, Department of Neurology
Neurologist-in-Chief
Boston Children's Hospital
Boston, Massachusetts
EDITOR: PART I: SECTIONS 1, 2, 3, 4, 5, 8, 12;
  PART II: SECTION 8

Kerry H. Levin, MD
Professor of Neurology
Cleveland Clinic Lerner College of Medicine
Case Western Reserve University
Chairman, Department of Neurology
Director, Neuromuscular Center
Cleveland Clinic
Cleveland, Ohio
EDITOR: PART I: SECTIONS 9, 10, 13;
  PART II: SECTIONS 4, 5, 6, 10, 11, 12

CONTRIBUTORS

Justin R. Abbatemarco, MD
Staff Physician
Mellen Center for Multiple Sclerosis
Neurological Institute
Cleveland Clinic
Cleveland, Ohio
PLATES 10.17–10.18

Mohammad Ammar Abdulrazzak, MD
Endovascular Surgical Neuroradiology
Cerebrovascular Center
Cleveland Clinic Foundation
Cleveland, Ohio
PLATES 9.20–9.21

Albert Aboseif, DO
Resident Physician
Department of Neurology, Neurological Institute
Cleveland Clinic Foundation
Cleveland, Ohio
PLATES 10.21–10.22

Harold P. Adams Jr, MD
Professor Emeritus
Department of Neurology
Division of Cerebrovascular Diseases
Carver College of Medicine
University of Iowa
Iowa City, Iowa
PLATES 9.41–9.45

Anas Alrohimi, MD
Endovascular Surgical Neuroradiology Fellow
Cerebrovascular Center, Neurological Institute
Department of Neurology
Cleveland Clinic
Cleveland, Ohio
PLATES 9.1–9.6

Moein Amin, MD
Neuroimmunology Fellow
Neurological Institute
Cleveland Clinic
Cleveland, Ohio
PLATES 10.3–10.5

Elizabeth Barkoudah, MD
Instructor in Neurology
Co-director, Cerebral Palsy and Spasticity
  Center
Program Director, Neurodevelopmental Disabilities
  Residency Program
Boston Children's Hospital
Boston, Massachusetts
PLATES 1.5–1.8, 1.10–1.12, 1.15–1.17, 1.23, 1.26–1.27

Robert A. Bermel, MD
Director, Mellen Center for Multiple Sclerosis
Neurological Institute
Cleveland Clinic
Cleveland, Ohio
PLATES 10.1, 10.3–10.5

Francois Bethoux, MD
Chairman, Department of Physical Medicine
  and Rehabilitation
Professor of Physical Medicine and Rehabilitation
Cleveland Clinic Lerner College of Medicine
Cleveland Clinic Foundation
Cleveland, Ohio
PLATES 9.47–9.50

Brian P. Brennan, MD, MMSc
Medical Director
Obsessive-Compulsive Disorders Institute
McLean Hospital
Belmont, Massachusetts;
Assistant Professor of Psychiatry
Harvard Medical School
Boston, Massachusetts
PLATES 4.8, 4.10

Andrew Blake Buletko, MD
Vascular Neurologist
Cleveland Clinic
Cleveland, Ohio
PLATES 9.26–9.27

Rahul Chandra, MD
Fellow, Vascular Neurology
Cleveland Clinic Foundation
Cleveland, Ohio
PLATES 9.9–9.11

Claudia Chaves, MD
Associate Professor of Neurology
Tufts University
Boston Massachusetts;
Staff Neurologist
Newton Wellesley Hospital
Newton, Massachusetts
PLATES 9.12–9.19

Jeffrey A. Cohen, MD
Hazel Prior Hostetler Endowed Chair
Professor of Neurology
Cleveland Clinic Lerner College of Medicine
Director, Experimental Therapeutics
Mellen Center for Multiple Sclerosis
Cleveland, Ohio
PLATE 10.14

Yasmin Cole-Lewis, PhD, MPH
Attending Psychologist, Department of Psychiatry
  and Behavioral Sciences
Boston Children's Hospital
Instructor of Psychology, Department of Psychiatry
Harvard Medical School
Boston, Massachusetts
PLATE 4.28

Hilary S. Connery, MD, PhDE
Clinical Director
Division of Alcohol, Drugs and Addiction
McLean Hospital
Belmont, Massachusetts;
Assistant Professor of Psychiatry
Harvard Medical School
Boston, Massachusetts
PLATES 4.14–4.19

Devon S. Conway, MD, MS
Staff Neurologist
Mellen Center for Multiple Sclerosis
Neurological Institute
Cleveland Clinic Foundation
Cleveland, Ohio
PLATES 10.8–10.11

Cristina Cusin, MD
Associate Professor in Psychiatry
Director, Ketamine Clinic
Psychiatrist, Depression Clinical and Research
  Program
Massachusetts General Hospital
Boston, Massachusetts
PLATES 4.2, 4.6–4.7

Jeremy K. Cutsforth-Gregory, MD
Associate Professor of Neurology
Mayo Clinic College of Medicine and Science
Rochester, Minnesota
PLATES 13.1–13.8, 13.10–13.19

James E. Eaton, MD
Cognitive Behavioral Neurology Fellow
Vanderbilt University Medical Center
Nashville, Tennessee
PLATES 2.1–2.31

Serena Fernandes, MD
Psychiatrist
Boston Children's Hospital
Boston, Massachusetts
PLATE 1.28

Robert Fox, MD
Staff Neurologist, Mellen Center for Multiple Sclerosis
Vice-Chair for Research, Neurological Institute
Cleveland Clinic
Cleveland, Ohio
PLATE 10.12

Oliver Freudenreich, MD
Co-director, Psychosis Clinical and Research Program
Massachusetts General Hospital
Boston, Massachusetts
PLATE 4.13

Heather J. Fullerton, MD, MAS
Professor of Neurology and Pediatrics
UCSF Benioff Children's Hospital
University of California, San Francisco
San Francisco, California
PLATE 9.46

Néstor Gálvez-Jiménez, MD, MSc, MHSA, MJur
Pauline M. Braathen Endowed Chair
Professor of Medicine (Neurology)
Cleveland Clinic Lerner College of Medicine;
Clinical Professor of Neurology
Herbert Wertheim College of Medicine
Florida International University
Miami, Florida;
Affiliate Professor of Clinical Biomedical Science
Charles E. Schmidt College of Medicine
Florida Atlantic University
Boca Raton, Florida
PLATES 7.1–7.17, 7.19

Joao Gomes, MD
Head, Neurointensive Care
Cerebrovascular Center
Cleveland Clinic
Cleveland, Ohio
PLATES 9.28–9.29, 9.31

Adriana Graciela Grau Chaves, MD
Department of Neurology
Cleveland Clinic Florida
Weston, Florida
PLATES 7.1–7.17, 7.19

Rahma Hida, PhD
Attending Psychologist
Department of Psychiatry and Behavioral Sciences
Boston Children's Hospital
Boston, Massachusetts
PLATES 4.32–4.33

Gregory L. Holmes, MD
Neurologist
Physician Leader, Neurology
Professor and Chair, Neurological Sciences
University of Vermont College of Medicine
Burlington, Vermont
PLATES 3.1–3.13

Shazam Hussain, MD
Professor of Neurology, Cleveland Clinic Lerner
College of Medicine
Director, Cerebrovascular Center
Vice Chair of Operations, Neurological Institute
Staff, Department of Neurology
Cleveland Clinic
Cleveland, Ohio
PLATES 9.1–9.6

Imari-Ashley P. Isaken, PhD
Staff Psychologist
Department of Psychiatry and Behavioral Sciences
Boston Children's Hospital
Instructor of Psychology
Department of Psychiatry and Behavioral Sciences
Harvard Medical School
Boston, Massachusetts
PLATE 4.9

Carlos S. Kase, MD
Emeritus Professor of Neurology
Boston University School of Medicine
Boston, Massachusetts;
Adjunct Professor of Neurology
Emory University School of Medicine
Atlanta, Georgia
PLATES 9.30, 9.38–9.40

Milissa L. Kaufman, MD, PhD
Assistant Professor of Psychiatry
McLean Hospital
Harvard Medical School
Director, Dissociative Disorders and Trauma
Research Program
Medical Director, Hill Center for Women
Medical Director, Outpatient Trauma Clinic
McLean Hospital
Belmont, Massachusetts
PLATES 4.11–4.12, 4.22–4.23

G. Abbas Kharal, MD, MPH
Assistant Professor of Neurology
Lerner College of Medicine
Cleveland Clinic
Cleveland, Ohio
PLATES 9.9–9.11

Zeshaun Khawaja, MD, MBA
Medical Director, Telestroke
Cerebrovascular Center
Cleveland Clinic
Cleveland, Ohio
PLATES 9.20–9.21

Kathryn Kieran, MSN, NP-BC
Instructor, Mental Health Nursing
MGH Institute of Health Professions
Charlestown, Massachusetts
PLATES 4.11–4.12, 4.22–4.23

Amy Kunchok, MD, PhD
Neurologist
Mellen Center for Multiple Sclerosis
Neurological Institute
Cleveland Clinic Foundation
Cleveland, Ohio
PLATES 10.19–10.22

Sidonie Ibrikji, MD
Vascular Neurologist
Cleveland Clinic Foundation
Cleveland, Ohio
PLATES 9.26–9.27

Anthony-Samuel LaMantia, PhD
Professor
Director, Center for Neurobiology Research
Fralin Biomedical Research Institute
Virginia Tech
Roanoke, Virginia
PLATES 1.1–1.4, 1.9, 1.13–1.14, 1.18–1.22, 1.24–1.25

Susan M. Linder, DPT, PhD
Assistant Staff, Physical Medicine & Rehabilitation
Associate Professor of Medicine, Cleveland Clinic
Lerner College of Medicine
Director of Clinical Research, Physical Medicine and
Rehabilitation
Cleveland Clinic
Cleveland, Ohio
PLATES 9.47–9.50

Jonathan Lipton, MD, PhD
Assistant Professor of Neurology
Boston Children's Hospital
Boston, Massachusetts
PLATES 5.1–5.22

Mei Lu, MD, PhD, EMBA
Neurologist, Cerebrovascular Center
Cleveland Clinic
Cleveland, Ohio
PLATES 9.7–9.8

Christine Lu-Emerson, MD
Director, Maine Medical Center Brain Tumor Program
Division Director of Neurology at Maine Medical
Center
Portland, Maine;
Clinical Assistant Professor of Neurology
Tufts School of Medicine
Boston, Massachusetts
PLATES 12.1–12.22

Kenneth J. Mack, MD, PhD
Division Chair
Child and Adolescent Neurology
Mayo Clinic
Rochester, Minnesota
PLATE 13.9

Ahmad Mahadeen, MD
Clinical Neuroimmunology Fellow
Mellen Center for Multiple Sclerosis
Neurological Institute
Cleveland Clinic Foundation
Cleveland, Ohio
PLATE 10.14

Kedar R. Mahajan, MD, PhD
Staff Neurologist
Mellen Center for Multiple Sclerosis
Neurological Institute
Cleveland Clinic
Cleveland, Ohio
PLATES 10.12–10.13

Ashutosh Mahapatra, MD
Endovascular Surgical Neuroradiology Fellow
Cerebrovascular Center, Neurological Institute
Cleveland Clinic
Cleveland, Ohio
PLATES 9.1–9.6

Marisa McGinley, DO, MSc
Neurologist
Mellen Center for Multiple Sclerosis
Neurological Institute
Cleveland Clinic
Cleveland, Ohio
PLATES 10.6–10.7

Sara Medina-DeVilliers, PhD
Psychology Attending
Department of Psychiatry and Behavioral Sciences
Boston Children's Hospital
Boston, Massachusetts
PLATE 4.27

Annalisa Morgan, MD
Resident Physician
Department of Neurology, Neurological Institute
Cleveland Clinic Foundation
Cleveland, Ohio
PLATES 10.17–10.18, 10.19–10.20

Brandon Moss, MD
Associate Staff Neurologist
Neurological Institute
Cleveland Clinic
Cleveland, Ohio
PLATES 10.15–10.16

Ruta M. Nonacs, MD, PhD
Staff Psychiatrist
Massachusetts General Hospital
Boston, Massachusetts
PLATE 4.3

Ryan O'Connor, MD
Attending Psychiatrist
Boston Children's Hospital
Boston, Massachusetts
PLATE 4.29

Daniel Ontaneda, MD, PhD
Associate Professor of Neurology
Cleveland Clinic
Cleveland, Ohio
PLATES 10.3–10.5

Joel M. Oster, MD
Associate Professor of Neurology
Director of EEG Laboratory and Epilepsy Service
Sleep Medicine Physician, Neurology and Pulmonary
    Medicine/Sleep Disorders Center
Tufts Medical Center
Boston, Massachusetts
PLATES 5.23–5.24

Sherry Paden, PsyD
Attending Psychologist, Inpatient Psychiatry Service
Department of Psychiatry and Behavioral Sciences
Boston Children's Hospital
Boston, Massachusetts
PLATE 4.20

Abhi Pandhi, MD
Endovascular Surgical Neuroradiology Fellow
Cerebrovascular Center
Neurological Institute
Cleveland Clinic
Cleveland, Ohio
PLATES 9.1–9.6

Alan K. Percy, MD
Professor of Pediatrics (Neurology) Emeritus
Sarah K. Bateh Endowed Professor for Rett
    Syndrome
University of Alabama at Birmingham
Birmingham, Alabama
PLATES 1.29–1.30, 8.19–8.20

Joseph Pleen, DO
Assistant Professor of Neurology
University of Kansas Medical Center
Kansas City, Kansas
PLATES 2.1–2.31

Joelle Reese, MA, CCC-SLP
Clinical Specialist, Rehabilitation
Cleveland Clinic Mercy Hospital
Canton, Ohio
PLATES 9.47–9.50

Mary R. Rensel, MD, FAAN, ABIHM
Director of Wellness and Pediatric Multiple Sclerosis
Mellen Center for Multiple Sclerosis
Cleveland Clinic
Cleveland, Ohio
PLATE 10.2

Carrie (Beth) E. Robertson, MD
Associate Professor of Neurology
Mayo Clinic College of Medicine and Science
Rochester, Minnesota
PLATES 13.1–13.8, 13.10–13.19

Shenandoah Robinson, MD, FAAP, FACS
Professor of Neurosurgery
Division of Pediatric Neurosurgery
Johns Hopkins University School of Medicine
Baltimore, Maryland
PLATES 1.5–1.8, 1.10–1.12, 1.15–1.17, 1.23, 1.26–1.27

Hannah J. Roeder, MD, MPH
Clinical Assistant Professor
Department of Neurology
Division of Cerebrovascular Diseases
Carver College of Medicine
University of Iowa
Iowa City, Iowa
PLATES 9.41–9.45

Karen L. Roos, MD
John and Nancy Nelson Professor Emerita
Professor Emerita, Neurological Surgery
Department of Neurology
Indiana University School of Medicine
Indianapolis, Indiana
PLATES 11.1–11.24

Andrew N. Russman, DO
Staff Physician, Vascular Neurology
Medical Director, Comprehensive Stroke Center
Cerebrovascular Center
Cleveland Clinic
Cleveland, Ohio
PLATES 9.22–9.25

Chase Samsel, MD
Attending Psychiatrist
Department of Psychiatry and Behavioral Sciences
Boston Children's Hospital;
Affiliate Staff
Psychosocial Oncology and Palliative Care
Dana-Farber Cancer Institute;
Assistant Professor of Psychiatry
Harvard Medical School
Boston, Massachusetts
PLATES 1.28, 4.1, 4.9, 4.20, 4.24–4.25, 4.27–4.33

Clifford B. Saper, MD, PhD
James Jackson Putnam Professor
Department of Neurology
Beth Israel Deaconess Medical Center
Harvard Medical School
Boston, Massachusetts
PLATES 5.1–5.22, 5.33–5.34

Jeremy D. Schmahmann, MD, FAAN, FANA, FANPA
Ataxia Center, Cognitive Behavioral Neurology Unit
Laboratory for Neuroanatomy and Cerebellar
    Neurobiology
Department of Neurology
Massachusetts General Hospital and Harvard
    Medical School
Boston, Massachusetts
PLATES 8.1–8.18

Rodney C. Scott, MD, PhD
Division Chief, Pediatric Neurology
Nemours Children's Health
Wilmington, Delaware
PLATES 3.1–3.13

Magdy Selim, MD, PhD
Professor of Neurology
Beth Israel Deaconess Medical Center/Harvard
    Medical School
Boston, Massachusetts
PLATES 9.35–9.37

Ah Lahm Shin, MD
Psychiatry Attending
Simches Division of Child and Adolescent Psychiatry
McLean Hospital
Belmont, Massachusetts
PLATE 4.30

Ann K. Shinn, MD
Research Psychiatrist
Schizophrenia and Bipolar Disorder Program
McLean Hospital
Belmont, Massachusetts;
Assistant Professor of Psychiatry
Harvard Medical School
Boston, Massachusetts
PLATES 4.4–4.5

Renee Sorrentino, MD
Clinical Assistant Professor
Department of Psychiatry
Harvard Medical School
Boston, Massachusetts
PLATE 4.21

Russell H. Swerdlow, MD
Gene and Marge Sweeney Professor
Department of Neurology
University of Kansas Medical Center
Kansas City, Kansas
PLATES 2.1–2.31

Robert C. Tasker, MBBS, MD
Harvard Medical School
Department of Anesthesiology, Critical Care & Pain
  Medicine
Department of Anesthesia (Pediatrics)
Boston Children's Hospital
Boston, Massachusetts
PLATES 6.1–6.9, 14.9

Samantha Marie Taylor, MD
Child and Adolescent Psychiatry Clinical Fellow
Department of Psychiatry and Behavioral Sciences
Boston Children's Hospital
Boston, Massachusetts
PLATES 4.24–4.25

Gabor Toth, MD
Professor of Neurology, Cleveland Clinic Lerner
  College of Medicine
Director, Neuroendovascular Intervention Fellowship
Cerebrovascular Center, Neurological Institute
Staff, Department of Neurology
Cleveland Clinic
Cleveland, Ohio
PLATES 9.1–9.6

Nicholas A. Tritos, MD, DSc, MMSc
Staff Neuroendocrinologist
Massachusetts General Hospital
Associate Professor of Medicine
Harvard Medical School
Boston, Massachusetts
PLATES 5.25–5.32

Kevin K. Tsang, PsyD
Psychology Attending
Department of Psychiatry and Behavioral Sciences
Boston Children's Hospital
Boston, Massachusetts
PLATE 4.31

Barbara Voetsch, MD, PhD, FAHA
Assistant Professor of Neurology
Tufts University School of Medicine
Boston, Massachusetts;
Director, Acute Stroke Services
Co-director, Comprehensive Stroke Center
Lahey Hospital and Medical Center
Burlington, Massachusetts
PLATES 9.32–9.34

Patrick Y. Wen, MD
Professor of Neurology
Harvard Medical School
Boston, Massachusetts
PLATES 12.1–12.22

Mark A. Whealy, MD
Assistant Professor of Neurology
Mayo Clinic College of Medicine and Science
Rochester, Minnesota
PLATES 13.1–13.8, 13.10–13.19

Jack Wilberger, MD
Professor of Neurosurgery
Drexel University College of Medicine
Pittsburgh, Pennsylvania
PLATES 14.1–14.8, 14.10–14.17

John W. Winkelman, MD, PhD
Chief, Sleep Disorders Clinical Research Program
Departments of Psychiatry and Neurology
Massachusetts General Hospital
Boston, Massachusetts
PLATE 4.26

Charles R. Wulff, MD
Attending Psychiatrist
Department of Psychiatry and Behavioral Sciences
Boston Children's Hospital
Instructor of Psychiatry
Harvard Medical School
Boston, Massachusetts
PLATE 4.1

CONTRIBUTORS TO SECOND EDITION

We acknowledge the work of contributors to the previous edition.

EDITORS-IN-CHIEF

H. Royden Jones, MD†
Ted M. Burns, MD†
Michael J. Aminoff, MD, DSc, FRCP
Scott L. Pomeroy, MD, PhD

CONTRIBUTORS

Harold P. Adams Jr, MD
Barry G.W. Arnason, MD
Elizabeth Barkoudah, MD
Christina A. Brezing, MD
Jeffrey M. Burns, MD, MS
Louis R. Caplan, MD
Claudia Chaves, MD
Daniel O. Claassen, MD, MS
Hilary Connery, MD, PhD
Cristina Cusin, MD
Fred Michael Cutrer, MD
David R. DeMaso, MD
Jamie M. Dupuy, MD
Lori R. Eisner, PhD
Oliver Freudenreich, MD, FAPM
Heather J. Fullerton, MD, MAS

Sandro Galea, MD, DrPH
Néstor Gálvez-Jiménez, MD, MSc, MSHA, FACP
Georgina Garcia, MD
Raghav Govindarajan, MD
Paul T. Gross, MD
Gregory L. Holmes, MD
Kinan Hreib, MD, PhD
Patricia Ibeziako, MD
Adil Javed, MD, PhD
Justin Johnston, MS
Carlos S. Kase, MD
Milissa L. Kaufman, MD, PhD
Alex Sogomon Keuroghlian, MD, MSc
Karestan C. Koenen, PhD
Daniel Honore Lachance, MD
Anthony-Samuel LaMantia, PhD
Jonathan Lipton, MD, PhD
Christine Lu-Emerson, MD
Kenneth J. Mack, MD, PhD
Ruta Nonacs, MD, PhD
Darren P. O'Neill, MD
Joel M. Oster, MD
Ayca Deniz Ozel, MD
Alan K. Percy, MD

Roy H. Perlis, MD, MSc
Dennis Roberts, MD
Carrie (Beth) E. Robertson, MD
Shenandoah Robinson, MD
Karen L. Roos, MD
Clifford B. Saper, MD, PhD
Jeremy Schmahmann, MD
Rod C. Scott, MD, PhD
Andrea L. Seek, MD
Magdy Selim, MD, PhD
V. Michelle Silvera, MD
Andrew M. Southerland, MD, MSc
Jerry W. Swanson, MD
Russell H. Swerdlow, MD
Robert C. Tasker, MA, AM, MBBS, FRCP, MD
Christine B. Thomas, MD
Nicholas A. Tritos, MD, DSc
Barbara Voetsch, MD, PhD
Heather J. Walter, MD, MPH
Patrick Y. Wen, MD
Jack Wilberger, MD, FACS
John W. Winkelman, MD, PhD
Curtis W. Wittmann, MD
Yuval Zabar, MD

†Deceased.

CONTENTS OF COMPLETE VOLUME 7— NERVOUS SYSTEM: TWO-PART SET

CONTENTS

Contents

NORMAL AND ABNORMAL DEVELOPMENT

Plate 1.1

Brain: PART I

INITIAL SPECIFICATION OF THE NERVOUS SYSTEM: THE EMBRYO AT 18 DAYS

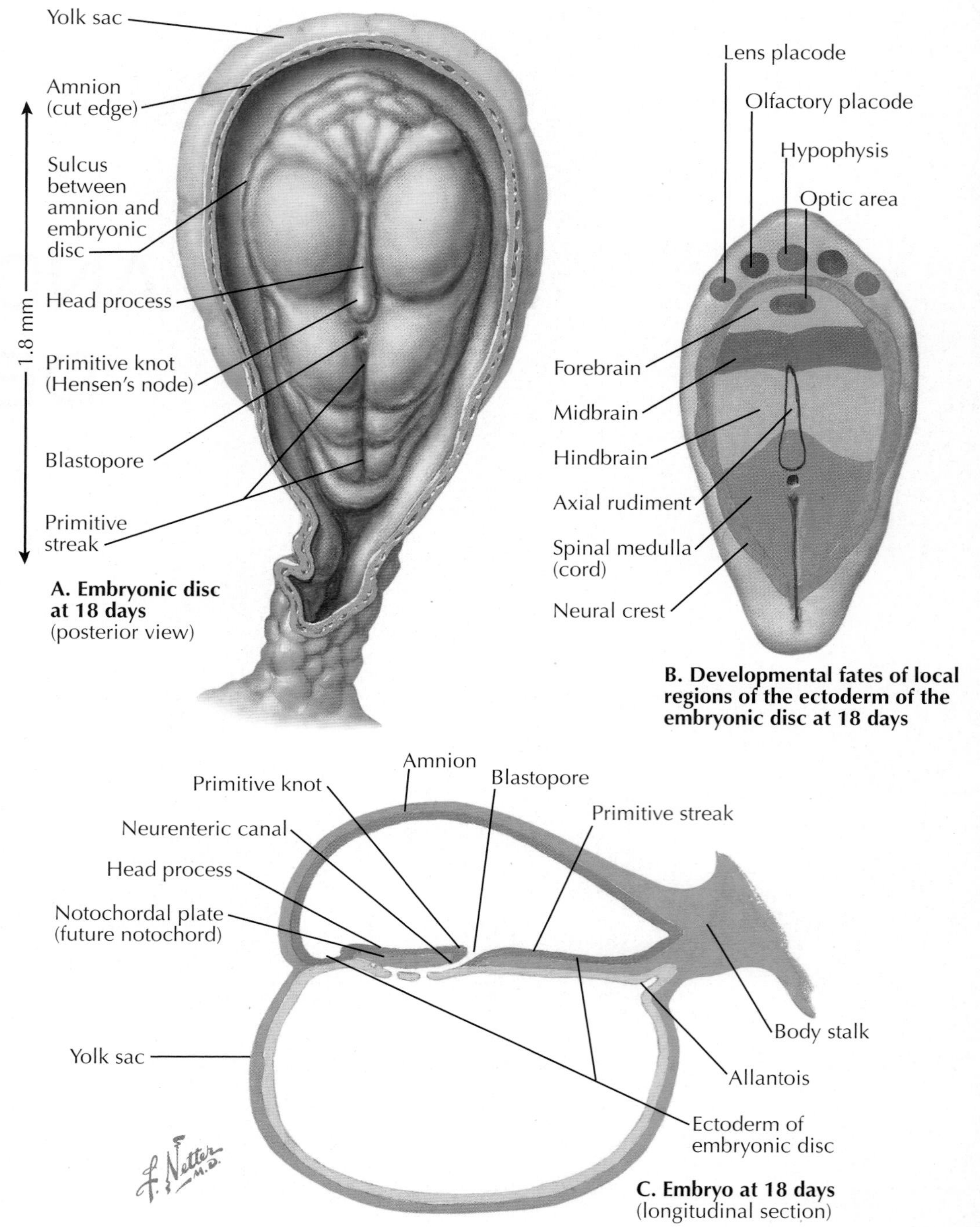

After implantation, the embryo is a single cell layer called the inner cell mass. The inner cell mass sits at the bottom of a fluid-filled cavity defined by the key extraembryonic membrane, the *amnion.* Beneath the embryo is another cavity, the *yolk sac,* lined with a cell layer called the embryonic *hypoblast,* some of which will go on to form the *allantois,* an additional extraembryonic membrane. Cells from the inner cell mass adjacent to the hypoblast constitute a second embryonic layer, the *epiblast,* that will form most of the embryo. At this point in development, approximately 18 days after fertilization/implantation, epiblast cells define the *embryonic disc.* Once formed, the embryonic disc undergoes a series of cell movements known as *gastrulation.* The key movement is the local proliferation, accumulation, and ingression of epiblast cells that form first the *primitive knot* (or Hensen's node), then the *primitive streak,* which defines the midline axis of the embryo. The cells that have migrated "into" the embryo (inward streaming of these cells further divides the epiblast) from the primitive knot, now interposed between the epiblast and the hypoblast, coalesce to form a distinct cell layer, the *mesoderm.* The position of these cells as the "middle" (meso) layer of the embryo defines the remaining epiblast cells on top of these mesodermal cells as *ectoderm* (ecto: outside) and the hypoblast cells that are underneath as *endoderm* (endo: inside). A subset of ectodermal cells will form the entire central nervous system (CNS) and peripheral nervous system (PNS). This subset of cells is defined by their proximity to mesodermal cells that coalesce first to form the *notochordal plate* and then the *notochord* at the midline of the embryo. Notochord formation and subsequent changes in overlying ectoderm precede *neurulation,* the process that initially specifies the nervous system and consolidates the embryonic axes: anterior, posterior, medial, lateral, dorsal, and ventral.

The notochord becomes a source of signaling molecules released by notochord cells that act on overlying ectoderm. These signals both instruct the overlying ectodermal cells to become neural stem cells capable of giving rise to neurons and glia of the mature CNS and PNS and protect these early neural stem cells (collectively, the *neuroectoderm*) from additional signals in the embryo that transform more lateral ectodermal cells into skin and other derivatives. At this point, the fate of ectodermal cells, particularly that of the visibly thickened sheet of cells above the notochord called the *neural plate,* can be mapped fairly precisely. The neural plate will give rise to nearly all neurons and glia of the CNS and PNS. In addition, stem cells found in local regions of the cranial ectoderm will go on to form sensory specializations, including the *olfactory placode* and *lens placode,* as well as endocrine tissue, the *hypophysis.*

The neural plate will become further divided into regions that will give rise to functionally distinct populations of neurons, as well as additional ectodermal, mesodermal, and endodermal cells in locations adjacent to the neural plate. These regions of the CNS include the *forebrain* (cerebral cortex, hippocampus, basal ganglia, and basal forebrain regions such as

the amygdala, olfactory bulb, and thalamus), *midbrain* (superior and inferior colliculi and tegmental areas), *hindbrain* (cerebellum and brainstem), and *spinal cord.* In addition, neuroectodermal cells at the margin of the neural plate—farthest from the notochord and its signals—become a specialized population of neural stem cells called the *neural crest.* Neural crest cells eventually delaminate from the neuroectoderm and migrate throughout the embryo, where they make sensory ganglia and sympathetic and parasympathetic ganglia of the PNS. Neural crest cells also migrate into the developing viscera and generate the *enteric nervous system,* a network of peripheral neurons that control visceral motor function, as well as immune and stress responses. In addition, neural crest cells contribute to the adrenal glands and make pigment cells, cranial bones, teeth, and connective tissue. This geometric

division of the neuroectoderm into a "fate map" for early populations of neural stem cells at distinct locations reflects a more fundamental molecular process. Because of variations in local signals exchanged between the notochord, neuroectoderm, and additional mesodermal, endodermal, and ectodermal cells in locations defined by the embryonic axes established during gastrulation, local changes in patterns of gene expression arise to distinguish cells that will generate the forebrain, midbrain, hindbrain, and spinal cord. These "regional genes" are primarily transcription factors that influence the subsequent expression of downstream genes that confer local neuronal identities. Thus the combination of cell movements and cell-cell signaling during early embryogenesis establishes a spatial and molecular template for the construction of the entire CNS and PNS.

Yolk sac

Amnion (cut edge)

Sulcus between amnion and embryonic disc

Head process

Primitive knot (Hensen's node)

Blastopore

Primitive streak

1.8 mm

A. Embryonic disc at 18 days (posterior view)

Lens placode

Olfactory placode

Hypophysis

Optic area

Forebrain

Midbrain

Hindbrain

Axial rudiment

Spinal medulla (cord)

Neural crest

B. Developmental fates of local regions of the ectoderm of the embryonic disc at 18 days

Amnion

Primitive knot   Blastopore

Neurenteric canal   Primitive streak

Head process

Notochordal plate (future notochord)

Yolk sac

Body stalk

Allantois

Ectoderm of embryonic disc

C. Embryo at 18 days (longitudinal section)

Plate 1.2   Normal and Abnormal Development

INITIAL FORMATION OF THE BRAIN AND SPINAL CORD: THE EMBRYO AT 20 TO 24 DAYS

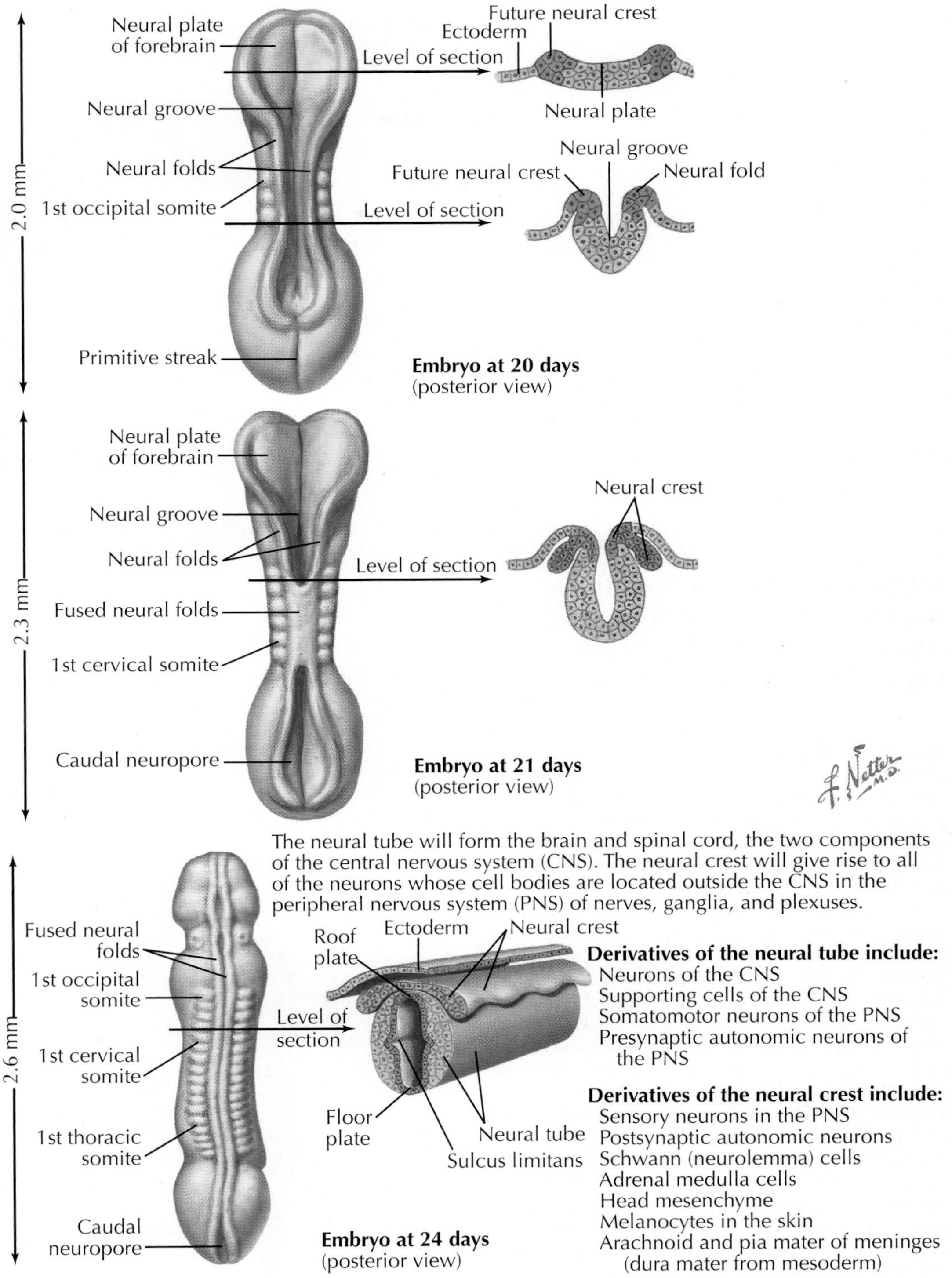

Neurulation, which relies upon the establishment of the midline mesoderm, including the notochord during gastrulation, transforms the neural plate into a tube of neural stem cells: the *neural tube.* Neurulation is accompanied by elaboration of mesodermal cells lateral to the notochord into *somites* that will form the axial skeleton and musculature and visceral differentiation by the endoderm. These events cooperate to yield an embryonic nervous system that consists of a tube surrounding a fluid-filled cavity that will constitute *the brain ventricles* (see below) and the *central canal* of the spinal cord. The geometric relationship between the neural plate and underlying notochord is the primary determinant of neural tube formation. By day 20 of development, the neural plate has thickened and flexed upward from the midline, right above the notochord, defining what will become the ventral (anterior) midline of the neural tube. The neural crest, initially specified at the lateral (alar) margins of the neural plate, is translocated to the dorsal (posterior) midline as the lateral neural plate forms a tube.

By embryonic day 21, the neural tube in the midsection of the embryo has closed; the neural folds fuse, and the underlying neuroectoderm encloses a fluid-filled cavity that becomes the spinal cord central canal. The neural crest delaminates at the posterior midline. This epithelial (cell sheets) to mesenchymal (loosely arrayed, motile cells between the sheets) transition of neural crest cells is much like the epithelial-to-mesenchymal transitions that occur in many cancers of mature epithelial tissues. For the neural crest, however, this transition begins a highly regulated process of migration to multiple peripheral locations where neural crest precursors divide and differentiate into sensory ganglia (cranial and posterior root), autonomic ganglia, enteric neurons, pigment cells, components of the posterior aorta, cranial bones, and connective tissues. As the midneural tube forms, the anterior and posterior neural plate has not yet reached the point where lateral margins meet and fuse at the dorsal (posterior) midline. The midline "hinge point" where neural tube formation begins is visible as the *neural groove* anteriorly and the *rhomboid sinus* posteriorly, and the forebrain neural plate and the posterior spinal cord remain open to the extraembryonic environment.

Within another 3 days, by embryonic day 24, the neural tube is closed from the anterior end (where the brain will form) throughout much of the length of the spinal cord, with the exception of an opening at the *rhomboid sinus* or *posterior neuropore.* At this stage, the neural tube has begun to acquire additional signs of differentiation that prefigure genesis of neurons with distinct functions. First, based upon the location of either the notochord ventrally or the alar region and neural crest where the neural tube fuses dorsally, a ventral and dorsal population of neuroectodermal cells becomes specialized to provide signals to the rest of the neural tube neural stem cells that constitute the developing nervous system. The neural tube cells above the notochord at the ventral (anterior) midline constitute the *floor plate,* and those at the fusion of the neural folds at the dorsal (posterior) midline become the *roof plate.* Floor plate and roof plate cells secrete signals that influence neighboring cells in the neural tube, such as sonic hedgehog (floor plate) and bone morphogenetic proteins (roof plate), peptide signals that regulate

Embryo at 20 days (posterior view)

Embryo at 21 days (posterior view)

The neural tube will form the brain and spinal cord, the two components of the central nervous system (CNS). The neural crest will give rise to all of the neurons whose cell bodies are located outside the CNS in the peripheral nervous system (PNS) of nerves, ganglia, and plexuses.

Derivatives of the neural tube include:
Neurons of the CNS
Supporting cells of the CNS
Somatomotor neurons of the PNS
Presynaptic autonomic neurons of the PNS

Derivatives of the neural crest include:
Sensory neurons in the PNS
Postsynaptic autonomic neurons
Schwann (neurolemma) cells
Adrenal medulla cells
Head mesenchyme
Melanocytes in the skin
Arachnoid and pia mater of meninges (dura mater from mesoderm)

Embryo at 24 days (posterior view)

neuronal identity, proliferation, and differentiation. These signals further distinguish the presumptive spinal cord and hindbrain into *anterior/basal* and *posterior/alar* regions separated by a midline groove referred to as the *sulcus limitans* (this structure is not always easy to see).

These geometrically defined domains of neural stem cells generate functionally distinct classes of neurons, which are most clearly defined in the spinal cord. The neural stem cells of the anterior/basal (ventral) region, influenced primarily by floor plate signals, give rise to motor neurons that project to peripheral muscles and

autonomic ganglia and interneurons that modulate the output of motor neurons. Those in the posterior/alar (dorsal) region, influenced primarily by roof plate signals, generate sensory projection and interneurons that relay and process incoming information from peripheral sensory ganglia. Gradients of signals from the floor plate and roof plate elicit additional local expression of transcription factors and other determinants in neighboring neural stem cells. These factors define the capacity of the stem cells to generate distinct classes of sensory or motor projection neurons and interneurons.

Plate 1.3

Brain: PART I

CENTRAL NERVOUS SYSTEM AT 28 DAYS

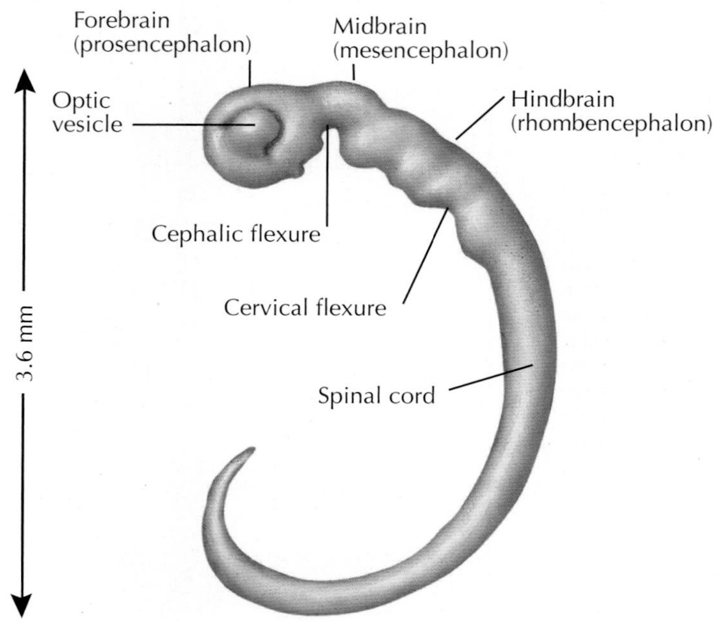

Forebrain (prosencephalon)
Midbrain (mesencephalon)
Optic vesicle
Hindbrain (rhombencephalon)
Cephalic flexure
Cervical flexure
Spinal cord
3.6 mm

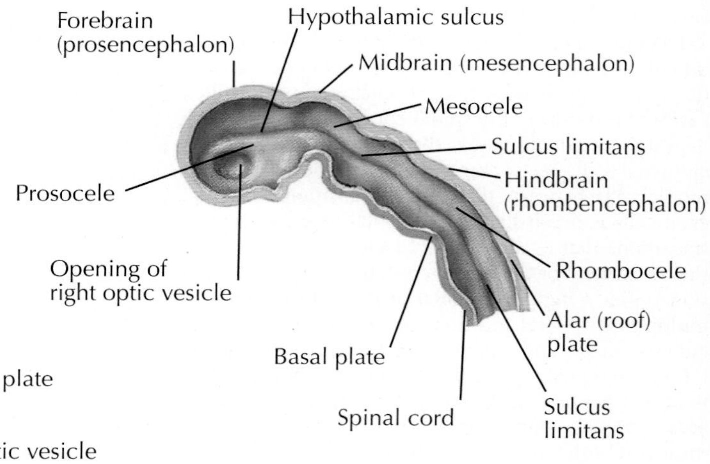

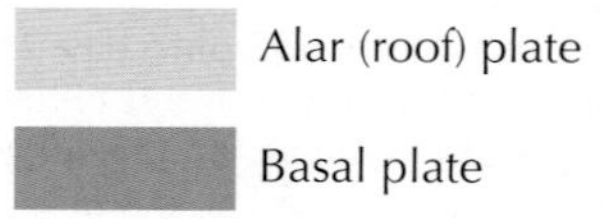

MORPHOGENESIS OF THE BRAIN, SPINAL CORD, AND PERIPHERAL NERVOUS SYSTEM: THE EMBRYO FROM 28 THROUGH 36 DAYS

Within an additional 4 days, the neural tube closes completely, and the developing nervous system undergoes additional changes that define neural stem cell populations that generate all of the distinct structures of the mature brain and PNS. These changes are seen anatomically as a series of bulges, bends, and grooves that distinguish specific regions of the developing nervous system from the anterior to posterior end. At the anterior end of the closed neural tube, the neuroepithelium expands into a hollow globe called the *prosencephalon*. Neural stem cells of the prosencephalon are specified to generate all of the neurons that will constitute the *forebrain*. Subsequently, two bilaterally symmetric structures emerge from the lateral/anterior aspect of the prosencephalon (a region that will subsequently be called the *diencephalon;* see below). These are the *optic vesicles* that generate all of the neural cells of the retina. Immediately posterior to the prosencephalon, the neural tube bends at a point referred to as the *cephalic flexure.* This bending begins the process by which the brain and the head become distinct from the spinal cord and the rest of the body. The neural stem cells in the neural tube in the region of the cephalic flexure become specified to generate *midbrain* structures (also referred to as the mesencephalon).

The region of the neural tube posterior to the midbrain undergoes a dramatic series of morphogenetic changes that transform it into the *rhombencephalon.* The most noticeable event is the establishment of a series of repeated bulges and grooves along the anterior/posterior axis that constitute a series of transient domains referred to collectively as *rhombomeres.* The neural stem cells in each rhombomere acquire distinct patterns of gene expression based upon their location. These distinctions then facilitate local genesis of motor neurons that give rise to cranial motor nerves and to sensory relay neurons that will constitute cranial sensory relay nuclei that provide the targets for peripheral cranial sensory inputs to the brainstem. The region of

the brainstem where most cranial motor neurons and sensory relay nuclei are found is called the *medulla oblongata,* or *myelencephalon.* The dorsal/alar region of the anterior rhombencephalon will generate the *cerebellum,* also known as the *metencephalon.* The relationship between rhombomeres and the developing structures of the head is quite precise. The neural crest that migrates from the neural tube in the region of each rhombomere (note that the neural crest neither arises nor

migrates from the prosencephalon) establishes cranial target structures that are often innervated by motor neurons generated in the rhombomere from which that neural crest originates. Similarly, cranial ganglia derived from the neural crest that migrates from distinct rhombomeres have a specific relationship with target nuclei generated within the relevant rhombomere. Thus this anterior-posterior organization of the rhombencephalon is essential for coordinating development of

Forebrain (prosencephalon)
Hypothalamic sulcus
Midbrain (mesencephalon)
Mesocele
Sulcus limitans
Hindbrain (rhombencephalon)
Prosocele
Rhombocele
Opening of right optic vesicle
Basal plate
Alar (roof) plate
Spinal cord
Sulcus limitans

Sagittal section

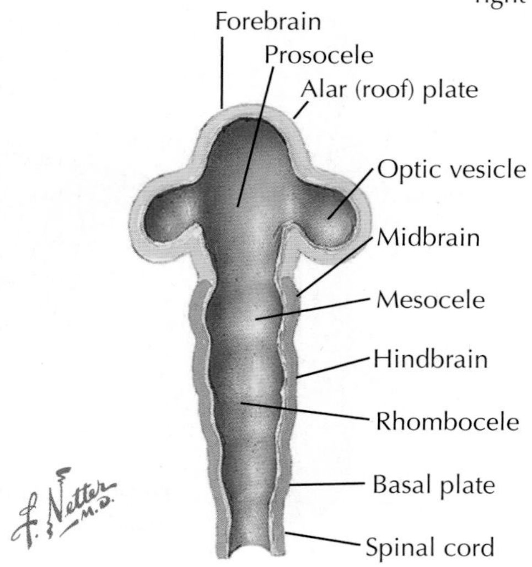

Forebrain
Prosocele
Alar (roof) plate
Optic vesicle
Midbrain
Mesocele
Hindbrain
Rhombocele
Basal plate
Spinal cord

Frontal section
(anterior to sulcus limitans)

Alar (roof) plate

Basal plate

Plate 1.4

Normal and Abnormal Development

CENTRAL NERVOUS SYSTEM AT 36 DAYS

Cranial n. V (trigeminal) (sensory and motor)

Cranial n. IV (trochlear) (motor)

Midbrain (mesencephalon)

Cranial n. III (oculomotor) (motor)

Forebrain (prosencephalon) — Diencephalon / Telencephalic vesicle

Cranial n. VI (abducens) (motor)

Cranial n. VII (facial) (sensory and motor)

Hindbrain (rhombencephalon)

Cranial n. VIII (vestibulocochlear) (sensory)

Cranial n. IX (glossopharyngeal) (sensory and motor)

Cranial n. X (vagus) (sensory and motor)

Cranial n. XI (accessory) (motor)
Cranial part
Spinal part

Cranial n. XII (hypoglossal) (motor)

1st cervical n. (sensory and motor)

Infundibulum

Optic cup

Central nervous system; cranial and spinal nerves at 36 days

1st thoracic n. (sensory and motor)

Coccygeal n. (sensory and motor)

1st lumbar n. (sensory and motor)

1st sacral n. (sensory and motor)

8.0 mm

MORPHOGENESIS OF THE BRAIN, SPINAL CORD, AND PERIPHERAL NERVOUS SYSTEM: THE EMBRYO FROM 28 THROUGH 36 DAYS (Continued)

cranial and oropharyngeal structures as well as their innervation.

Within an additional 8 days of development (36 days), the basic topography of the entire nervous system has been established, as have most of the component regions that then grow and differentiate throughout the balance of embryogenesis. The prosencephalon becomes further subdivided into two *telencephalic vesicles* (collectively called the *telencephalon*) that will give rise to the bilaterally symmetric structures of the forebrain: the cerebral cortical hemispheres, the hippocampi, the basal ganglia, the basal forebrain nuclei (including the amygdala), and the olfactory bulbs. The remainder of the prosencephalon, posterior to the telencephalic vesicles, becomes the *diencephalon,* which, in addition to the neural retina, will generate the epithalamus (dorsal structures known as the habenula), thalamus (relay nuclei that project to the cerebral cortex), and hypothalamus (motor/endocrine control nuclei that regulate visceral function, reproduction, and homeostasis). The mesencephalon, rhombencephalon, and myelencephalon differentiate further so that *cranial motor nerves* (darker blue, upper panel of Plate 1.4), *sensory ganglia,* and associated cranial *sensory nerves* (lighter pink, Plate 1.4) become visible along the anterior to posterior extent of the midbrain and hindbrain. In parallel, motor nerves, sensory ganglia, and associated sensory nerves of the rest of the body become visible along the spinal cord.

While the neural tube acquires additional regional identity that prefigures the generation of the mature neurons and glia in distinct brain regions, the space enclosed by the neural tube becomes further defined as the *ventricular system.* The individual ventricles of the ventricular system will be filled with a distinctive fluid—cerebrospinal fluid (CSF)—that provides specific signaling molecules to neural stem cells during development and then homeostatic signaling molecules and an

Lamina terminalis

Median telocele (3rd ventricle)

Telencephalic vesicle

Lateral telocele (lateral ventricle)

Alar plate

Diocele (3rd ventricle)

Optic stalk

Optic cup

Infundibular recess

Diencephalon

Mesencephalon

Mesocele (cerebral aqueduct)

Basal plate

Metencephalon (cerebellum, pons)

Metacele (4th ventricle)

Myelencephalon (medulla oblongata)

Myelocele (4th ventricle)

Spinal cord

Central canal

Rhombencephalon

Frontal section (anterior to sulcus limitans)

Metencephalon (cerebellum, pons)

Alar plate

Basal plate

Sulcus limitans

Mesencephalon

Mesocele (cerebral aqueduct)

Diencephalon

Diocele (3rd ventricle)

Opening of right telencephalic vesicle (lateral telocele)

Metacele (4th ventricle)

Thin roof of myelencephalon (medulla oblongata)

Myelocele (4th ventricle)

Spinal cord

Central canal

Hypothalamic sulcus

Infundibulum

Opening of right optic stalk

Lamina terminalis

Sagittal section

Alar (roof) plate

Basal plate

Derivatives of neural crest

appropriate ionic balance for electrical signaling for the mature nervous system. Initially, at 28 days of embryonic development, the ventricular spaces are referred to as the *prosocele, mesocele,* and *rhombocele,* corresponding to the primitive regions of the neural tube that surround them. Within 8 days, the ventricular system has become more elaborate, in parallel with morphogenesis of the forebrain, midbrain, and hindbrain. There are now two lateral ventricles enclosed by the telencephalic

vesicles, a *diocele* that will become the third ventricle, a *mesocele* that will become the cerebral aqueduct, and a *metacele* and *myelocele* that will collectively grow into the fourth ventricle. The ventricular space enclosed by the developing spinal cord is now defined as the *central canal.* Thus by approximately 36 days—a bit more than 1 month into the 9-month gestation period—the fetus has acquired all of the major regions of the brain and the anatomic divisions of the ventricular system.

Plate 1.5

Brain: PART I

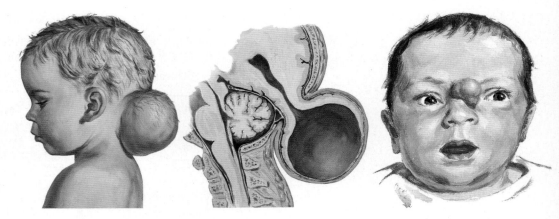

Occipital encephalocele

Frontal encephalocele

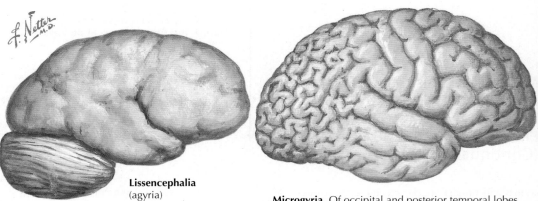

Lissencephalia
(agyria)

Microgyria. Of occipital and posterior temporal lobes

DEFECTIVE NEURAL TUBE FORMATION

The process of neurulation, including neural tube closure, is the first target of pathogenesis that specifically compromises the developing nervous system. Neural tube defects—most frequently failure of neural tube closure—can be caused by a number of factors, including single-gene mutations, aneuploid chromosomal anomalies, toxic exposures to pharmaceuticals, chemicals and drugs of abuse, maternal diabetes, and dietary deficits (most notably low levels of folic acid). Failure of cranial neural tube closure results in either *anencephaly* or an *encephalocele* (see Plate 1.5), whereas a defective caudal closure results in *myelomeningocele* (see Plate 1.8). Onset of anencephaly, a fatal maldevelopment characterized by lack of a majority of the forebrain, is by day 24. The skull vault is absent, and the brain is a highly vascular and poorly differentiated mass. Ultrasound examination and an elevated alpha-fetoprotein level in maternal blood and amniotic fluid indicate the diagnosis prenatally. Risk of recurrence is 5%.

An encephalocele is a protrusion of a portion of the brain or meninges through a skull defect. Although an encephalocele usually occurs in the occipital region in patients from Europe and North America, it can develop frontally or in the nasal passages, especially in

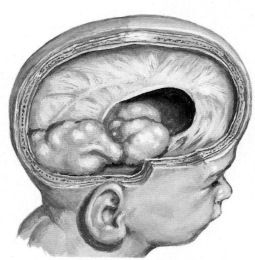

Hydranencephaly cranial cavity filled with cystic sac.
Only remnants of basal ganglia and posterior lobe.

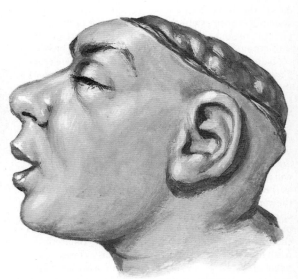

Anencephaly

children in Southeast Asia (see Plate 1.5). The herniated brain tissue is connected through a narrow isthmus. With occipital encephaloceles, there may be associated abnormalities of the cerebellum and midbrain. Meckel-Gruber syndrome includes a posterior encephalocele, microcephaly, microphthalmus, cleft lip and palate, polydactyly, and polycystic kidneys. This syndrome is inherited in an autosomal recessive manner, whereas for parents of a child with simple encephalocele, the

risk of recurrence is 5%. *Myelomeningocele* results from failure of caudal closure of the neural tube, with an 80% incidence in the lumbar region. Because closure of the central canal is essential to subsequent development of the rostral CNS, myelomeningocele also causes numerous associated brain anomalies. Prenatally, fetal ultrasonography is used to diagnose a myelomeningocele. Postnatally, magnetic resonance imaging (MRI) is particularly valuable in delineating the extent of the

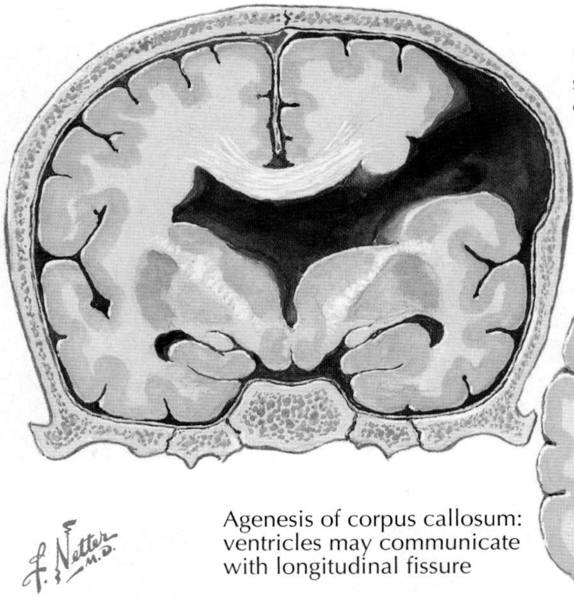

Plate 1.6

Normal and Abnormal Development

Porencephaly, with absence of
septum pellucidum and thinning
of overlying skull

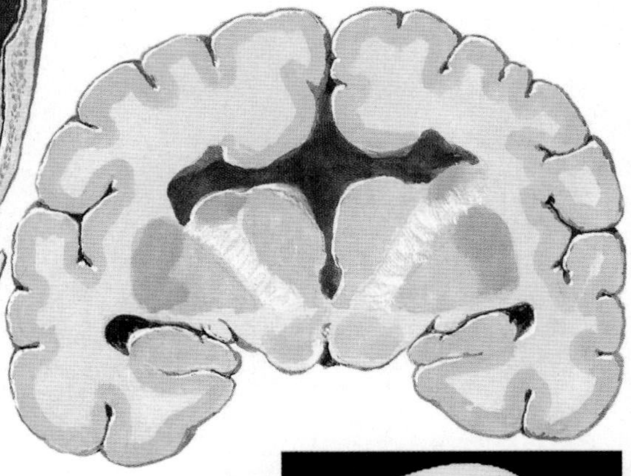

Agenesis of corpus callosum:
ventricles may communicate
with longitudinal fissure

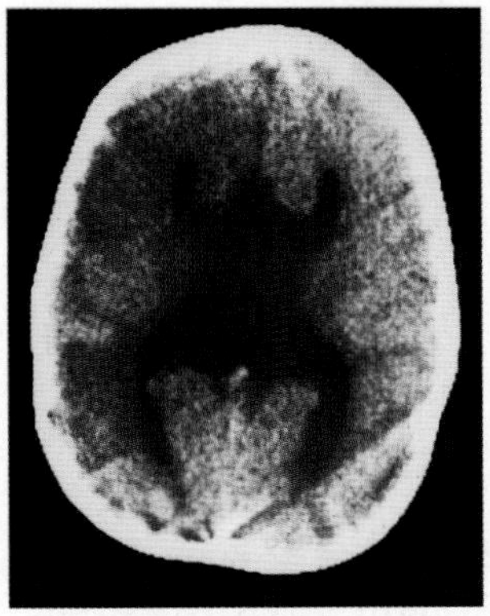

CT scan showing agenesis
of corpus callosum

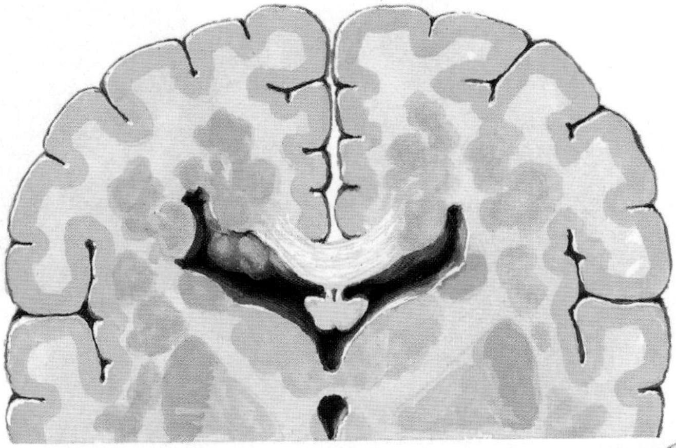

Heterotopic gray matter: islands of
gray matter within white matter
in centrum ovale; in subependymal
area, with projections into ventricles;
and in insular regions

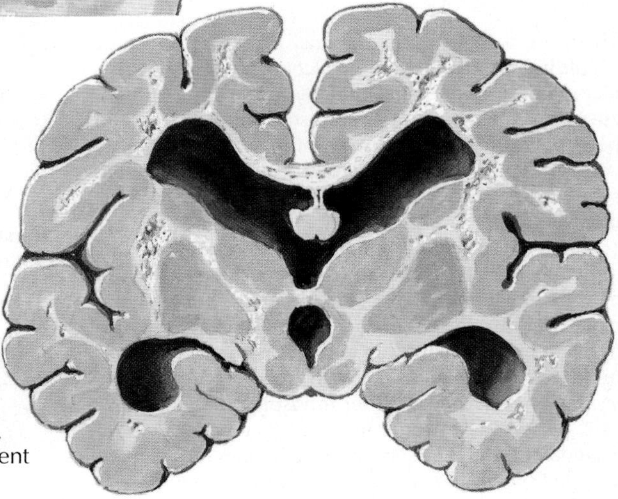

DEFECTIVE NEURAL TUBE FORMATION (Continued)

Perinatal telencephalic
leukoencephalopathy:
scarcity of white matter,
with resultant enlargement
of ventricles

structural abnormalities. All affected infants require neurosurgical intervention. The prognosis for sensorimotor function depends on the degree of CNS involvement, which may be difficult to assess in the neonate.

The most common CNS malformation is *holoprosencephaly* (arrhinencephalia). Holoprosencephaly results from incomplete development and septation of the midline CNS structures. It may be isolated or associated with other brain defects and occurs with varying degrees of severity. The most severe form results in a single ventricle, an absent olfactory system, hypoplastic optic nerves, or even a single "cyclopean" eye. The corpus callosum is absent, and the cortex is malformed. Potential facial anomalies include a single eye (cyclops) and a single nasal protuberance (proboscis), but in less severe cases, defects include ocular hypotelorism, microphthalmus, a flat nose, and a median cleft lip and palate. Ultrasound examination indicates the prenatal diagnosis, and MRI scans can delineate the extent of the defects. Early death is predictable in severe forms. Chromosomal abnormalities (trisomy 13–15, trisomy 18) are present in 50% of cases. In a small percentage of holoprosencephalic cases (~7%), genes related to sonic

hedgehog signaling are mutated. Increased awareness of chromosomal anomalies and single genes associated with holoprosencephaly makes genetic counseling important for families who have a child with holoprosencephaly.

Several other clinical conditions characterized by congenital failure of fusion of the midline structures of the spinal column are grouped under the general classification of *spinal dysraphism*. These various manifestations

of the dysraphic state span a clinical continuum, from the mildest forms, such as asymptomatic and unseen bony abnormalities (spina bifida occulta), to cutaneous lesions that can suggest an associated tethered cord (dimple, subcutaneous lipoma or hemangioma), to the most severe and disabling congenital malformations of the spinal structures (myelomeningocele). Early postnatal imaging with MRI has transformed the management of infants with these lesions.

Plate 1.7

Brain: PART I

Spina bifida occulta

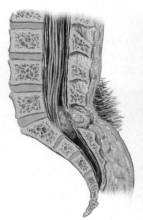

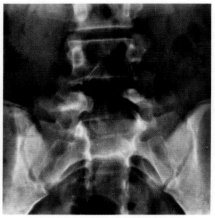

X-ray film. Showing deficit of lamina of sacrum (spina bifida occulta).

Dermal sinus

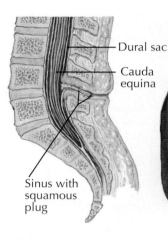

— Dural sac

— Cauda equina

Sinus with squamous plug

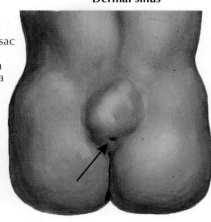

Fat pad overlying spinal bifida occulta. Tuft of hair or only skin dimple may be present, or there may be no external manifestation. Dermal sinus is also present in this case (*arrow*).

Spinal Dysraphism

SPINA BIFIDA OCCULTA

The more benign forms of spinal dysraphism include occult bony abnormalities unaccompanied by any displacement of spinal canal contents and with or without cutaneous stigmata. In these cases, there is failure of bony fusion between the two laminae of the involved vertebra (Plate 1.7). Spina bifida occulta is of no clinical significance when it occurs alone without intraspinal involvement.

Cutaneous stigmata of spina bifida occulta include dimples, dermal sinuses, subcutaneous lipomas, tufts of hair, hemangiomas, or asymmetric gluteal cleft. Cutaneous lesions may occur in isolation or herald an underlying tethered cord due to a low-lying conus or fat-infiltrated filum. Only a small subset of cutaneous lesions is associated with an intraspinal anomaly, and MRI performed within a few months of age can often exclude the diagnosis without radiation or sedation. *Tethered spinal cord syndrome* occurs when a hypertrophied filum terminale is too inflexible and causes progressive traction and relative caudal displacement of the conus medullaris as the spine grows. This traction can produce progressive ischemia in the conus medullaris and lead to symptoms of sphincter dysfunction and gait abnormalities. One-third of infants with a congenital tethered cord are likely to eventually develop neurologic dysfunction if the tethered cord is not treated. Prophylactic detethering by microsurgical sectioning of the filum terminale, ideally before 2 years of age, allows immediate ascent of the conus medullaris toward a more normal location within the spinal canal

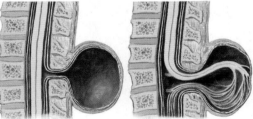

Meningocele

Meningomyelocele

Spina bifida. With central cicatrix.

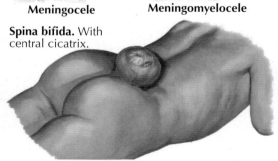

Chiari II malformation

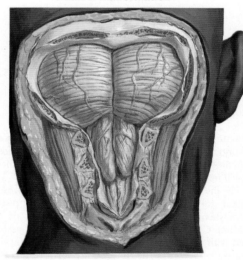

and minimizes the chance of development of neurologic deficits as the spine grows. For older children who have a late symptomatic presentation, treatment may minimize the further progression of neurologic deficits. If spina bifida occulta occurs in conjunction with a dermal sinus (an epithelium-lined tract linking the dural sac with the skin surface), there is a potential for communication between the skin and intraspinal contents and subsequent infection. Dermal sinuses located above the sacrococcygeal region should be removed

surgically after MRI imaging to evaluate for other associated lesions.

SPINA BIFIDA APERTA

Dysraphic conditions in which there are overt manifestations of the underlying bony defect are referred to as *spina bifida aperta* (Plate 1.7). Within this group, the progression of neurologic sequelae is defined, to a large extent, by the degree to which the contents of the spinal

Plate 1.8

Normal and Abnormal Development

Diastematomyelia

Dura mater

Spinal cord

Bony spur

Posterior view

Spinal Dysraphism

Body of vertebra

Spinal cord

Bony spur

Spinal nerve

Sectional view

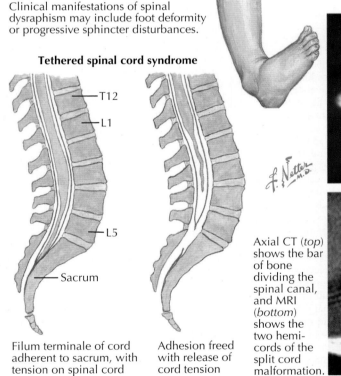

Midsagittal MRI shows Chiari II malformation with inferior displacement of the cerebellar tonsils and vermis into the cervical canal, and other typical findings of children with myelomeningocele, including partial agenesis of the corpus callosum, large massa intermedia, tectal beaking, inferiorly displaced torcular Herophili, and a small posterior fossa.

Clinical manifestations of spinal dysraphism may include foot deformity or progressive sphincter disturbances.

Tethered spinal cord syndrome

T12

L1

L5

Sacrum

Filum terminale of cord adherent to sacrum, with tension on spinal cord

Adhesion freed with release of cord tension

Axial CT (*top*) shows the bar of bone dividing the spinal canal, and MRI (*bottom*) shows the two hemicords of the split cord malformation.

SPINAL DYSRAPHISM (Continued)

canal are displaced from their normal location. In the case of a *meningocele*, the most benign form of spina bifida aperta, a meningeal cyst free of neural elements is extruded. Often, a meningocele can be completely removed surgically and the defect closed.

Diastematomyelia is a congenital malformation in which the spinal cord is split into two divisions, or hemicords. It is frequently associated with a midline cutaneous tuft of hair, and all infants with a worrisome tuft should be screened with an MRI. Frequently, a bony or cartilaginous septum separates the divided sections. Patients with a split cord malformation are at risk of developing associated scoliosis and progressive myelopathy as the spine grows. Surgical excision of the midline septum can halt the deteriorating condition and, in some cases, lead to restored function.

A far more severe variant of spina bifida aperta is *myelomeningocele*, in which the spinal cord or nerve roots, or both, protrude through the posterior bony and cutaneous defects due to failed closure of the posterior neuropore. The severity of deficits from a myelomeningocele correlates with its location along the spinal canal, with increasing deficits occurring with more rostral lesions. The neurologic deficits are due to abnormal in utero development throughout the entire CNS. Postnatal closure of the myelomeningocele in the term infant is performed within a few days of birth to minimize the risk of meningitis and is associated with low morbidity. Prenatal fetal closure may be an option for a select group of patients and often reduces the severity of hindbrain herniation.

Prenatal folate supplementation has markedly decreased both the incidence of infants born with myelomeningocele and lesion severity. Infants with sacral and low lumbar lesions often achieve some degree of ambulation, and approximately 80% can achieve social bladder and bowel continence. Approximately half of infants with a lumbar or sacral myelomeningocele will develop hydrocephalus that requires surgical treatment (see Plate 1.7). Most of these infants will have an associated Chiari II malformation, with displacement of the cerebellar vermis into the cervical canal, but only a few percent will become symptomatic at any point. Children are at risk for developing the tethered cord syndrome as the myelomeningocele scar adheres to the repair site while the spine grows. All repaired myelomeningoceles will appear adherent to some degree on MRI, and the diagnosis of a tethered cord in this population is made clinically. Although multidisciplinary care is needed throughout the life span of children born with a myelomeningocele, many will become independent productive adults with a good quality of life.

Plate 1.9

Brain: PART I

FETAL BRAIN GROWTH IN THE FIRST TRIMESTER

After initial brain morphogenesis is complete and neural crest migration has established the PNS (see Plate 1.4), several bendings, invaginations, and evaginations transform the developing brain. The addition of neurons via *neurogenesis,* which begins in the first trimester, underlies these morphogenetic movements. Neurogenesis reaches a maximum during midgestation to late gestation and ceases (with few exceptions) shortly after birth. Accordingly, as more mature brain morphology emerges, neurons that will form brain circuits differentiate for a lifetime of electrical signaling.

At 49 days of age, the brain and spinal cord undergo further bending that situates both appropriately in the developing head and trunk. The *cephalic flexure* moves the diencephalon and telencephalon nearly parallel with the hindbrain. The *pontine flexure* anticipates the location of the cerebellum and pons, and the *cervical flexure* positions the spinal cord parallel to the anterior-posterior body axis. At this stage, telencephalic and diencephalic landmarks are visible: olfactory bulbs in the telencephalon; the optic cup displaced laterally from the diencephalon as it generates the neural retina; the infundibulum (hypophysis), the rudimentary stalk of the pituitary gland; and the epiphysis, which forms the pineal gland.

Within 1.5 months, differential growth yields an even more mature embryonic brain and spinal cord. The *cerebral hemispheres* (or neopallium) grow disproportionately from the telencephalon primarily due to addition of neural stem cells that generate neurons of the mature cerebral cortex. Dysregulation of this process has dramatic consequences. Mutations that result in *microcephaly*—dramatic reduction of the size of the cerebral hemisphere and other brain structures—occur in genes that influence this expansion of cortical neural stem cells. Disproportionate cerebral hemisphere growth makes the diencephalon a "deep" structure, occluded from view. Diencephalic subdivisions, including the *thalamus, epithalamus* (habenular nuclei and pineal gland), *hypothalamus,* and *posterior pituitary* (neurohypophysis), are only seen by dissection, imaging, or histologic sectioning.

The hindbrain also undergoes dramatic changes. The dorsal (posterior) tectum and ventral (anterior) tegmentum of the mesencephalon become distinct: a groove or sulcus divides the *superior* and *inferior* colliculi of the tectum. The superior colliculus integrates visual information and motor commands for eye and head movements, and the inferior colliculus localizes sound in register with head movements. The posterior rhombencephalon expands dramatically as the rudimentary *cerebellum* becomes visible. The cerebellum is derived from stem cells in or near the roof of the fourth ventricle, as well as progenitors that migrate from other rhombencephalic and mesencephalic locations. Local neurogenesis, as well as migration of additional progenitors, results in dramatic cerebellar growth. The ventral (anterior) rhombencephalon becomes the rudimentary pons, which expands dramatically as axons from the cerebral cortex innervate pontine relay neurons that project to the cerebellum.

Spinal cord differentiation during this developmental period reflects distinct functional demands of arms and legs versus trunk and midline structures. Posterior to the cervical flexure, the cervical enlargement is broader

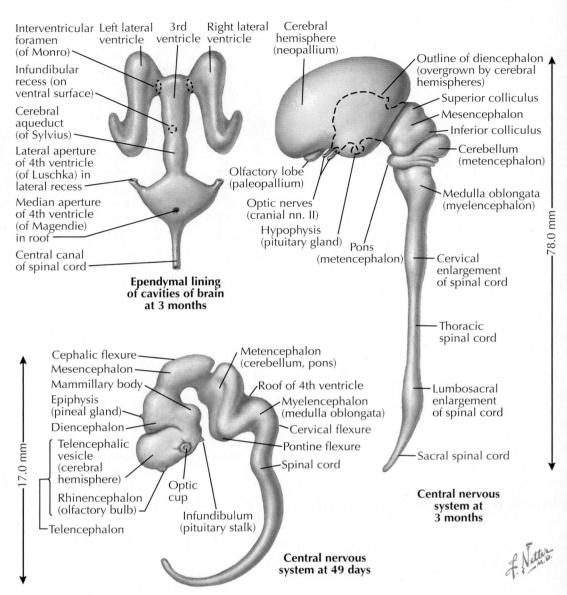

Interventricular foramen (of Monro)
Left lateral ventricle
3rd ventricle
Right lateral ventricle
Cerebral hemisphere (neopallium)
Infundibular recess (on ventral surface)
Cerebral aqueduct (of Sylvius)
Lateral aperture of 4th ventricle (of Luschka) in lateral recess
Median aperture of 4th ventricle (of Magendie) in roof
Central canal of spinal cord

Ependymal lining of cavities of brain at 3 months

Outline of diencephalon (overgrown by cerebral hemispheres)
Superior colliculus
Mesencephalon
Inferior colliculus
Cerebellum (metencephalon)
Olfactory lobe (paleopallium)
Optic nerves (cranial nn. II)
Hypophysis (pituitary gland)
Pons (metencephalon)
Medulla oblongata (myelencephalon)
Cervical enlargement of spinal cord

78.0 mm

Thoracic spinal cord

Lumbosacral enlargement of spinal cord

Sacral spinal cord

Central nervous system at 3 months

Cephalic flexure
Mesencephalon
Mammillary body
Epiphysis (pineal gland)
Diencephalon
Telencephalic vesicle (cerebral hemisphere)
Rhinencephalon (olfactory bulb)
Telencephalon
Optic cup
Infundibulum (pituitary stalk)
Metencephalon (cerebellum, pons)
Roof of 4th ventricle
Myelencephalon (medulla oblongata)
Cervical flexure
Pontine flexure
Spinal cord

17.0 mm

Central nervous system at 49 days

because it includes larger numbers of motor and sensory relay neurons that innervate or receive inputs from muscles and sensory receptors in the shoulders, arms, and hands. The spinal cord then narrows, and this region, the *thoracic cord,* includes motor and sensory neurons that innervate or receive sensory inputs from axial musculature, as well as preganglionic neurons that project to the autonomic ganglia of the sympathetic chain for central regulation of the sympathetic branch of the autonomic nervous system. The spinal cord expands again in the lumbar enlargement, reflecting larger numbers of motor and sensory relay neurons dedicated to the legs and feet. Finally, the narrow posterior *sacral cord* innervates and receives information from the pelvic and gluteal muscles.

As brain morphogenesis advances, the ventricles, defined initially by the space enclosed by the neural tube, become highly differentiated. The dramatic growth of the cerebral hemispheres is matched by growth of two bilaterally symmetric *lateral ventricles.* Their "C" shape reflects development of "deep" telencephalic structures, including the hippocampus and basal ganglia. Continuity between the lateral and *third ventricles* (surrounded by the diencephalon) occurs at the intraventricular foramen of Monro. Occluding this

opening leads to one type of noncommunicating hydrocephalus (see below). CSF trapped in the lateral ventricles causes secondary expansion of the cerebral hemispheres and overlying cranium (a second form, communicating hydrocephalus, reflects impaired reabsorption of CSF). The third ventricle also has a modest invagination, the infundibular recess, that reflects the position of the pituitary gland. The cerebral aqueduct, surrounded by the mesencephalon, and the fourth ventricle, defined by the rhombencephalon, become well defined. Occlusion of the cerebral aqueduct—aqueductal stenosis—is the most common noncommunicating hydrocephalus. In the fourth ventricle, the foramen of Luschka and Magendie establish continuity between the ventricles and subarachnoid space between the arachnoid and pia, the innermost meningeal layer. These apertures permit CSF, produced primarily by the choroid plexus, to flow into the subarachnoid space to mechanically cushion the brain and distribute signaling molecules to the developing meninges and external surface of the developing brain. Occlusion of these foramina, which is rare, also leads to noncommunicating hydrocephalus. The fourth ventricle narrows in the medulla, defining the central canal that extends most of the length of the spinal cord.

Plate 1.10

Normal and Abnormal Development

CRANIOSYNOSTOSIS

The growth of the brain is matched by the flexible growth of the cranial bones to establish a mechanism to expand the skull vault coincident with increased brain volume. The cranial bones, mostly generated by neural crest–derived chondrogenic and osteogenic precursors, are arranged as "plates" with elastic joints between each plate referred to as *cranial sutures*. *Craniosynostosis* implies a premature closure of one or more cranial sutures (see Plate 1.10). Early fusion of bone plates results in a progressively dysmorphic cranial shape. True craniosynostosis occurs in 1 of every 2000 infants, predominates in males, and manifests in nonsyndromic and syndromic forms. Normally, the metopic, or frontal, suture closes before birth; the posterior fontanelle, at the union of the lambdoid and sagittal sutures, closes by 3 months; and the anterior fontanelle, at the junction of the coronal, sagittal, and metopic sutures, closes by 18 months. After a suture is fused, growth occurs parallel to that suture; that is, growth is inhibited at 90 degrees to the suture. The fusion itself is felt as a ridge. Cranial sutures cannot be separated by increased intracranial pressure after 12 years of age.

Nonsyndromic craniosynostosis occurs much more frequently than syndromic. The most common premature closure occurs in the sagittal suture, which leads to *scaphocephaly, dolichocephaly,* or elongated head. The next most common premature closure is found in the *coronal suture,* which may be either unilateral or bilateral. If unilateral, it causes a unilateral ridge, with a pulling up of the orbit, flattening of the frontal area, and prominence near the zygoma on the affected side, which produces a quizzical expression. If premature coronal closure is bilateral, *brachycephalia,* which is manifested by an abnormally broad skull, is the result. Metopic craniosynostosis causes *trigonocephaly,* with a pointed frontal bone, hypotelorism, and prominent temporal hollowing. True lambdoid synostosis, which can also be unilateral or bilateral, is exceedingly rare, with an incidence less than 1 in 100,000. *Turricephaly,* a towering cranial vault due to multiple suture closure, is quite rare and disfiguring. Some infants will have prominent ridges along sutures without the other typical cranial findings, and these ridges will spontaneously resolve with time.

Syndromic craniosynostosis usually is autosomal dominant. Crouzon disease, with closure of multiple sutures and the associated facial anomalies of hypertelorism, proptosis, and choanal atresia, is known as *craniofacial dysostosis.* Intelligence is normal, but premature suture closure can cause elevated intracranial pressure. In *acrocephalosyndactyly,* or Apert syndrome, the head is elongated as a result of premature closure of all sutures; the orbits are shallow, causing exophthalmos; and either syndactyly or polydactyly is present. Saethre-Chotzen, Pfeiffer, and Carpenter have also identified syndromes of acrocephalosyndactyly that include various combinations of synostosis, syndactyly, and other anomalies. Syndromic craniosynostosis can be associated with hydrocephalus.

Conditions that can be confused with craniosynostosis include *microcephaly* and *deformational plagiocephaly.* Microcephaly from lack of brain growth is not typically accompanied by a disfigured cranial shape.

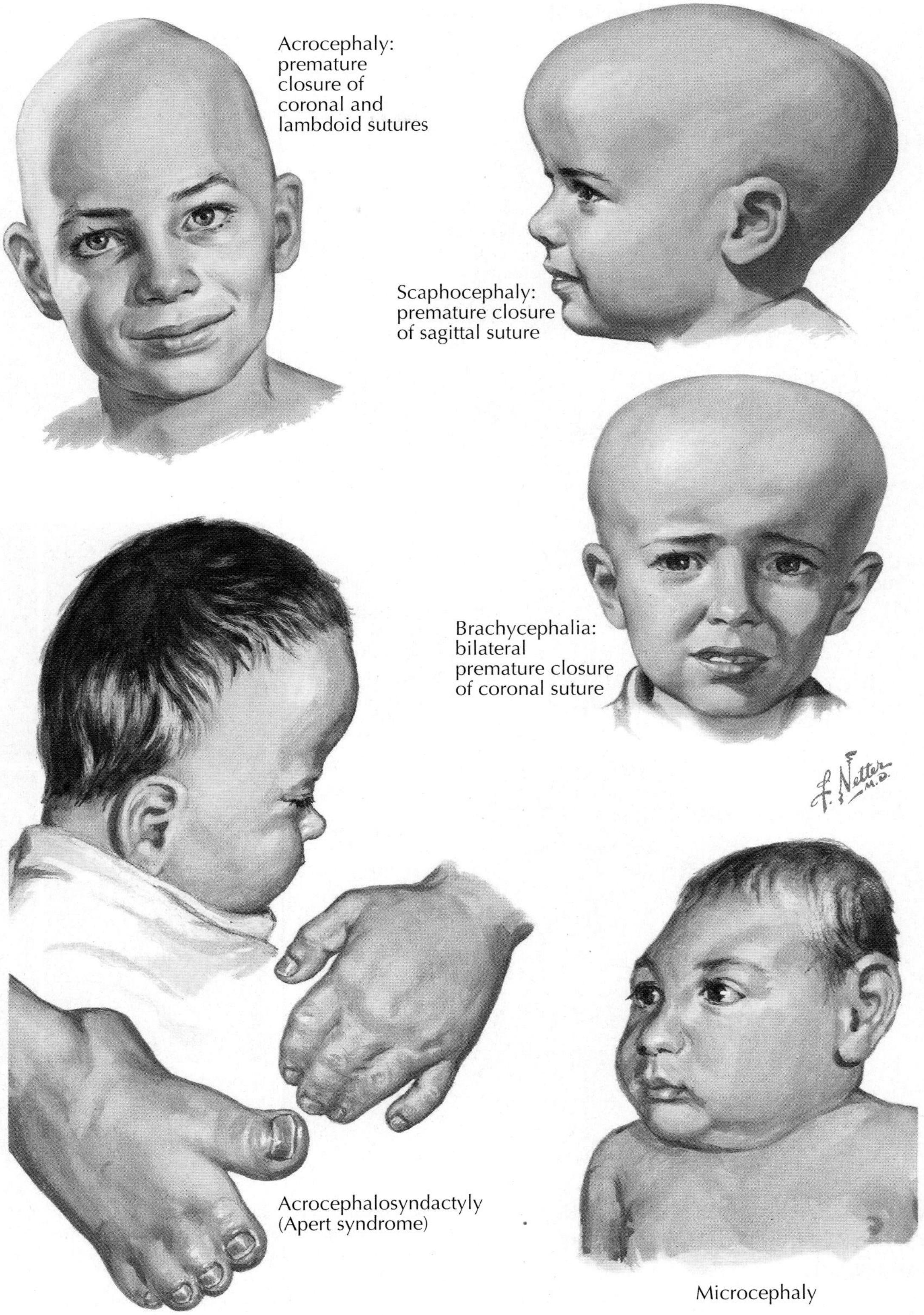

Acrocephaly: premature closure of coronal and lambdoid sutures

Scaphocephaly: premature closure of sagittal suture

Brachycephalia: bilateral premature closure of coronal suture

Acrocephalosyndactyly (Apert syndrome)

Microcephaly

Posterior deformational plagiocephaly is very common and currently occurs in approximately 1 in 10 infants. The baby tends to lie on one area of the skull, which causes flattening in the affected area, anterior displacement of the unilateral ear, and ipsilateral frontal and contralateral parietal bossing, with an overall parallelogram shape. Some infants have associated torticollis. Most infants will have spontaneous improvement with exercises; very severe cases may need treatment with a cranial orthosis.

The diagnosis of craniosynostosis is made by clinical examination in most cases. Appropriate radiographic examinations are typically only needed as a roadmap for surgical repair. Treatment for true craniosynostosis is surgical, with either endoscopic or open techniques. Early referral optimizes the opportunity to use minimally invasive techniques. Treatment of syndromic and multiple-suture craniosynostosis typically requires multiple procedures by an experienced multidisciplinary craniofacial team during early childhood.

Plate 1.11

Brain: PART I

Extracranial Hemorrhage or Edema in Newborn

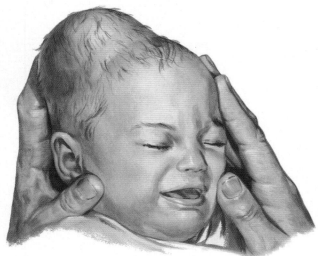

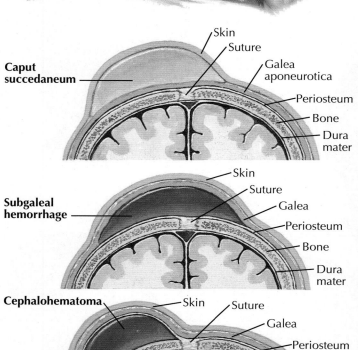

Caput succedaneum

Skin
Suture
Galea aponeurotica
Periosteum
Bone
Dura mater

Subgaleal hemorrhage

Skin
Suture
Galea
Periosteum
Bone
Dura mater

Cephalohematoma

Skin
Suture
Galea
Periosteum
Bone
Dura mater

Skull Fractures in Newborn

Depressed ("ping-pong") fracture

Growing skull fracture, or leptomeningeal cyst, results from an unrepaired dural laceration in the context of a growing cranium. Plain radiographs show the initial fracture after birth, and subsequent skull defect after several months (*arrows*). CT and MRI images demonstrate the extracranial cyst, skull defect, and underlying parenchymal loss.

EXTRACRANIAL HEMORRHAGE AND SKULL FRACTURES IN THE NEWBORN

Modern obstetric practice has decreased the incidence of trauma to the neonate that is clearly associated with primiparity, large infant size, difficult or breech delivery, and use of forceps.

Caput succedaneum, an edematous swelling that may be hemorrhagic, is seen in vaginal deliveries. It may transilluminate, is soft, pits, is usually at the vertex over suture lines, and resolves rapidly.

Subgaleal hemorrhage, which usually results from shearing forces tearing veins, occurs between the galea aponeurotica and the periosteum of the skull. It spreads widely, crosses suture lines, may dissect over the forehead and even into an orbit, and may take weeks to resolve. Neonates should be followed closely for symptomatic anemia.

Cephalohematoma is a subperiosteal hemorrhage associated with a linear skull fracture in about 5% of cases. It may result from the use of forceps, can also be related to mechanical factors in the pelvis and the shearing forces of active labor, and palpates like a depressed fracture. Rarely, these hematomas calcify instead of resorbing. Most calcified hematomas will spontaneously resolve as the skull grows and incorporates the area; surgery is not indicated.

SKULL FRACTURES

Neonatal skull fractures may be classified as linear, depressed, or occipital osteodiastasis. *Linear fracture* may be associated with cephalohematoma or, in traumatic deliveries, with epidural and subdural hemorrhage. Most heal without complication. Rarely, fractures become diastatic and are associated with a leptomeningeal cyst due to associated dural and meningeal tears that enlarge with brain growth.

Depressed ("ping-pong") fractures are of little clinical significance. Most are associated with the use of forceps, but some are related to intrauterine trauma against pelvic prominences after automobile collisions and falls, and also in active labor. Surgical elevation may be required and often can be performed with minimally invasive techniques.

Occipital osteodiastasis is seen in breech deliveries. The associated dural sinuses may be ruptured, causing a subdural hemorrhage of the posterior fossa. Surgical drainage is rarely necessary.

Plate 1.12

Normal and Abnormal Development

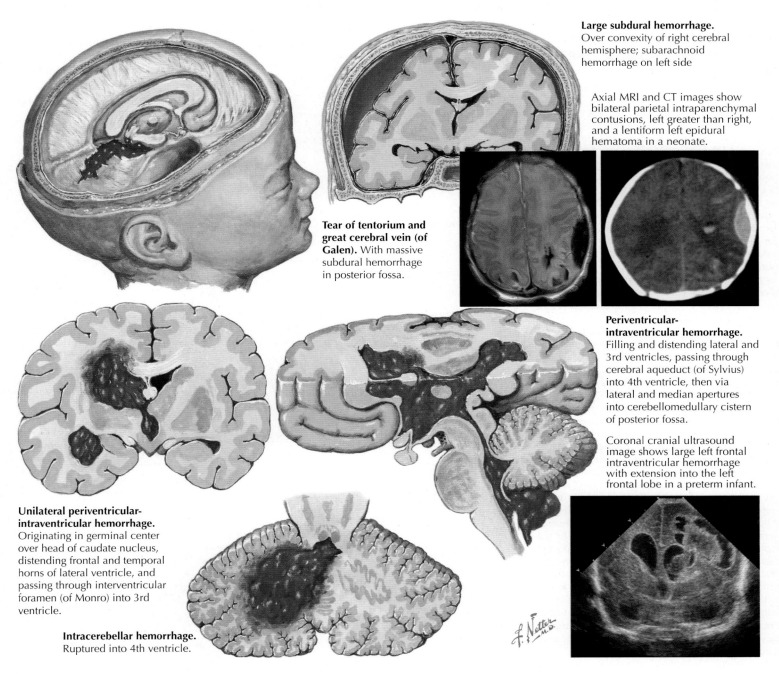

Large subdural hemorrhage. Over convexity of right cerebral hemisphere; subarachnoid hemorrhage on left side

Axial MRI and CT images show bilateral parietal intraparenchymal contusions, left greater than right, and a lentiform left epidural hematoma in a neonate.

Tear of tentorium and great cerebral vein (of Galen). With massive subdural hemorrhage in posterior fossa.

Periventricular-intraventricular hemorrhage. Filling and distending lateral and 3rd ventricles, passing through cerebral aqueduct (of Sylvius) into 4th ventricle, then via lateral and median apertures into cerebellomedullary cistern of posterior fossa.

Coronal cranial ultrasound image shows large left frontal intraventricular hemorrhage with extension into the left frontal lobe in a preterm infant.

Unilateral periventricular-intraventricular hemorrhage. Originating in germinal center over head of caudate nucleus, distending frontal and temporal horns of lateral ventricle, and passing through interventricular foramen (of Monro) into 3rd ventricle.

Intracerebellar hemorrhage. Ruptured into 4th ventricle.

INTRACRANIAL HEMORRHAGE IN THE NEWBORN

Intracranial hemorrhage in the neonate is classified by location and in order of frequency as (1) periventricular-intraventricular, (2) subarachnoid, (3) subdural, or (4) posterior fossa hemorrhage. All neonates should be followed closely for symptomatic anemia.

Periventricular-intraventricular hemorrhage (IVH) originates in the germinal matrix near the lateral ventricles and typically is observed in infants born preterm before 34 weeks' gestation (Plate 1.12). In preterm infants, the inherent friability of the germinal matrix is often complicated by cardiopulmonary compromise during birth and physiologic stresses of adjusting to the extrauterine environment in the early neonatal period. Massive bleeding, now quite rare, precipitates a bulging fontanelle, respiratory difficulties, tonic posturing, seizures, anemia, and, ultimately, multisystem failure. Minor bleeding detected with serial cranial ultrasonography is now more common. Some preterm infants will develop ventriculomegaly without cranial growth or elevated intracranial pressure, consistent with hydrocephalus ex vacuo from encephalomalacia. Approximately 15% of preterm infants with IVH will require surgical intervention for symptomatic hydrocephalus. Long-term neurologic deficits, including cerebral palsy, epilepsy, cognitive delay, and behavioral abnormalities, are common in preterm infants with IVH. In full-term infants, IVH typically occurs secondary to deep central venous thrombosis, and approximately half of these infants will develop early or late hydrocephalus. Term infants with IVH are also prone to chronic neurologic deficits, including epilepsy, cognitive delay, and behavioral abnormalities.

Subarachnoid hemorrhage may be caused by asphyxia or by forces of normal delivery. In full-term infants, it may be asymptomatic or associated with focal or generalized seizures, with no focal deficits. *Subdural hemorrhage* results from tears in the falx cerebri and tentorium, rupture of bridging veins over the hemispheres, or occipital osteodiastasis in breech delivery. Causes include excessive molding forces during delivery, the infant's size, and difficult extractions. Symptoms are acute or subacute hemiparesis, focal seizures, and ipsilateral pupillary abnormalities. Surgical drainage is the appropriate treatment in select cases. Cranial ultrasonography rarely provides adequate information, and either a rapid computed tomography (CT) or MRI scan is needed for management decisions.

Posterior fossa hemorrhage can result from tentorial trauma or occipital osteodiastasis. Either a rapid CT or MRI scan is often needed for management decisions, although high-resolution cranial ultrasound imaging via mastoid windows can now visualize the posterior fossa. Surgical drainage is rarely indicated.

Plate 1.13

Brain: PART I

External Development of the Brain in the Second and Third Trimesters

By the sixth month of gestation, the cerebral hemispheres acquire several features that prefigure the division of the cortical surface into cytoarchitectonic areas (regions with different neuron densities and varying thickness of the six cortical cell layers) that will define functional regions of the cortex. Four distinct domains, or *lobes,* define cortical territories at this time. The *frontal lobe* is most anterior; it eventually includes cortical areas devoted to motor control, language production (left hemisphere only in most individuals), and *executive function*—the capacity, moment by moment, to integrate perceptions of external stimuli with internal representations of motivations, goals, and memories to plan appropriate complex behavioral responses. Midway along the anterior-posterior axis, the *central* (also known as the rolandic) *sulcus* divides the frontal and more posterior *parietal lobe,* which mediates somatosensation and attention. This anatomic landmark is one of the earliest local furrowings that defines the *sulci* (grooves) and *gyri* (bulges) that reflect the elaborate folding of the mature cerebral cortex.

The central sulcus defines two essential, functionally distinct cortical regions. The *precentral gyrus* on the anterior bank is the location of the *primary motor cortex.* Neurons of the primary motor cortex send axons directly to brainstem and spinal cord motor neurons that innervate muscles or to adjacent interneurons that synapse upon these motor neurons. The *postcentral gyrus* on the posterior bank is the location of the *primary somatosensory cortex.* The primary somatosensory cortex receives topographically mapped inputs that represent somatosensory information from the entire body surface from thalamic sensory relay nuclei. The remainder of the parietal lobe, posterior to the postcentral gyrus, is devoted to sensory integration and attention. The *occipital lobe,* marked by the *parietooccipital sulcus,* is devoted exclusively to representation and processing of vision. Finally, anterior to the *lateral sulcus,* the anterior extension of the hemisphere defines the *temporal lobe,* including cortical regions that integrate information about the identity of visual stimuli, auditory information, and, in the left hemisphere of most individuals, the representation of "lexical" language (the brain's "dictionary" of words). The initial growth of the frontal, parietal, occipital, and temporal lobes results in "operculation," or covering of cortical tissue called the *insula.* The cortex of the insula becomes specialized for visceral and homeostatic control and the representation of taste information.

The dramatic growth of the cerebral hemispheres is accompanied by differentiation of the cerebellum and medulla. By the end of the sixth month of gestation, the cerebellum expands with furrows and ridges that eventually become the highly folded folia of the cerebellar cortex (note: a cortex is the outer sheet of cells that invests any organ). The pons is distinct, consisting of axons from the cortex that project to neurons in the pontine nuclei that then send axons to the cerebellar cortex. The medulla also becomes furrowed and ridged, but for a different reason. The *pyramid,* a prominent ridge on the ventral (anterior) medulla, reflects growth of axons from motor cortical neurons to the brainstem and spinal cord. By the end of gestation, the pyramid is adjacent to a more lateral ridge, the *olive.* The olive reflects accumulation of

neurons into the olivary nucleus; olivary neurons selectively innervate the extensive dendritic arbors of Purkinje cells.

Finally, further elaboration of the ventricular system accompanies these morphogenetic transformations. The ventricular system is best depicted in a "cast" of space within the brain and spinal cord, as if the ventricles were filled with plaster in the absence of any neural tissue. The key changes in ventricular shape reflect differential growth of brain regions that correspond to each ventricular division. The lateral ventricles grow disproportionately and acquire further anatomic definition. The *anterior horn* extends into the frontal lobe,

with the caudate nucleus of the basal ganglia as its floor. The *inferior horn* extends into the temporal lobe; on its anterior and medial surface is the hippocampus. The *posterior horn* extends into the occipital lobe. The shape and size of the additional ventricular spaces also change substantially. The third ventricle becomes a narrow midline space, further indented by the thalamus on each side (the thalamic impression), as well as a foramen surrounding the intrathalamic adhesion. In addition, the third ventricle is indented by the optic chiasm at the optic recess, the pineal gland at the pineal and suprapineal recess, and the pituitary gland at the infundibular recess.

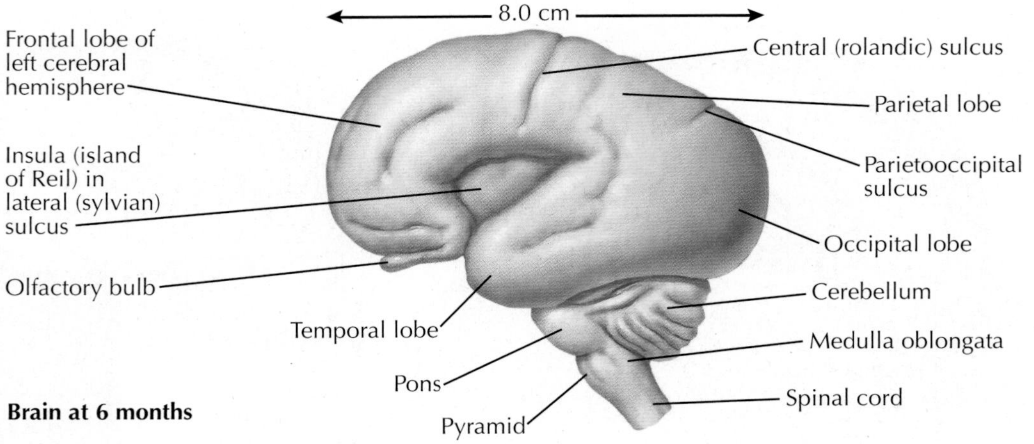

Brain at 6 months

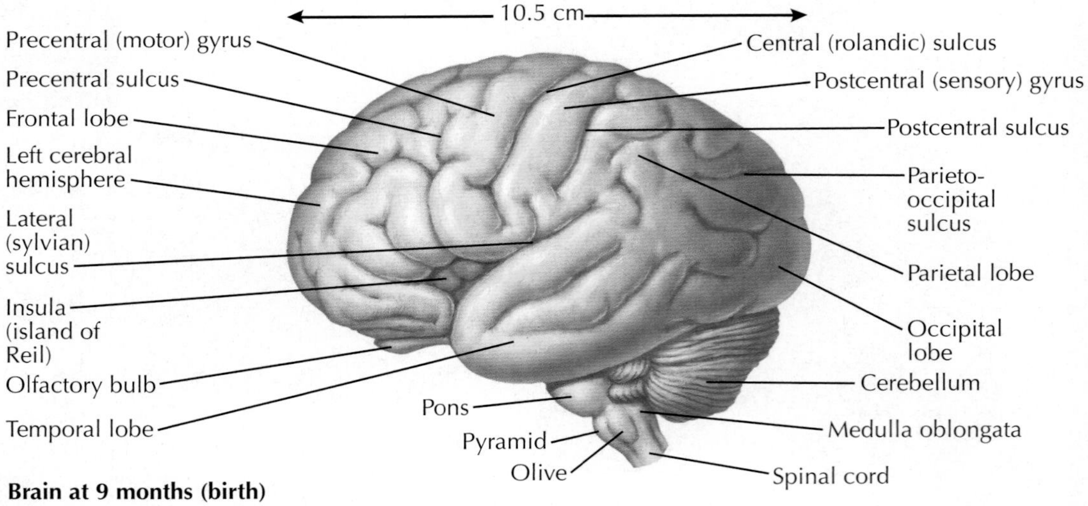

- 8.0 cm
- Frontal lobe of left cerebral hemisphere
- Insula (island of Reil) in lateral (sylvian) sulcus
- Olfactory bulb
- Temporal lobe
- Pons
- Pyramid
- Central (rolandic) sulcus
- Parietal lobe
- Parietooccipital sulcus
- Occipital lobe
- Cerebellum
- Medulla oblongata
- Spinal cord

Brain at 9 months (birth)

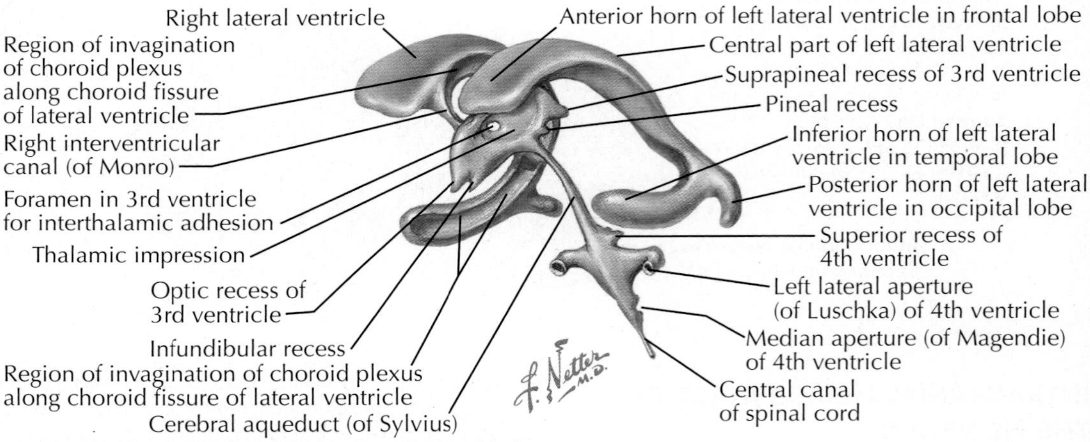

- 10.5 cm
- Precentral (motor) gyrus
- Precentral sulcus
- Frontal lobe
- Left cerebral hemisphere
- Lateral (sylvian) sulcus
- Insula (island of Reil)
- Olfactory bulb
- Temporal lobe
- Pons
- Pyramid
- Olive
- Central (rolandic) sulcus
- Postcentral (sensory) gyrus
- Postcentral sulcus
- Parieto-occipital sulcus
- Parietal lobe
- Occipital lobe
- Cerebellum
- Medulla oblongata
- Spinal cord

Ventricular system of the brain at 9 months (birth)

- Right lateral ventricle
- Region of invagination of choroid plexus along choroid fissure of lateral ventricle
- Right interventricular canal (of Monro)
- Foramen in 3rd ventricle for interthalamic adhesion
- Thalamic impression
- Optic recess of 3rd ventricle
- Infundibular recess
- Region of invagination of choroid plexus along choroid fissure of lateral ventricle
- Cerebral aqueduct (of Sylvius)
- Anterior horn of left lateral ventricle in frontal lobe
- Central part of left lateral ventricle
- Suprapineal recess of 3rd ventricle
- Pineal recess
- Inferior horn of left lateral ventricle in temporal lobe
- Posterior horn of left lateral ventricle in occipital lobe
- Superior recess of 4th ventricle
- Left lateral aperture (of Luschka) of 4th ventricle
- Median aperture (of Magendie) of 4th ventricle
- Central canal of spinal cord

Plate 1.14

Normal and Abnormal Development

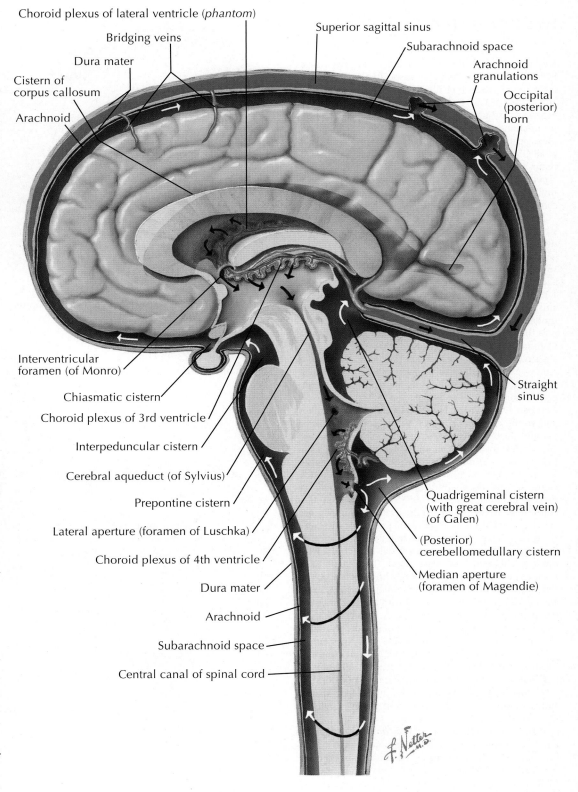

Choroid plexus of lateral ventricle (*phantom*)

Bridging veins

Dura mater

Cistern of
corpus callosum

Arachnoid

Superior sagittal sinus

Subarachnoid space

Arachnoid
granulations

Occipital
(posterior)
horn

Straight
sinus

Quadrigeminal cistern
(with great cerebral vein)
(of Galen)

(Posterior)
cerebellomedullary cistern

Median aperture
(foramen of Magendie)

Interventricular
foramen (of Monro)

Chiasmatic cistern

Choroid plexus of 3rd ventricle

Interpeduncular cistern

Cerebral aqueduct (of Sylvius)

Prepontine cistern

Lateral aperture (foramen of Luschka)

Choroid plexus of 4th ventricle

Dura mater

Arachnoid

Subarachnoid space

Central canal of spinal cord

Mature Brain Ventricles

Few anatomic features of the mature brain reflect brain development more directly than the brain ventricles. This continuous system of fluid-filled chambers is the same space that was defined by the closure of the neural tube. Subsequent morphogenesis modifies this space; nevertheless, its relationship to the original neural tube lumen is clear. CSF, which is produced in the mature brain by the choroid plexus found in the lateral, third, and fourth ventricles, circulates throughout this space in the adult (as well as the embryonic) brain. The proteins and ions in the CSF vary over the course of development and in the adult, providing a dynamic set of signals to support the maturing and mature brain. The ventricular space also has a series of continuities with the subarachnoid space so that CSF can bathe the external and deep (or ventricular) surfaces of the brain.

In the adult brain, the two mature cerebral hemispheres surround the lateral ventricles. These two ventricles, the largest of the ventricular chambers, have three extensions into distinct regions of the cerebral hemispheres. The *anterior horns* extend into the frontal lobes, the *inferior horns* extend into the temporal lobe (including adjacent to the hippocampus), and the *posterior horns* extend into the occipital lobes. The *atrium* is the junction of the anterior, posterior, and temporal horns. The relationship between the anterior horns of the lateral ventricles—the corpus callosum posteriorly, the caudate nucleus anterolaterally (defining the ventral aspect of the lateral ventricles), and the third ventricle and thalamus—is shown in the lower panel of Plate 1.13. The lateral ventricles remain continuous with the third ventricle via the intraventricular foramen of Monro (the curved black arrow shows the continuity between lateral and third ventricles provided by the foramen of Monro). The third ventricle extends the anterior to posterior length of the diencephalon.

The third ventricle is continuous with the *cerebral aqueduct,* which travels through the mature mesencephalon. The cerebral aqueduct connects to the *fourth*

ventricle, which is adjacent to the cerebellum and pons, and extends into the upper medulla. The fourth ventricle has a significant bilateral extension, the *lateral recess,* which opens into the inferior cerebellar peduncle. The fourth ventricle also has several specialized continuities with the subarachnoid space to facilitate the circulation and drainage of CSF, which maintains the integrity of cells from the exterior surface of the brain, as well as at the ventricular zone, and helps maintain the ionic balance of interstitial fluid in brain tissue.

The two *lateral apertures* (also known as the foramen of Luschka) are continuous with the subarachnoid space at the lateral aspect of the pontocerebellar junction (near the inferior cerebellar peduncle), and the *median aperture,* located at the midline where the two lateral recesses originate, is continuous with the *cerebellomedullary cistern* (also referred to as the cisterna magna). Indeed, there is a distributed system of cisterns throughout the subarachnoid space that provides reservoirs of CSF.

Plate 1.15

Brain: PART I

HYDROCEPHALUS

Hydrocephalus results in the enlargement of ventricles. Symptomatic hydrocephalus associated with elevated intracranial pressure results most often from decreased absorption of CSF or blockage of outflow through the ventricular system (see Plate 1.15). Sustained excess CSF production is quite rare and usually due only to choroid plexus papilloma, a choroid plexus tumor. Enlargement of all CSF spaces, including the ventricles, that is due to brain atrophy (or encephalomalacia) is termed *hydrocephalus ex vacuo*. The etiology of hydrocephalus can be multifactorial, and the clinical course and management can change throughout the lifetime.

Symptomatic hydrocephalus is subdivided into obstructive and nonobstructive etiologies. Obstructive hydrocephalus is due to blockage of CSF flow by a congenital malformation, such as aqueductal stenosis or suprasellar arachnoid cyst, or by an acquired condition, such as a ventricular tumor that obstructs flow (Plate 1.15). Communicating (or nonobstructive) hydrocephalus was originally defined before modern imaging modalities by the ability to recover dye initially injected into the lateral ventricle from the lumbar thecal space. Communicating hydrocephalus is due to impaired CSF absorption through the arachnoid villi and occurs most commonly secondary to intraventricular or subarachnoid hemorrhage, trauma, meningitis, or leptomeningeal tumor spread.

When symptomatic hydrocephalus occurs in infants and young children, progressive macrocephaly occurs because the cranial sutures are not yet fused. Head circumference measurement and assessment of the fontanel and cranial suture splay are routine components of the neurologic examination (see Plate 1.16). Other causes of macrocephaly in infants are *benign enlargement of subarachnoid space* (BESS) and extraaxial fluid collections. BESS usually occurs in the setting of familial macrocephaly, is asymptomatic except for the excessively large head circumference, and has a characteristic imaging pattern of frontal extraaxial collections without any suggestion of mass effect. The infant has a normal neurologic examination without other symptoms or signs of elevated intracranial pressure. Extraaxial fluid collections associated with elevated intracranial pressure have other etiologies, including meningitis and subdural hematomas from abusive head trauma and rare metabolic disorders. Elevated intracranial pressure in infants, including from advanced symptomatic hydrocephalus or extraaxial fluid collections, is often characterized by lethargy, irritability, poor oral intake, engorged scalp veins, a full fontanel and splayed sutures, and downward deviation of the eyes, referred to as "sunset eyes."

Imaging with CT or MRI can facilitate the diagnosis and management of patients with suspected hydrocephalus. Patients with suspected elevated intracranial pressure from hydrocephalus need imaging with CT or MRI before any intervention that might change the CSF dynamics, such as a lumbar puncture. Current MRI sequences can suggest points of blockage or demonstrate flow through the aqueduct of Sylvius. The coronal brain section shown in the illustration indicates that the hydrocephalus, in this instance, is caused either by obstruction of an outflow pathway distal to the third ventricle or is a form of communicating hydrocephalus, in which case the fourth ventricle would also be dilated.

Symptomatic hydrocephalus in older children and adults is similarly divided into obstructive and nonobstructive etiologies, and this guides management

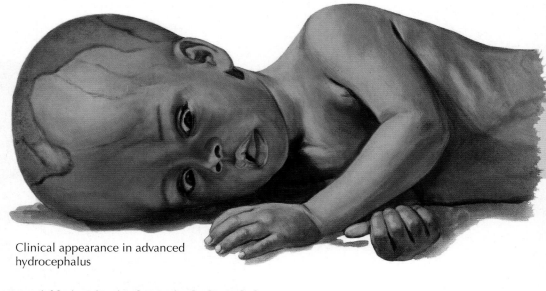

Clinical appearance in advanced hydrocephalus

Potential lesion sites in obstructive hydrocephalus

1. Interventricular foramen (of Monro)
2. Cerebral aqueduct (of Sylvius)
3. Lateral apertures (of Luschka)
4. Median aperture (of Magendie)

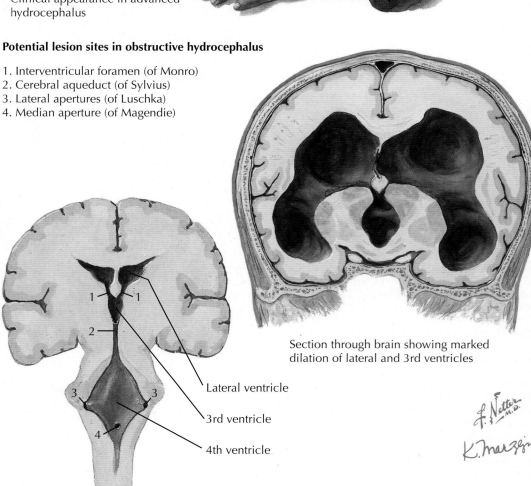

Section through brain showing marked dilation of lateral and 3rd ventricles

Lateral ventricle
3rd ventricle
4th ventricle

decisions. Clinically, patients with symptomatic hydrocephalus are often lethargic, with headache, emesis, and other features of elevated intracranial pressure, including papilledema and cranial nerve palsies. *Idiopathic intracranial hypertension,* or pseudotumor cerebri, is characterized by elevated intracranial pressure without ventriculomegaly. Patients typically present with headache, vision loss, and diplopia and may require urgent intervention to minimize vision loss.

Normal pressure hydrocephalus (NPH) is a well-described syndrome in older adults that is associated with neurologic symptoms and signs without markedly elevated intracranial pressure. Initial symptoms are progressive dementia, gait disorders, and urinary incontinence. Brain imaging shows ventricular dilation, and the condition must be differentiated from ventricular dilation secondary to brain atrophy. A high-volume lumbar puncture can be diagnostic, although other clinicians prefer to use an isotope cisternogram to trace the CSF circulation (remove cisternogram images). In carefully selected patients with NPH, symptoms improve or resolve after the CSF shunt insertion (see Plate 1.16).

Plate 1.16

Normal and Abnormal Development

SURGICAL TREATMENT OF HYDROCEPHALUS

The treatment of hydrocephalus depends on the etiology and factors such as the patient's age, comorbidities, and anatomy. When hydrocephalus is secondary to a tumor or cyst blocking CSF outflow pathways, tumor removal or cyst fenestration may suffice. Most patients with communicating or obstructive hydrocephalus, however, require a CSF diversion procedure to compensate for impaired absorption or blockage. Successful CSF diversion procedures can halt progressive ventricular dilation and elevation of intracranial pressure and can frequently lead to improvement in neurologic function. CSF diversion can be accomplished by endoscopic procedures that bypass an obstruction or by insertion of a shunt to move CSF to an alternate site for eventual absorption into the bloodstream.

Transient hydrocephalus can be temporarily treated with an external ventriculostomy or lumbar drain. These temporary drainage systems allow constant monitoring of the amount and character of CSF drainage, which can be quite helpful in patients with a limited neurologic examination. For obstructive hydrocephalus, the CSF diversion must occur above the blockage. In preterm infants, temporary treatment of symptomatic hydrocephalus is achieved with a ventriculosubgaleal shunt that drains the CSF into a subgaleal pocket or into a ventricular access device with a reservoir. Once the preterm infant achieves an adequate size, typically at 2 to 3 months of age, a more permanent CSF diversion procedure is performed, if needed.

Endoscopic procedures for CSF diversion include endoscopic third ventriculostomy, cyst fenestration, choroid plexus coagulation, and other procedures. The success of these procedures depends on multiple factors, including patient selection and specific anatomic details. The primary benefit of endoscopic procedures is the avoidance of implantation of shunt components that may later malfunction, become infected, or induce shunt dependence. Endoscopic procedures for CSF diversion can have late failure, and all patients after endoscopic procedures continue to require chronic neurosurgical supervision similar to patients with shunts.

The most common shunt system used is a ventriculoperitoneal shunt with a valve. Shunt components are made from silicone rubber material, and some are impregnated with antibiotic to decrease the risk of infection. The ventricular catheter tip is targeted to the frontal horn of a lateral ventricle from either a frontal or parietooccipital trajectory. As the catheter exits the skull in the subcutaneous space, it is connected to a valve. Some surgeons use an intervening reservoir. The goal of the valve is to minimize overdrainage with subsequent collapse of the ventricular system and formation of life-threatening subdural hematomas. Various types of valves have been devised; none among them have been proven superior in a well-designed multicenter trial. Shunt tubing can also contain a valve at the distal tip. The subcutaneous distal shunt tubing is inserted into the peritoneal cavity, where the peritoneum absorbs the CSF back into systemic veins. Adequate tubing is placed in infants to decrease the chance that a lengthening procedure will be required. Alternate distal tubing sites include the right atrium or the pleural cavity. Lumboperitoneal shunts are used in select patients. Occasionally, it is necessary to obtain CSF from a patient with a shunt or to inject antibiotics or chemotherapy into the ventricular system instead of via a lumbar puncture. Rarely, contrast material may also be injected to identify loculations within the

SHUNT PROCEDURE FOR HYDROCEPHALUS

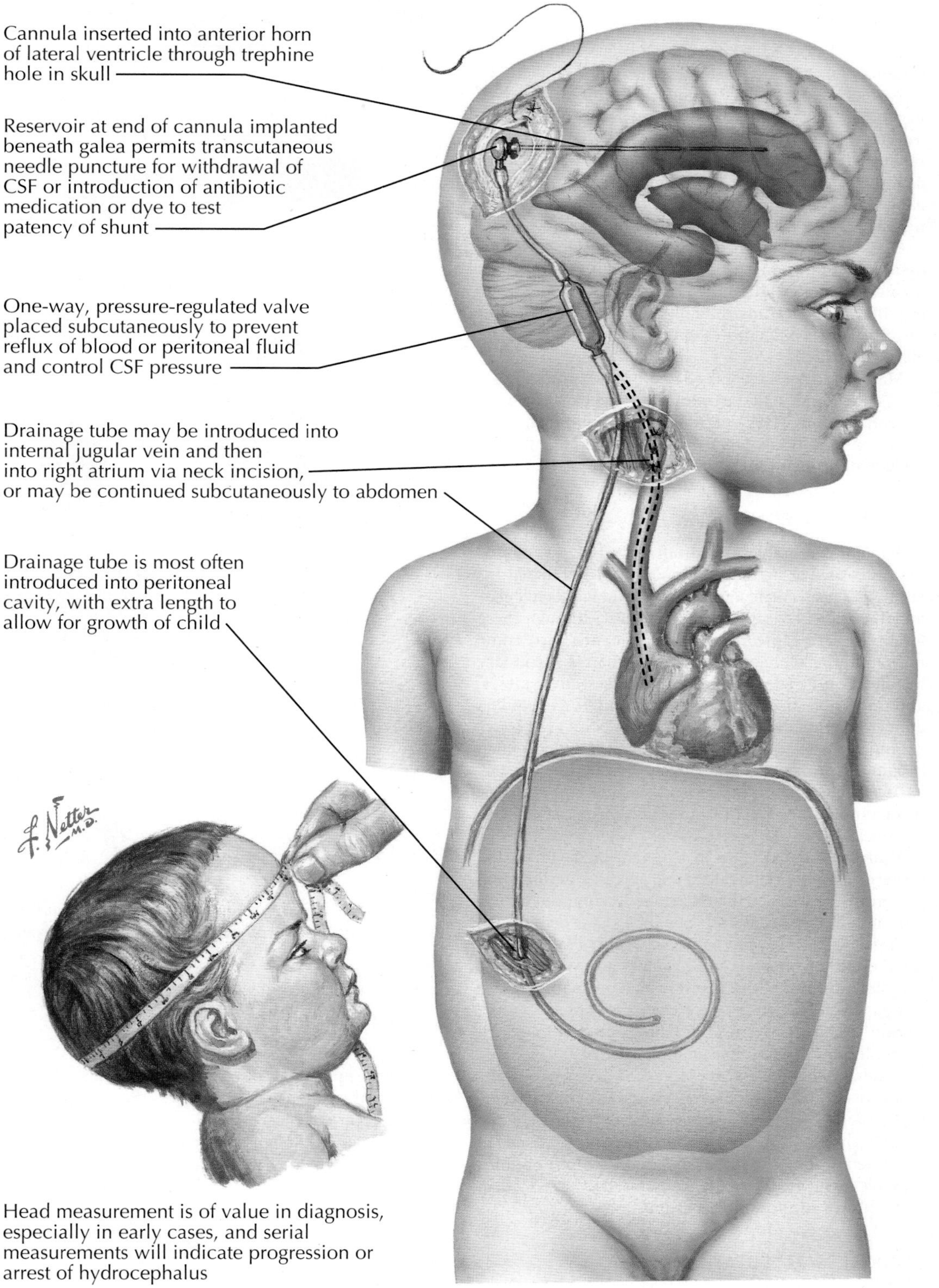

Cannula inserted into anterior horn of lateral ventricle through trephine hole in skull

Reservoir at end of cannula implanted beneath galea permits transcutaneous needle puncture for withdrawal of CSF or introduction of antibiotic medication or dye to test patency of shunt

One-way, pressure-regulated valve placed subcutaneously to prevent reflux of blood or peritoneal fluid and control CSF pressure

Drainage tube may be introduced into internal jugular vein and then into right atrium via neck incision, or may be continued subcutaneously to abdomen

Drainage tube is most often introduced into peritoneal cavity, with extra length to allow for growth of child

Head measurement is of value in diagnosis, especially in early cases, and serial measurements will indicate progression or arrest of hydrocephalus

ventricular cavity. Any manipulation of a shunt by a non-neurosurgeon should be performed only in direct collaboration with a neurosurgeon.

The long-term success of the CSF diversion procedure depends on the continued patency of the shunt or endoscopic opening. Failure of an endoscopic fenestration can lead to the same symptoms and signs of neurologic decline as a shunt failure. Once shunted, patients who may have previously absorbed a portion of their CSF may become completely dependent on the shunt for CSF diversion. The clinical presentation of a patient with failure of

the CSF diversion procedure may or may not mimic the symptoms at the time of the diagnosis of hydrocephalus and initial treatment. The symptoms and signs of failure and period of illness may depend on the type of failure, the etiology of hydrocephalus, and the patient's age. The most common cause of shunt malfunction is proximal catheter occlusion. Many patients with CSF diversion failure will present with recurrence of ventriculomegaly. Of importance, 10% to 20% of children presenting with a shunt malfunction will have no apparent change in the ventricular size compared with a baseline imaging study.

Plate 1.17

Brain: PART I

CEREBRAL PALSY

Cerebral palsy (CP) is caused by a broad group of developmental, genetic, metabolic, ischemic, infectious, and other etiologies that produce a common group of neurologic phenotypes. It is defined as a central motor dysfunction affecting muscle tone, posture, and movement that is attributed to nonprogressive disturbances in the developing brain. Although nonprogressive, CP is not static in evolution but rather dynamic due to factors such as growth, CNS maturation, and aging.

CP is a descriptive diagnosis and manifests as motor defects that range in severity. Associated disorders may include intellectual disability, epilepsy, visual and hearing difficulties, feeding difficulties, and orthopedic deformities. Other diagnoses should be excluded before CP is diagnosed.

Many children have CP related to birth trauma (see Plates 1.11 and 1.12) attributed to hypoxic-ischemic encephalopathy (HIE). Low oxygen combined with impaired blood flow is particularly damaging and can include other neurologic symptoms such as seizures.

CEREBRAL LESIONS

Five major cerebral lesions result from HIE: (1) neuronal necrosis, (2) status marmoratus, (3) watershed infarcts, (4) periventricular telencephalic leukoencephalopathy, and (5) focal ischemic lesions. Although these lesions describe the neuropathologic findings, some may underlie damage to the CNS that is secondary to infection, trauma, vascular diseases, dysgeneses, and migration disorders. In *neuronal necrosis*, hypoxia damages neural cells throughout the CNS.

Status marmoratus affects the basal ganglia, which become shrunken with a whitish, marble-like appearance. Affected infants are most often full term with initial hypotonia (see Plate 1.17), followed by spasticity and dyskinesias.

Watershed infarcts due to hypotension begin in the posterior parietooccipital area and spread anteriorly and posteriorly. Watershed infarcts are most common in full-term infants and result in spastic diplegia or hemiplegia.

Periventricular telencephalic leukoencephalopathy is most common in premature infants and often affects the centrum ovale. Minor lesions lead to white matter atrophy, whereas more severe lesions appear cystic. Minor lesions can cause learning disabilities, with severe lesions causing spastic diplegia.

Focal ischemic lesions are large and occur in specific blood vessel distributions, most often the middle cerebral artery. Probable causes are hypoxic-ischemic events, emboli, and thromboses. The large damaged area often becomes cavitated and develops into a porencephalic cyst. Occasionally, a cyst causes mass effect and requires surgical intervention.

CLINICAL MANIFESTATIONS OF CEREBRAL PALSY

The two main types of CP are spastic and extrapyramidal. These classifications are based on the type and distribution of motor abnormalities, which are divided into subtypes.

Spastic cerebral palsy involves damage to cortical areas responsible for voluntary movements, which contributes to spasticity. Subtypes include hemiplegia, quadriplegia, diplegia, triplegia, and rarely monoplegia.

Hemiplegia typically affects term infants, with most causes arising from maldevelopment and neonatal stroke. A hypotonic limb is initially noted, with subsequent spasticity (the arm more often than the leg).

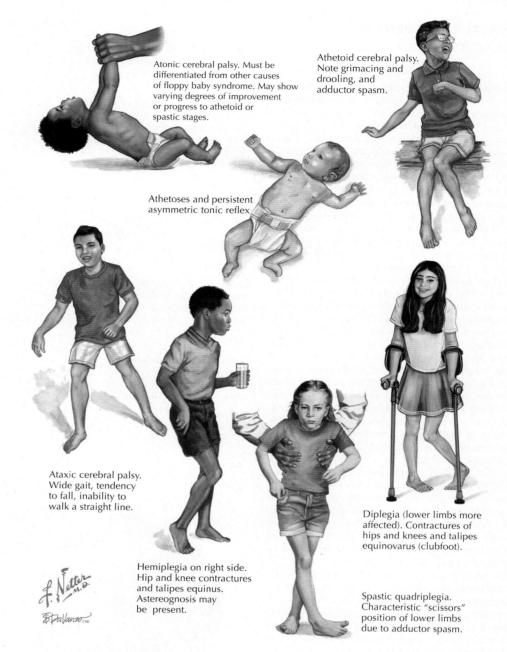

Atonic cerebral palsy. Must be differentiated from other causes of floppy baby syndrome. May show varying degrees of improvement or progress to athetoid or spastic stages.

Athetoid cerebral palsy. Note grimacing and drooling, and adductor spasm.

Athetoses and persistent asymmetric tonic reflex

Ataxic cerebral palsy. Wide gait, tendency to fall, inability to walk a straight line.

Hemiplegia on right side. Hip and knee contractures and talipes equinus. Astereognosis may be present.

Diplegia (lower limbs more affected). Contractures of hips and knees and talipes equinovarus (clubfoot).

Spastic quadriplegia. Characteristic "scissors" position of lower limbs due to adductor spasm.

Quadriplegia, the most severe form, can affect all infants with a range of etiologies, from hypoxic or traumatic perinatal cerebral injuries to developmental abnormalities. Although spastic quadriplegia is usually evident early, hypotonia may manifest initially. Individuals typically have severe comorbidities, including epilepsy, intellectual disability, and pseudobulbar palsy.

Diplegia primarily affects the legs, causing spasticity with scissoring. This affects both term and preterm infants and, in the latter, is often associated with periventricular leukomalacia (PVL). Hand function and cognition are relatively intact.

Monoplegia is the involvement of any one of the four limbs of the body, but it usually affects the arms.

Triplegia is formed from a combination of spastic diplegia and a hemiplegia. This can be seen in preterm infants who develop PVL, resulting in diplegia and a unilateral intraventricular hemorrhage causing a concurrent hemiplegia.

Extrapyramidal cerebral palsy results from damage typically to the subcortical areas responsible for movement, coordination, and balance, with intelligence spared in most. Subtypes are named according to the type of movement.

Ataxia affects term infants and can result in hypotonia, difficulty with balance and coordination, or slower movements.

Dyskinesias are most often due to HIE. Infants are hypotonic, with persistence of primitive motor patterns (arching, tonic neck reflexes) that preclude orderly motor development. Involuntary movements, including dystonia and/or choreoathetosis, become more consistent with dyskinetic CP.

TREATMENT

Evaluation and treatment of CP demand a multidisciplinary approach. Treatment goals focus on maximizing daily function and independence and target the child's multiple medical, social, psychologic, educational, and therapeutic needs.

Treatment of spasticity and dyskinesias includes rehabilitation strategies, pharmacology, and surgical (orthopedic and neurosurgical) options.

Plate 1.18

Normal and Abnormal Development

Establishing Cellular Diversity in the Embryonic Brain and Spinal Cord

The morphogenetic transformation of the embryonic brain from a neural tube during the early first trimester to an organ that resembles the adult brain by the end of gestation is ultimately driven by ongoing neural stem cell proliferation, neurogenesis, and differentiation. This "histogenesis" depends on the specification and accumulation of neural stem cells with distinct capacities to generate diverse classes of neurons and glial cells in brain regions specified during earlier stages of development. Subsequently, these stem cells, based on their position in the anterior-posterior and dorsal-ventral axes of the neural tube, as well as their access to both local and circulating signals, establish identity that is maintained in their postmitotic progeny. Thus the position of neural stem cells in the developing brain is a key determinant of the ultimate organization of each brain region. This relationship can be used to understand the basic adult organization of the entire CNS.

Neural stem cells that give rise to mature brain neurons and glia, with few exceptions, comprise a layer of cells that lines the ventricular space of the neural tube throughout its entire anterior-posterior extent. This layer, known either as the *ependymal layer* or *ventricular zone* of the developing neuroepithelium, is the primary location of true neural stem cells: the proliferative cells in the nervous system that divide symmetrically and slowly to yield additional stem cells that have the capacity to generate all of the cell types in that region. A distinct type of proliferative cell, the *intermediate or transit amplifying progenitor* (also called a *basal progenitor* in the developing cerebral cortex), is found in the mantle layer (also known as the intermediate zone). In addition, many newly postmitotic neurons are also found in the mantle layer. Finally, the outermost region of the neural tube epithelium is referred to as the *marginal layer*, or *marginal zone*. The marginal zone has some postmitotic neurons and glia and some nascent axonal and dendritic processes from local differentiating neurons. In the spinal cord and hindbrain (medulla and mesencephalon), the marginal zone is also usually the site of axon pathways that grow from other regions of the brain to innervate local target neurons. Thus these three neuroepithelial layers or zones—ependymal/ventricular, mantle/intermediate, and marginal—maintain local neural stem cells, facilitate neurogenesis, and support initial neuronal differentiation.

The neural tube also acquires regional distinctions in the posterior-anterior axis that reflect the ultimate division of the spinal cord, hindbrain, mesencephalon, and diencephalon into sensory and motor regions that either receive inputs from peripheral sensory receptors and relay this information to additional brain regions or send axons to skeletal muscles or autonomic ganglia to regulate behavior and homeostasis. From the most posterior aspect of the spinal cord through the anterior end of the diencephalon, the neural tube becomes divided into *posterior* or *alar* and *anterior* or *basal plates*. In most vertebrates, except for bipedal primates, including humans, the posterior and anterior axes of the spinal cord are actually parallel to the dorsal and ventral body axes. Thus the alar plate is often referred to as the dorsal neural tube, and the basal plate is referred to as the ventral neural tube. These zones are distinguished from one another by a local groove, called the *sulcus limitans,* that indents the ependymal/ventricular zone. Thus in the spinal cord, medulla, mesencephalon, and diencephalon, alar plate derivatives become sensory relay zones or distinct sensory relay nuclei. In spinal cord, the sensory relay zone is referred to as the *posterior horn* and eventually becomes highly laminated in register with different classes of sensory input. In the medulla, the posterior plate gives rise to sensory coordinating, or relay, nuclei for the cranial nerves. In the mesencephalon, the posterior plate gives rise to the superior and inferior colliculi, which receive input either directly from the eye (superior) or indirectly from the auditory nerve (inferior). These two nuclei are crucial for integrating sensory information with the initiation of motor commands. Finally, in the diencephalon, the posterior plate gives rise to all of the thalamic sensory coordinating, or relay, nuclei for the senses: vision (lateral geniculate nucleus), audition (medial geniculate nucleus), somatosensation (anterobasal complex), taste (anterobasal complex), and olfaction (medioposterior nucleus). As development proceeds, the dorsal (posterior) spinal cord, medulla, mesencephalon, and diencephalon become the location of *axon tracts* that carry sensory afferent axons.

The basal plate yields groups of neurons whose axons project directly to striated muscles (skeletal motor neurons), autonomic ganglia (preganglionic motor neurons), and cranial muscles (cranial motor neurons). The position of various anterior plate derivatives along the anterior-posterior axis, from the spinal cord through medulla and mesencephalon, determines the type of motor neuron that is generated. Thus throughout the entire spinal cord, most of the motor neurons in the anterior (ventral) horn or column are skeletal motor neurons. In addition, in the thoracic spinal cord, preganglionic motor (or visceral) neurons are generated in the lateral horn, approximately in the region of the sulcus limitans. In the medulla, there is a variety of cranial motor nuclei that have cranial motor nerves that project to the muscles of the head and neck, the jaws, the tongue, and the eyes. Their medial to lateral position identifies them as either skeletal motor neurons or branchial motor neurons that project to cranial and oropharyngeal muscles. In the mesencephalon, there are a number of tegmental nuclei that influence motor function (including the ventral tegmental area, which has dopaminergic neurons), as well as the red nucleus, whose neurons project to skeletal motor neurons that regulate, among other things, gross arm movements. Finally, the basal plate of the diencephalon becomes a collection of motor control nuclei of the hypothalamus that projects to preganglionic, visceral motor neurons in the brainstem and spinal cord that regulate a broad range of homeostatic and reproductive functions. The mantle zone of each region of the anterior plate develops into distinctive axon tracts that primarily carry axons of motor control neurons that project from higher centers (like the mesencephalon or hypothalamus) to motor neurons in the medulla and spinal cord.

Thus based on the position of neural stem cells in the ependymal/ventricular layer of the entire rudimentary spinal cord, medulla, mesencephalon, and diencephalon, there is an orderly specification of distinct sensory and motor neurons that serve distinct regions of the body: the trunk, limbs, and viscera for the spinal cord; the head, neck, and viscera for the medulla; the mesencephalon; and the diencephalon. This specification relies on the establishment of centers that provide molecular signals to the posterior/alar and anterior/basal plate from the posterior spinal cord through the anterior mesencephalon. At the ventral (anterior) midline is the *floor plate,* a thin region of neuroepithelial cells established based upon their proximity to the notochord that secretes the key signaling molecule sonic hedgehog as well as several other signals to establish motor neuron identity. At the posterior midline is the *roof plate,* which provides multiple signals that similarly influence the genesis and differentiation of sensory neurons. These include bone morphogenetic proteins (BMPs), wingless/integration (WNT) signals, and retinoic acid. Accordingly, the basic neuroanatomy and functional organization of the spinal cord, medulla, mesencephalon, thalamus, and hypothalamus reflect the developmental position and molecular signaling history of neural stem cells in the alar and basal plate that generate the neurons of each brain region.

Plate 1.18 continued on next page

Plate 1.18

Spinal Cord

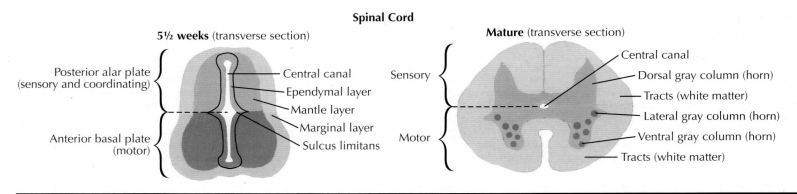

5½ weeks (transverse section)

Posterior alar plate (sensory and coordinating)
Anterior basal plate (motor)

Central canal
Ependymal layer
Mantle layer
Marginal layer
Sulcus limitans

Mature (transverse section)

Sensory
Motor

Central canal
Dorsal gray column (horn)
Tracts (white matter)
Lateral gray column (horn)
Ventral gray column (horn)
Tracts (white matter)

Medulla Oblongata

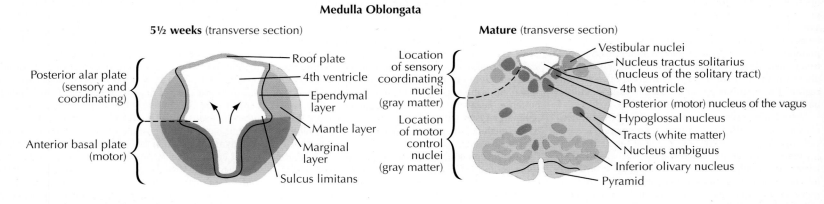

5½ weeks (transverse section)

Posterior alar plate (sensory and coordinating)
Anterior basal plate (motor)

Roof plate
4th ventricle
Ependymal layer
Mantle layer
Marginal layer
Sulcus limitans

Mature (transverse section)

Location of sensory coordinating nuclei (gray matter)
Location of motor control nuclei (gray matter)

Vestibular nuclei
Nucleus tractus solitarius (nucleus of the solitary tract)
4th ventricle
Posterior (motor) nucleus of the vagus
Hypoglossal nucleus
Tracts (white matter)
Nucleus ambiguus
Inferior olivary nucleus
Pyramid

Mesencephalon

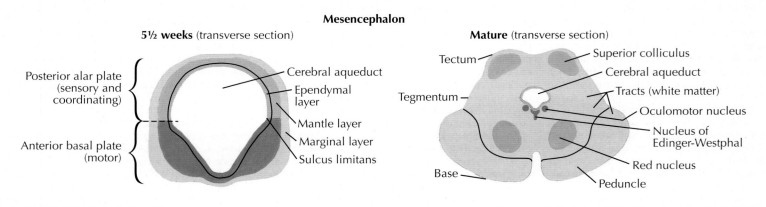

5½ weeks (transverse section)

Posterior alar plate (sensory and coordinating)
Anterior basal plate (motor)

Cerebral aqueduct
Ependymal layer
Mantle layer
Marginal layer
Sulcus limitans

Mature (transverse section)

Tectum
Tegmentum
Base

Superior colliculus
Cerebral aqueduct
Tracts (white matter)
Oculomotor nucleus
Nucleus of Edinger-Westphal
Red nucleus
Peduncle

Diencephalon

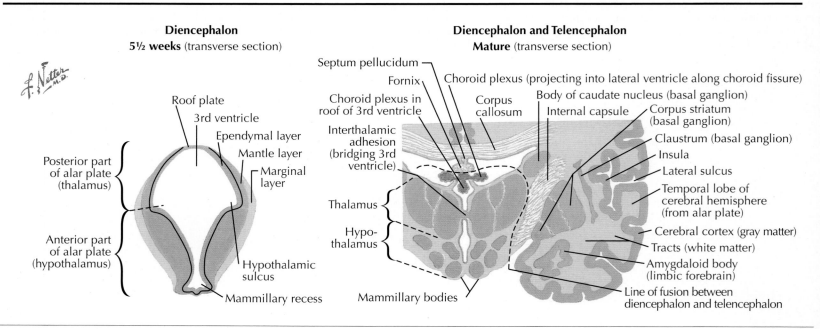

5½ weeks (transverse section)

Posterior part of alar plate (thalamus)
Anterior part of alar plate (hypothalamus)

Roof plate
3rd ventricle
Ependymal layer
Mantle layer
Marginal layer
Hypothalamic sulcus
Mammillary recess

Diencephalon and Telencephalon

Mature (transverse section)

Septum pellucidum
Fornix
Choroid plexus in roof of 3rd ventricle
Interthalamic adhesion (bridging 3rd ventricle)
Thalamus
Hypothalamus
Mammillary bodies

Choroid plexus (projecting into lateral ventricle along choroid fissure)
Corpus callosum
Internal capsule
Body of caudate nucleus (basal ganglion)
Corpus striatum (basal ganglion)
Claustrum (basal ganglion)
Insula
Lateral sulcus
Temporal lobe of cerebral hemisphere (from alar plate)
Cerebral cortex (gray matter)
Tracts (white matter)
Amygdaloid body (limbic forebrain)
Line of fusion between diencephalon and telencephalon

Plate 1.19

Normal and Abnormal Development

GENERATION OF NEURONAL DIVERSITY IN THE SPINAL CORD AND HINDBRAIN

Morphogenesis ultimately reflects the establishment of distinct neuronal and glial cell classes in appropriate numbers and positions throughout the neural tube. In the spinal cord and hindbrain, the basic relationships between neural stem cells and their progeny are well established. These relationships define cell lineages, broadly, for the spinal cord and hindbrain. The key distinctions that establish *lineages*—the range of cell types generated by specific classes of neural stem cells—are position in the neural tube of the stem cells and the way in which the final positions of postmitotic progeny are established.

The neural stem cells in the spinal cord and hindbrain can be divided into four broad classes: motor neurons and related interneuron progenitors, sensory relay neurons and related interneuron progenitors, glial cell progenitors, and neural crest progenitors. There are key distinctions for each of these four classes. The first two stem cell classes, motor and sensory progenitors, have the capacity to give rise to both projection neurons with long axons that connect either the spinal cord with muscles and autonomic ganglia (motor) or send their axons from the spinal cord to higher brain regions to relay sensory information (sensory). These stem cells can also give rise to multiple classes of interneurons, whose axons remain close to the position of the interneuron cell body and which tend to make local inhibitory synapses to modulate the excitability of motor or sensory projection neurons. For these classes of neural stem cells (and related intermediate progenitors), most cell division happens in the ventricular/marginal zone. The newly generated neuroblasts are then displaced over small distances so that they acquire an appropriate

position in the dorsal or anterior horn. In the hindbrain, there is some local cell migration between distinct anterior-posterior locations (defined by the segmental organization of rhombomeres that prefigures the morphogenesis of the hindbrain) that leads to greater diversity of cells within cranial nerve motor or sensory relay nuclei. Additional neural stem cells in the spinal cord and hindbrain generate multiple classes of glia. These stem cells are indistinguishable from the neurepithelial progenitors that give rise to neurons, and indeed they are mostly multipotent: they give rise to neurons as well as glial cells.

The specification and subsequent generation and differentiation of glial progeny are distinct from those of neurons. For the most part, the three primary classes of glia—astrocytes, oligodendroglial cells (see below), and radial glia—are generated later than the neurons of the spinal cord and hindbrain. Astrocytes are further differentiated into two classes: (1) protoplasmic astrocytes, which are found primarily adjacent to neuronal cell bodies and their processes, where they collectively constitute the neuropil (gray matter) and (2) fibrous astrocytes, which are found primarily in axon tracts (white matter) and whose processes often contact blood vessels. Radial glia resemble neuroepithelial progenitors and indeed may be indistinguishable from these cells in many ways. A small number of radial glial cells remain in the mature ependymal zone in many regions, and these cells, when placed in appropriate cell culture conditions, can generate neurons as well as astrocytes and oligodendroglial cells. Thus spinal cord and hindbrain radial glial cells are likely neural stem cells. Oligodendroglial cells interact with axons to generate the myelin sheaths that ensure efficient conduction of action potentials (see Plate 1.21). Many of the earliest oligodendroglial precursors are generated initially at the anterior midline and rely on some of the same secreted signaling molecules and transcription factors that also influence motor neuron determination and

differentiation. Subsequently, however, oligodendroglial precursors are found throughout the developing and mature brain, and they can either retain their progenitor capacity (and, in some cases, when isolated and cultured, can give rise to neurons as well as glia) or generate local myelinating oligodendroglia.

The fourth class of neural stem cell, generated from the neural tube that gives rise to the spinal cord, hindbrain, and midbrain, is the neural crest progenitor. These neural crest stem cells generate intermediate progenitors or give rise to postmitotic neuroblasts that actively move, or migrate, short distances from the neural tube and then reaggregate to form the sensory ganglia, including posterior root ganglia and most of the cranial nerves. Sensory ganglion cells have a single cell body with a single process that bifurcates into a peripheral receptor process and a central presynaptic process. This polarity facilitates generating receptor potentials in the periphery that subsequently initiate action potentials in the axon branch that projects into the CNS, where sensory information is then relayed via synapses made by this axon, or central process, of the sensory ganglion cell. Neural crest–derived neuroblasts also coalesce to form the autonomic ganglia of the sympathetic chain and the more widely distributed parasympathetic ganglia. Finally, neural crest–derived neuroblasts give rise to the neurosecretory adrenal chromaffin cells found in the adrenal medulla. The neural crest also gives rise to significant populations of migrating progenitor cells that divide further at their destinations. These include mesenchymal neural crest cells that populate the head and craniofacial primordia and that give rise to the meninges (arachnoid, pia, and dura), some local blood vessel–associated cells, and multiple skeletal elements, including teeth and cranial bones. In addition, pigment cells in the epidermis are derived from migratory neural crest progenitors. Finally, Schwann cells, the major class of peripheral glial cells that have characteristics similar to oligodendroglia in the CNS, are derived from the neural crest.

Plate 1.19 continued on next page

Plate 1.19

Brain: PART I

SOMATIC AND AUTONOMIC NEURON FORMATION

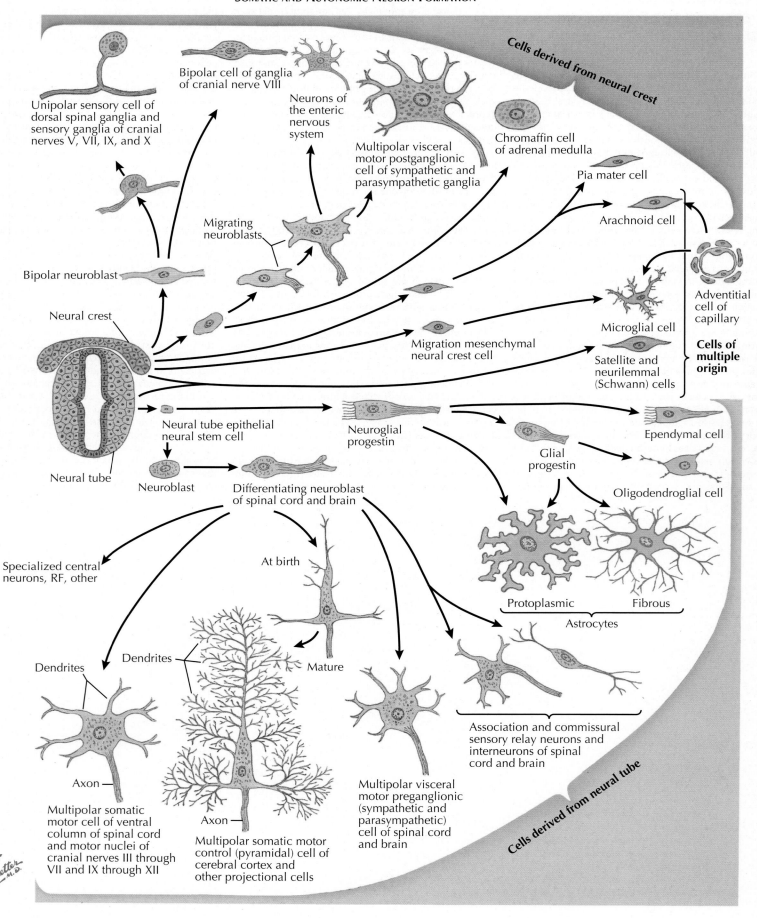

Cells derived from neural crest

Bipolar cell of ganglia of cranial nerve VIII

Neurons of the enteric nervous system

Unipolar sensory cell of dorsal spinal ganglia and sensory ganglia of cranial nerves V, VII, IX, and X

Multipolar visceral motor postganglionic cell of sympathetic and parasympathetic ganglia

Chromaffin cell of adrenal medulla

Pia mater cell

Arachnoid cell

Migrating neuroblasts

Bipolar neuroblast

Adventitial cell of capillary

Neural crest

Microglial cell

Cells of multiple origin

Migration mesenchymal neural crest cell

Satellite and neurilemmal (Schwann) cells

Neural tube epithelial neural stem cell

Neuroglial progestin

Ependymal cell

Glial progestin

Neural tube

Neuroblast

Differentiating neuroblast of spinal cord and brain

Oligodendroglial cell

Specialized central neurons, RF, other

At birth

Protoplasmic   Fibrous

Astrocytes

Dendrites

Dendrites

Mature

Axon

Association and commissural sensory relay neurons and interneurons of spinal cord and brain

Multipolar somatic motor cell of ventral column of spinal cord and motor nuclei of cranial nerves III through VII and IX through XII

Axon

Multipolar somatic motor control (pyramidal) cell of cerebral cortex and other projectional cells

Multipolar visceral motor preganglionic (sympathetic and parasympathetic) cell of spinal cord and brain

Cells derived from neural tube

f. Netter M.D.

Plate 1.20

Normal and Abnormal Development

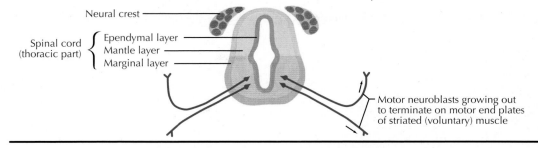

Differentiation and Growth of Neurons at 26 Days

Neural crest

Spinal cord (thoracic part) {
Ependymal layer
Mantle layer
Marginal layer

Motor neuroblasts growing out to terminate on motor end plates of striated (voluntary) muscle

CIRCUIT FORMATION IN THE SPINAL CORD

Cellular diversity provides the foundation for the next essential step of nervous system development: the construction of interconnected networks of neurons that serve specific behavioral functions. These networks are referred to as *neural circuits,* and their identity reflects the molecular distinctions between neuron classes and between the growth, adhesion, and recognition molecules that mediate elaboration of axons, dendrites, and synapses. This process is remarkably well understood for the construction of circuits that mediate motor control, relay of sensory information in the spinal cord, and local sensory-motor integration for segmental reflex control. As described above, sensory relay neurons and related interneurons are generated from the alar plate, motor neurons and related interneurons are generated from the basal plate, and peripheral sensory ganglion cells are generated from the neural crest. Each of these cell classes will become interconnected in distinct circuits. For these circuits to form, there must be clear rules, mediated by local *chemoattractant* and *chemorepulsive* cues, for where each neuron class can extend its axons and dendrites. In addition, there are temporal gradients of neuronal differentiation so that some neuron classes grow their axons and dendrites earlier (as early as 26 days of gestation), and, within a few days, other neuron classes will begin to extend their processes. Thus the construction of circuits from the newly generated neurons in the spinal cord relies on time of origin of neurons, neuronal position, and time of axon or dendritic growth.

The direction of growth chosen by axons from different neuron classes must be exquisitely regulated to ensure proper connectivity within spinal cord circuits. Thus motor neurons, whose axons are the earliest to grow out of the spinal cord, are directed to an exit point lateral and anterior, based on chemoattractant signals that guide them there and cell surface adhesion molecules that facilitate their exit from the CNS. Additional cell adhesion molecules maintain the appropriate trajectory for these axons and facilitate the formation of a coherent nerve. Chemorepulsive signals prevent axons from growing aberrantly into inappropriate nonmuscle targets. Accordingly, motor axons grow to their skeletal muscle and autonomic ganglia targets with great fidelity.

The parallel growth of several classes of sensory neuron axons within the spinal cord illustrates the complexity—and remarkable precision—of the relationship between cell position, axon guidance, and molecular signals that attract or repel subsets of axons. Sensory relay neurons or interneurons generated from the alar plate either extend axons across the anterior midline and then into the spinothalamic tract or into the motor column on the same side to make local reflex connections (like those necessary for withdrawal in response

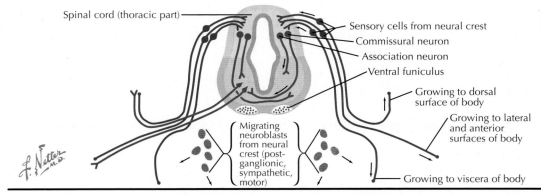

Differentiation and Growth of Neurons at 28 Days
(right side of diagram shows newly acquired neurons only)

Spinal cord (thoracic part)

Sensory cells from neural crest
Commissural neuron
Association neuron
Ventral funiculus

Growing to dorsal surface of body

Growing to lateral and anterior surfaces of body

Migrating neuroblasts from neural crest (postganglionic, sympathetic, motor)

Growing to viscera of body

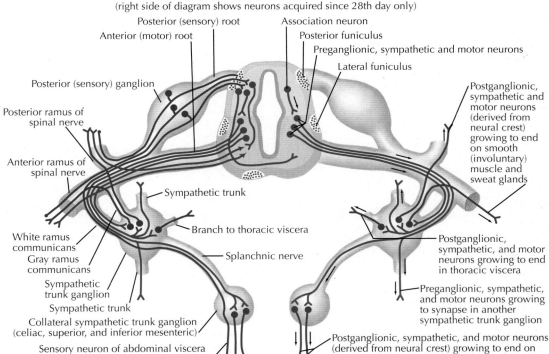

Differentiation and Growth of Neurons at 5 to 7 Weeks
(right side of diagram shows neurons acquired since 28th day only)

Posterior (sensory) root
Anterior (motor) root
Association neuron
Posterior funiculus
Preganglionic, sympathetic and motor neurons
Lateral funiculus

Posterior (sensory) ganglion

Posterior ramus of spinal nerve

Anterior ramus of spinal nerve

Postganglionic, sympathetic and motor neurons (derived from neural crest) growing to end on smooth (involuntary) muscle and sweat glands

Sympathetic trunk

White ramus communicans
Gray ramus communicans
Sympathetic trunk ganglion
Sympathetic trunk

Branch to thoracic viscera

Splanchnic nerve

Collateral sympathetic trunk ganglion (celiac, superior, and inferior mesenteric)
Sensory neuron of abdominal viscera (cell body in dorsal ganglion)

Postganglionic, sympathetic, and motor neurons growing to end in thoracic viscera

Preganglionic, sympathetic, and motor neurons growing to synapse in another sympathetic trunk ganglion

Postganglionic, sympathetic, and motor neurons (derived from neural crest) growing to end on glands and smooth (involuntary) muscle

to painful stimuli). Clearly, there need to be discriminating sets of signals: one set that attracts spinothalamic relay axons to the anterior midline and then maintains them on the contralateral side and one set that attracts interneuron axons to the anterior horn and prevents them from extending past the midline. The signals that guide sensory axons to their midline crossing point include sonic hedgehog, the vascular endothelial growth factor, and an adhesion molecule, netrin, that apparently constrains the growth of the axons along the marginal zone of the spinal cord. The signals

that ensure that a spinal cord sensory relay axon crosses the midline and does not cross back include a secreted chemorepulsive molecule called *slit*, which, based upon binding to its receptor *robo* on the sensory axons, signals that these axons should not cross back once they have crossed the midline. Thus pathways for relaying pain and temperature are generated by precise molecular mechanisms that attract axons to the ventral midline, guide them across, and then maintain them on the contralateral side of the spinal cord, brainstem, thalamus, and cortex.

Plate 1.21

Brain: PART I

SHEATH AND SATELLITE CELL FORMATION

Two postganglionic autonomic neurons of a sympathetic or parasympathetic ganglion

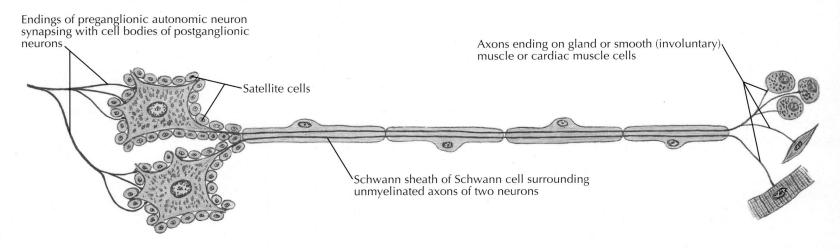

Endings of preganglionic autonomic neuron synapsing with cell bodies of postganglionic neurons

Satellite cells

Axons ending on gland or smooth (involuntary) muscle or cardiac muscle cells

Schwann sheath of Schwann cell surrounding unmyelinated axons of two neurons

Somatic or visceral sensory neuron of a spinal ganglion or sensory ganglion of cranial nerves V, VII, IX, or X

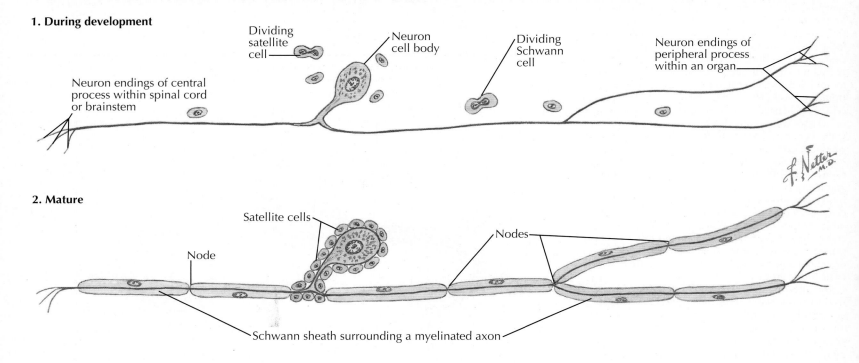

1. During development

Dividing satellite cell

Neuron cell body

Dividing Schwann cell

Neuron endings of peripheral process within an organ

Neuron endings of central process within spinal cord or brainstem

2. Mature

Satellite cells

Nodes

Node

Schwann sheath surrounding a myelinated axon

MAKING PERIPHERAL NERVES AND CENTRAL TRACTS

Another essential aspect of establishing cellular diversity in the nervous system is the differentiation of distinct classes of glial cells that associate themselves with developing axons as these axons and glia form large axon pathways, or *tracts,* in the CNS. Similar glial cells are found in the PNS, where they are derived from the neural crest and are essential for the differentiation of peripheral axon pathways or *nerves.* Many peripheral and central glial cells generate *myelin* to ensheathe axons and enhance their conduction of action potentials. In peripheral nerves, *Schwann cells* establish a clear relationship with *unmyelinated axons,* which are surrounded by Schwann cell processes. Each Schwann cell usually ensheathes more than one axon of this type. Most axons of postganglionic autonomic (sympathetic and parasympathetic) neurons are unmyelinated. Numerous layers of the cell membrane of Schwann cells wrap myelinated axons of the PNS. A single Schwann cell typically forms a segment of myelin sheath for only one peripheral axon.

Oligodendrocytes in the CNS form myelin sheaths by processes similar to those used by Schwann cells. In an action similar to the continuous wrapping of a bolt of cloth, the oligodendroglial cell membrane becomes wrapped around the axon many times. As the wrapping occurs, the oligodendroglial cytoplasm retracts or is extruded so that the two layers of the cell's plasma membrane, which originally were separated by cytoplasm, come together and fuse. Except for small islands of cytoplasm, which may be trapped between the fused membranes, the fusion is complete. The cell membrane of the myelinating oligodendrocyte, like cell membranes elsewhere, is composed of alternate layers of lipid and protein molecules.

These relationships between Schwann cells and oligodendroglial cells are closely associated with the functional capacity of the relevant axons. Unmyelinated neurons have a low conduction velocity and show fatigue (diminished firing after a repeated volley of depolarizing action potentials) earlier, whereas myelinated neurons fire rapidly and have a long period of activity before fatigue occurs. Axons that extend from neurons that ultimately are capable of

Plate 1.22

Normal and Abnormal Development

DEVELOPMENT OF MYELINATION AND AXON ENSHEATHMENT

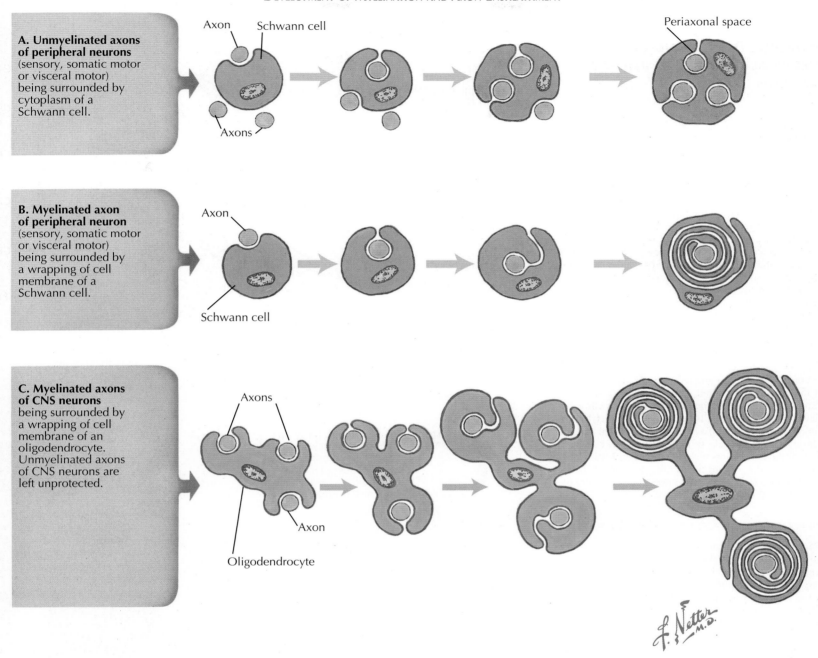

A. Unmyelinated axons of peripheral neurons (sensory, somatic motor or visceral motor) being surrounded by cytoplasm of a Schwann cell.

Axon   Schwann cell   Periaxonal space   Axons

B. Myelinated axon of peripheral neuron (sensory, somatic motor or visceral motor) being surrounded by a wrapping of cell membrane of a Schwann cell.

Axon   Schwann cell

C. Myelinated axons of CNS neurons being surrounded by a wrapping of cell membrane of an oligodendrocyte. Unmyelinated axons of CNS neurons are left unprotected.

Axons   Axon   Oligodendrocyte

MAKING PERIPHERAL NERVES AND CENTRAL TRACTS (Continued)

rapid transmission of impulses become fully functional at about the time their axons become completely insulated with a myelin sheath. In general, the motor neurons of cranial nerves become myelinated before their sensory counterparts. The sensory axons of the trigeminal nerve and the cochlear division of the vestibulocochlear nerve begin to acquire myelin only in the fifth and sixth months of development. The optic nerve axons begin to be sheathed at birth, and myelination is completed by the end of the second week after birth.

Another type of cell, which is derived from both the neural crest and the wall of the neural tube and which participates in covering the neurons of the PNS, is the *satellite cell*. Satellite cells completely encapsulate the cell bodies of sensory neurons in the sensory ganglia of both the cranial and spinal nerves and also the postganglionic neurons of the sympathetic and parasympathetic ganglia. Finally, there is a specialized glial cell that shares properties of Schwann and satellite cells but is only found immediately adjacent to the unmyelinated axons of the

olfactory nerve. These axons originate from receptor neurons in the sensory or *olfactory epithelium* of the nose that are continually replaced throughout life and thus must regrow into the olfactory bulb in the CNS and make new synapses. These olfactory ensheathing cells are apparently specialized to support the constant regrowth of the axons and the establishment of new connections in the CNS. Accordingly, there is great interest in these cells as a substrate for improved axon growth in other regions of the CNS after injury.

Plate 1.23

Brain: PART I

BRACHIAL PLEXUS AND/OR CERVICAL NERVE ROOT INJURIES AT BIRTH

The maturation and myelination of peripheral nerves, including cranial nerves, are not complete at birth. Thus these axons, not yet fully protected by myelin, associated glial cells, and connective tissue, are susceptible to perinatal injury. Brachial plexus injuries in the newborn now occur much less commonly, although the incidence is still approximately 1 in 1000 live births. The injury results from traction forces in delivering the shoulder in vertex deliveries and delivering the head in breech deliveries. The associated obstetric factors are occipitoposterior or transverse presentation, the use of oxytocin, shoulder dystocia, and large babies (weighing more than 3500 g) with low Apgar scores.

Brachial birth palsy is believed to be secondary to stretching of the plexus by traction, with the nerve roots being anchored by the spinal column and cord. In less severe lesions, only the myelin sheath may be damaged, which is evidenced by swelling and edema that may, in turn, damage the myelin. If only a small segment of the axon is affected, or if it is stretched but not ruptured, quick repair and recovery are likely. However, if the axon is interrupted, repair can take a very long time, considering that the rate of axonal growth is believed to be 1 mm/day. If the axon is completely ruptured, recovery is unlikely. Bilateral brachial injuries almost always indicate spinal involvement, and avulsion of the nerve roots may be evident on MRI. Upper brachial plexus injuries involve the junction of the C5 and C6 roots (Erb point), and lower injuries involve the junction of the C8 and T1 roots.

UPPER BRACHIAL PLEXUS INJURY (ERB PALSY)

This is the most common brachial plexus injury, affecting muscles supplied by C5 and C6 and accounting for 90% of the total incidence. An *asymmetric Moro response* is usually the first indication of the injury. The upper extremity assumes the "waiter's tip" position: the shoulder is adducted and internally rotated; the elbow is extended; and the forearm is pronated, with the hand in flexion. A mild sensory loss may develop over the lateral aspect of the shoulder and arm, but it is rather difficult to detect. Associated fractures of the clavicle or humerus must be ruled out, and fluoroscopic examination should be carried out to exclude the rare diaphragmatic paralysis caused mainly by a C4 lesion.

LOWER BRACHIAL PLEXUS INJURY (KLUMPKE PALSY)

A pure lower brachial plexus injury is quite uncommon, and most cases of Klumpke palsy involve the more proximal muscles supplied by C7 or C8. An *absent grasp reflex* is the most prominent clinical feature. Involvement of sympathetic fibers from T1 causes Horner syndrome (ptosis, miosis, anhidrosis). A significant sensory deficit is usually present. Infants and children may sometimes traumatize their fingers unwittingly, with occasionally severe results such as loss of a fingertip. Prognosis for full recovery in these infants is poor. The upper extremity often remains small and distally foreshortened.

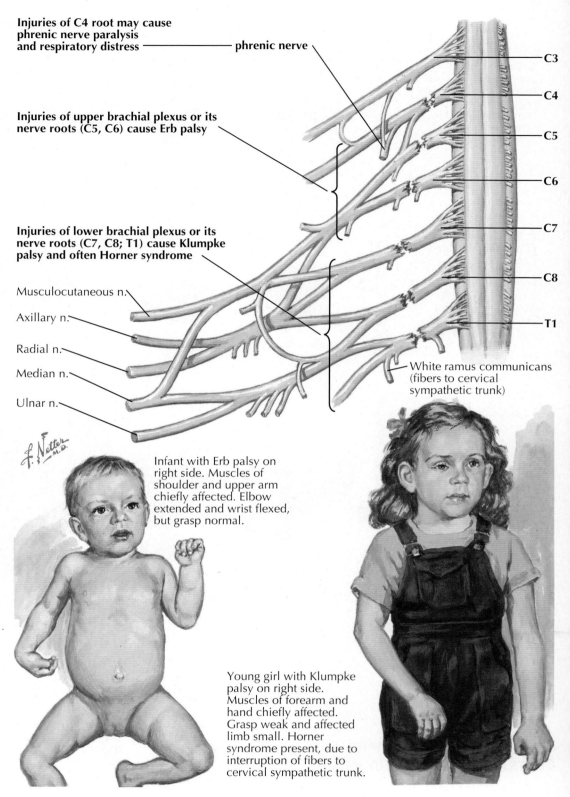

Injuries of C4 root may cause phrenic nerve paralysis and respiratory distress — phrenic nerve

Injuries of upper brachial plexus or its nerve roots (C5, C6) cause Erb palsy

Injuries of lower brachial plexus or its nerve roots (C7, C8; T1) cause Klumpke palsy and often Horner syndrome

Musculocutaneous n.
Axillary n.
Radial n.
Median n.
Ulnar n.

C3
C4
C5
C6
C7
C8
T1

White ramus communicans (fibers to cervical sympathetic trunk)

Infant with Erb palsy on right side. Muscles of shoulder and upper arm chiefly affected. Elbow extended and wrist flexed, but grasp normal.

Young girl with Klumpke palsy on right side. Muscles of forearm and hand chiefly affected. Grasp weak and affected limb small. Horner syndrome present, due to interruption of fibers to cervical sympathetic trunk.

TREATMENT

In all cases of brachial plexus injury, a thorough evaluation is indicated. The limb should be placed in its best functional position, that is, across the chest, not abducted, and flexed. Gentle, passive, range-of-motion exercise should be initiated within 7 to 10 days of birth, and physical or occupational therapy should be continued throughout at least the first year of life. Hand and wrist splints can be used as necessary. Most infants will experience marked recovery of function in the first few months. If no recovery is observed, electromyography can be useful to determine the extent of the injury. For infants with persistent severe injury and no evidence of improvement at 4 to 6 months of age, MRI may be helpful in determining whether the infant will benefit from a brachial plexus repair with nerve grafts. Although brachial plexus repair does not restore normal function, it can provide carefully selected infants with functional improvement. After the child is 5 to 6 years of age, muscle transfers may be helpful.

Plate 1.24

Normal and Abnormal Development

MORPHOGENESIS AND REGIONAL DIFFERENTIATION OF THE FOREBRAIN

The forebrain, unlike the spinal cord, does not receive signals from the notochord and somites. Thus its regional differentiation depends on distinct mechanisms that result in the growth and differentiation of the two telencephalic vesicles into the cerebral cortex, hippocampus, basal ganglia, basal forebrain nuclei (including the amygdala), and the olfactory bulb. After the anterior neural tube has closed, a population of neural crest–derived mesenchymal cells migrate into the head and surround the newly formed prosencephalic vesicle. These mesenchymal cells are a key source of inductive signals, including retinoic acid, and play a similar role in forebrain patterning to that of the notochord and somites in the spinal cord and hindbrain. These mesenchymal cells signal directly to the forebrain neuroepithelium to influence the establishment of additional signaling centers in the neuroepithelium itself. The intrinsic forebrain signaling centers resemble the floor plate and roof plate of the spinal cord and hindbrain. There is a ventral-medial source of sonic hedgehog and a dorsal-medial source of BMPs as well as WNTs that influence further regional and cellular differentiation. In addition, there is an anterior/ventral-medial domain that produces fibroblast growth factor (FGF) signals. Thus the interaction between mesenchyme and forebrain neuroepithelium and establishment of intrinsic signaling forebrain centers is essential for establishing the foundations of forebrain regional differentiation.

Based on their proximity to anteromedial and anterior sonic hedgehog and FGF signals or posteromedial BMP and WNT signals, the telencephalic vesicles become divided into anterior and posterior territories based on differential expression of multiple transcription factors. The posterior territory is referred to as the *pallium*. It generates the *cerebral cortex (neopallium)* as well as the *hippocampus and pyriform cortex (archipallium)*. The anterior territory is referred to as the *ganglionic eminences*. These structures generate the *corpus striatum* or *basal ganglia* as well as nuclei of the basal forebrain, including the amygdala. Finally, at the ventral and anterior aspect of each telencephalic vesicle, the olfactory bulbs evaginate and extend anteriorly.

The division of the forebrain into the telencephalic vesicles is accompanied by the elaboration of the choroid plexus that emerges at the posterior midline. At this region, *choroidal veins and arteries,* generated from angiogenic mesenchymal cells outside the brain, are adjacent to the posterior neuroepithelium. Subsequently, these blood vessels continue to grow in close apposition to a very attenuated neural-derived epithelium. Together, the blood vessels and this attenuated forebrain epithelium constitute the *choroid plexus* of the lateral ventricles. Thus in the adult brain, the choroid plexus serves as an interface between systemic circulation and the CSF that fills the ventricular system to maintain ionic balance and deliver molecular signals for homeostatic control. In the embryo, the choroid plexus is apparently one of several tissues (including the posterior and anterior domains that produce sonic hedgehog, BMPs, and WNTs) that secrete signaling molecules into the embryonic CSF to influence neural stem cell proliferation and differentiation. Thus the CSF

is an essential source of molecular instruction for neural stem cell proliferation and specification in the forebrain, influenced by molecules secreted dynamically by the choroid plexus as it develops.

Subsequently, once neurogenesis and neuronal differentiation begin in the forebrain, a series of axon pathways, referred to collectively as the *cerebral commissures,* emerge to cross the midline, much like those that cross the midline in the spinal cord and hindbrain. These include the *corpus callosum, hippocampal*

commissure, and *anterior commissure.* The growth of these axon pathways from one telencephalic vesicle to the other involves similar molecules and mechanisms to those that influence the midline crossing of sensory axons that constitute the spinothalamic pathway. In addition to netrin, slit and its robo receptor, members of the Ephrin/Eph receptor family of adhesion molecules, seem to be essential for the development of the cerebral commissures, as does the calcium-independent adhesion molecule L1.

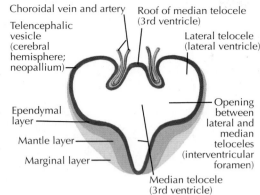

Forebrain at 7 Weeks
(transverse section)

Choroidal vein and artery · Roof of median telocele (3rd ventricle) · Telencephalic vesicle (cerebral hemisphere; neopallium) · Lateral telocele (lateral ventricle) · Ependymal layer · Opening between lateral and median teloceles (interventricular foramen) · Mantle layer · Marginal layer · Median telocele (3rd ventricle)

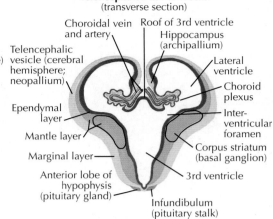

Telencephalon at 7½ Weeks
(transverse section)

Choroidal vein and artery · Roof of 3rd ventricle · Hippocampus (archipallium) · Telencephalic vesicle (cerebral hemisphere; neopallium) · Lateral ventricle · Choroid plexus · Ependymal layer · Inter-ventricular foramen · Mantle layer · Corpus striatum (basal ganglion) · Marginal layer · 3rd ventricle · Anterior lobe of hypophysis (pituitary gland) · Infundibulum (pituitary stalk)

Forebrain at 2 Months
(coronal section; anterior view)

Epiphysis (pineal gland) · Cerebral hemisphere (neopallium, cut edge) · Diencephalon · Hippocampus (archipallium) · Roof of 3rd ventricle · Choroid plexus · Choroid fissure · Thalamus · Lateral ventricle · Corpus striatum (basal ganglion) · Interventricular foramen · Optic (nerve) stalk · 3rd ventricle · Lamina terminalis

Telencephalon at 2½ Months
(right anterior view)

Right cerebral hemisphere (neopallium, cut edge) · Left cerebral hemisphere (neopallium) · Hippocampus (archipallium) · Choroid plexus protruding into right lateral ventricle along choroid fissure · Corpus striatum (basal ganglion) · Interventricular foramen · Opening of cavity of right olfactory lobe · Olfactory lobes (paleopallium)

Right Cerebral Hemisphere at 3 Months
(medial aspect)

Corpus callosum · Medial surface of right cerebral hemisphere (neopallium) · Commissure of fornix (hippocampal commissure) · Choroidal vessels passing to choroid plexus, which protrudes into right lateral ventricle along choroid fissure · Fornix · Anterior commissure · Hippocampus (archipallium) · Lamina terminalis · Stria terminalis · Olfactory lobe (paleopallium) · Thalamus (cut surface) · 3rd ventricle · Line of division between diencephalon and telencephalon

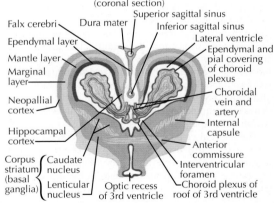

Cerebral Hemispheres at 3 Months
(coronal section)

Falx cerebri · Dura mater · Superior sagittal sinus · Inferior sagittal sinus · Ependymal layer · Lateral ventricle · Mantle layer · Ependymal and pial covering of choroid plexus · Marginal layer · Neopallial cortex · Choroidal vein and artery · Hippocampal cortex · Internal capsule · Corpus striatum (basal ganglia) { Caudate nucleus / Lenticular nucleus } · Optic recess of 3rd ventricle · Anterior commissure · Interventricular foramen · Choroid plexus of roof of 3rd ventricle

Plate 1.25

Brain: PART I

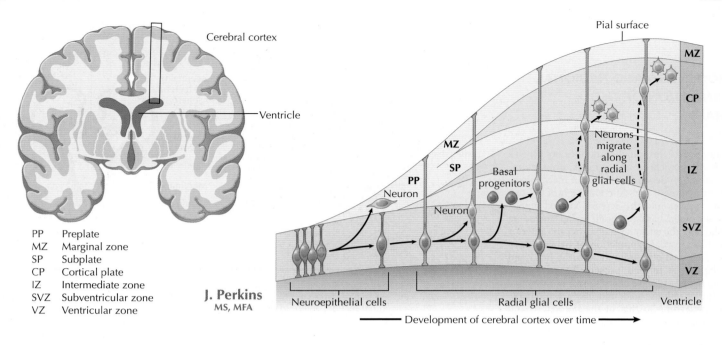

Cerebral cortex

Ventricle

Pial surface

MZ

CP

Neurons migrate along radial glial cells

IZ

MZ

SP

PP

Neuron

Basal progenitors

SVZ

Neuron

VZ

PP   Preplate
MZ   Marginal zone
SP   Subplate
CP   Cortical plate
IZ   Intermediate zone
SVZ   Subventricular zone
VZ   Ventricular zone

J. Perkins
MS, MFA

Neuroepithelial cells   Radial glial cells   Ventricle

→ Development of cerebral cortex over time →

Neurogenesis and Cell Migration in the Developing Neocortex

Most, if not all, cortical neurons are generated in or near the ventricle and migrate radially to the cortex that forms on top of the neuroepithelial precursors. Cortical neural stem cells, called *radial glia*, maintain cell bodies at the ventricular zone, where they divide symmetrically and slowly. Cortical radial glia also give rise to rapidly and asymmetrically dividing intermediate or basal progenitors that become slightly displaced into the subventricular zone, where they generate postmitotic cortical projection or pyramidal neurons. The cortical neurons have long axons that extend from the location of their cell body to other regions of the cortex, the basal ganglia and forebrain, thalamus, brainstem, and spinal cord. They also have apical and basal dendrites extending from their cell bodies that reflect their pyramidal shape.

Radial glial cells in the developing cerebral cortex serve a dual function. Their long processes directed toward the pia provide a migratory guide for newly postmitotic neurons from the ventricular and subventricular zones into the cortical plate, where they disengage from the radial glial processes and differentiate. Further constraints reflect the time when cortical neurons undergo their final cell division. Cortical projection neurons "born" first (become postmitotic earliest) form the *preplate*, the earliest histologic indicator of cortical differentiation. The preplate divides into the *marginal zone*, which becomes layer I of the cortex, and the transient *subplate*, which influences subsequent development of additional cortical layers. Early generated marginal zone and subplate neurons provide signals that influence migration and initial axon growth. Some early generated marginal zone neurons remain in layer I as Cajal-Retzius cells. Subplate neurons fare less

well. A few become interstitial subcortical white matter neurons; however, most die postnatally.

The earliest-born neurons of the cortex itself migrate through the preplate, splitting it into the marginal zone and subplate, thus constituting layer VI of the cortex. Each successive cortical projection neuron cohort, mostly generated during the last two-thirds of gestation in humans, migrates past earlier-born neighbors to their final positions. Thus there is an "inside-out" gradient of cortical neurogenesis that parallels the six layers of the cortex: early born neurons are deepest (layers V and VI), and those born last, except for Cajal-Retzius cells, are superficial (layers II and III). These distinctions are accompanied by differences in which cortical neurons send their axons dendritic differentiation and connectivity. Thus radial migration and the inside-out neurogenesis gradient together produce cortical projection neurons: these neuron axons extend to other cortical regions or subcortical targets and use the excitatory neurotransmitter glutamate.

Surprisingly, the other major class of cortical neurons, *interneurons* or local circuit neurons that use the inhibitory neurotransmitter γ-aminobutyric acid (GABA), is not generated within the developing cortex from radial glia. Instead, interneuron progenitors are found in two anterior forebrain domains: the medial and caudal ganglion eminences. These progenitors yield postmitotic GABAergic neuroblasts within the ganglion eminences that migrate into the neocortex. Initially, this migration is tangential, that is, parallel to the plane of the cortical sheet. When these neurons reach the cortical area where they will differentiate, they migrate radially in much the same way as projection neurons, using radial glial guides. Neural progenitors in the ganglionic eminences also generate the GABAergic projection neurons that will differentiate in the caudate nucleus, the putamen, and the globus pallidus.

The *hippocampus* is generated in much the same way as the cerebral cortex. A part of the ventricular zone that generates hippocampal interneurons, called the

subgranular zone, retains neural stem cells that give rise to additional hippocampal interneurons throughout life. The functional significance of these neurons, if any, remains uncertain. In the *olfactory bulb,* projection neurons (mitral cells) are also generated locally, and GABAergic interneurons migrate from the lateral ganglion eminence by a distinct migratory route called the *rostral migratory stream.* In some mammals, the rostral migratory stream remains in place and guides newly generated neurons from a proliferative zone called the *anterior subventricular zone* to the olfactory bulb, perhaps throughout life. The human brain, however, lacks a rostral migratory stream after birth, and it is unlikely that new olfactory interneurons are generated long into postnatal life. In the cerebellum, interneurons (glutamatergic rather than GABAergic) are generated from a proliferative layer immediately beneath the pia, called the *external granule cell layer.* The postmitotic granule cells then migrate back into the rudimentary cerebellum, past Purkinje cells (cerebellar projection neurons, generated locally), using a glial guide, the Bergmann glia, to facilitate migration. Thus, in several brain regions, projection neurons and interneurons are generated in distinct proliferative zones, followed by migration that brings these neurons together to form circuits.

This complex developmental history makes the neocortex and other forebrain regions vulnerable to developmental changes, with a potential impact on disease. Behavioral disorders, from autism and attention deficit/hyperactivity disorder (ADHD) to bipolar disorder and schizophrenia, may reflect, in part, changes in neurogenesis and migration. Cortical development demands exquisite precision so that neurons are generated at the right times and get to the right places. Small but significant disruptions could lead eventually to subtle but significant alterations of cortical circuits and the social, communicative, and cognitive behaviors they subserve. These hypotheses, which unite a spectrum of psychiatric diseases into a continuum of disorders of development of cortical connectivity, remain to be thoroughly tested.

Plate 1.26

Normal and Abnormal Development

NEURONAL PROLIFERATION AND MIGRATION DISORDERS

The complexity and duration of cortical neurogenesis and migration make the cortex a particularly vulnerable target for disruptions that result in a broad range of brain disorders. These include a variety of epilepsies, intellectual disability, and potentially disorders such as autism and ADHD. Many of these disorders and the cell biologic and genetic analyses that better defined their pathogenesis as disruptions of cortical neuronal proliferation and migration took advantage of structural imaging of the cortex. MRI identifies anatomic irregularities in the size, shape, and gyral and sulcal patterns of the cortical hemispheres. Nevertheless, a "normal" MRI scan does not rule out microscopic localized gyral malformations or, most important, significant defects of the cortical layers and heterotopias of neurons that are initially destined for one cortical layer but, due to altered migration, are found in an aberrant laminar location. Clearly, such disruptions of cortical neurogenesis and migration must result in altered circuits that lack the capacity to mediate maximally adaptive behaviors.

DEFECTIVE PROLIFERATION

A decrease in neuronal number may lead to *microcephaly* (microencephaly vera), whereas an increase may result in *megalencephaly*. Prenatal influences, including familial factors, are paramount in each abnormality. Microcephaly may be caused by a variety of genetic and environmental etiologies. It may be isolated or associated with other anomalies. Primary microcephaly results from a developmental insult giving rise to a reduced neuronal population. Secondary microcephaly occurs from an injury or insult to a previously normal brain.

Megalencephaly is classified as either anatomic or metabolic. It may be associated with neurofibromatosis, achondroplasia, or cerebral gigantism. Familial megalencephaly, the most common and benign form, is usually inherited through the father. Excessive postnatal growth also occurs often, suggesting hydrocephalus. Measurements of the parental head circumference and MRI scans showing normal ventricles aid in diagnosis. Approximately 70% of infants with microcephaly and 30% of those with megalencephaly have developmental defects.

DEFECTIVE MIGRATION

After proliferation in the subependymal region, neurons migrate to the cortex. The neurons appear to follow radial glial cells like raindrops on telephone wires. Early migrations form the deepest cortical layers, and later migrations form the more superficial layers, ultimately forming a six-layer cortex. The cellular complement is greatest in the outer cortical layers, leading to an increased surface area, with buckling causing gyri to begin to appear between 26 and 28 weeks and to become increasingly complex in the final trimester. If the normal complement of neurons is absent, gyral formation does not take place, and *lissencephaly* (smooth brain, agyria) results (see Plate 1.5). An abnormally thick gyral formation is known as *pachygyria*. In this anomaly, the cortex lacks the six-layer configuration. Cerebral *heterotopias* appear to result from defective neuronal migration and subsequent accumulation of aberrant neurons anywhere between the ependyma and cortex (see Plate 1.5). Significant numbers of such heterotopias occurring in isolation are likely to result in some

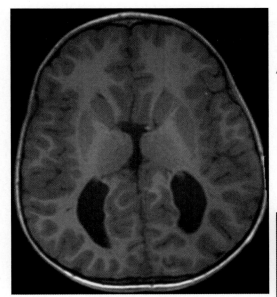

Agenesis of the corpus callosum

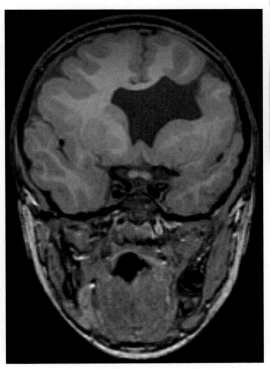

Lissencephaly, posterior predominant

Left schizencephaly

Images courtesy P. Ellen Grant, MD, Associate Professor of Radiology, Harvard Medical School.

degree of intellectual disability. Most of the disorders of migration discussed previously have associated heterotopias. The presence of multiple small gyri having no resemblance to a normal gyral pattern, along with deranged lamination of the cortical mantle, is called *polymicrogyria* (see Plate 1.5). *Schizencephaly* is characterized by an abnormal cleft that joins the cortex and the ventricles. It is usually bilateral but can be unilateral. Malformed gyri (polymicrogyria) are aligned radially around the cleft.

Agenesis of the corpus callosum, partial or complete, is often accompanied by disorders stemming from defective neuronal migration. This results in developmental defects, seizures, mental retardation, and occasional hydrocephalus (see Plate 1.5). The diagnosis may be suggested by ocular hypertelorism, an antimongoloid slant to the eyes, and other midline facial defects. Aicardi syndrome, a sporadically occurring abnormality seen in female infants, is associated with retinal defects that suggest chorioretinitis, infantile spasms, hypsarrhythmia, and severe psychomotor retardation. Agenesis is one of the most common anomalies diagnosed by MRI in "idiopathic" psychomotor retardation (see Plates 1.5 and 1.6).

Plate 1.27

Brain: PART I

DEVELOPMENTAL DYSLEXIA

Developmental dyslexia, or developmental reading disorder, is defined as a significant impairment in the development of reading and related skills, such as spelling, writing, and reading comprehension, due to problems with phonologic processing despite adequate intelligence and conventional instruction. This disorder frequently occurs in association with other specific learning disabilities, such as disturbances in auditory comprehension, expressive language, articulation, and visual discrimination. It is the most commonly identified learning disorder, now felt to affect the sexes equally, and is often present in siblings and other family members.

Because the primary deficit in developmental dyslexia is in reading and writing, the abnormality is usually not identified until the first few years of grade school, the time when children begin to read. Most parents are not aware of any disorder in their child before this stage. Because it is common and affects skills recently acquired by humans, developmental dyslexia may have had certain advantages in preliterate societies, because dyslexic persons often have enhanced visual-spatial and artistic skills.

ETIOLOGIC THEORIES

Early investigators postulated that developmental dyslexia was caused by a lesion in the left angular gyrus, an area of the brain in which a lesion in adults produces word blindness. Later, Orton (1925) felt that the disorder was caused by equipotential visual association areas in the two cerebral hemispheres actively competing with each other, with one side seeing a mirror image of the other. Orton was particularly impressed with reversals of letters and letter sequences in words, the inconsistency of these errors, and the ability of some dyslexic students to read better with the aid of a mirror. Emotional problems and improper instruction were also thought to cause dyslexia.

More recent investigations, including CT, computed-evoked electroencephalographic studies, and postmortem studies of the brain, have all provided evidence of a structural basis for dyslexia. MRI has demonstrated a variety of structural changes in the corpus callosum, left temporal lobes, thalamus, caudate, inferior frontal gyrus, and cerebellum (Pennington, 1999; Eliez, 2000; Robichon, 2000; Leonard, 2001; Rae, 2002; Brown, 2011; Elnakib, 2012).

Historically, Drake (1968) noted abnormally formed gyri in the parietal regions and *ectopic neurons* in the white matter, arrested during their migration to the cerebral cortex. Examination of a second brain by Galaburda and Kemper (1979) showed cerebral cortical abnormalities characterized by focal and verrucose dysplasia in the sensory speech area (Wernicke's area) and language-dominant left cerebral hemisphere. The third brain examined showed only verrucose dysplasia almost exclusively confined to the left cerebral hemisphere (Kemper, 1984). Thus examination of all three brains has demonstrated minor malformations.

Analysis of human malformations and animal models indicates that the focal and verrucose dysplasia probably arise during the later stages of neuronal migration to the cerebral cortex and appear to result from the migration of neurons into focal areas of cortical destruction. In humans, neuronal migration to the cerebral cortex occurs from the eighth week to approximately week 16 of gestation. Consistent with this timing is the presence of ectopic neurons in the white matter in two of the three brains examined. The nature of this postulated

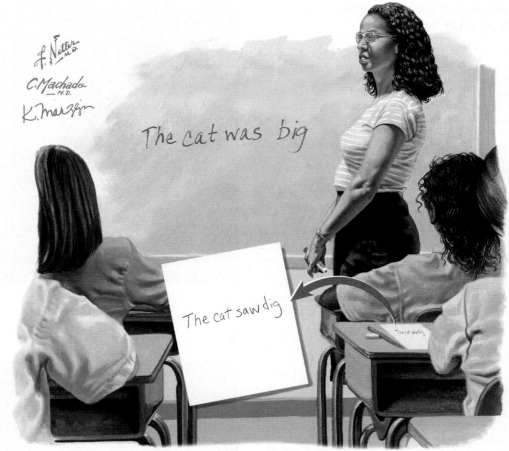

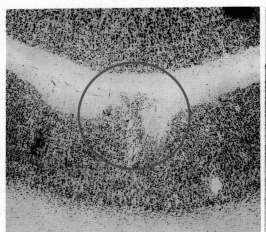

Child reverses letters (writes "d" for "b") and sequence of letters in words (writes "saw" for "was")

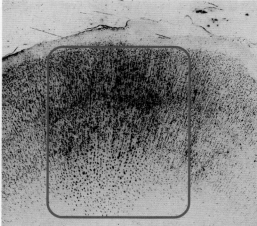

Verrucose dysplasia, with focal accumulation of neurons in layer I of cerebral cortex

Focal dysplasia, with abnormally large neurons extending into white matter of brain

destructive process is unknown. Geschwind and Behan (1982) have noted a significant clustering of dyslexia, left-handedness, autoimmune disease, and migraine in persons related to each other, indicating an association among these traits.

Currently, it is believed that developmental dyslexia is a disorder of network connections, as demonstrated by Vandermosten (2012). By using MRI tractography, adults with dyslexia were noted to have a reduction in the left arcuate fasciculus, which connects the posterior temporal and frontal areas. This may represent an area of decreased myelination.

TREATMENT

Early identification and evaluation of dyslexia are essential for proper treatment. The optimal educational approach is multisensory, including phonemic awareness and enhanced phonologic processing, where virtually all respond. However, given that dyslexia is a lifelong disorder, many continue to struggle into adulthood when presented with new or less familiar words, in reading comprehension settings, or with reading fluency. Treatment should be aimed at enabling those to overcome deficits where possible and to learn strategies to circumvent and compensate for difficulties that cannot be overcome.

Plate 1.28

Normal and Abnormal Development

AUTISM SPECTRUM DISORDER

Autism spectrum disorder (ASD) is a neurodevelopmental disorder characterized by challenges in several areas of development, including communication and social interaction, with restricted interests and repetitive behaviors that affect the child's ability to function. With recent increasing prevalence rates, ASD is now estimated to occur in 1.5% of children in the United States and other developed countries, across all racial, ethnic, and socioeconomic groups. Boys are affected four times more often than girls. Its increasing prevalence may be due to increased awareness, expansion of diagnostic criteria, or genetic or environmental factors such as advanced parental age, low birth weight, or fetal exposure to infections or toxins. The pathophysiology of ASD is not well understood, but it is believed to involve abnormalities in the synaptic functioning and organization of the brain, affecting structures and pathways that relate to social relatedness and communication.

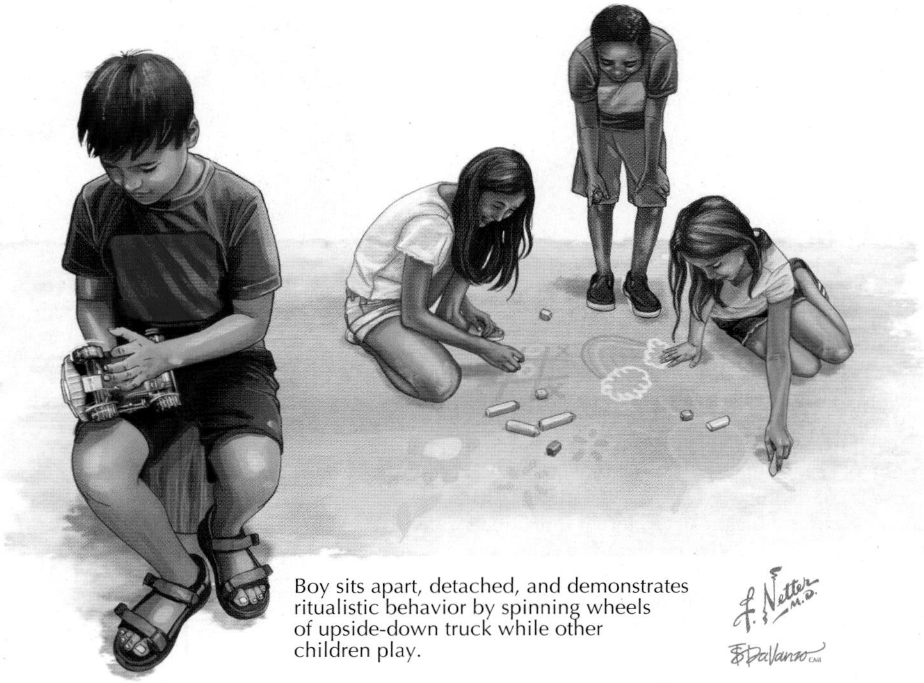

CLINICAL PRESENTATION

The essential features of ASD are persistent deficits in social communication and social interaction and restricted, repetitive patterns of behavior, interests, or activities. These symptoms are present from early childhood and impair daily functioning. The behavioral presentation varies based on severity of the deficits, developmental level, age, and associated supports to compensate, hence the existence of a spectrum. Verbal social communication deficits may range from complete lack of language, to stilted and overly literal language, to language that lacks social reciprocity. Nonverbal social communication deficits may include absent or atypical use of eye contact, gestures, prosody, facial expressions, and body language. A young child may not smile or point or may fail to follow a parent's eye gaze or pointing finger. Deficits may be present in initiating or engaging in social interactions, sharing of emotions and feelings, and/or attempts to mirror others' social behaviors. This can result in poor or absent peer friendships, lack of shared social play or make-believe play, or use of inappropriate social behavior that is potentially perceived as rude or disruptive.

ASD also involves restricted, repetitive patterns of behavior, interests, or activities. Children may have repetitive behaviors such as hand flapping or repetitive speech. They may have rigid adherence to routines and become agitated with small changes or transitions to other activities. Interests are often atypical in focus and intensity and can involve unusual objects such as elevators or repetitively spinning the wheels of a toy car.

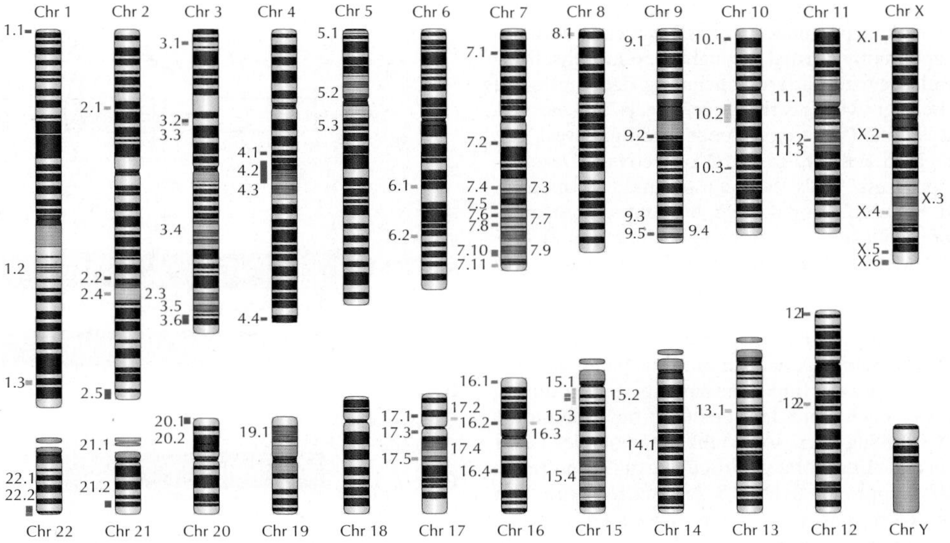

Boy sits apart, detached, and demonstrates ritualistic behavior by spinning wheels of upside-down truck while other children play.

A schematic summary of association and linkage studies of ASD, organized by chromosome. Purple bands indicate a chromosomal region that shows a linkage with ASD. Red and yellow bars (parallel to the chromosome) correspond to losses/gains in copy number, respectively, that are observed in people with ASD when compared with matched controls. Green bars correspond to genes that are observed to modulate the risk for ASD (either through a rare syndrome or genetic association): light green and dark green bars represent locations of candidate genes. *From Abrahams BS, Geschwind DH: Nat Rev Genet. 2008;9:341-355.*

DIAGNOSIS

Ideally, a multidisciplinary team of expert clinicians, including a child psychologist, speech pathologist, and a medical professional with developmental expertise (e.g., a child psychiatrist, developmental behavioral pediatrician, neurodevelopmental pediatrician, or child neurologist), should conduct the evaluation. The evaluation should include assessment of cognitive, communication, family, and other domains; a physical examination and direct behavioral observation; reports from multiple people who know the child well; and possible use of diagnostic instruments such as the Autism Diagnosis Interview–Revised or the Autism Diagnostic Observation Schedule. Symptoms must have been present in early childhood, are usually recognized between 12 to 24 months, and may be associated with regression in social behaviors or language

during the first 24 months. An ASD diagnosis in children often co-occurs with other conditions such as intellectual disability (30%), epilepsy (up to 50%), language disorders, and gastrointestinal disorders. Increasingly, genetic testing after diagnosis allows for identification of single-gene disorders or genetic variations associated with ASD in up to 15% to 20% of cases.

TREATMENT

Autism is a neurodevelopmental condition and not a temporal ailment that can be cured. Interventions are tailored to a child's specific needs and focus on reducing symptoms; improving cognitive, social, and communication abilities; and maximizing daily functioning. A treatment plan can include early intervention services,

highly structured behavioral therapies such as applied behavioral analysis, language and social skills training, and educational support. Some children may also benefit from medication therapy for associated symptoms, such as stimulants for hyperactivity, atypical antipsychotics for aggression, or antidepressants for depression or anxiety.

COURSE

ASD is a lifelong condition, although for some individuals, the degree of symptom severity may decrease with age or with intensive interventions. Childhood IQ, early language/communication ability, and involved family and educational supports are positively correlated with better communication, social skills, and functioning.

Plate 1.29

Brain: PART I

Rett Syndrome

Rett syndrome (RTT) is a neurodevelopmental disorder first noted around 1960 by the Austrian developmental pediatrician Andreas Rett and the Swedish child neurologist Bengt Hagberg. RTT, due principally to mutations in *MECP2* gene (coding for methyl-CpG-binding protein 2), which is located at Xq28, is the leading genetic cause of severe intellectual disability in females. Its incidence is approximately 1 in 10,000 female births. RTT remains a clinical diagnosis as not all individuals meeting diagnostic criteria have an identified mutation. Diagnosis is based on defined clinical criteria, which include a frank regression followed by the partial or complete loss of spoken language and fine motor skills, absent or abnormal gait, and hand stereotypies. Atypical RTT is based on meeting two of the four main criteria above, as well as 5 of 11 supportive criteria.

After a normal pregnancy and delivery, early development is apparently normal through age 6 months; however, subtle deviant patterns, including deceleration of normal head growth as early as age 6 weeks to 3 months, low muscle tone (hypotonia), poor feeding, a weak cry, and decreased activity, occur retrospectively. Developmental progress stalls between 6 and 18 months, followed, between 1 and 4 years, by frank regression of fine motor skills and communication function, including loss of acquired language with poor visual and aural interactions, irritability, and low interest, suggesting autism.

Concomitantly, stereotyped hand movements, including hand-wringing, hand-mouthing, hand-clapping or patting, or unusual finger movements, appear during wakefulness. Each child develops their own repertoire, generally evolving over time. Subtle stereotypies occur in the feet and circumorally. Although gait is acquired in about 80%, approximately 20% of children with Rett syndrome require assistance. It is subsequently lost in about 25% to 35%, becoming considerably dyspraxic in the remainder, with broad-based, semipurposeful patterns, toe-walking, or retropulsion. Overall, about 70% are able to walk, 20% of whom require assistance.

After the early period of autistic-like behaviors, an increasingly interactive phase emerges, typically by age 3 to 5 years. Here the child becomes very responsive to external stimuli, with intensive eye gaze and markedly improved receptive communication skills. However, expressive language remains poor. Their inability to speak or engage in volitional fine motor functions makes intellectual assessment difficult. Improved communication is possible through picture boards and advanced computer-based technologies. Although cognitive function remains stable, gradual slowing of motor skills occurs in adulthood, with increasing rigidity and dystonic posturing of ankles and feet.

Multiple associated medical problems are common. Bruxism is prominent, especially before age 10 years. Periodic breathing, consisting of breath-holding, hyperventilation, or a combination, occurs in more than 90%. This trait is prominent between ages 5 and 15 years and is exacerbated by unfamiliar or stressful circumstances, including large crowds or new surroundings.

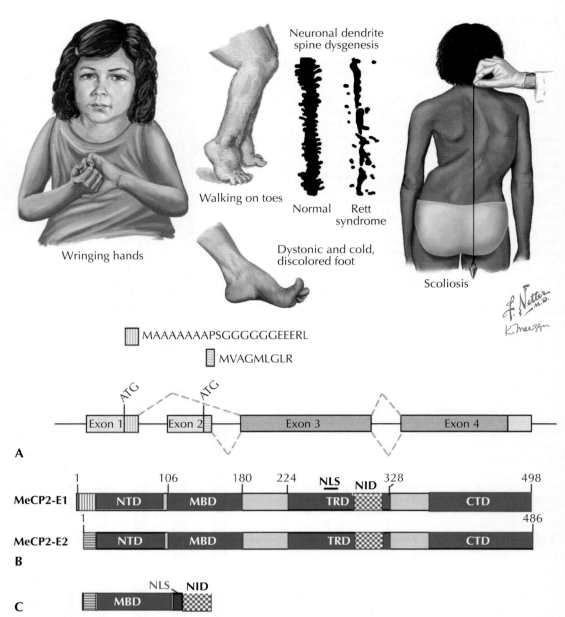

MAAAAAAAPSGGGGGGEEERL

MVAGMLGLR

MECP2 gene and protein isoforms and structural domains. **A,** Schematic illustration of the *MECP2* gene exons (not drawn to scale) and alternative splicing pattern that generates the two protein isoforms, MeCP2-E1 and MeCP2-E2. MeCP2-E1 is encoded by exons 1, 2, and 4, whereas MeCP2-E2 is encoded by exons 2, 3, and 4. The amino acid sequence of the N-terminus ends of the two isoforms is also shown. MeCP2-E1 has a 21–amino acid region missing in the E2 isoform, whereas MeCP2-E2 has a 9–amino acid region missing in the E1 isoform. **B,** Major structural domains of *MECP2*. CTD = C-terminal domain, MBD = methylated-DNA binding domain, TRD = transcription repression domain, NTD = N-terminus domain, NID = NCOR1-interacting domain, and NLS = nuclear localization domain. **C,** Schematic representation of the severely truncated MeCP2-E2 construct used in the study by Tillotson et al. (2017). An SV-40 NLS (in red) was inserted to ensure nuclear localization. *(From D'Mello SR. MECP2 and the biology of MECP2 duplication syndrome. J Neurochem. 2021;159:29–60.)*

Gastrointestinal dysfunction includes disordered chewing and swallowing, gastroesophageal reflux, delayed stomach emptying, constipation, gallbladder dysfunction, and impaired growth, all related to the neurobiologic underpinnings of the syndrome. The incidence of epilepsy and scoliosis increases throughout childhood and adolescence, ultimately occurring in 80% to 90% in this population.

Seizures are infrequent before age 2 years, after which they may be generalized or partial and usually managed effectively. Many children have unusual behaviors ("vacant spells") that are difficult to distinguish from epilepsy. Thus video electroencephalographic monitoring is required to establish the presence of seizures. Scoliosis becomes evident by age 4 years, with greater severity in children with significant hypotonia and who cannot maintain independent upright posture. Surgery is required in 18% to 20%, greatly improving the overall quality of life. Bracing is used with greater frequency; its effectiveness has been inadequately

Plate 1.30

Normal and Abnormal Development

RETT SYNDROME (Continued)

evaluated, however. Feet and hands are generally small, unusually cold, and discolored. With increasing age, parkinsonian features, including hypomimia (decreased facial expression), tremor, and rigidity occur. Rigidity is common past the age of 10 to 15 years and should be distinguished from spasticity. Osteopenia and osteomalacia are noted frequently and may lead to nontraumatic fractures in up to 30%. Prolonged QTc intervals are seen in up to 20% of individuals. A gastrostomy or gastrojejunostomy tube is present in one-third of individuals due to inability to swallow safely or insufficiently to meet caloric requirements. Growth failure and poor muscle development occur in most (~90%), with greater muscle growth in those with retained hand function and independent gait.

Unexplained sudden death occurs, possibly related to unwitnessed seizures, respiratory failure, or prolonged QT syndrome. With increasing appreciation of the underlying medical issues, including optimizing nutritional health, physical activity, and socialization, general well-being has improved remarkably.

Clinical involvement and overall progression may vary broadly. Two females with the same mutation may differ greatly in their level of involvement. This is thought to be based primarily on X chromosome inactivation but can also be related to their genetic background and the opportunities to engage with their environment at home and at school.

Average longevity is greater than 50 years.

PATHOPHYSIOLOGY

At present, more than 96% of those with RTT have a mutation in the *MECP2* gene (coding for methyl-CpG-binding protein 2), located at Xq28. MeCP2, a member of a family of methyl-binding proteins, is an epigenetic regulator of a large and increasing number of genes, including *BDNF* (brain-derived neurotrophic factor) and *CRH* (corticotrophin-releasing hormone). Reduced growth of dendrites and their spines is present throughout the cerebral hemispheres (an explanation for deceleration of head growth) and brainstem. Neurotransmitter function is impaired, with an imbalance between excitatory (principally glutamatergic) and inhibitory (chiefly GABAergic) expression. Conditional knockout mouse models indicate the diverse functional impact in specific neural centers. For example, knockout of GABAergic function in the forebrain, sparing the brainstem, results in an absence of periodic breathing abnormalities.

In general, RTT is a sporadic condition with recurrence in a family being less than 0.1%. In 85% or more of affected individuals, new mutations derive from paternal germ lines. In the small number of familial cases, the mother carries the gene but is normal or shows mild cognitive impairment or a learning disability due principally to favorable skewing of X chromosome inactivation. The differential diagnosis includes autism, Angelman syndrome, CDKL5 deficiency disorder, FOXG1 disorder, and other neurodevelopmental disorders.

Symptoms in males with mutations in *MECP2* range from those of a progressive disorder to intellectual delay. The abnormal gene is expressed in all cells, unlike in females, and the degree of involvement depends on the specific mutation. Males with *MECP2* mutations coupled with Klinefelter syndrome (47XXY) or somatic mosaicism may have typical RTT syndrome, as they have two X chromosomes, as in females. Duplication of *MECP2* produces a quite distinctive disorder that is modified by the inclusion of other genes in the duplication. These males have significant issues, including prominent epilepsy later in childhood, whereas their mothers, 70% (or more) of whom carry the same duplication, appear normal but may have significant obsessive-compulsive behaviors and evidence of depression.

At present, substantial research is being conducted in mouse models of RTT/*MECP2* mutants, and a number of clinical trials are ongoing. Replacing the defective gene is currently under study and is the ultimate goal.

Typical fronto-occipital growth pattern in females

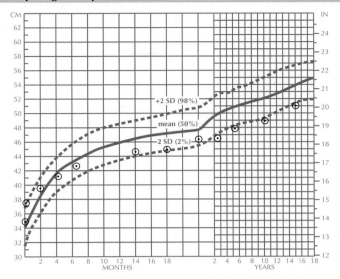

Typical height and weight growth pattern in females ages 2 to 20 years

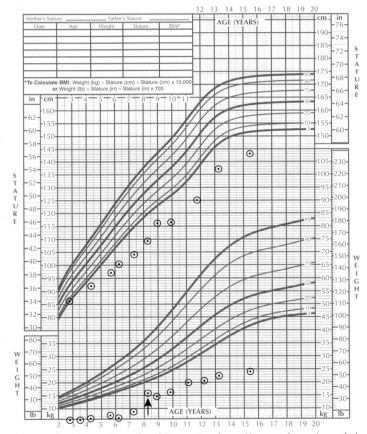

Base graphs from Centers for Disease Control and Prevention. https://www.cdc.gov/growthcharts/clinical_charts.htm.

CEREBRAL CORTEX AND NEUROCOGNITIVE DISORDERS

Plate 2.1

Brain: PART I

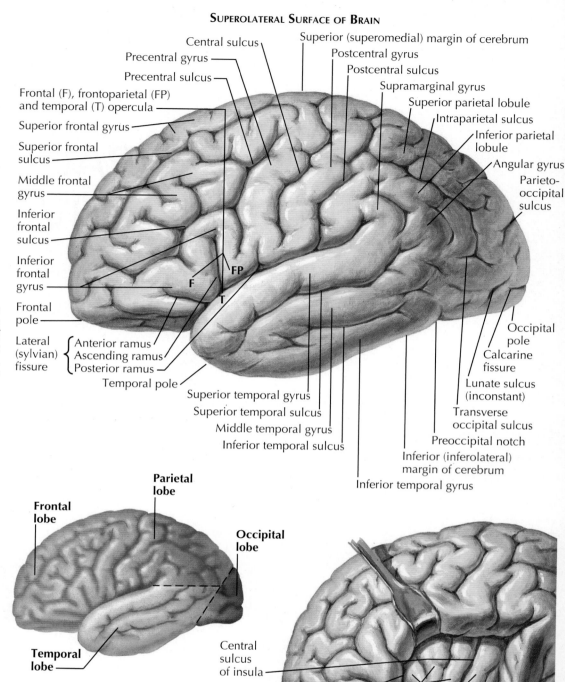

SUPEROLATERAL SURFACE OF BRAIN

Central sulcus
Precentral gyrus
Precentral sulcus
Frontal (F), frontoparietal (FP) and temporal (T) opercula
Superior frontal gyrus
Superior frontal sulcus
Middle frontal gyrus
Inferior frontal sulcus
Inferior frontal gyrus
Frontal pole
Lateral (sylvian) fissure { Anterior ramus / Ascending ramus / Posterior ramus }
Temporal pole
Superior temporal gyrus
Superior temporal sulcus
Middle temporal gyrus
Inferior temporal sulcus
Superior (superomedial) margin of cerebrum
Postcentral gyrus
Postcentral sulcus
Supramarginal gyrus
Superior parietal lobule
Intraparietal sulcus
Inferior parietal lobule
Angular gyrus
Parieto-occipital sulcus
Occipital pole
Calcarine fissure
Lunate sulcus (inconstant)
Transverse occipital sulcus
Preoccipital notch
Inferior (inferolateral) margin of cerebrum
Inferior temporal gyrus

Parietal lobe
Frontal lobe
Occipital lobe
Temporal lobe

Central sulcus of insula
Circular sulcus of insula
Insula { Short gyri / Limen / Long gyrus }

F. Netter M.D.

SURFACES OF THE CEREBRUM

The cerebrum is divided into right and left hemispheres by a longitudinal fissure. Each hemisphere has three surfaces—superolateral, medial, and inferior—all of which have irregular fissures, or sulci, demarcating convolutions, or gyri. Although there are variations in arrangement between the two hemispheres in the same brain and in those from different persons, a basic similarity in the pattern allows the parts of the brain to be mapped and named.

SUPEROLATERAL SURFACE

On the superolateral surface, two sulci, the lateral and the central, can be easily identified. The _lateral (sylvian) sulcus_ has a short stem between the orbital surface of the frontal lobe and the temporal pole; in life, the lesser wing of the sphenoid bone projects into it. At its outer end, the stem divides into anterior, ascending, and posterior branches. The anterior and ascending rami are each about 2.5 cm long; the former runs horizontally into the inferior frontal gyrus, and the latter runs vertically. The posterior ramus is about 7.5 cm long and inclines upward as it extends backward to end in the supramarginal gyrus, which is part of the inferior parietal lobule. These rami separate triangular areas of cortex called _opercula_, which cover a buried lobe of cortex, the _insula_.

The _central (rolandic) sulcus_ proceeds obliquely downward and forward from a point on the superior border almost halfway between the frontal and occipital poles. It is sinuous and ends above the middle of the posterior ramus of the lateral sulcus. Its upper end usually runs onto the medial surface of the cerebrum and terminates in the paracentral lobule.

The _parieto-occipital sulcus_ is situated mainly on the medial surface of the cerebrum, but it cuts the superior margin and appears for a short distance on the superolateral surface about 5 cm in front of the occipital pole. At about the same distance from the occipital pole on the inferior margin, there is a shallow indentation, the _preoccipital notch,_ produced by a small ridge on the upper surface of the tentorium cerebelli.

The above features divide the cerebrum into frontal, parietal, occipital, and temporal lobes. The _frontal lobe_ lies in front of the central sulcus and anterosuperior to the lateral sulcus. The _parietal lobe_ lies behind the central sulcus, above the posterior ramus of the lateral sulcus and in front of an imaginary line drawn between the parieto-occipital sulcus and the preoccipital notch.

The _occipital lobe_ lies behind this same imaginary line. The _temporal lobe_ lies below the stem and posterior ramus of the lateral sulcus and is bounded behind by the lower part of the aforementioned imaginary line.

Frontal Lobe

The superolateral surface of the frontal lobe is traversed by three main sulci and is thus divided into four gyri. The _precentral sulcus_ runs parallel to the central sulcus, separated from it by the _precentral gyrus,_ the great cortical somatomotor area. The _superior_ and _inferior frontal sulci_ curve across the remaining part of the surface, dividing it into superior, middle, and inferior frontal gyri.

Parietal Lobe

The parietal lobe has two main sulci, which divide it into three gyri. The _postcentral sulcus_ lies parallel to the central sulcus, separated from it by the _postcentral gyrus,_ the great somatic sensory cortical area. The

Plate 2.2   Cerebral Cortex and Neurocognitive Disorders

SURFACES OF THE CEREBRUM (Continued)

remaining, larger part of the superolateral parietal surface is subdivided into superior and inferior parietal lobules (gyri) by the *intraparietal sulcus,* which runs backward from near the midpoint of the postcentral sulcus and usually extends into the occipital lobe, where it ends by joining the transverse occipital sulcus.

Occipital Lobe

The outer surface of the occipital lobe is less extensive than that of the other lobes and has a short *transverse occipital sulcus* and a *lunate sulcus;* the latter demarcates the visuosensory and visuopsychic areas of the cortex. The *calcarine sulcus* notches the occipital pole.

Temporal Lobe

The temporal lobe is divided by *superior* and *inferior temporal sulci* into superior, middle, and inferior temporal gyri. The sulci run backward and slightly upward, in the same general direction as the posterior ramus of the lateral sulcus, which lies above them. The superior sulcus ends in the lower part of the inferior parietal lobule, and the superjacent cortex is called the angular gyrus. The superior temporal gyrus contains the auditosensory and auditopsychic areas.

Insula

The insula is a sunken lobe of cortex, overlaid by opercula and buried by the exuberant growth of adjoining cortical areas. It is ovoid in shape and is surrounded by a groove, the *circular sulcus* of the insula. The apex is inferior, near the anterior (rostral) perforated substance, and is termed the *limen* of the insula. The insular surface is divided into larger and smaller posterior parts by the *central sulcus* of the insula, which is roughly parallel to the central sulcus of the cerebrum. Each part is further subdivided by minor sulci into short and long insular gyri. The claustrum and lentiform nucleus lie deep to the insula.

MEDIAL SURFACE OF CEREBRAL HEMISPHERES

The medial surfaces of the cerebral hemispheres are flat, and, although separated for most of their extent by the longitudinal fissure and falx cerebri, they are connected in parts by the cerebral commissures and by the structures bounding the third ventricle.

Corpus Callosum

The corpus callosum is the largest of the cerebral commissures and forms most of the roof of the lateral ventricle. In a median sagittal section, it appears as a flattened bridge of white fibers, and its central part, or *trunk,* is convex upward. The anterior end is recurved to form the *genu,* which tapers rapidly into the *rostrum.* The expanded posterior end, or *splenium,* overlies the midbrain and adjacent part of the cerebellum. The corpus callosum is about 10 cm long and 2.5 cm wide between the points where it sinks into the opposing hemispheres in the depths of the corpus callosal sulcus. Its fibers diverge to all parts of the cerebral cortex.

Fornix

Below the splenium and trunk of the corpus callosum are the symmetric arching bundles (crura of the fornix) that meet to form the body of the fornix and separate again to become the *columns* of the fornix, curving downward to the mammillary bodies. The body of the fornix lies in the roof of the third ventricle, and the tela choroidea is subjacent; the lateral fringed margins of this double fold of pia mater are the choroid plexuses of the central parts of the lateral ventricles, and an

MEDIAL SURFACE OF BRAIN

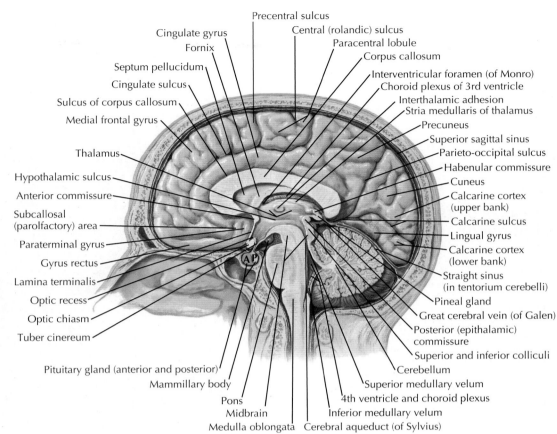

Plate 2.3

Brain: PART I

INFERIOR SURFACE OF BRAIN

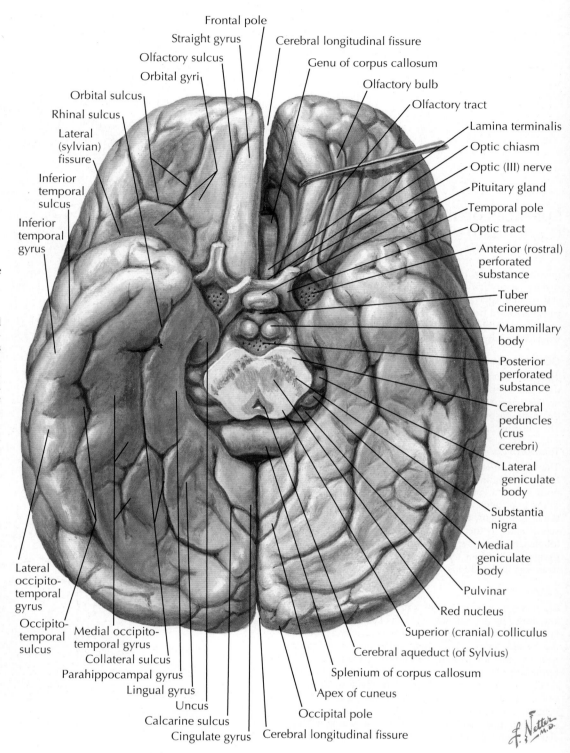

Frontal pole
Straight gyrus
Olfactory sulcus
Orbital gyri
Orbital sulcus
Rhinal sulcus
Lateral (sylvian) fissure
Inferior temporal sulcus
Inferior temporal gyrus
Cerebral longitudinal fissure
Genu of corpus callosum
Olfactory bulb
Olfactory tract
Lamina terminalis
Optic chiasm
Optic (III) nerve
Pituitary gland
Temporal pole
Optic tract
Anterior (rostral) perforated substance
Tuber cinereum
Mammillary body
Posterior perforated substance
Cerebral peduncles (crus cerebri)
Lateral geniculate body
Substantia nigra
Medial geniculate body
Pulvinar
Red nucleus
Superior (cranial) colliculus
Cerebral aqueduct (of Sylvius)
Splenium of corpus callosum
Apex of cuneus
Occipital pole
Cerebral longitudinal fissure
Cingulate gyrus
Calcarine sulcus
Uncus
Lingual gyrus
Parahippocampal gyrus
Collateral sulcus
Medial occipito-temporal gyrus
Occipito-temporal sulcus
Lateral occipito-temporal gyrus

SURFACES OF THE CEREBRUM (Continued)

extension from the underside of the fold in the midline forms the choroid plexus of the third ventricle.

Cingulate Sulcus

The cingulate sulcus is easily identified on the medial surface, lying parallel to the corpus callosum. It begins below the genu of the corpus callosum and ends above the posterior part of the trunk by turning upward to cut the superior margin of the hemisphere. Opposite the middle of the trunk is another vertical branch sulcus, and the area of cortex between these ascending sulci is the *paracentral lobule,* which contains parts of the motor and sensory cortical areas. The cingulate sulcus separates the *medial frontal* and *cingulate gyri,* and below the genu and rostrum of the corpus callosum are small *parolfactory sulci* separating the *subcallosal (parolfactory) areas* and *paraterminal gyrus.*

Posterior Medial Surface

The posterior part of the medial surface has two deep sulci. The upper *parieto-occipital sulcus* inclines backward and upward to cut the superior border. The lower *calcarine sulcus* extends forward from the occipital pole to end beneath the splenium of the corpus callosum, and the isthmus of cortex between them connects the cingulate and parahippocampal gyri. The wedge-shaped region between the parieto-occipital and calcarine sulci is the *cuneus,* and the area between the parieto-occipital sulcus and the paracentral lobule is the *precuneus.* The main visuosensory area is located in the walls of the calcarine sulcus and in the adjacent cortex.

INFERIOR SURFACE OF CEREBRAL HEMISPHERE

The inferior surface is divided by the stem of the lateral sulcus into the smaller orbital surface and larger tentorial surface.

The *orbital surface* rests on the roofs of the orbit and nose and is marked by an H-shaped *orbital sulcus,* as well as by a straight groove on the medial side, the *olfactory sulcus,* which lodges the olfactory bulb and tract. The orbital sulcus demarcates the *orbital gyri;* the small convolution medial to the olfactory sulcus is the *straight gyrus.*

The *tentorial surface* lies partly on the floor of the middle cranial fossa and partly on the tentorium cerebelli.

It has two anteroposterior grooves, the *collateral* and *occipitotemporal sulci.* Both run almost directly forward from the occipital pole to the temporal pole; like other sulci, they may be subdivided, and the anterior end of the collateral sulcus is called the *rhinal sulcus.* The *parahippocampal* and *lingual gyri* lie medial to the collateral sulcus. The *dentate gyrus,* a narrow fringe of cortex with transverse markings, occupies the groove between the parahippocampal gyrus and the fimbria of

the hippocampus. The anterior end of the parahippocampal gyrus becomes recurved to form the *uncus,* which is partly occupied by the cortical olfactory area. The *medial occipitotemporal gyrus* is fusiform in shape and lies between the collateral and occipitotemporal sulci. The *lateral occipitotemporal gyrus* lies lateral to the occipitotemporal sulcus and is continuous with the *inferior temporal gyrus* around the inferior margin of the hemisphere.

Plate 2.4

Cerebral Cortex and Neurocognitive Disorders

CEREBRAL CORTEX: FUNCTION AND ASSOCIATION PATHWAYS

In humans, the cerebral cortex is highly developed, and the complexity of the interhemispheric and intrahemispheric connections parallels this degree of development. The cerebral cortex has definite areas related to specific neurologic functions, either for primary sensory reception or for complex integrated activity.

ASSOCIATION PATHWAYS

When one cortical area is activated by a stimulus, other areas also respond. This is due to the rapid activity along a large number of precisely organized, reciprocally acting association pathways. The pathways may be very short, linking neighboring areas and running only within the gray matter, or they may be longer (arcuate) bundles, passing through the white matter to connect gyrus to gyrus or lobe to lobe within a cerebral hemisphere–intrahemispheric connection. Other commissural bundles conduct interhemispheric activity. The most prominent are the *corpus callosum,* a large band of fibers that lies immediately beneath the cingulum; the *anterior commissure,* which connects both temporal lobes; and the *hippocampal commissure (commissure of the fornix),* which connects the right and left hippocampus.

The reciprocal activity of the connections in the cerebral cortex ensures the coordination of sensory input and motor activity, as well as the regulation of higher function. For example, for the appreciation and integration of visual information, the primary visual sensory area of the occipital cortex is linked to the visual association areas. These visual centers are connected by intrahemispheric fibers to the ipsilateral parietal cortex, as well as to other areas, such as the temporal lobe, for further integrated activity. The right and left parietal and posterior temporal areas, in turn, are connected by the corpus callosum.

PREFRONTAL CORTEX

The prefrontal cortex (which includes the three frontal gyri, the orbital gyri, most of the medial frontal gyrus, and approximately half of the cingulate gyrus) is concerned with focused attention, impulse inhibition, prospective memory, cognitive flexibility, and complex social behaviors. This area receives numerous connections from the temporal and parietal lobes via pathways in the cingulum, a bundle of long association fibers lying within the cingulate gyrus. Bilateral lesions of the prefrontal area produce a loss of concentration, decreased intellectual ability, and memory and judgment deficits.

MOTOR AND SENSORY CORTICES

The primary motor cortex and the primary *somatosensory cortex* occupy contiguous parts of the frontal and parietal lobes, and the *premotor cortex* lies just anterior to the primary motor cortex. They are primarily concerned with the initiation, activation, and performance of *motor activity,* as well as the reception of *primary sensation* of the body. Lesions of the somatosensory cortex result in contralateral paralysis and loss of somatosensory reception or perception.

PARIETAL LOBE

The parietal lobe is primarily concerned with the interpretation and integration of information from sensory areas; that is, the visual areas and the somatosensory cortex.

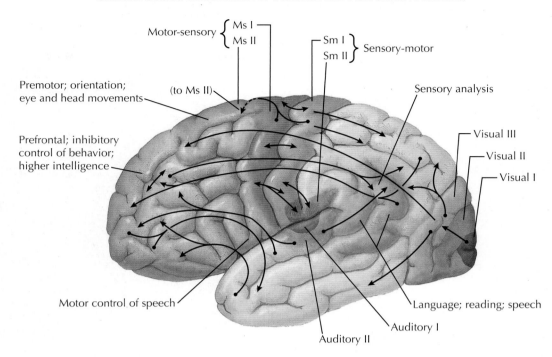

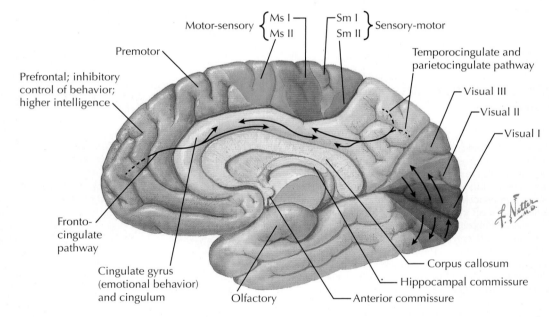

Lesions in the parietal lobe result in sensory ataxia, a loss of general awareness, defective recognition of sensory impulses, and a lack of interpretation of spatial relationships.

OCCIPITAL LOBE

Lesions of the striate cortex (the primary visual area) on one side result in contralateral hemianopsia, whereas lesions of the secondary regions of the visual cortex cause a lack of ability to interpret visual impulses.

TEMPORAL LOBE

The *posterior part of the temporal lobe* is concerned with the reception and interpretation of auditory information and with some aspects of pattern recognition and higher visual coordination; the interconnections of the auditory and visual segments of the occipital, temporal, and parietal lobes make this a highly integrated function. The *anterior part of the temporal lobe* is concerned with visceral motor activity and certain aspects of behavior. Lesions here may be manifested by psychomotor seizures or, if they occur in the region of the uncus, by uncinate "fits" characterized by alteration of consciousness and hallucinations of taste and odor.

LESIONS

In general, lesions of primary receptive areas produce identifiable deficits. A lesion in a specific area of the cerebral cortex may produce a deficit far beyond the functional identity of that particular area because the complex interconnections beneath that cortical region may be damaged.

Plate 2.5

Brain: PART I

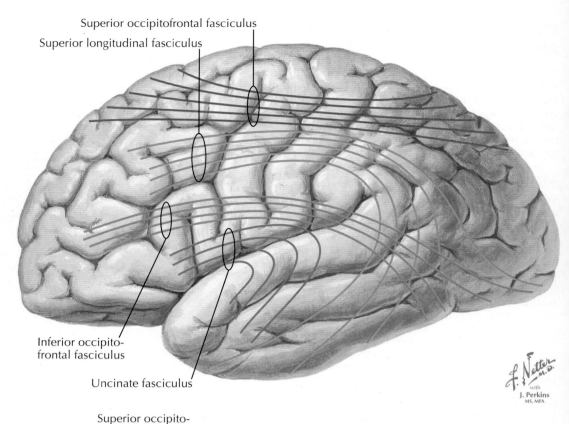

Superior occipitofrontal fasciculus
Superior longitudinal fasciculus

Inferior occipito-
frontal fasciculus

Uncinate fasciculus

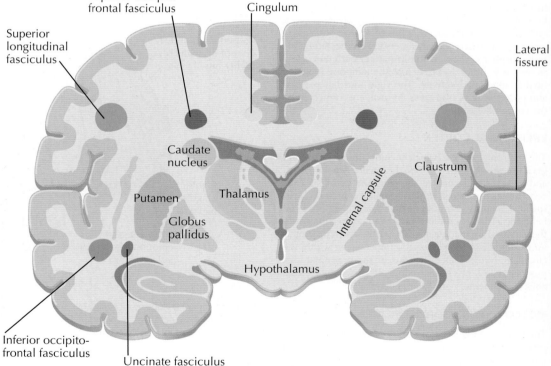

Superior occipito-
frontal fasciculus

Cingulum

Superior
longitudinal
fasciculus

Lateral
fissure

Caudate
nucleus

Claustrum

Putamen

Thalamus

Internal capsule

Globus
pallidus

Hypothalamus

Inferior occipito-
frontal fasciculus

Uncinate fasciculus

MAJOR CORTICAL ASSOCIATION BUNDLES

Association fibers are predominantly located in the cerebral white matter and connect intrahemispheric cortical regions. There are two main types of association fibers, and they are differentiated by size and function. Short association fibers known as arcuate fibers (or "U fibers") connect adjacent gyri, thus allowing for communication between neighboring cortical regions. Long association fibers provide the architectural basis for large-scale neurocognitive networks. These networks connect more widespread cortical regions and are visualized as "bundles" of fibers that allow communication between primary and association cortical regions. For instance, the *superior longitudinal fasciculus* (SLF) (which has three major bundles, I, II, and III) allows communication between the parietal and frontal lobes. In particular, the SLF I allows information from the superior parietal lobe, or motor cortex, to be relayed to the supplementary motor cortex. SLF II connects the caudal parietal region with the prefrontal lobes, thus allowing an individual to have a visual perception of space. SLF III connects rostral parietal areas with the frontal opercular region (the region that controls facial movements), thus enabling an individual to imitate an action. Other long association fibers include the *fronto-occipital fasciculus,* which links the posterior and medial parietal and occipital areas; *the uncinate fasciculus* (or the anterior limbic fiber bundle), which connects the temporal lobe and frontal lobes; the *inferior longitudinal fasciculus,* which connects the temporal lobe to the occipital and parietal regions; and the *cingulum bundle* (or the posterior limbic fiber bundle), which stretches from the frontal lobe to the parahippocampal gyrus. The *cingulum bundle* enables monoamines

(dopamine, norepinephrine, and serotonin), along with cholinergic projections, to travel to widespread cortical targets.

Lesions to cortical association bundles can provide clinical relevance to fiber pathway tracts and cortical origins and destinations. For instance, a patient who develops acute damage to the *uncinate fasciculus* and

right anterior frontal cortex (e.g., from a stroke) will have a "disconnection" between the temporal and frontal lobes. This individual may develop amnesia for experiences predating the stroke, along with impairment of self-awareness of personal experiences across time (this clinical finding is also known as a disruption of autonoetic consciousness).

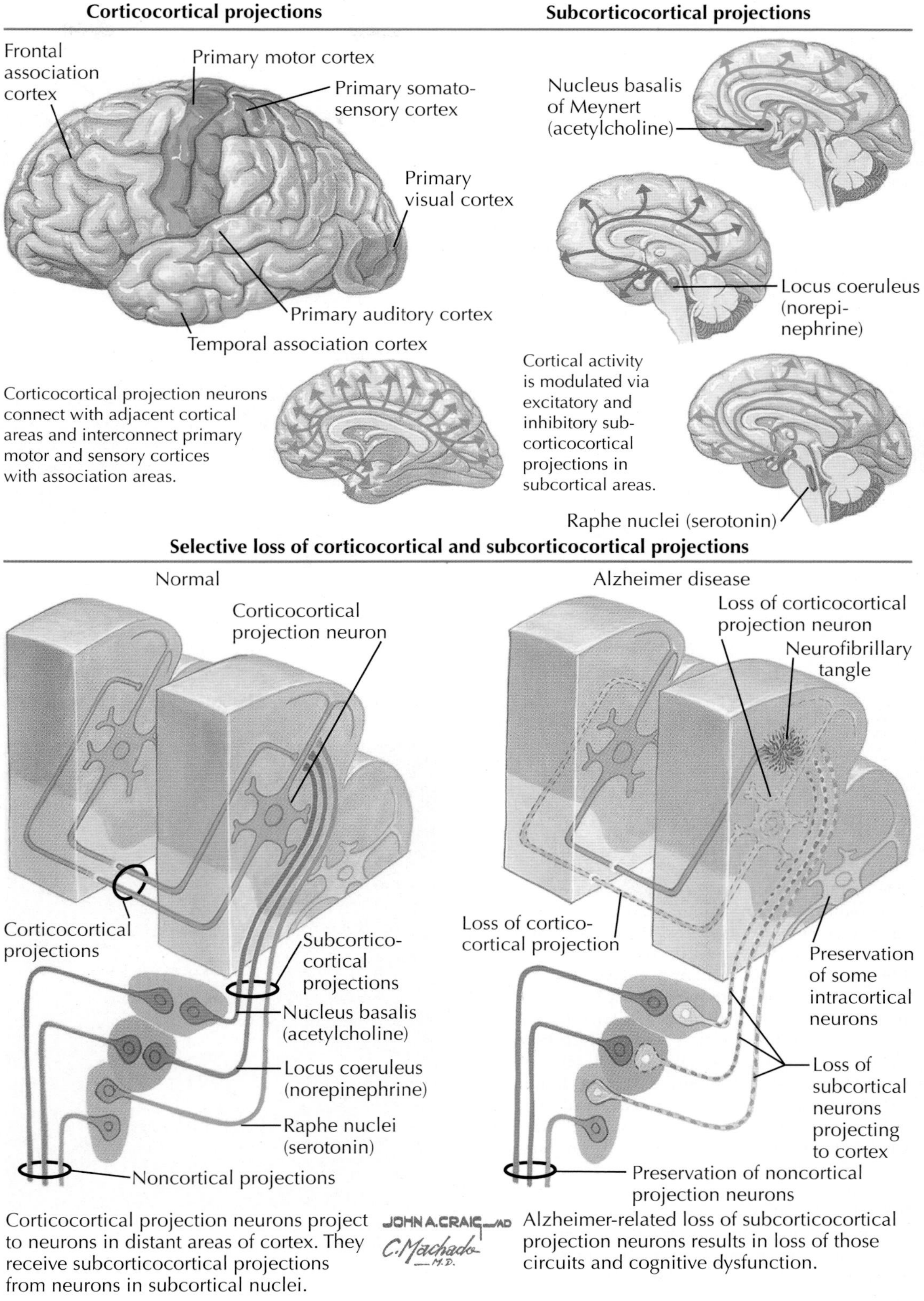

Plate 2.6

Cerebral Cortex and Neurocognitive Disorders

Corticocortical projections

Frontal association cortex
Primary motor cortex
Primary somato-sensory cortex
Primary visual cortex
Primary auditory cortex
Temporal association cortex

Corticocortical projection neurons connect with adjacent cortical areas and interconnect primary motor and sensory cortices with association areas.

Subcorticocortical projections

Nucleus basalis of Meynert (acetylcholine)
Locus coeruleus (norepinephrine)

Cortical activity is modulated via excitatory and inhibitory sub-corticocortical projections in subcortical areas.

Raphe nuclei (serotonin)

Selective loss of corticocortical and subcorticocortical projections

Normal

Corticocortical projection neuron
Corticocortical projections
Subcortico-cortical projections
Nucleus basalis (acetylcholine)
Locus coeruleus (norepinephrine)
Raphe nuclei (serotonin)
Noncortical projections

Corticocortical projection neurons project to neurons in distant areas of cortex. They receive subcorticocortical projections from neurons in subcortical nuclei.

JOHN A.CRAIG _MD
C.Machado _M.D.

Alzheimer disease

Loss of corticocortical projection neuron
Neurofibrillary tangle
Preservation of some intracortical neurons
Loss of cortico-cortical projection
Loss of subcortical neurons projecting to cortex
Preservation of noncortical projection neurons

Alzheimer-related loss of subcorticocortical projection neurons results in loss of those circuits and cognitive dysfunction.

CORTICOCORTICAL AND SUBCORTICOCORTICAL PROJECTION CIRCUITS

The cerebral white matter consists of myelinated axons that link cortical areas with both cortical and subcortical regions. There exist three main categories of efferent fibers from a cortical area: association fibers, striatal fibers, and commissural/subcortical fibers. Corticocortical projections allow both adjacent and distant cortical regions to communicate, whereas cortico-subcortical projections allow reciprocal communication between cortical regions and subcortical structures. These subcorticocortical projections connect the cortex to the thalamus, the pontocerebellar system, brainstem, and spinal cord.

CORTICOCORTICAL CIRCUITS

Local short association fibers, or U fibers, connect adjacent cortical gyri and lie beneath the sixth cortical layer. Neighborhood association fibers traverse longer distances than U fibers but still connect nearby cortical regions. Long association fibers travel within the same hemisphere and connect more distant cortical regions. These include the superior, middle, and inferior longitudinal fasciculi, arcuate fasciculus, extreme capsule, fronto-occipital fasciculus, uncinate fasciculus, and cingulum bundle (see Plate 2.5).

SUBCORTICOCORTICAL CIRCUITS

Striatal fibers describe fiber groups that connect cortical regions to the striatum (the caudate and putamen). For instance, these fibers allow cortical motor control. The commissural bundle is a collection of fibers that travel from a cortical region to the opposite hemisphere via the corpus callosum or anterior commissure. Subcortical fibers travel via the internal capsule to diencephalic structures (e.g., thalamus) and brainstem (e.g., pons). The origins of the subcorticocortical cell bodies are laminae V and VI. Cortical activity is modulated via

excitatory and inhibitory projections in subcortical areas. For instance, diffuse cortical cholinergic projections to the cortex arise from the nucleus basalis of Meynert, and norepinephrine projections arise from the locus coeruleus.

In the case of Alzheimer disease, a loss of corticocortical projection neurons is associated with neurofibrillary tangle formation. This indicates a "disconnection"

of adjacent cortex and cortical association areas. The disconnection of subcorticocortical circuits is evident in the reduction of cholinergic projections throughout the cortex, resulting in reduced acetylcholine levels in the cortex. This observation led to the development of the first effective therapies for Alzheimer disease, acetylcholinesterase inhibitors, which boost acetylcholine levels in the brain.

Plate 2.7

Brain: PART I

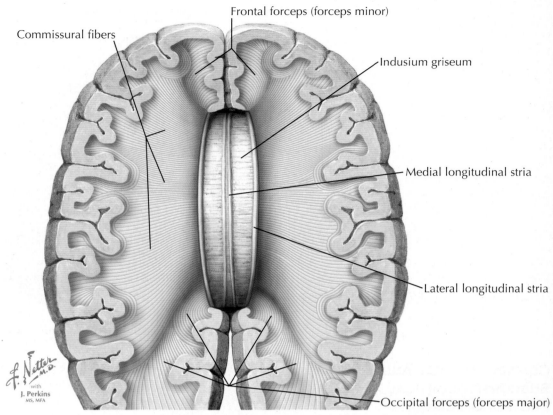

Commissural fibers

Frontal forceps (forceps minor)

Indusium griseum

Medial longitudinal stria

Lateral longitudinal stria

Occipital forceps (forceps major)

Schematic view of the lateral extent of major components of the corpus callosum

CORPUS CALLOSUM

The corpus callosum is the major commissure of the forebrain, connecting homologous cortical regions of the two cerebral hemispheres. The corpus callosum is divided into anterior and posterior parts, known as the genu and splenium, respectively. The genu includes fibers of the frontal forceps (forceps minor) interconnecting frontal areas. Posteriorly, the splenium includes the occipital forceps (forceps major), interconnecting the parietal, occipital, and temporal lobes. A corpus callosotomy, a surgical lesioning of the corpus callosum, has been performed in patients with medication-refractory epilepsy. The goal of this surgery is to prevent seizure spread from one hemisphere to another.

Agenesis of the corpus callosum (ACC) is a congenital birth defect characterized by an absence of a corpus callosum. This condition can occur in isolation (with little to no impact on cognitive performance) or can occur as part of abnormalities such as Dandy-Walker syndrome, Arnold-Chiari malformation, schizencephaly, holoprosencephaly, Andermann syndrome, or Aicardi syndrome. Midline facial defects often accompany ACC.

COLOR IMAGING BY DIFFUSION TENSOR IMAGING

Diffusion-weighted imaging measures the rate of water diffusion in brain tissue, measured using an apparent diffusion constant. Diffusion tensor imaging is used to measure the "anisotropy" or randomness of water

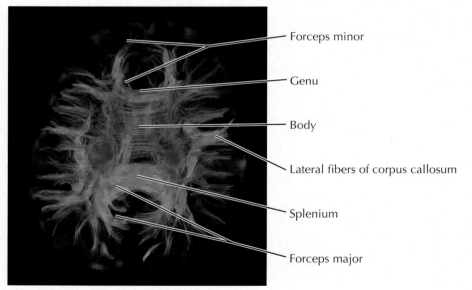

Forceps minor

Genu

Body

Lateral fibers of corpus callosum

Splenium

Forceps major

Color imaging of the corpus callosum, by diffusion tensor imaging, axial view. *From Felten DL, O'Banion MK, Maida MS. Netter's Atlas of Neuroscience, 4th ed. Elsevier; 2022.*

diffusion. The degree of anisotropy is called fractional anisotropy (FA), and it is measured from 0 to 1, where 0 is unrestricted and 1 is fully restricted and diffuses along only one axis. Due to the properties of white matter, parallel bundles of axons and the myelin sheaths allow for a certain orientation of water diffusion. Water diffuses more rapidly in the aligned direction and more slowly perpendicular to this direction. This enables

"visualization" of white matter tracts based on the calculated FA values. To discriminate the direction of different fiber bundles, a color scheme is adopted in which green represents an anterior-posterior direction, red a left-right direction, and blue a superior-inferior direction. In these images of the corpus callosum, components of this major commissural bundle are represented in red.

Plate 2.8

Cerebral Cortex and Neurocognitive Disorders

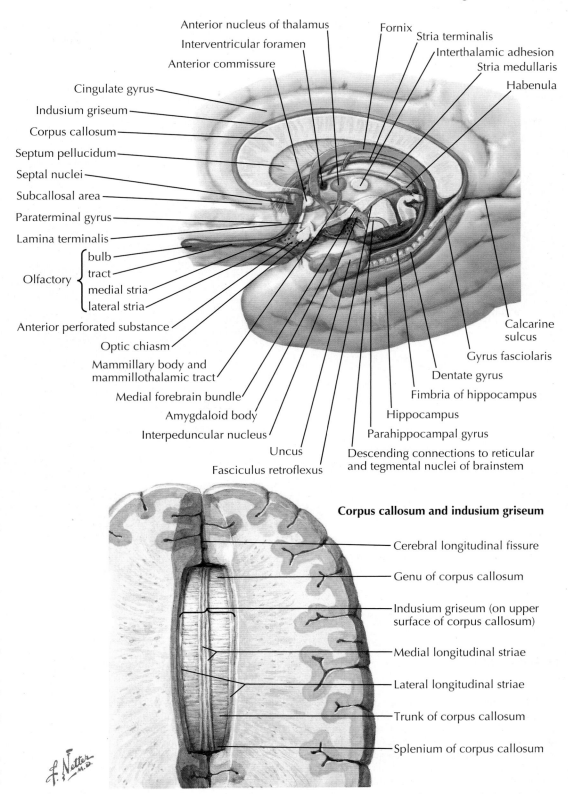

Anterior nucleus of thalamus
Interventricular foramen
Anterior commissure
Cingulate gyrus
Indusium griseum
Corpus callosum
Septum pellucidum
Septal nuclei
Subcallosal area
Paraterminal gyrus
Lamina terminalis
Olfactory {
bulb
tract
medial stria
lateral stria
}
Anterior perforated substance
Optic chiasm
Mammillary body and mammillothalamic tract
Medial forebrain bundle
Amygdaloid body
Interpeduncular nucleus
Fasciculus retroflexus
Uncus

Fornix
Stria terminalis
Interthalamic adhesion
Stria medullaris
Habenula
Calcarine sulcus
Gyrus fasciolaris
Dentate gyrus
Fimbria of hippocampus
Hippocampus
Parahippocampal gyrus
Descending connections to reticular and tegmental nuclei of brainstem

Corpus callosum and indusium griseum

Cerebral longitudinal fissure
Genu of corpus callosum
Indusium griseum (on upper surface of corpus callosum)
Medial longitudinal striae
Lateral longitudinal striae
Trunk of corpus callosum
Splenium of corpus callosum

RHINENCEPHALON AND LIMBIC SYSTEM

The *rhinencephalon* is a term that describes quite literally the "nose" or "smell" regions of the brain. The *limbic system* refers to the structures and tracts involved with emotion, memory formation, and autonomic and endocrine response to emotional stimuli. The terms rhinencephalon and limbic system are sometimes used synonymously, but the rhinencephalon refers to olfactory structures and related pathways. Located in the medial and inferior surface of the forebrain, these parts include the olfactory bulb, tract and striae, the anterior perforated substance, the uncus, the hippocampus, the dentate gyrus, the gyrus fasciolaris, the indusium griseum, the habenular trigone, the subcallosal area, the paraterminal gyrus, the fornix, and the amygdaloid body as direct olfactory afferents project to the amygdala. The olfactory pathway is described and illustrated in Plate 5.8.

The limbic forebrain refers to the areas that are functionally and anatomically connected structures that relate to emotion, motivation, and self-preservation. The limbic system is thought to be a major substrate for regulation of emotional responsiveness and behavior, for individualized reactivity to sensory stimuli and internal stimuli, and for integrated memory tasks. The main regions of the limbic forebrain include the hypothalamus, amygdala, hippocampus, and limbic cortex (prefrontal cortex and orbital frontal cortex). The hippocampal formation and amygdala send axonal projections through the forebrain, via the fornix and stria terminalis, respectively, to the hypothalamus and septal region. The amygdala also has a more direct pathway to the hypothalamus via the anterior amygdalofugal pathway. The septal nuclei lie rostral to the hypothalamus and send axons to the habenular nuclei via the stria medullaris thalami.

PIRIFORM AREA

The anterior (rostral) perforated substance, the uncus, the anterior end of the dentate gyrus, and the anterior part of the parahippocampal gyrus medial to the rhinal sulcus are often referred to as the piriform area. These regions function to give perception of smell.

The *anterior perforated substance* is continuous with the paraterminal gyrus and separated from the anterior part of the globus pallidus of the lentiform nucleus by the anterior (rostral) commissure, ansa lenticularis, and ansa peduncularis; posteromedially, it blends into the tuber cinereum.

The *indusium griseum* is a thin layer of gray matter spread over the upper surface of the corpus callosum.

Anteriorly, it curves around the genu and rostrum to merge with the paraterminal gyri; laterally, it becomes continuous with the cortex of the cingulate gyrus; and posteriorly, it passes over the splenium to blend with the dentate and parahippocampal gyri through the narrow gyrus fasciolaris. Two slender strands of white fibers, the *medial* and *lateral longitudinal striae,* are embedded in the indusium griseum.

Plate 2.9

Brain: PART I

MAJOR AFFERENT AND EFFERENT CONNECTIONS OF THE HIPPOCAMPAL FORMATION

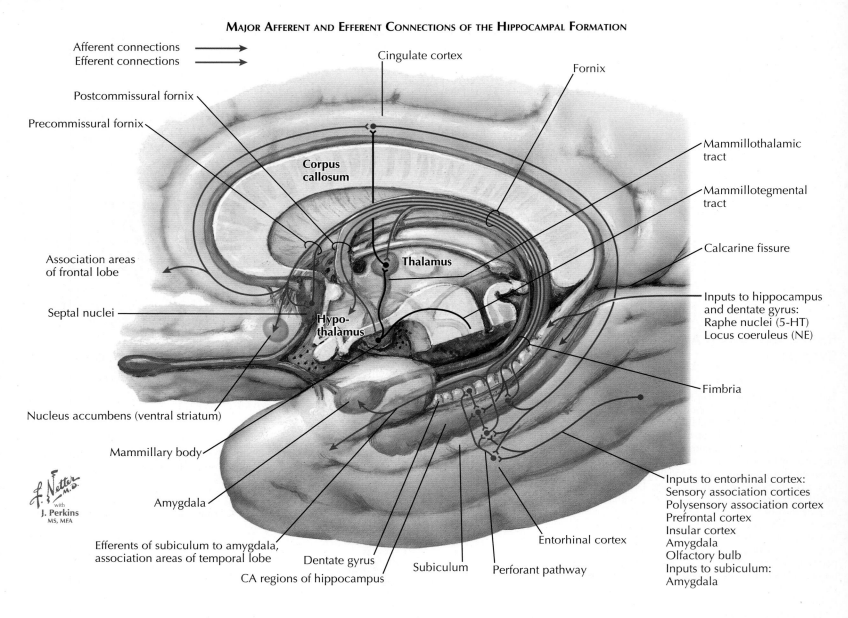

Afferent connections →
Efferent connections →

Cingulate cortex

Fornix

Postcommissural fornix

Precommissural fornix

Mammillothalamic tract

Mammillotegmental tract

Corpus callosum

Calcarine fissure

Association areas of frontal lobe

Thalamus

Inputs to hippocampus and dentate gyrus:
Raphe nuclei (5-HT)
Locus coeruleus (NE)

Septal nuclei

Hypo-thalamus

Nucleus accumbens (ventral striatum)

Fimbria

Mammillary body

Amygdala

Inputs to entorhinal cortex:
Sensory association cortices
Polysensory association cortex
Prefrontal cortex
Insular cortex
Amygdala
Olfactory bulb
Inputs to subiculum:
Amygdala

Efferents of subiculum to amygdala, association areas of temporal lobe

Dentate gyrus

Entorhinal cortex

CA regions of hippocampus

Subiculum

Perforant pathway

HIPPOCAMPUS

The hippocampus, the posterior part of the dentate gyrus, and the indusium griseum are sometimes grouped together as the hippocampal formation. In humans, the attenuated gray and white structures of this formation are produced by the enormous enlargement of the corpus callosum, which encroaches upon the parahippocampal and dentate gyri and the hippocampi, thus expanding them.

The *hippocampus* is a part of the marginal cortex of the parahippocampal gyrus that has been invaginated, or rolled, into the floor of the inferior horn of the lateral ventricle by the exuberant growth of the nearby temporal cortex. The curved hippocampal eminence is composed mostly of gray matter, and its anterior end is expanded and grooved like a paw, the *pes hippocampi*. Axons conveying efferent impulses from the pyramidal cells of the hippocampus form a white layer on its surface, the *alveus,* and then converge toward its medial edge to form a white strip, the *fimbria.* The

hippocampus is an important part of the olfactory apparatus in lower animals; in humans, few or no secondary olfactory fibers end in it. However, it possesses substantial connections with the hypothalamus, which regulates many visceral activities that influence emotional behavior, and with temporal lobe areas reputedly associated with memory.

The *dentate gyrus* (dentate fascia) is a crenated fringe of cortex occupying the narrow furrow between the fimbria of the hippocampus and the parahippocampal gyrus. Anteriorly, this fringe fades away on the surface of the uncus, and posteriorly, it becomes continuous with the indusium griseum through the gyrus fasciolaris.

The hippocampus contains pyramidal cells in regions CA1 and CA3 that project via the efferent fornix to the septal nuclei and hypothalamus. The subiculum receives input from the hippocampal pyramidal cells and also projects via the fornix to the mammillary nuclei and anterior nucleus of the thalamus. It is connected reciprocally with the amygdala and sends axons to cortical association areas of the temporal lobe. The

dentate gyrus contains granule cells that project to the pyramidal cells of the hippocampus and subiculum and receive hippocampal input. The afferent connections to the hippocampal formation include the cerebral association cortices, prefrontal cortex, cingulate cortex, insular cortex, amygdaloid nuclei, and olfactory bulb via projections to the entorhinal cortex. Afferent cholinergic axons from septal nuclei traverse the fornix to provide the dentate gyrus and hippocampal CA regions.

There exist several clinical conditions where damage unique to the hippocampal formation occurs. CA1 neurons are particularly susceptible to ischemic conditions as seen in cardiorespiratory arrest. Also, patients with temporal lobe epilepsy can experience CA1 neuronal loss. The most common clinical scenario affecting the hippocampal formation is Alzheimer disease (AD). AD is pathologically associated with neuronal cell loss, neurofibrillary tangles, neuritic amyloid plaques, and granule vacuolar degeneration of the hippocampal region. AD is discussed in more detail in Plates 2.24 to 2.26.

Plate 2.10

Cerebral Cortex and Neurocognitive Disorders

HIPPOCAMPUS AND FORNIX

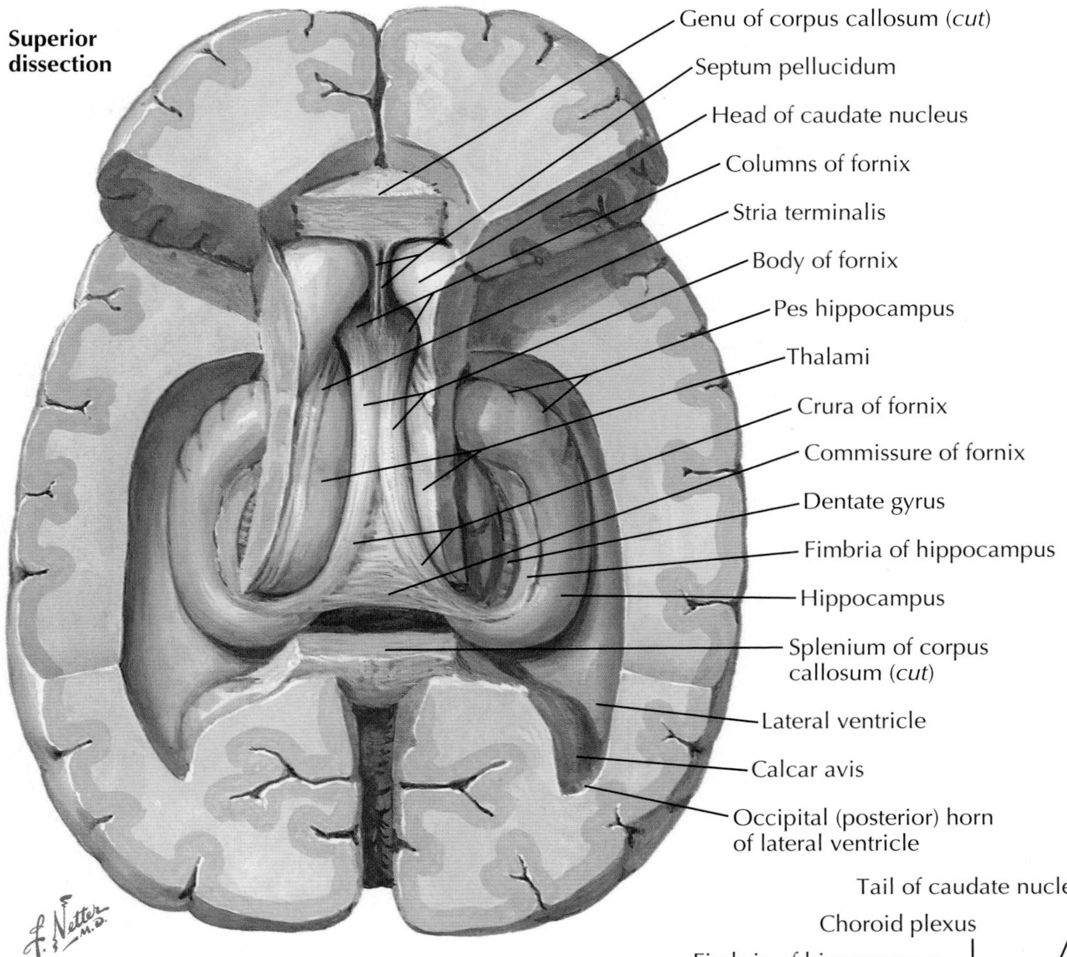

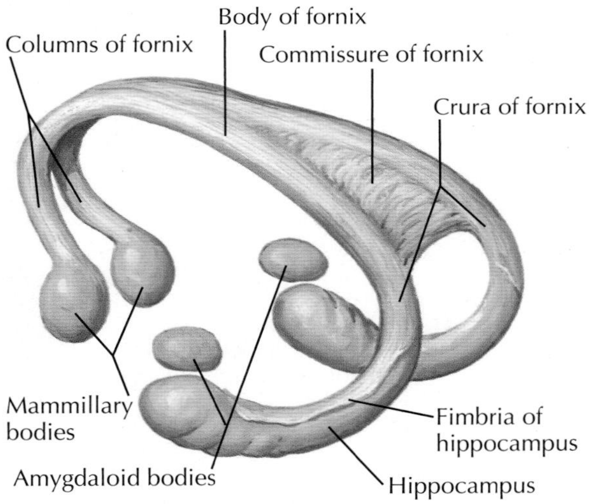

Superior dissection

- Genu of corpus callosum (*cut*)
- Septum pellucidum
- Head of caudate nucleus
- Columns of fornix
- Stria terminalis
- Body of fornix
- Pes hippocampus
- Thalami
- Crura of fornix
- Commissure of fornix
- Dentate gyrus
- Fimbria of hippocampus
- Hippocampus
- Splenium of corpus callosum (*cut*)
- Lateral ventricle
- Calcar avis
- Occipital (posterior) horn of lateral ventricle

FORNIX

The fornix is an almost circular arrangement of white fibers conveying the great majority of the hippocampal efferents to the hypothalamus and carrying commissural fibers to the opposite hippocampus and habenular trigone. The fornix rises out of the fimbria of the hippocampus, which turns upward beneath the splenium of the corpus callosum and above the thalamus to form the *crura* (posterior columns) of the fornix. Anterior to the *commissure* of the fornix, the two crura unite for a variable distance in the midline and create the triangular body of the fornix. The free lateral edges of the fornix help bind the choroid fissure, through which the pia mater of the tela choroidea becomes invaginated into the lateral ventricles.

Above the interventricular foramina, the two halves of the body of the fornix separate to become the (anterior) columns of the fornix. As each column descends, it sinks into the corresponding lateral wall of the third ventricle; the majority of its fibers end in the *mammillary body,* although some also pass to other hypothalamic nuclei.

The fornix is the main efferent pathway from the hippocampus to the hypothalamus. Fibers ending in the mammillary body form synapses around its cells. The axons of these cells pass upward in the mammillothalamic tract to the homolateral anterior thalamic nucleus, from which they are relayed to the cingulate gyrus. The fornix is a key structure in the Papez circuit, which is described later.

OTHER STRUCTURES

The *habenular trigone* is a small area found bilaterally between the posterior end of the thalamus, the superior

- Columns of fornix
- Body of fornix
- Commissure of fornix
- Crura of fornix
- Fimbria of hippocampus
- Hippocampus
- Mammillary bodies
- Amygdaloid bodies

Fornix: schema

- Tail of caudate nucleus
- Choroid plexus
- Fimbria of hippocampus
- Optic tract
- Hippocampal sulcus
- Dentate gyrus
- Hippocampus
- Alveus of hippocampus
- Temporal (inferior) horn of lateral ventricle

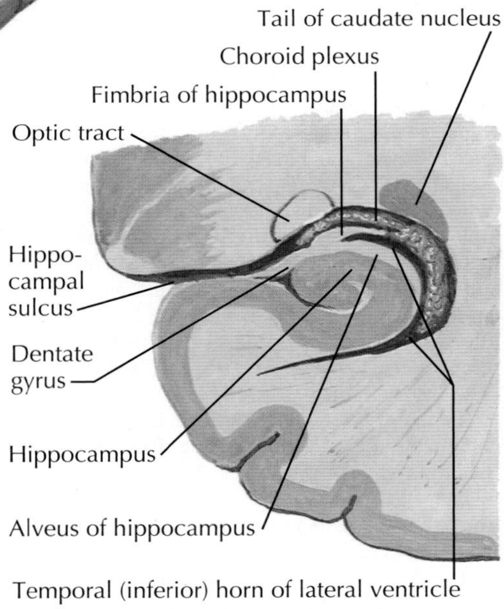

Coronal section: posterior view

(cranial) colliculus, and the stalk of the pineal gland. Each trigone overlies a *habenular nucleus,* which receives afferent fibers via the *stria medullaris* of the thalamus (stria habenularis), a fine strand demarcating the superior and medial surfaces of the thalamus. This stria conveys fibers from the anterior perforated substance, the paraterminal gyrus and subcallosal area, and perhaps other fibers detached from the stria terminalis near the interventricular foramen. Most of these fibers end in the homolateral habenular nucleus, but some

decussate in the small habenular commissure lying above the stalk of the pineal gland. The fresh relay of fibers arising in the habenular nucleus passes by way of the fasciculus retroflexus to the *interpeduncular nucleus* in the posterior (interpeduncular) perforated substance. Efferent fibers from the interpeduncular nucleus then descend in or near the medial longitudinal fasciculus to be distributed to tegmental and reticular nuclei in the brainstem. The *amygdaloid body* is described in Plate 2.11.

Plate 2.11

Brain: PART I

HORIZONTAL BRAIN SECTIONS SHOWING THE BASAL GANGLIA

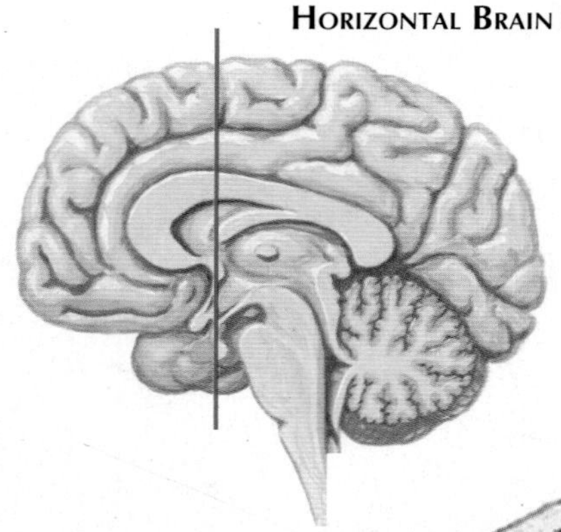

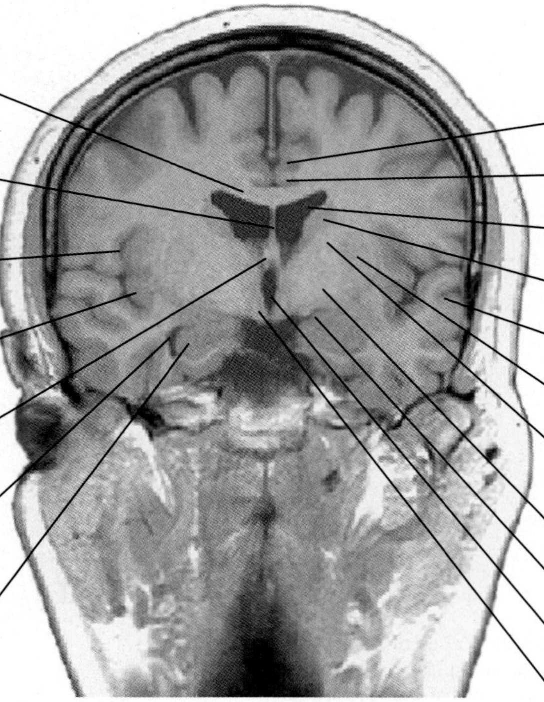

Level of section (amygdala, anterior limb of internal capsule)

Body of corpus callosum

Septum pellucidum

Lateral fissure

Insular cortex

Columns of fornix

Inferior horn of lateral ventricle

Amygdala

Cingulate cortex

Cingulum

Body of lateral ventricle

Body of caudate nucleus

Temporal lobe

Putamen

Genu/anterior limb of internal capsule

Globus pallidus

Optic tract

3rd ventricle

Hypothalamus

From Felten DL, O'Banion MK, Maida MS. Netter's Atlas of Neuroscience, 4th ed. Elsevier; 2022.

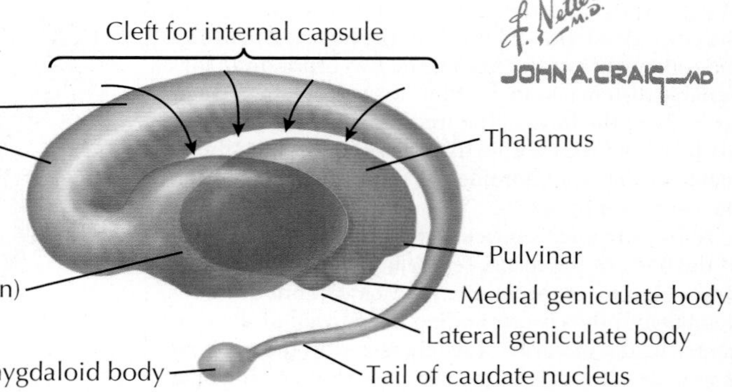

Cleft for internal capsule

Caudate nucleus { Body / Head

Lentiform nucleus (globus pallidus medial to putamen)

Amygdaloid body

Thalamus

Pulvinar

Medial geniculate body

Lateral geniculate body

Tail of caudate nucleus

Schematic illustration showing interrelationship of thalamus, lentiform nucleus, caudate nucleus, and amygdaloid body (viewed from side)

AMYGDALA

The amygdala is an almond-shaped complex located in the medial temporal lobe and contains approximately 13 nuclei. The three main regions are the corticomedial nuclei, basolateral nuclei (both receive afferents and project axons to target structures), and central nucleus (which provides mainly efferent projections to the brainstem). Afferent connections to the amygdala originate from cortical and thalamic areas and hypothalamic and brainstem areas. Its function is to provide emotional relevance to external and internal sensory information and to provide a behavioral and emotional response, particularly a fearful and aversive response, to a sensory input.

The majority of afferent information arises from the glutamatergic projections arising from pyramidal neurons in layer V of the cortex. These projections largely travel ipsilaterally via the extreme capsule. Information from sensory association areas and memory-related structures, such as the hippocampus, is relayed via cortical and thalamic inputs. Autonomic and behavioral inputs arise from the hypothalamus and brainstem.

Afferents to the corticomedial nuclei arrive primarily from subcortical limbic sources, including the olfactory bulb, septal nuclei, and hypothalamic nuclei (ventromedial, lateral hypothalamic area); the thalamus (intralaminar nuclei); the stria terminalis; and excessive numbers of autonomic nuclei and monoamine nuclei of the brainstem. Afferents to the basolateral nuclei arrive mainly from the cortical areas, including extensive sensory association cortices, the prefrontal cortex, the cingulate cortex, and the subiculum.

In the late 1930s, Klüver and Bucy described a behavioral syndrome characterized by hypersexuality, hyperorality, excessive exploration of visual stimuli (hypermetamorphosis), visual agnosia, apathy, and withdrawal. They linked this behavior to bilateral amygdaloid complex lesions. This syndrome has been described in patients with neurodegenerative diseases, such as Alzheimer disease and frontotemporal dementia. Because the amygdala processes sensory information for emotional relevance, it is not surprising that atypical emotional responses, such as anger, aggressive behavior, and even apathy, can evolve in these patients. Damage to the hypothalamic connectivity of the amygdala is responsible for hyperphagia, hypersexuality, and overeating/obesity. Likewise, alterations of the visual association cortical afferent projections to the amygdala result in hypermetamorphosis and visual agnosia (patients cannot recognize facial expressions that indicate fear).

Plate 2.12   Cerebral Cortex and Neurocognitive Disorders

Cerebral regions associated with hypothalamus

Premotor area — Motor area (4)
Cingulate gyrus — Somatosensory area
Fornix — Corpus callosum
Thalamus — Hippocampus
Mammillary body — Hippocampal gyrus
Prefrontal area — Visual area
Olfactory bulb
Orbital cortex
Rhinal system 1
Rhinal system 2
Amygdaloid complex
Rhinal system 3

Rhinencephalic and isocortical regions presumably concerned in emotional and visceroautonomic functions

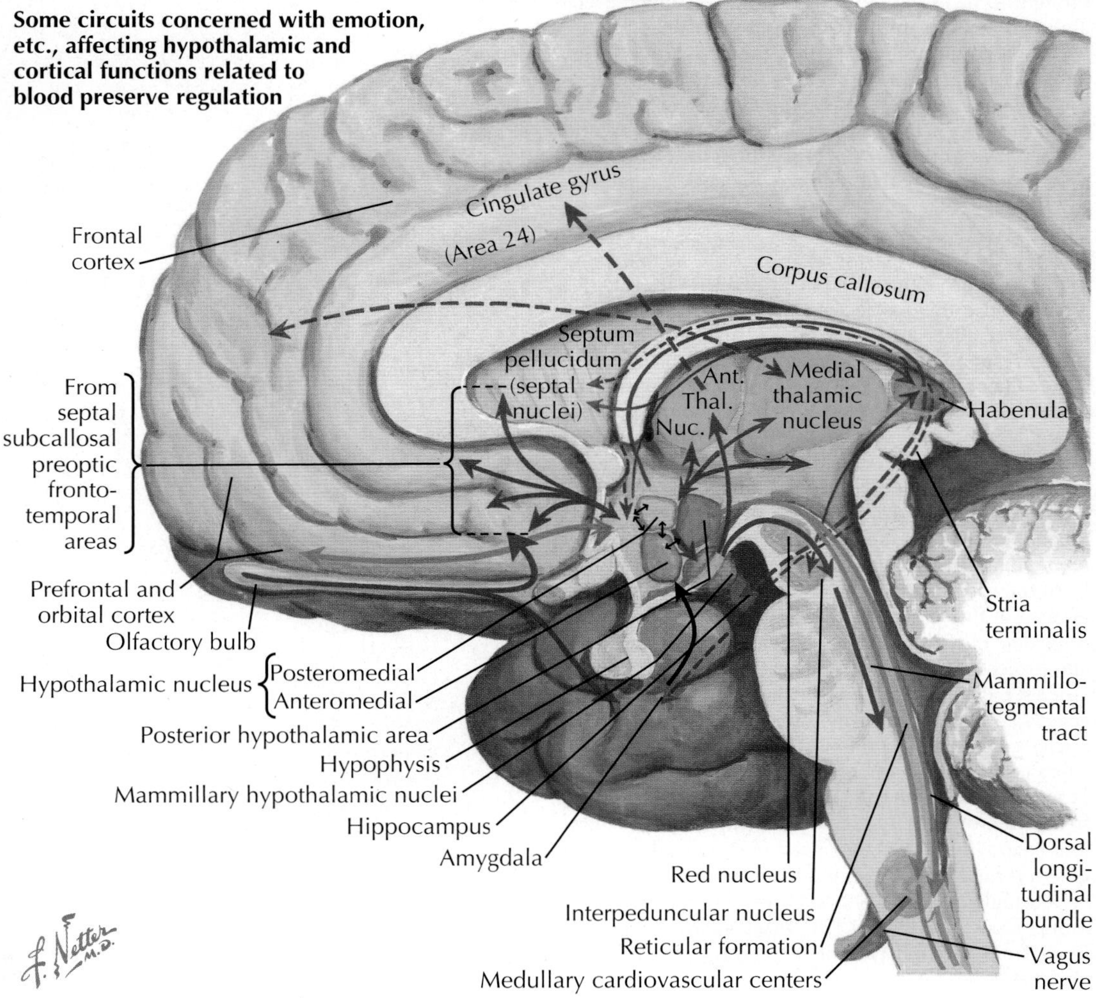

FOREBRAIN REGIONS ASSOCIATED WITH HYPOTHALAMUS

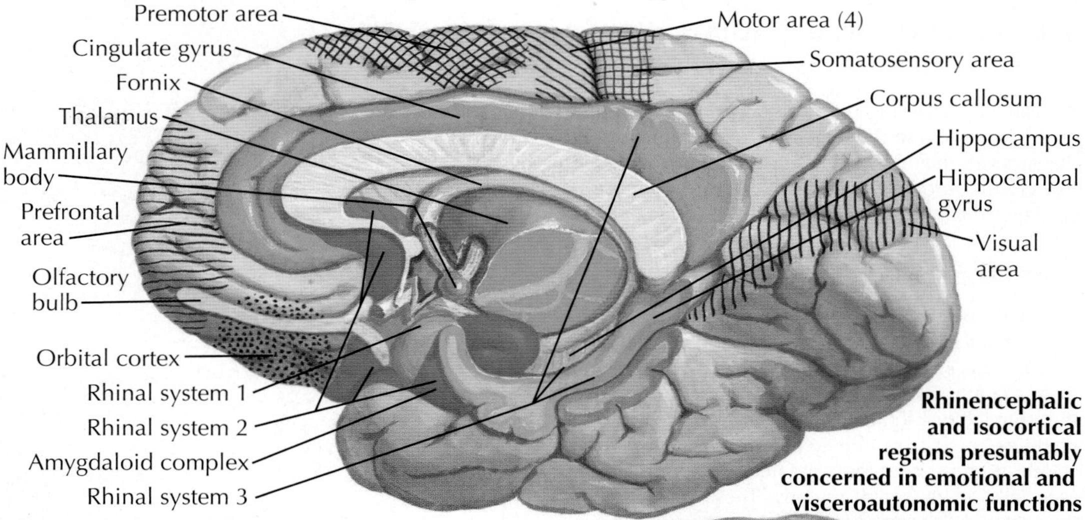

The cerebral cortex influences the "autonomic" neurovisceral outflow and the neurohumoral output of the endocrine glands, as can be demonstrated experimentally by stimulating the orbitofrontal cortex of the cingulate gyrus to produce respiratory, cardiovascular, and digestive responses, as well as certain emotional reactions. The responses are less marked than those produced by stimulating the hypothalamus but are still striking; some of them, moreover, do not depend on the integrity of the hypothalamus, a fact that suggests mediation by corticoreticular fibers to lower "centers." In humans, subjective emotional experiences are associated with autonomic discharges (e.g., tachycardia, increased blood pressure, blushing) and changes in endocrine activity (e.g., stress-induced amenorrhea or anorexia nervosa).

Behavioral changes produced by cortical ablations, such as prefrontal lobotomy, are well known. Other such changes, varying from mania and hyperphagia to apathy, aphagia, and somnolence, result from lesions to certain parts of the hypothalamus.

Thus hypothalamic circuitry is tied into countless other circuits in the cerebral cortex, limbic system, brainstem reticular formation, and other parts of the diencephalon. These circuits are poorly understood, but rich connections with the frontotemporal and cingulate cortex, septal/preoptic areas, amygdala, anterior mesencephalic tegmentum, and numerous thalamic nuclei (midline, intralaminar, medial posterior, anterior, etc.) have been demonstrated.

Some of these connections are indicated schematically in the illustration. Connections between the orbital cortex of the frontal lobe and the hypothalamus have been demonstrated in certain mammals. Indirect connections with the prefrontal areas through the medial posterior thalamic nucleus are well established. The hypothalamus is linked with the cingulate gyrus by way of the anterior thalamic nuclei and with the hippocampal formation via the fornix. The amygdala has reciprocal connections with the hypothalamus through the anterior amygdalofugal pathway. Additional amygdalo-hypothalamic connections run through the stria terminalis.

The hypothalamus also receives input, through reticulo-hypothalamic fiber systems departing from the main reticulo-thalamic stream, from the great sensory systems. Through this offshoot, the responses evolved through thalamocortical feature analysis are paralleled by responses in the visceral realm. The limbic (border) structures of the cerebral hemisphere also participate in these responses: the olfactory bulb, amygdala, frontotemporal cortex, septal nuclei, hippocampal formation, and limbic lobe. Stimulation of limbic structures can

Some circuits concerned with emotion, etc., affecting hypothalamic and cortical functions related to blood preserve regulation

Frontal cortex
Cingulate gyrus (Area 24)
Corpus callosum
Septum pellucidum (septal nuclei)
Ant. Thal. Nuc.
Medial thalamic nucleus
Habenula
From septal subcallosal preoptic frontotemporal areas
Prefrontal and orbital cortex
Olfactory bulb
Hypothalamic nucleus { Posteromedial / Anteromedial }
Posterior hypothalamic area
Hypophysis
Mammillary hypothalamic nuclei
Hippocampus
Amygdala
Red nucleus
Interpeduncular nucleus
Reticular formation
Medullary cardiovascular centers
Stria terminalis
Mammillo-tegmental tract
Dorsal longitudinal bundle
Vagus nerve

produce respiratory and vascular changes, and psychotropic drugs, such as mescaline, apparently exert some of their effects on the limbic system.

The stria medullaris thalami and medial forebrain bundle deserve mention: the former bypasses the hypothalamus, and the latter runs right through it. The *stria medullaris thalami* connect the medial olfactory area, amygdala, and preoptic area with the habenular nucleus, from which fibers pass to the interpeduncular

region. The *medial forebrain bundle* links the anteromedial olfactory areas with the preoptic areas, hypothalamus, and mesencephalic tegmentum. A diffuse system of fine fibers, it pervades the lateral hypothalamic area and is the key fiber tract of the hypothalamus. Lastly, fibers of the fornix end in both medial and lateral mammillary nuclei, as well as in the hypothalamus anterior to the mammillary region. A few fibers pass caudally into the mesencephalon.

Plate 2.13

Brain: PART I

THALAMOCORTICAL RADIATIONS

All pathways carrying information from the periphery or the brainstem to the neocortex relay in the nuclei of the *posterior thalamus*. These nuclei can be divided into two groups on the basis of their structure, connections, and function.

NONSPECIFIC NUCLEI

The first group includes the *midline (median)* and *intralaminar nuclei* and the medial portion of the *ventral anterior nucleus*. These nuclei receive ascending input from the mesencephalic reticular formation and from the spinal cord (paleospinothalamic tract) and descending input from the cerebral cortex. They project widely, both to other thalamic nuclei and to the cortex, especially to its frontal regions. These projections are thought to be essential in regulating the general excitability of neurons in the thalamus and cortex.

Another nucleus included in the first group is the *reticular nucleus,* which overlies the lateral surface of the thalamus. Neurons of this nucleus, which receive input from collaterals of thalamocortical fibers and project back to the thalamus, are thought to constitute a feedback pathway that regulates thalamic excitability.

SPECIFIC NUCLEI

The second group of nuclei is termed the "specific nuclei" because they project to restricted regions of the cortex (see Plate 2.13). The major specific nuclei and the corresponding cortical regions to which they project are illustrated in matching colors. One set of specific nuclei are the sensory relay nuclei. The *ventral posterolateral* and *ventral posteromedial nuclei* receive their input from somatosensory relay neurons via the medial lemniscus, trigeminal lemnisci, and the neospinothalamic tract. They project to the primary (Sm I) and secondary (Sm II) somatosensory cortex. The *ventral posterointermediate nucleus* (not shown) receives input from the vestibular system and projects to the vestibular area in the parietal lobe (see Plate 2.13). The *lateral geniculate nucleus* receives its input from the optic tract and projects to the primary visual area in the occipital lobe (see Plate 2.13). The principal part of the *medial geniculate nucleus* receives input from auditory relay nuclei and projects to the primary auditory area in the supratemporal transverse gyrus (see Plate 2.13).

A second set of specific nuclei is involved in the control of motor activity. The *ventral lateral* and *ventral intermedial nuclei* and the lateral portion of the *ventral anterior nucleus* receive input from the cerebellum and basal ganglia, respectively, and project to the precentral motor areas (see Plate 2.13). These areas also receive input from the oral part of the ventral posterolateral nucleus.

The *anterior dorsal* (the least prominent of the anterior group of nuclei) and the *medial dorsal nuclei* are specifically related to the limbic system, which regulates emotional and autonomic activity (see Plates 2.8 and 2.13). The anterior dorsal nucleus receives input from the hippocampus relayed via the mammillothalamic tract and projects to the cingulate gyrus. The medial dorsal nucleus receives input from the hypothalamus and amygdala and projects to the frontal lobe.

The remaining specific nuclei are related to association areas of the cortex involved in higher integrative mechanisms. They include the *lateral dorsal* and *lateral*

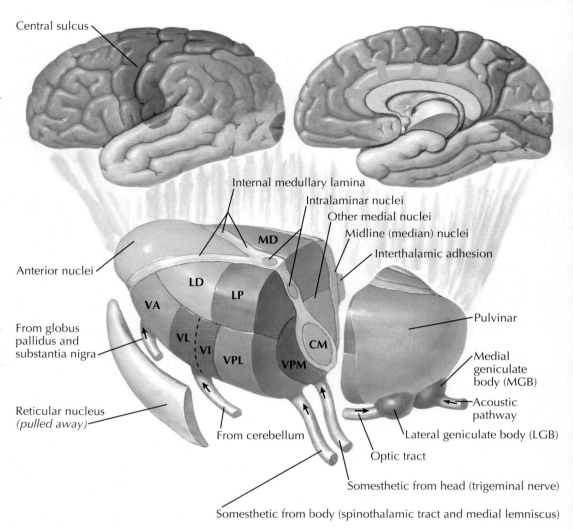

Central sulcus

Internal medullary lamina

Intralaminar nuclei

Other medial nuclei

Midline (median) nuclei

Interthalamic adhesion

MD

Anterior nuclei

LD

LP

VA

Pulvinar

From globus pallidus and substantia nigra

VL

VI

CM

VPL

VPM

Medial geniculate body (MGB)

Reticular nucleus *(pulled away)*

Acoustic pathway

From cerebellum

Lateral geniculate body (LGB)

Optic tract

Somesthetic from head (trigeminal nerve)

Somesthetic from body (spinothalamic tract and medial lemniscus)

Thalamic nuclei

CM	Centromedian
LD	Lateral dorsal
LP	Lateral posterior
MD	Medial dorsal
VA	Ventral anterior
VI	Ventral intermedial
VL	Ventral lateral
VPL	Ventral posterolateral
VPM	Ventral posteromedial

posterior nuclei and the *pulvinar complex*. The medial, magnocellular part of the *medial geniculate nucleus,* which receives widespread convergent input from many afferent systems, should probably also be included in this category.

CORTICAL CONNECTIONS

In addition to receiving the ascending input described above, all of the thalamic nuclei receive descending input from the cerebral cortex, principally from the cortical regions to which they project (see Plate 2.13). These descending projections serve as a two-way feedback system between each cortical area and its thalamic relay nucleus.

Not all of the nuclei of the posterior thalamus project to the cerebral cortex. One important nucleus without a cortical projection is the *centromedian nucleus,* which communicates only with the basal ganglia.

Plate 2.14

Cerebral Cortex and Neurocognitive Disorders

NEURONAL STRUCTURE AND SYNAPSES

NEURONAL STRUCTURE

A typical neuron of the central nervous system (CNS) consists of three parts: dendritic tree, cell body (soma), and axon.

The highly branched *dendritic tree* has a much greater surface area than the remainder of the neuron and is the receptive part of the cell. Incoming synaptic terminals make contact directly with the dendritic surface or with the small spines (gemmules) that protrude from it. The membrane potential induced in the dendrites spreads passively onto the cell soma, which allows all inputs acting on the neuron to summate in controlling the rate of neuronal discharge through the axon.

The *soma* contains the various organelles that control and maintain neuronal structure: nucleus, Golgi apparatus, lysosomes, ribosomes, mitochondria, and smooth and rough endoplasmic reticula. The rough endoplasmic reticulum, studded with ribosomes, is called the *Nissl substance* because of its characteristic blue staining with Nissl stain. The *ribosomes* are the site of synthesis of neuronal proteins; as in other cells, the ribonucleic acid templates that control protein structure are transcribed from patterns in the nuclear deoxyribonucleic acid. The soma membrane is also covered with synaptic endings separated by glial processes. Because of their proximity to the origin of the axon, these synaptic endings have an especially potent effect on the rate of discharge of the neuron.

In humans, the *axon* can extend for several feet. Such lengths pose supply problems because the neuron must transport proteins and other synthesized substances as far as the axon terminals. Certain key substances are transported, at a rate as high as 400 mm/day, by rapid axonal transport, a process probably associated with the microtubules that originate in the soma and run the length of the axon. Other soluble and particulate substances move by *slow axonal transport* at a rate of 1 to 4 mm/day, aided partly by the peristalsis-like motion of the axon.

The axon originates from a conical projection (axon hillock) on the soma (as shown in Plate 2.14) or on one of the proximal dendrites. The axon membrane is specialized for the transmission of action potential. Because of its shape and high excitability, the initial segment of the axon is usually the site of action potential generation. The action potential then spreads down the axon and back to the soma and proximal dendrites. Because of the low excitability of the dendrites, the impulse usually does not spread very far into the dendritic tree. At its distal end, the axon divides into numerous branches, which end in synapses.

TYPES OF NEURONAL SYNAPSES

The most common CNS synapses are those between axon terminals and dendrites (axodendritic) or between axon terminals and somata (axosomatic). *Axodendritic synapses* take several forms. Spine synapses are of particular interest, because they may be the site of morphologic changes accompanying learning. *Axosomatic synapses* are of the simple type shown in example A. Synaptic interconnections between a number of neurons

occur within structures of a complex organization, such as the cerebellar glomerulus, although all synapses within the glomerulus are axodendritic.

Axons also form *axoaxonic synapses* with other axon terminals, and these are responsible for the phenomenon of presynaptic inhibition. Axoaxonic synapses are also seen in the efferent vestibular system and in connection with motor neuron dendrites and other terminals ending on those dendrites.

The CNS also contains several, less common types of synapses. *Dendrodendritic synapses* are found in the

olfactory bulb. In the internal plexiform layer of the retina, synaptic interactions involve *synaptic triads* of bipolar, amacrine, and ganglion cell processes.

Other synapses are those formed between the peripheral axonal processes of sensory neurons and *sensory receptor cells*, as in the inner ear. Here, the axon terminal forms the postsynaptic element that is depolarized by the presynaptic sensory cell.

There are also specialized axosomatic synapses formed by efferent motor axons on muscle (motor end plates) and by autonomic axons on secretory cells.

Structure of a neuron (pyramidal cell of cerebral motor cortex)

Labels: Dendrites; Dendritic spines (gemmules); Rough endoplasmic reticulum (Nissl substance); Ribosomes; Mitochondrion; Nucleus; Nucleolus; Axon hillock; Axon; Neurotubules; Golgi body; Lysosome; Cell body (soma); Axosomatic synapse; Glial (astrocyte) process; Axodendritic synapse

F. Netter M.D. with J. Perkins MS, MFA

Types of synapses

A. Simple axodendritic or axosomatic synapse — Axon; Glial process; Dendrite or cell body

B. Dendritic spine synapse — Axon; Dendrite; Dendritic spine (gemmule)

C. Dendritic crest synapse — Axon

D. Simple synapse plus axoaxonic synapse

E. Combined axoaxonic and axodendritic synapse

F. Varicosities ("boutons en passant")

G. Dendrodendritic synapse — Dendrite; Dendrodendritic synapse

H. Reciprocal synapse

I. Serial synapse

J. Cerebellar glomerulus — Granule cell dendrites; Glial capsule; Golgi cell axon; Golgi cell dendrite; Mossy cell axon

K. Inner plexiform layer of retina — Ganglion cell; Bipolar cell axon; Müller cell (supporting); Amacrine cell processes

Plate 2.15

Brain: PART I

CHEMICAL SYNAPTIC TRANSMISSION

Chemical synaptic transmission proceeds in three steps: (1) the release of the transmitter substance from the bouton in response to the arrival of an action potential, (2) the change in the ionic permeabilities of the postsynaptic membrane caused by the transmitter, and (3) the removal of the transmitter from the synaptic cleft. Depending on the type of permeability changes produced in the second step, synaptic activation may have either an excitatory or an inhibitory effect on the postsynaptic cell.

Synaptic transmitter substances are concentrated in *synaptic vesicles* within the bouton. Although the exact mechanism of its release is unknown, it appears that the transmitter substance is released in packets, or quanta, of 1000 to 10,000 molecules at a time and that the probability of release of these quanta increases with the degree of depolarization of the terminal membrane. Thus the intense depolarization caused by an action potential actuates the nearly simultaneous release of a large number of quanta. A reasonable hypothesis to account for the quantal nature of transmitter release is that the contents of an entire vesicle are discharged at once into the synaptic cleft, perhaps by the process of *exocytosis*.

After their release, transmitter molecules diffuse across the synaptic cleft and combine with specific receptor molecules in the postsynaptic membrane. This combination gives rise to a change in the ionic permeability of the postsynaptic membrane and results in a flow of ions down their electrochemical potential gradients. This ionic flow is not synchronous with the arrival of the action potential in the terminal but begins after a *synaptic delay* of 0.3 to 0.5 msec, which is the time required for transmitter release and diffusion and for the completion of reactions within the postsynaptic membrane, which alter membrane permeability.

The direction of current flow produced by transmitter action depends on which ionic permeabilities are altered. In an *excitatory synapse*, the transmitter causes an increase in the permeability of the postsynaptic membrane to sodium ions (Na^+) and potassium ions (K^+). Because of their respective concentration gradients across the neuronal membrane (see Plate 2.15), Na^+ tends to move into the postsynaptic cell, and K^+ moves out of it. The negative potential of the neuronal cytoplasm, however, assists the inward flow of positive ions and slows their outward flow so that the combined electrochemical force for Na^+ influx greatly exceeds that for K^+ efflux. Thus the predominant ionic movement across the postsynaptic membrane is an inward flow of Na^+. As shown, the resulting current flow causes a shift of the postsynaptic cell membrane potential in the depolarizing direction. This depolarizing potential change, which is called an *excitatory postsynaptic potential* (EPSP), brings the postsynaptic cell closer to its threshold for action potential initiation.

In an *inhibitory synapse*, transmitter action causes an increase of the postsynaptic membrane's permeability to K^+ and chloride ions (Cl^-) but not to Na^+. Because Cl^- is approximately at electrochemical equilibrium across the neuronal membrane, the major ionic movement is an outward flow of K^+. The resulting current flow is in the opposite direction to that of the current flow in an excitatory synapse and gives rise to a shift of the postsynaptic cell membrane potential in the hyperpolarizing direction. This hyperpolarizing potential

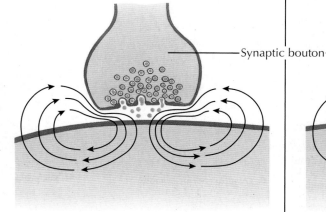

When impulse reaches excitatory synaptic bouton, it causes release of a transmitter substance into synaptic cleft. This increases permeability of postsynaptic membrane to Na^+ and K^+. More Na^+ moves into postsynaptic cell than K^+ moves out, due to greater electrochemical gradient.

At inhibitory synapse, transmitter substance released by an impulse increases permeability of the postsynaptic membrane to Cl^-. K^+ moves out of postsynaptic cell, but no net flow of Cl^- occurs at resting membrane potential.

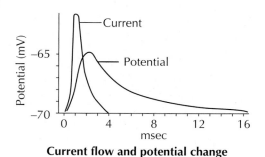

Resultant net ionic current flow is in a direction that tends to depolarize postsynaptic cell. If depolarization reaches firing threshold, an impulse is generated in postsynaptic cell.

Resultant ionic current flow is in direction that tends to hyperpolarize postsynaptic cell. This makes depolarization by excitatory synapses more difficult—more depolarization is required to reach threshold.

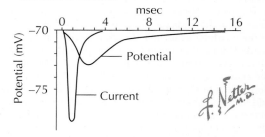

Current flow and potential change

Current flow and potential change

change, which is called an *inhibitory postsynaptic potential*, moves the membrane potential away from the threshold for action potential initiation. The increased ionic permeability of the postsynaptic membrane also contributes to the inhibitory effect by tending to "short out" any membrane depolarization occurring simultaneously.

The ionic current and the resulting membrane potential change have different time courses because

the synaptic current charges the membrane capacitance, which then discharges passively over a period of 10 to 15 msec. The short duration of the synaptic current is the consequence of the removal of transmitter from the synaptic cleft. This removal is accomplished in part by passive diffusion and in part by specific mechanisms that lead to transmitter uptake by surrounding cells or transmitter breakdown by enzymatic degradation.

Plate 2.16

Cerebral Cortex and Neurocognitive Disorders

SUMMATION OF EXCITATION AND INHIBITION

Summation of excitation and inhibition is the vital principle on which the functioning of the CNS is based. The illustration shows the various intracellular potential changes observed during temporal and spatial summation of excitation and inhibition as voltage-versus-time tracings similar to those produced by an oscilloscope.

The principle of summation relates to the fact that a neuron typically has a large number of synaptic terminals (boutons) ending upon it; alone, each bouton is capable of producing only a small synaptic potential. The small EPSP produced by a single excitatory terminal is not sufficient to depolarize the motor neuron to its threshold point. For suprathreshold depolarization to be produced, either temporal or spatial summation of excitation must take place.

Temporal summation occurs when a burst of action potentials reaches a nerve fiber terminal. If the terminal is excitatory, the first action potential in the burst produces a depolarizing EPSP in the motor neuron that begins to decay toward the resting potential. Before the decay is complete, another action potential arrives in the terminal and evokes a second EPSP. The depolarization caused by this EPSP adds to the residual depolarization remaining from the first EPSP and moves the membrane potential closer to the threshold level. Finally, the EPSP evoked by a third action potential adds its depolarization to that produced by the first two to drive the membrane potential past the threshold level and to trigger an action potential in the motor neuron. Thus because of temporal summation, a burst of action potentials in an excitatory fiber is able to evoke the firing of a target neuron, even though the individual EPSPs evoked by single action potentials are too small to produce a suprathreshold depolarization. In a similar manner, the inhibitory postsynaptic potentials produced by a burst of action potentials in an inhibitory fiber can summate to produce a large hyperpolarizing potential.

Spatial summation involves the activation of two or more terminals at approximately the same time. When such synchronous activation occurs, the inward and outward currents evoked by excitatory and inhibitory terminals summate to produce a net shift in the membrane potential of the target cell. If two excitatory terminals are activated, the net membrane potential shift will be a depolarization approximately equal to the sum of the EPSPs that would be evoked by each terminal acting alone; this combined depolarization exceeds the threshold level and triggers an action potential. If, in addition to the two excitatory terminals, an inhibitory terminal is also activated, the net depolarization will be reduced by an outward flow of current at the inhibitory synapse. Under these conditions, additional excitation is required to produce a suprathreshold depolarization.

Spatial summation plays a vital role in the interaction of patterns of activity originating in various neuronal pathways. For example, in the case of the effect of central motor tone on the reflex evoked by muscle stretch, the stretch produces a volley of action potentials in the group Ia fibers from the stretched muscle. The synaptic action of the Ia fiber terminals evokes medium-to-large EPSPs in motor neurons supplying the stretched muscle and small EPSPs in motor neurons supplying synergistic muscles. If the body is in a relaxed state, only the motor neurons receiving large EPSPs will discharge

action potentials, causing a small twitch of the stretched muscle; the remaining motor neurons, which receive EPSPs too small to evoke firing, constitute the *subliminal fringe* of the stretch reflex. If the body is in an active state, central nervous pathways will produce a steady excitatory input to the motor neurons involved in the stretch reflex. Thus many of the neurons in the subliminal fringe will receive sufficient additional

excitation to cause them to fire, and muscle stretch may result in a vigorous contraction of that muscle and its synergists. In a similar way, motor neurons that fall within the subliminal fringe of two different reflexes may be fired when both reflexes occur together. This kind of reflex interaction by spatial summation helps to adapt reflex patterns to meet the demands of different external conditions.

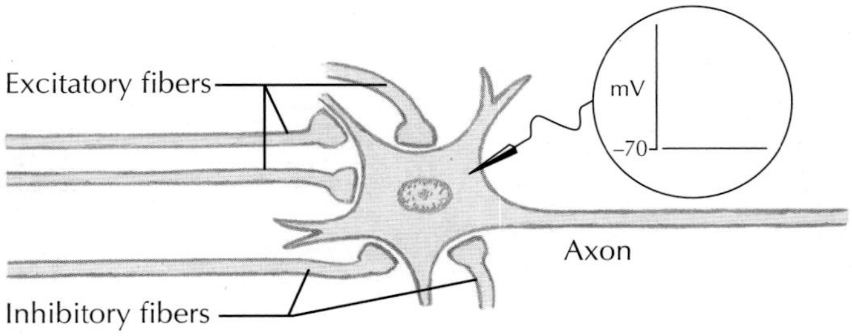

A. Resting state: motor nerve cell shown with synaptic boutons of excitatory and inhibitory nerve fibers ending close to it

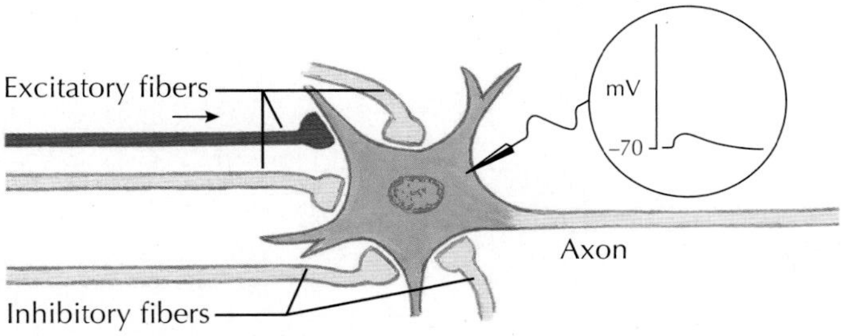

B. Partial depolarization: impulse from one excitatory fiber has caused partial (below firing threshold) depolarization of motor neuron

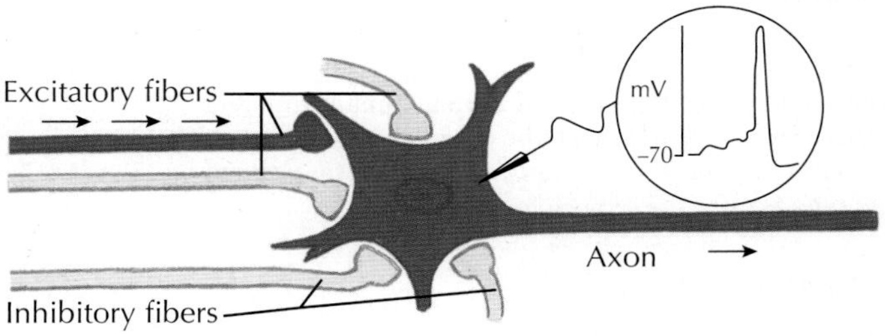

C. Temporal excitatory summation: a series of impulses in one excitatory fiber together produce a suprathreshold depolarization that triggers an action potential

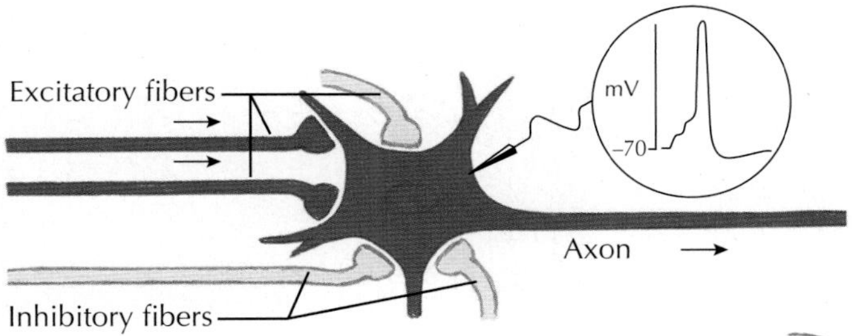

D. Spatial excitatory summation: impulses in two excitatory fibers cause two synaptic depolarizations that together reach firing threshold triggering an action potential

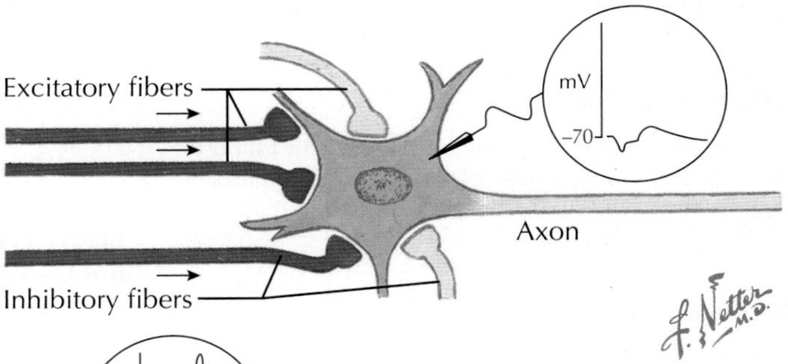

E. Spatial excitatory summation with inhibition: impulses from two excitatory fibers reach motor neuron but impulses from inhibitory fiber prevent depolarization from reaching threshold

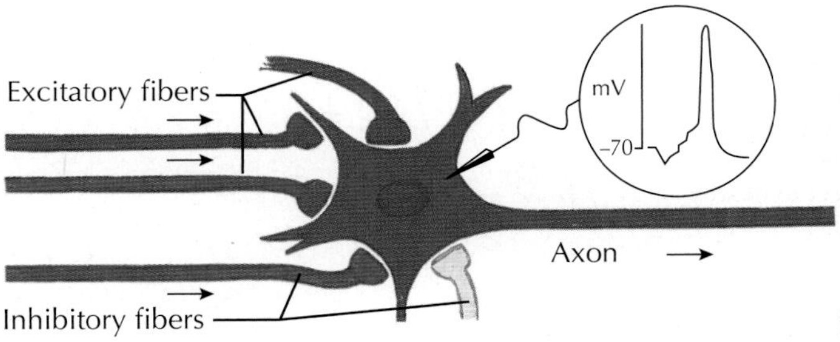

E. (continued): motor neuron now receives additional excitatory impulses and reaches firing threshold despite a simultaneous inhibitory impulse; additional inhibitory impulses might still prevent firing

■ Axon(s) activated in each scenario

Plate 2.17

Brain: PART I

Types of Neurons in Cerebral Cortex

The six layers of the cerebral cortex contain different types of neurons, which can be broadly classified as *interneurons, association neurons,* and *efferent (projection) neurons.*

INTERNEURONS

Interneurons have axons that do not leave the cortex and may be of several kinds. The most common are *stellate* (star-shaped), or *granule, cells,* which have symmetrically branching dendritic trees and short axons that end upon nearby neurons. These cells are especially prevalent in layer IV, which is accordingly named the "granule cell layer." Other interneurons are *horizontal cells,* which are found in layer I; *Martinotti cells,* which are located in deeper layers and send axons toward the cortical surface; and the small *pyramidal cells* of layers II and III, which send axons to deeper layers.

ASSOCIATION NEURONS

Association neurons are small pyramidal cells found in the deep parts of layer III or in the superficial parts of layer V; they send axons through the white matter to other regions of the cortex.

EFFERENT NEURONS

Efferent neurons leave the cortex to innervate structures in the brainstem or spinal cord and originate from the *giant pyramidal (Betz) cells* in layer V or from spindle-shaped cells in layer VI. In addition to their main axons, which leave the cortex, efferent neurons may also have collateral axons, which project to nearby cortical neurons for association.

AFFERENT FIBERS

Two major classes of nerve fibers bring information to the cortex. *Specific cortical afferent fibers,* which originate in corresponding thalamic relay nuclei, project to layer IV to end in a highly branched terminal arborization. *Nonspecific cortical afferent fibers,* which originate in the thalamus or in other areas of the cortex and ascend through the entire depth of the cortical gray matter, give off terminal branches in all layers. Specific afferent fibers may thus activate granule cells and efferent neurons of layers III, V, and VI (via their dendrites in layer IV), whereas nonspecific afferents may influence all classes of cortical neurons. Neurons activated by incoming fibers relay information to other cortical neurons via intrinsic connections within the cortex.

CORTICAL ORGANIZATION

An important aspect of the flow of information mediated by cortical neurons is that it occurs predominantly in a vertical direction across the six cortical layers. With the exception of the horizontal cells of layer I, there are very few cortical neurons that relay activity laterally over any significant distance. The vertical cell axons and dendrites are arranged within the cortex in columns of neurons that have similar properties. These columns are approximately 0.5 to 1.0 mm wide and extend across all six cortical layers. In the sensory cortex, neurons within an individual column all respond to the same stimulus; within the motor cortex, the activity of all neurons in one column is related to the activity of a single muscle or muscle group. These columns, as well as the underlying vertical neural organization, appear to represent one of the central features of information processing by the cerebral cortex.

Black—cell bodies and dendrites
Brown—axons of interneurons and association neurons
Red—axon of efferent neurons

Cortical interneurons

Cortical association neurons

Efferent neurons

Key for Abbreviations
a Horizontal cell
b Martinotti cell
c Chandelier cell
d Aspiny granule cell
e Spiny granule cell
f Stellate (granule) cell
g Small pyramidal cell of layers II, III
h Small pyramidal association cell
i Small pyramidal association and projection cells of layer V
j Large pyramidal projection cell (Betz cell)

Plate 2.18

Cerebral Cortex and Neurocognitive Disorders

NEURONS AND GLIAL CELLS

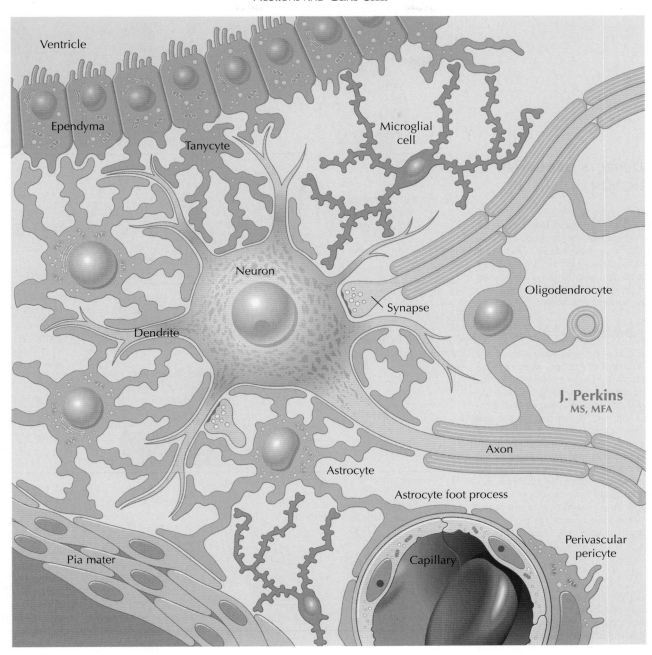

Ventricle

Ependyma

Tanycyte

Microglial
cell

Neuron

Dendrite

Synapse

Oligodendrocyte

J. Perkins
MS, MFA

Axon

Astrocyte

Astrocyte foot process

Pia mater

Perivascular
pericyte

Capillary

ASTROCYTES

Astrocytes provide structural isolation of neurons and their synapses and provide ionic (K^+) sequestration, trophic support, and support for growth and signaling functions to neurons. Oligodendroglia provide myelination of axons in the CNS. Microglia are scavenger cells that participate in phagocytosis, inflammatory responses, cytokine and growth factor secretion, and some immune reactivity in the CNS. Perivascular cells participate in similar activities at sites near the blood vessels. Schwann cells provide myelination, ensheathment, trophic support, and actions that contribute to the growth and repair of peripheral neurons. Activated T lymphocytes normally can enter and traverse the

CNS for immune surveillance for a period of approximately 24 hours.

Recent years have witnessed a growing appreciation for functional roles astrocytes play within the CNS. It increasingly appears to be the case that astrocytes are integral to brain energy utilization. For example, at glutamate synapses astrocytes take up the glutamate that is released into the synaptic space by the presynaptic neuron. The glutamate is imported into the astrocyte along with a sodium cation. The sodium cation, in turn, is removed from the astrocyte by the action of the plasma membrane adenosine triphosphate (ATP)-dependent Na^+-K^+ pump. This consumes ATP, which activates astrocyte glycolysis, and, in turn, this stimulates glucose uptake from neighboring capillaries. By consuming more glucose through glycolysis, the astrocyte restores

its energy supply but, in the process, also generates lactate. Astrocyte-generated lactate is then exported to the recently activated synapse neurons to help meet its increased energy needs. This relationship defines what is called the "astrocyte-neuron lactate shuttle hypothesis" and suggests that the classic bipartite synapse of a presynaptic and postsynaptic neuron might more accurately be thought of as a tripartite synapse consisting of a presynaptic neuron, postsynaptic neuron, and associated astrocyte. It is also important to note that glutamate absorbed by the synaptic astrocyte is recycled back to the presynaptic neuron. This is accomplished by converting it to glutamine before releasing it into the extracellular space. The presynaptic neuron is able to take up the glutamine, and once it is back inside the neuron, the glutamine is converted back to glutamate.

Plate 2.19

Brain: PART I

A. *Appearance and interpersonal behavior*
Pleasant, neatly dressed, good spirits

Depressed, sloppily dressed, careless

Belligerent

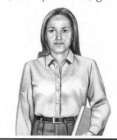
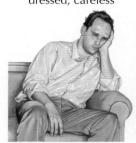
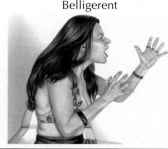

TESTING FOR DEFECTS OF HIGHER CORTICAL FUNCTION

It is useful to test functions that can be localized to individual brain regions because abnormalities on these tests can help localize a neuroanatomic defect and thereby suggest a specific etiology. Screening for disorders of higher cortical function can be completed within the context of an office visit, whereas extensive examinations can take up to several hours.

TEST LANGUAGE FUNCTION

Judge the fluency of the patient's language. Note whether language is effortful or not and whether there are mistakenly spoken phonemes or mistakes in grammar. Evaluate comprehension by testing the patient's ability to follow simple or complex commands. Determine whether the patient can repeat, read, write, and name. Some people may express themselves well and understand what is said yet still have a language problem. More sensitive approaches that could prove useful in this setting include counting how many animals the patient can name in 1 minute (a test of semantic fluency). In most people language is a relatively left brain–mediated cognitive domain, so inability to perform any of these tasks indicates dysfunction of the perisylvian region of the dominant, usually left, cerebral hemisphere.

TEST MEMORY

Memory is often thought of as long versus short term, but these are potentially misleading terms. What is referred to as short-term memory is really memory stored in "buffer" storage, particularly the posterolateral prefrontal cortices. Long-term memory is information stored in the brain "hard drive," which requires function of the medial temporal structures such as the hippocampus. These different problems can be distinguished by giving the patient information to encode, ensuring that information has entered the buffer memory, and then distracting the patient. Later on, determine whether the information is still available to the patient. Good preservation and easy accessing of the information suggest intact memory "retention," whereas good preservation that requires cueing implies a deficit of "retrieval."

B. *Language*

Doctor: "Write me a brief paragraph about your work."

Good

Defective

C. *Memory*

Doctor: "Here are three objects: a pipe, a pen, and a picture of Abraham Lincoln. I want you to remember them, and in 5 minutes, I will ask you what they were."

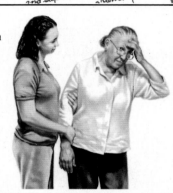

5 minutes later:
Patient: "I'm sorry, I can't remember. Did you show me something?"

D. *Constructional praxis and visual-spatial function*

Doctor: "Draw me a simple picture of a house."

Good   Abnormal

"Draw a clock face for me."

Good   Abnormal

E. *Reverse counting and spelling*

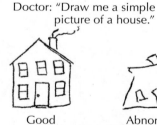

Doctor: "Count backward from 20 by 3s."
Patient: "17...15...16, ...17...18..."

Doctor: "Spell the word 'world' backward for me."
Patient: "W..L..R..D."

TEST VISUAL-SPATIAL FUNCTIONS

Have the patient draw a clock, house, daisy, or bicycle and check for organization, angulation, and asymmetry. Also ask the patient to copy a simple design. If the drawings indicate abnormal visual-spatial orientation, the patient may have parietal lobe dysfunction. Importantly, difficulty with such tasks can reflect frontal, occipital, or temporal lobe dysfunction.

TEST ABILITY TO CONCENTRATE

Ask the patient to recite in reverse a series of numbers or to subtract 7s serially from 100. Also observe the patient's degree of alertness and orientation, manner of dress, and grooming and note whether the patient is happy, sad, or indifferent and how the patient relates to others. Such objective observations are an important part of a complete neurologic examination.

TEST EXECUTIVE FUNCTION

Determine whether the patient can shift from one set to another, perform actions in a sequence, think abstractly, and calculate. For example, asking the patient how much money is "two quarters, two dimes, and two nickels" screens several of these skills. Executive dysfunction suggests a lesion of the posterolateral prefrontal cortex or a disconnection between this area and other brain regions.

Plate 2.20

Cerebral Cortex and Neurocognitive Disorders

Afferent and efferent cortical connections of entorhinal cortex

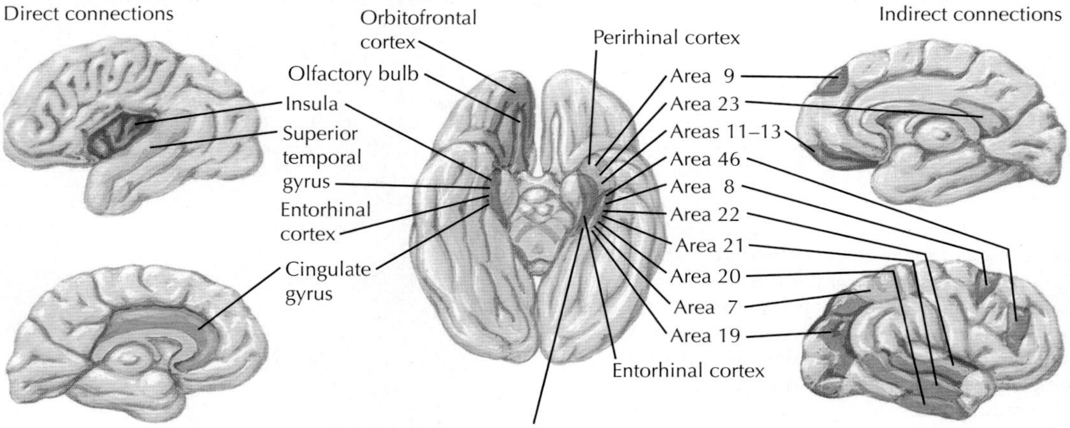

Direct connections

Indirect connections

Orbitofrontal cortex
Olfactory bulb
Insula
Superior temporal gyrus
Entorhinal cortex
Cingulate gyrus

Perirhinal cortex
Area 9
Area 23
Areas 11–13
Area 46
Area 8
Area 22
Area 21
Area 20
Area 7
Area 19
Entorhinal cortex

Entorhinal cortex is a major source of projections to hippocampus (major processing center for recent memory). Polysensory association cortices project directly to entorhinal cortex or indirectly via perirhinal cortex or parahippocampal gyrus. Association cortices receive reciprocal projections from entorhinal cortex. Area numbers refer to Brodmann classifications.

Possible processing circuit for recent memory

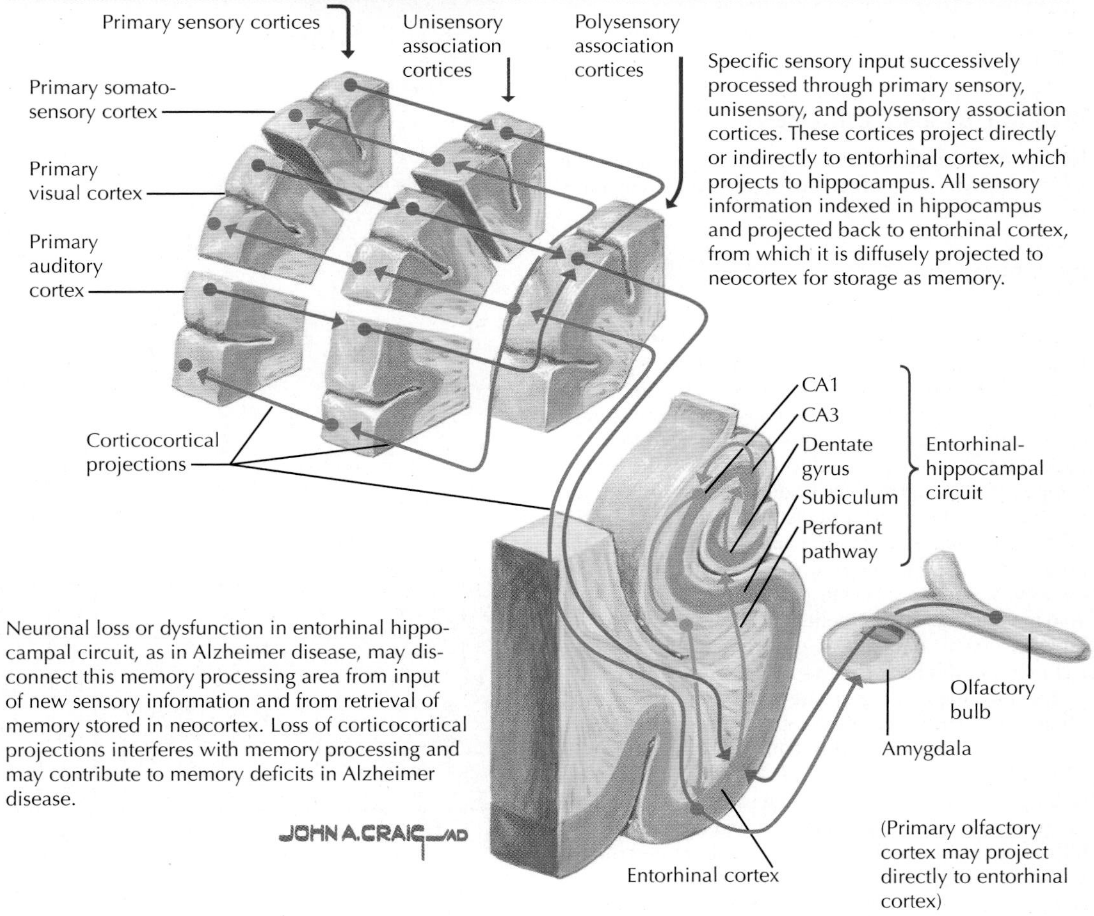

Primary sensory cortices
Unisensory association cortices
Polysensory association cortices

Primary somato-sensory cortex
Primary visual cortex
Primary auditory cortex

Corticocortical projections

CA1
CA3
Dentate gyrus
Subiculum
Perforant pathway

Entorhinal-hippocampal circuit

Specific sensory input successively processed through primary sensory, unisensory, and polysensory association cortices. These cortices project directly or indirectly to entorhinal cortex, which projects to hippocampus. All sensory information indexed in hippocampus and projected back to entorhinal cortex, from which it is diffusely projected to neocortex for storage as memory.

Neuronal loss or dysfunction in entorhinal hippo-campal circuit, as in Alzheimer disease, may disconnect this memory processing area from input of new sensory information and from retrieval of memory stored in neocortex. Loss of corticocortical projections interferes with memory processing and may contribute to memory deficits in Alzheimer disease.

JOHN A. CRAIG—AD

Olfactory bulb

Amygdala

Entorhinal cortex

(Primary olfactory cortex may project directly to entorhinal cortex)

MEMORY CIRCUITS

Long-term memory is a term that encapsulates the brain's ability to store information. It is subdivided into two main types: explicit memory (also known as declarative memory) and implicit memory (also known as nondeclarative memory). Explicit memory refers to the acquisition of information about objects, stimuli, and information that is consciously noted and recallable. The mesial temporal lobe, which includes the *hippocampal formation* (CA1, CA3, and dentate gyrus) and *entorhinal cortex,* is the region responsible for this process. The hippocampal formation stores memories, and the entorhinal cortex mediates learning and memory via its interaction with the hippocampus and neocortex. For instance, neocortical information from a visual stimulus is translated via the entorhinal cortex to higher-order complex memory representations such that an emotion can trigger a visual memory. Layer II of the entorhinal cortex is the first region affected in AD. The memory circuit that integrates the mesial temporal lobe and hippocampal formation includes several pathways: the *perforant pathway* (input to the hippocampus from the entorhinal cortex), *Mossy fiber pathway* (dentate gyrus to CA3 region), *Schaffer collateral/associational commissural pathway* (from CA3 to CA1 region), and *CA1-subiculum-entorhinal cortex pathway* (the principal output of the hippocampus).

There are two main types of explicit memory: episodic and semantic memory. Episodic memory is likened to autobiographic memory, as an episode of one's life is recalled (remembering a certain vacation to the beach). Semantic memory refers to memory about facts and general knowledge that is unrelated to a specific experience (e.g., knowing that a zebra has stripes). Not surprisingly, CA1 and the subiculum undergo selective neuronal degeneration in AD. The loss of connections between the hippocampal formation and entorhinal cortical neurons, which project to the hippocampus via the perforant pathway, account for the clinical presentation of explicit memory problems in patients with AD. Implicit memory, on the other hand, is "unconscious," can sometimes be linked to an emotion, and can be procedural (e.g., remembering how to drive a car).

The study of one particular patient, H.M., provided significant insights into the formation of memory and the role of the mesial temporal structures in memory. H.M. underwent a bilateral resection of the medial temporal regions as part of an experimental treatment for medically refractory seizures. Subsequently, H.M. developed profound loss of personal memories but had preserved language, attention, procedural memory, and general intellectual ability.

Plate 2.21

Brain: PART I

AMNESIA

The term *amnesia* is used generally to describe impairment or loss of memory. It is often subclassified as being either retrograde or anterograde. With retrograde amnesia, memories that had previously been stored are no longer available. With anterograde amnesia, information occurring in real time does not enter long-term storage. Memory is a complex process comprising three different functions: (1) registration of information, (2) storage by reinforcement, and (3) retrieval.

REGISTRATION OF INFORMATION

If information is not registered initially, it will not be remembered later. Failure to register is the explanation for absentmindedness, probably the most common abnormality of memory.

STORAGE BY REINFORCEMENT

Repetition of information to be remembered or relating such information to other factors or events enhances later recall.

RETRIEVAL

To recall the information, a person must search the "memory bank" where it has been stored. Inability to recall information on request could result from a defect in any of the three aspects of memory function.

The key anatomic regions for registration and storage of memory traces are in an area often referred to as the Papez circuit, in which the fornix connects the hippocampus to the mammillary bodies, which, in turn, are connected to the anterior nuclei of the thalamus by the mammillothalamic tract. The anterior thalamic nuclei project to the cingulate gyri, which then connect with the hippocampus, completing the circuit. The memory system is primarily cholinergic. The left medial temporal lobe is most concerned with verbal memory and the right temporal lobe with visual recall.

The prototype of amnestic disorders is *Korsakoff syndrome,* seen in chronic alcoholism and other states of vitamin B deficiency. This syndrome affects the medial thalamus and mammillary bodies and is characterized by an inability to record new memories and recall events of the recent past. Some patients confabulate to fill in gaps in their memory. Any bilateral destructive lesion of the thalami and medial temporal lobes can cause a similar syndrome. Such lesions include gliomas that spread bilaterally over the fornix and splenium of the corpus callosum; bilateral posterior cerebral artery infarctions, often caused by embolism of the top of the basilar artery; and herpes simplex encephalitis, a viral disease with predilection for temporal lobe damage. Lesions within the Papez circuit affect the memory bank. The patient is unable to recall items despite being given cues or being asked to select the correct item to be recalled from a group of alternatives. Unilateral lesions of the left medial temporal lobe and thalamus can produce amnesia that may last up to 6 months.

Head trauma often disrupts functions of memory. The severity of a head injury or concussion is often

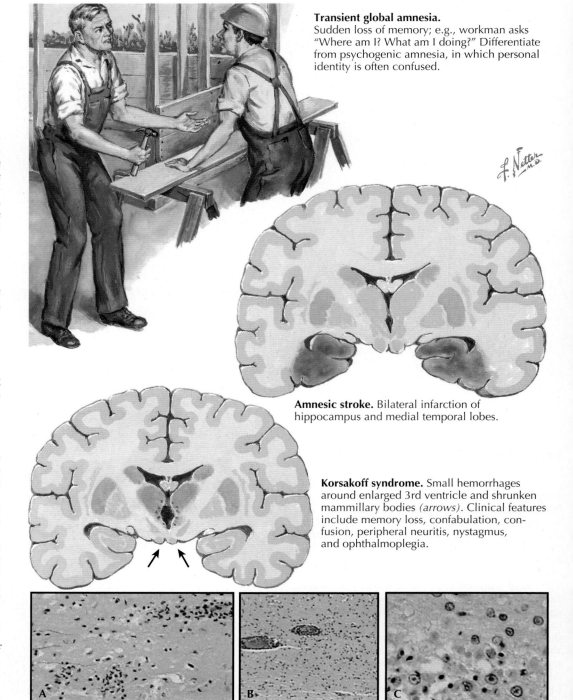

Transient global amnesia. Sudden loss of memory; e.g., workman asks "Where am I? What am I doing?" Differentiate from psychogenic amnesia, in which personal identity is often confused.

Amnesic stroke. Bilateral infarction of hippocampus and medial temporal lobes.

Korsakoff syndrome. Small hemorrhages around enlarged 3rd ventricle and shrunken mammillary bodies *(arrows)*. Clinical features include memory loss, confabulation, confusion, peripheral neuritis, nystagmus, and ophthalmoplegia.

Herpes simplex encephalitis. May also cause memory loss. Microglial nodules (**A**), perivascular lymphocyte cupping (**B**), and intranuclear inclusion bodies (**C**) in brain.

classified by the degree of *retrograde amnesia* that results; the longer the period of retrograde amnesia, the worse the injury. Persons sustaining a head injury may also experience a period of anterograde amnesia.

TRANSIENT GLOBAL AMNESIA

Transient global amnesia is a particularly common memory disorder. In this syndrome, the patient seems bewildered and asks repetitive questions about the environment and activities and, despite appropriate replies, asks the same questions moments later. The

patient cannot form new memories and is often unable to recall events of the past days, months, and even years. Speech, reading, writing, calculations, drawing, and copying are normal, as are the results of the rest of the neurologic examination. Behavior and memory usually return to normal within 24 hours, but the patient is never able to recall events during the period of amnesia. Occasionally, punctate areas of restricted diffusion are seen in the hippocampus on brain magnetic resonance imaging during, or shortly after, the event, suggesting transient ischemia. Such attacks may recur, but overall the cause of the syndrome remains obscure.

Plate 2.22   Cerebral Cortex and Neurocognitive Disorders

CLINICAL SYNDROMES RELATED TO SITE OF REGION

R   L

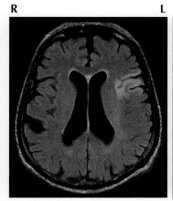
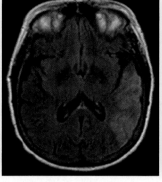
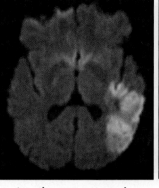
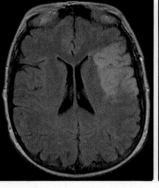
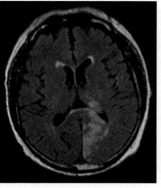

| Broca aphasia MRI-FLAIR | Wernicke aphasia | Angular gyrus-posterior temporal, inferior parietal | Global aphasia-T2 FLAIR | Alexia without agraphia |

	Broca aphasia	**Wernicke aphasia**	**Angular gyrus**	**Global aphasia**	**Alexia without agraphia**
Pronunciation, speech rhythm	Dysarthria, stuttering, effortful	Normal, fluent, loquacious	Normal	Very abnormal	Normal
Speech content	Missed syllables, ungrammatical, telegraphic	Use of wrong or nonexistent words	Often normal	Very abnormal	Normal
Repetition of speech	Abnormal but better than spontaneous	Abnormal	Normal	Very abnormal	Normal
Comprehension of spoken language	Normal	Very abnormal	Normal	Very abnormal	Normal
Comprehension of written language	Not as good as for spoken language	Abnormal but better than for spoken	Very abnormal	Very abnormal	Normal
Writing	Clumsy, ungrammatical, misspelled	Penmanship OK but misspelling and inaccuracies	Very abnormal, spelling errors	Very abnormal	Normal
Naming	Better than spontaneous speech	Wrong names	Often abnormal	Very abnormal	Normal
Other	Hemiplegia, apraxia	Sometimes hemianopsia and apraxia	Slight hemiparesis, trouble calculating, finger agnosia, hemianopsia	Hemiplegia	Abnormal reading

DOMINANT HEMISPHERE LANGUAGE DYSFUNCTION

Aphasia, a disorder of language usage and comprehension, should be distinguished from *dysarthria,* impaired articulation, and *mutism,* the absence of speech. Usually, the presence of aphasia accurately localizes dysfunction to the cerebral hemisphere concerned with speech.

To classify an aphasia, it is necessary to determine whether the patient can (1) speak fluently, with normal articulation and rhythm and without paraphasic, syntactic, or grammatical errors or use of circumlocutory phrases; (2) accurately repeat spoken sounds, words, and phrases; (3) understand spoken language,

as evidenced by accurate responses to spoken questions and ability to follow spoken commands (failure to follow a command may also be due to apraxia or paralysis and does not necessarily reflect poor comprehension); (4) consistently name common objects, presented visually, verbally, or tactilely; (5) read aloud accurately and with comprehension; (6) name words spelled aloud; and (7) write legibly and grammatically.

In *transcortical aphasia,* repetition of spoken language is preserved. *Transcortical motor aphasia* is a subtype in which there is a primary inability to produce spontaneous speech but the ability to understand spoken language is retained. *Transcortical sensory aphasia* is a subtype that is characterized by a failure to understand spoken language; a transcortical sensory aphasia usually indicates a lesion deep in the basal ganglia or in the paramedian frontal lobe.

Disconnection syndromes in general can present in fascinating, well-defined ways. One of the most famous language disconnection syndromes is the alexia without agraphia syndrome, in which patients can write but not read. This is most commonly seen as a consequence of left occipital strokes that damage the visual cortex on the left and also perturb the transfer of visual information from the right occipital visual cortex to the usually language-dominant left hemisphere. Patients with Gerstmann syndrome have difficulty with naming of fingers, left-right orientation, calculation, constructional drawing, and writing. The lesion is in the dominant hemisphere, causing the disorder either by disrupting language and semantic knowledge circuits within the angular gyrus or by creating a disconnection syndrome.

Plate 2.23

Brain: PART I

A. Constructional dyspraxia and spatial disorientation

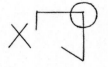
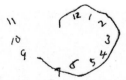
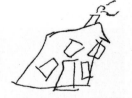

Clock face drawn by patient   Patient asked to copy ⟶ Draws this   House drawn by patient

NONDOMINANT HEMISPHERE HIGHER CORTICAL DYSFUNCTION

When it comes to stroke-induced lateralized deficits, patients with left-sided hemiplegia caused by damage to the nondominant right cerebral hemisphere frequently do not recover as well as patients with similar left hemisphere lesions, despite the fact that they are not aphasic. Return to the workplace and previous home and family participation occur less frequently after a stroke causing left-sided hemiplegia. Although disturbances of higher cortical function and behavior in patients with right hemisphere disease are more subtle, they are equally or more functionally disabling than the more obvious aphasia caused by left hemisphere disease. Deficits in right hemisphere disease include the following.

CONSTRUCTIONAL DYSPRAXIA

The right cerebral hemisphere, especially its inferior parietal lobe, is specialized for visual-spatial functions. Parietal lesions compromise the patient's ability to draw and copy figures and diagrams, reproduce block designs or figures made with sticks or tongue blades, read a map, and follow or give directions to a given destination. Spontaneous drawings are complex and contain all appropriate details, but proportions, angles, and picture relationships are inaccurate, and the left half of the drawing often is omitted or minimized. Copying a figure does not significantly improve the performance.

UNILATERAL SPATIAL NEGLECT

Patients with right hemisphere lesions, especially those involving the frontal or parietal lobe or thalamus, often neglect objects, people, or sounds on their left side. They may also not be able to adequately dress the left side of their body. When asked to read a headline or paragraph or examine a picture, they do not appreciate words or objects on the left. When instructed to bisect all lines on a piece of paper, patients with right hemisphere damage often divide the right side of the line and do not cross lines on the left side of the page. Similar spatial neglect of the right side after left hemisphere damage is unusual.

ANOSOGNOSIA AND BLUNTED EMOTIONAL RESPONSES

Patients who have right hemisphere damage often do not recognize or acknowledge an obvious left-sided hemiplegia. Not only do they verbally deny weakness or do not localize it to one side but they may fall when attempting to walk. Furthermore, even when they admit the deficit, these patients seem not to be appropriately concerned or distressed and generally are not discouraged about their uncertain future.

Testing of patients with right hemisphere lesions also shows that they have difficulty in appreciating the tone, mood, and emotional content of facial expressions or spoken language and miss nonlanguage cues. They also may be unable to invest their own voice or face with a given mood. Apathy and blunted recognition and transmission of emotional tone may hamper rehabilitation and resumption of an active goal-oriented life.

B. Neglect of left-sided stimuli

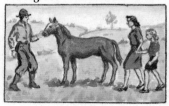

Patient shown picture ⟶ Sees this   Patient shown printed page ⟶ Sees this

C. Anosognosia
(unawareness of deficit)

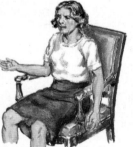

Patient with obvious left hemiplegia. Asked, "What is wrong with you?" Answers, "Nothing is wrong, I am perfectly all right."

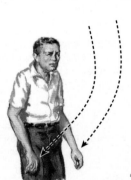

Not recognizing deficit, patient insists on trying to walk and falls but still fails to recognize deficit.

D. Motor impersistence

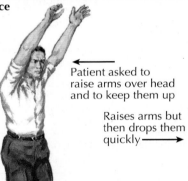

Patient asked to raise arms over head and to keep them up

Raises arms but then drops them quickly ⟶

E. Abnormal recognition of nonlanguage cues (facial expression, voice tone, mood)

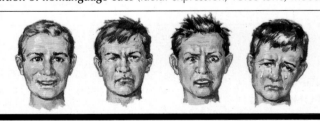

Patient shown picture. Asked, "Which is the happy face?"

Patient answers, "I don't know, they are all the same."

IMPERSISTENCE

Some patients with nondominant cerebral hemisphere damage are unable to persevere with a given task. A command that is quickly followed is just as quickly forgotten. When asked to keep their eyes closed, for example, or to cross off all A's on a page, they begin the task correctly but soon abandon it. Questions are often answered before the query is complete. Impulsive behavior with little forethought and poor perseverance is also functionally disabling.

OTHER DYSFUNCTIONS

Damage to the right cerebral hemisphere can also affect either the ability to perceive rhythm, pitch, or tonality or to read, write, or play music. Some patients have difficulty in recognizing familiar faces (prosopagnosia) and may be unable to visualize from memory the appearance of an object or a person. Loss of topographic recall of places and errors of localization or distance concerning buildings or geographic landmarks also occur.

Plate 2.24

Cerebral Cortex and Neurocognitive Disorders

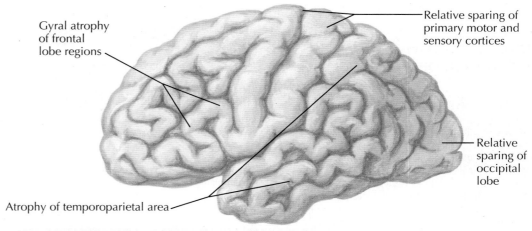

Gyral atrophy of frontal lobe regions

Relative sparing of primary motor and sensory cortices

Relative sparing of occipital lobe

Atrophy of temporoparietal area

Control

AD

PET imaging with florbetapir reveals the presence of amyloid plaque deposits in the brain of an individual with a clinical diagnosis of Alzheimer disease (shades of red) compared to a cognitively normal older adult with little to no evidence of amyloid (lighter red and yellow).

0.5   1.0   1.5   2.0   2.5

ALZHEIMER DISEASE: PATHOLOGY

Alzheimer disease (AD) is the most common neurodegenerative disorder and affects 10% of people older than 65 years and nearly 50% of those 85 years and older. The brain affected by AD has gross changes of brain atrophy accompanied by microscopic changes of amyloid plaques and neurofibrillary tangles.

The gross pathology of AD appears as enlargement of the ventricles and widening of the sylvian fissure secondary to cortical atrophy. Many convexal gyri are shrunken, and the sulci between these gyri are widened. The cerebral cortex may appear thin, and the basal ganglia are relatively small. The hippocampal region of the medial temporal lobe is affected early in the disease process, and prominent atrophy of this region is usually observed. This region is responsible for storing new information, and its degeneration is associated with the prominent short-term memory impairment that is characteristic of AD.

Microscopic examination of the affected regions reveals plaques and neurofibrillary tangles, the pathologic hallmarks of AD. Plaques are primarily composed of extracellular accumulation of insoluble amyloid protein. The amyloid hypothesis speculates that the accumulation of amyloid is the critical trigger leading to the pathologic changes in the brain of patients with AD and results in synapse loss, inflammation, neurofibrillary changes, and ultimately neuron death. Amyloid appears to accumulate years before the clinical symptoms and is associated with parallel worsening of brain atrophy. Neuroimaging techniques

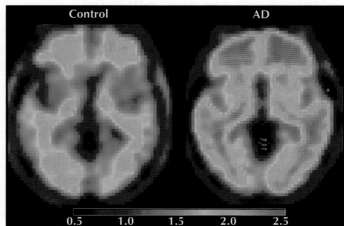

Hippocampal atrophy (more pronounced in older patients)

Gyral atrophy (more pronounced in younger patients)

Widening of sulci

Thinning of cortical mantle

Atrophy of olfactory bulbs and tracts

Ventriculomegaly, especially temporal horn of lateral ventricle

JOHN A. CRAIG—AD

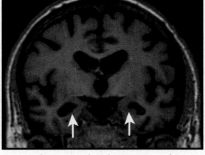

Coronal T1-weighted MRI scan showing atrophy of the hippocampus bilaterally (arrows), with enlargement of the temporal horns of the lateral ventricles. Global atrophy is evident with widening of the sulci and enlargement of subarachnoid spaces.

using positron emission tomography (PET) allow the presence and burden of amyloid deposits in the brain to be detected using radioligand labels. The molecular imaging of amyloid deposits has promise as a potential biomarker for AD and possibly may allow the identification of individuals who are still in the presymptomatic stages of the illness.

Neurofibrillary tangles are intracellular inclusions composed of aggregated tau proteins that normally

function to stabilize axonal microtubules. Tau protein found in neurofibrillary tangles is in an abnormal state of hyperphosphorylation, which occurs in conjunction with its dissociation from microtubules and clumping as paired helical filaments. Neurofibrillary tangles are a ubiquitous accompaniment of aging and accumulate in a predictable pattern. Individuals with AD tend to have more tangles, plaques, and neuron loss than individuals without dementia.

Plate 2.25

Brain: PART I

Alzheimer Disease: Distribution of Pathology

The pathologic diagnosis of AD is determined at autopsy based on the presence of its cardinal histopathologic features, neurofibrillary tangles, and amyloid plaques.

Neurofibrillary tangles (NFTs) are a ubiquitous accompaniment of aging and accumulate in a predictable fashion in typical AD. Accumulation of NFTs begins in the medial temporal lobe (amygdala and entorhinal cortex), gradually extending into the limbic system (hippocampus and cingulate cortices) and later throughout the entire isocortex. This stereotypic pattern of accumulation is used in pathologic staging of the disease (Braak staging). The pathologic staging of AD is based on the hierarchic pattern of the appearance of NFTs in various regions. There are two "presymptomatic" transentorhinal stages, where NFTs remain in the perirhinal cortex. In stage III, the NFTs involve the limbic regions and layer II of the entorhinal cortex. Stage IV AD is marked by more extensive NFTs in the limbic regions, entorhinal layer IV, and hippocampal CA1 region. These latter stages (III and IV) correspond clinically to mild cognitive impairment (MCI), not dementia. MCI represents an intermediate stage between normal aging and dementia. Typically, patients note subjective memory problems, the need to make lists, and short-term memory "slip ups," but these changes are not severe enough to interfere with day-to-day activities. As the pathologic stage of AD progresses, the NFTs accumulate in the inferotemporal, retrosplenial, and, eventually, association regions of the cortex, whereas the primary motor cortex is spared. In later stages, the clinical hallmarks of AD are present and include impairments in memory, judgment, orientation, language, and decision making.

Amyloid plaques are abundant in the cerebral cortex of individuals with AD but deposit in a less typical fashion. Amyloid deposition is commonly observed in leptomeningeal arteries as amyloid angiopathy. Autopsy studies and, more recently, amyloid imaging techniques have revealed that amyloid plaques begin to accumulate in the brain years, perhaps decades, before the emergence of clinically recognizable symptoms and are found in cortical regions that are highly metabolically active, such as the default-mode network that is active when an individual is at rest and not engaged in a specific cognitive task. Regions such as the precuneus and posterior cingulate, which have strong connections with the hippocampus, are among the areas affected earliest. Therapies directed toward altering amyloid formation, deposition, and clearance have been investigated for years with disappointing results. Recently monoclonal antibodies directed against amyloid beta have shown significant efficacy in reducing amyloid plaque levels in the brains of individuals with AD. Lecanumab and aducanumab are anti-amyloid antibody therapies that have been approved by the FDA and have shown some benefit in slowing disease progression in clinical trials. The long-term benefits of these therapies is an area of ongoing investigation.

Of interest, some NFT pathology is present in all older adults, although individuals with AD have a greater burden of NFTs and a much more widespread distribution throughout the isocortex. The CA1 region of the hippocampus and the entorhinal cortex are particularly susceptible to the accumulation of both plaques

In neocortex, primary involvement of association areas (especially temporoparietal and frontal) with relative sparing of primary sensory cortices (except olfactory) and motor cortices

JOHN A. CRAIG—MD
C. Machado—M.D.

Hippocampus

Nucleus basalis

Olfactory bulb

Amygdala

Locus coeruleus

Raphe nuclei

Pathologic involvement of limbic system and subcortical nuclei projecting to cortex

Dura mater

Pia-arachnoid

β-Amyloid peptide deposition in cortical and leptomeningeal arterioles

I
II
III
IV
V
VI

SP

NFT

Association cortex

In association cortex, neurofibrillary tangles (NFTs) and synaptic and neuronal loss predominate in layer V. Senile plaques (SPs) occur in more superficial layers.

CA2   CA4
CA3
CA1
Subiculum

Entorhinal cortex

Presubiculum

In hippocampus, neurofibrillary tangles, neuronal loss, and senile plaques primarily located in layer CA1, subiculum, and entorhinal cortex

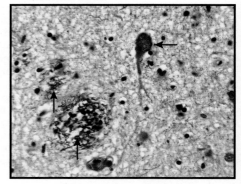

Characteristic pathologic findings in the brain of a patient with Alzheimer disease: neuritic plaque and neurofibrillary tangle. Neuritic plaques (bottom arrows) are extracellular deposits of amyloid in the brain. Neurofibrillary tangles (top arrow) are aggregates of hyperphosphorylated tau protein.

and tangles in the early stages of the disease. These regions are important for mediating the formation of memories, and their degeneration accounts for the prominent impairments in short-term memory observed in patients with AD.

Biochemical data from patients with AD reveal an early decrease in choline acetyltransferase and acetylcholinesterase, indicating dysfunction in the neural pathways that use acetylcholine as a neurotransmitter.

The number of neurons is reduced in the basal nucleus of Meynert, which has widespread cholinergic neuron innervations through most of the cerebral cortex. Selective degeneration of the basal forebrain cholinergic neurons results in a cholinergic deficit that contributes to AD symptoms. These findings led to the development of the first effective treatments in ameliorating the symptoms of AD, acetylcholinesterase inhibitors, which act by increasing acetylcholine levels in the brain.

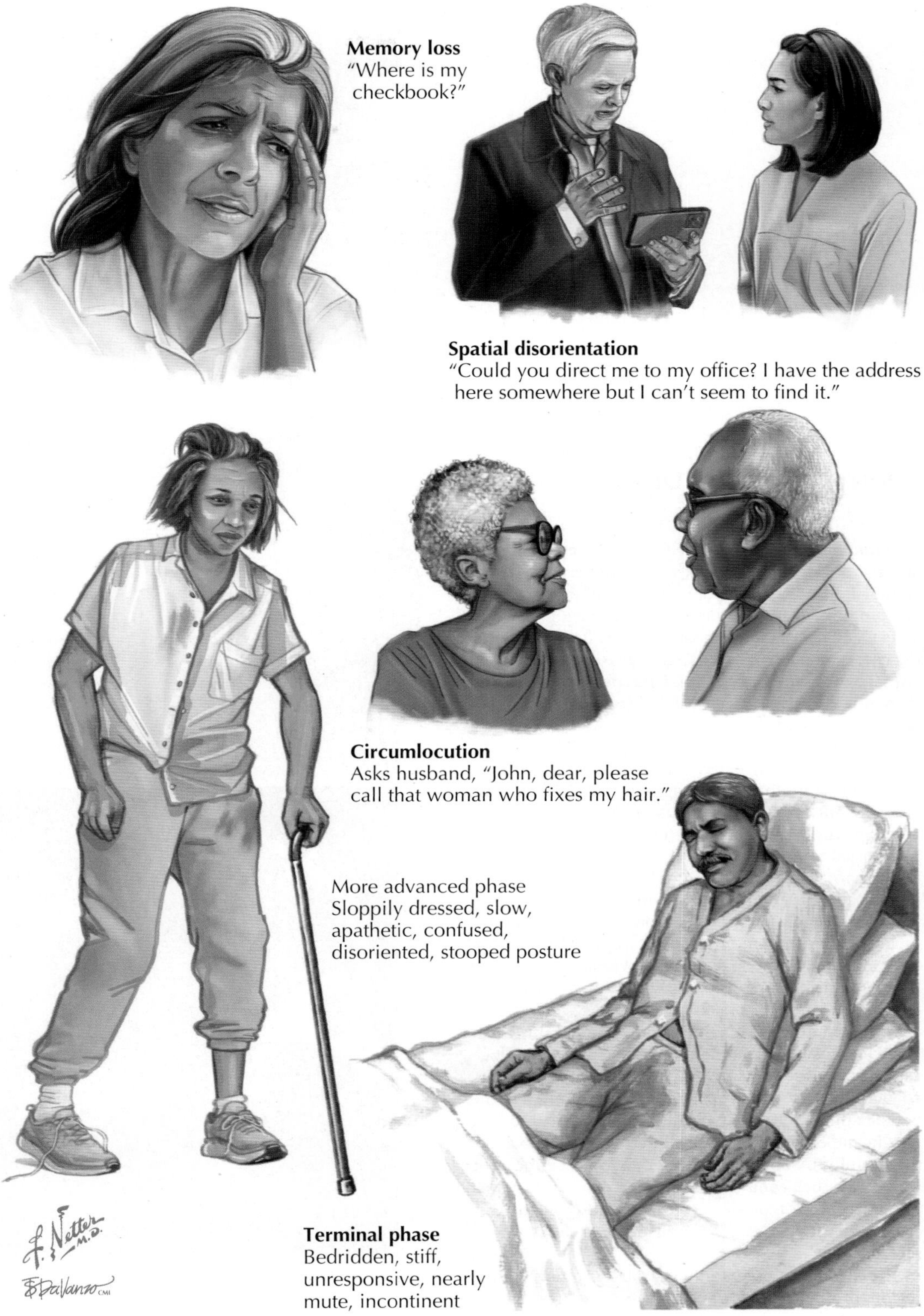

Plate 2.26

Cerebral Cortex and Neurocognitive Disorders

Alzheimer Disease: Clinical Manifestations, Progressive Phases

The earliest stages of AD are generally marked by changes in multiple domains of cognition, including memory, executive function, language, and visuospatial function. Of importance, these cognitive changes are often well compensated; individuals may still be independent in many activities in the community, and their symptoms may not be readily apparent in casual conversation. Observations from an attentive family member, relative, or friend describing cognitive changes interfering even mildly with the patient's usual function is a sensitive indicator of the earliest stages of AD.

1. *Memory loss:* The clinical hallmark of AD is memory loss. Patients may be forgetful of details of recent conversations and events. Family members frequently report that the patient asks repetitious questions or repeats stories, even in the same conversation. Patients have difficulty remembering appointments and taking their medications and tend to lose things more than before. These symptoms indicate hippocampal and mesial temporal dysfunction.

2. *Executive dysfunction:* Executive function is loosely defined as an ability to organize information and pursue goals. Subtle problems in executive function are often observed in the early stages as problems in planning and organizing. This may manifest as difficulty in managing a checkbook and the household finances or greater difficulty in following a recipe. Patients have more difficulty making decisions and solving problems and are now more likely to enlist the help of others.

3. *Decreased language facility:* Communication may be less precise than normal and contain more "filler" words and circumlocutory elements. Patients may have difficulty recalling names of people and places although they generally retain the ability to understand and repeat spoken language and do not make paraphasic errors, in contrast to patients with aphasia due to stroke. These symptoms usually reflect perisylvian dysfunction.

4. *Visuospatial dysfunction:* Patients may have navigational problems while driving and in the early stages often self-restrict their driving to the most familiar areas. Ultimately, spatial disorientation interferes with the ability to navigate even in the most familiar areas, such as the patient's neighborhood. These symptoms reflect parietal lobe dysfunction.

As the disease relentlessly progresses into the moderate stages, greater cognitive and functional decline reflects more widespread involvement of neocortical regions. Increasing difficulties with instrumental activities of daily living are prominent, such as cooking, cleaning, and dressing. Apraxia, a disorder of skilled movement despite intact strength, sensation, and coordination, develops as typical AD progresses but is not a prominent early feature. This may manifest as greater difficulty in using tools (such as silverware, unlocking a door with a key) and dressing in the proper sequence. Behavioral changes may be prominent. Patients may

Memory loss
"Where is my checkbook?"

Spatial disorientation
"Could you direct me to my office? I have the address here somewhere but I can't seem to find it."

Circumlocution
Asks husband, "John, dear, please call that woman who fixes my hair."

More advanced phase
Sloppily dressed, slow, apathetic, confused, disoriented, stooped posture

Terminal phase
Bedridden, stiff, unresponsive, nearly mute, incontinent

become increasingly apathetic and less interested in others and in their environment. They also lose interest in reading, television, and social gatherings. Less attention is paid to grooming and attire, and even formerly fastidious people allow their house, room, and belongings to become untidy and disorganized. Occasionally, agitated or belligerent behavior occurs.

In the *advanced stage* of AD, patients cannot perform the simple activities of daily living. They remain in bed unless they are helped up and require aid for dressing, eating, and toilet functions. They cannot venture out alone and become lost even in their home. They confuse night and day, and incontinence develops.

The course of the disease is usually from 7 to 12 years. In the terminal phase, patients are bedridden, mute, and stiff and ultimately succumb to medical complications such as pneumonia, urosepsis, or decubitus ulcers.

Plate 2.27

Brain: PART I

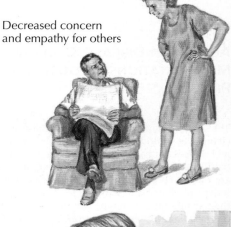

Decreased concern
and empathy for others

Atrophy of frontal
and/or temporal areas

Clinical
features
of frontal
lobe variant

Decrease
in speech

Oral fixation:
increased eating
causes weight
gain

Loss of
awareness
of personal
appearance
and hygiene

FRONTOTEMPORAL DEMENTIA

Frontotemporal dementia (FTD) is a heterogeneous spectrum of disorders marked by degeneration in the frontal and anterior temporal lobes, resulting in various symptoms of disturbed personality, behavior, and language. FTD is the third most common form of neurodegenerative dementia, ranking after AD and dementia with Lewy bodies, accounting for perhaps 5% of all dementia cases. FTD generally presents at a younger age than AD and has a mean age at onset of 58 years. There are several clinical phenotypes of FTD, with the most common being behavioral variant FTD (bvFTD), nonfluent-agrammatic primary progressive aphasia, and semantic variant primary progressive aphasia. Overlap syndromes can be seen with progressive supranuclear palsy or corticobasal syndrome.

Behavioral and personality changes are prominent early features in individuals with bvFTD, reflecting pathologic involvement of the frontal lobes. Symptoms include disinhibition, impulsivity, impaired judgment, and disturbed social skills. An individual with bvFTD may have inappropriate behavior, such as swearing, off-color jokes, and loss of social tact. Dietary habits may change, and an individual may only eat certain foods, particularly sweets. Family members may have to lock cabinets to prevent overeating. Prominent personality changes are disturbing to the patient's family, yet the patients themselves are typically unconcerned and lack insight and empathy regarding how these changes affect their families. Some individuals develop repetitious or compulsive behavior. Severe amnesia and visuospatial impairment are typically not present early in the disease, and patients may do well on bedside cognitive screens.

The language presentations of FTD vary based on the region of the brain primarily impacted. Nonfluent-agrammatic primary progressive aphasia primarily involves the inferior and middle gyri of the left frontal lobe, Broca's area. Neurodegeneration affecting Broca's area results in the loss of fluent speech and grammatical structure. Their speech has a halting quality due to frequent pauses for word-finding. Articles and connecting words, such as "the" and "with," may be dropped. Generally, comprehension is preserved early in the disease, but patients may have difficulty understanding grammatically complex sentences. Semantic variant primary progressive aphasia is secondary to degeneration of the anterior temporal lobe of the dominant hemisphere.

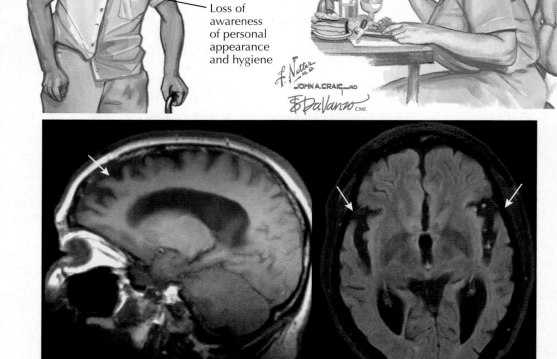

T1-weighted MRIs demonstrating significant atrophy in the frontal *(left)* and temporal lobes *(right)* in a patient with frontotemporal dementia

Patients develop impairment in semantics (word meaning), resulting in empty, fluent speech and a loss of speech comprehension. Speech may be effortless and without hesitancies, but little meaningful information is conveyed. Initially, they may use more common words to describe a range of objects. These patients have prominent comprehension problems (i.e., following commands) despite their fluent and effortless speech. As the disease progresses, complex visuoperceptual dysfunction, such as prosopagnosia and loss of visual object recognition, may develop, often referred to as semantic dementia.

Neuroimaging should be obtained to rule out the presence of structural lesions (e.g., stroke, tumor) and may reveal the presence of disproportionate atrophy in the frontal and temporal lobes. Additionally, functional imaging in the form of PET may reveal altered metabolic activity in the frontal and temporal lobes.

Plate 2.28

Cerebral Cortex and Neurocognitive Disorders

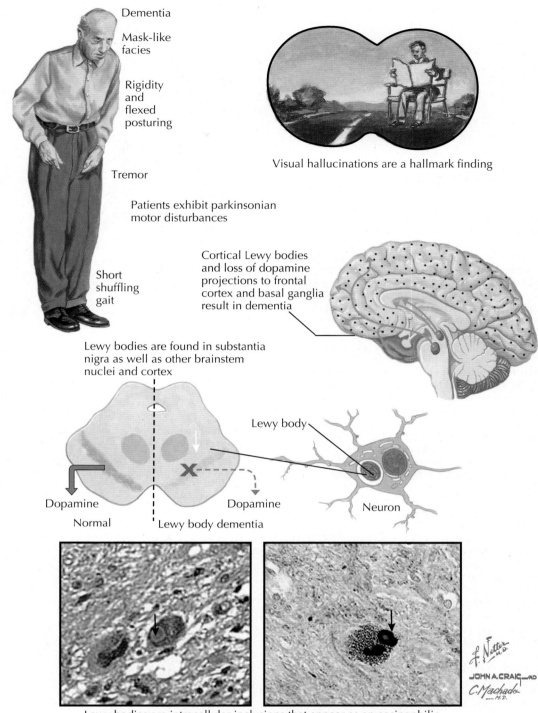

Dementia

Mask-like facies

Rigidity and flexed posturing

Tremor

Patients exhibit parkinsonian motor disturbances

Short shuffling gait

Visual hallucinations are a hallmark finding

Cortical Lewy bodies and loss of dopamine projections to frontal cortex and basal ganglia result in dementia

Lewy bodies are found in substantia nigra as well as other brainstem nuclei and cortex

Lewy body

Dopamine

Normal

Dopamine

Lewy body dementia

Neuron

Lewy bodies are intracellular inclusions that appear as an eosinophilic inclusion with a halo when stained with hematoxylin and eosin (left). Immunostaining techniques using antibodies to alpha-synuclein densely label Lewy bodies (right).

DEMENTIA WITH LEWY BODIES

Dementia with Lewy bodies (DLB) is the second most common cause of dementia, accounting for 10% to 15% of dementia cases. The pathologic hallmark of DLB is the presence of Lewy bodies in neurons of the brainstem, primarily the substantia nigra, and throughout the cerebral cortex. Lewy bodies are primarily composed of abnormal aggregations of the synaptic protein alpha-synuclein. Lewy body pathology and Alzheimer disease pathology (plaques and tangles) can co-occur.

In patients with DLB, the cognitive and functional decline of dementia is accompanied by a combination of clinical features that include visual hallucinations, parkinsonism, and fluctuating cognitive impairment. Visual hallucinations may present early in the clinical course and tend to persist throughout the course. Classically, the visual hallucinations are vivid images of animate objects (e.g., children, animals) as opposed to nonspecific visual phenomena; however, a spectrum of visual and other perceptual hallucinations can occur. Parkinsonism (rigidity, tremor, bradykinesia, gait abnormalities) develops in most patients with DLB at some time in the course of the disease and usually does not respond to levodopa. Severe sensitivity to neuroleptic medications—that is, dopamine-blocking agents—is a common finding. Individuals with DLB typically present with recurrent episodes of confusion on a background of progressive deterioration. The fluctuations in cognitive function manifest as shifting attention and levels of alertness that may vary over minutes, hours, or days.

Other features that are commonly observed in patients with DLB include additional neuropsychiatric symptoms of delusions, apathy, and anxiety. Rapid eye movement (REM) sleep behavior disorders are often prodromal to DLB and other synucleinopathies such as Parkinson disease. REM sleep behavior disorders are manifested complex motor behavior during the REM stage of sleep. This can be confirmed with polysomnography. Additionally, autonomic abnormalities are common in DLB and include orthostatic hypotension, constipation, and carotid sinus hypersensitivity. These abnormalities can result in "dizziness," presyncope, syncope, and falls as common aspects of the clinical presentation.

Plate 2.29

Brain: PART I

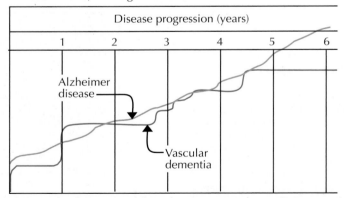

CLINICAL CHARACTERISTICS OF VASCULAR (MULTIINFARCT) DEMENTIA

Dementia, personality and mood changes

Cardiac and renal disease

Hypertension

Hyperreflexia

Babinski sign

Hemiparesis

Urinary frequency or urgency

Patients with symptoms of vascular dementia may have risk factors for stroke.

Bilateral infarcts usually required for development of dementia

Cortical infarcts may cause focal signs and symptoms related to area of cortex involved.

Arteriolar intra-cranial disease

Subcortical (lacunar) infarcts cause signs and symptoms of subcortical dementia.

Intracranial medium-size vessel disease

Extracranial large-vessel disease

JOHN A.CRAIG—AD
C.Machado—M.D.

Cerebrovascular disease results in multiple occlusions in cerebral vascular tree, causing scattered cortical and subcortical infarcts.

Disease progression (years)
1 2 3 4 5 6

Alzheimer disease

Vascular dementia

Clinical progression. Vascular dementia exhibits abrupt onset and stepwise progression in contrast to gradual onset and progression of Alzheimer disease.

VASCULAR DEMENTIA

Vascular dementia is interesting in that many of those who do have true vascular dementia are not diagnosed with it, whereas many who probably do not have vascular dementia are diagnosed with it. The most straightforward presentations are those in which there is a clear temporal relationship between a stroke and a cognitive deficit. For instance, an individual with normal cognition has a large vessel stroke that causes a combination of cognitive signs, such as aphasia and memory retrieval issues. If the patient cannot resume their pre-stroke day-to-day level of function because of these new cognitive deficits, the criteria for vascular dementia are met, but because the stroke so clearly caused the deficits, they are held by many to simply represent the consequences of a stroke (as opposed to a frank vascular dementia). On the other hand, some patients will present with a gradually progressive dementia, a retrieval-type memory deficit without preceding clinical strokes, and neuroimaging that shows subcortical changes consistent with small-vessel cerebrovascular disease, also referred to as *Binswanger disease.*

Vascular dementias can be subclassified depending on whether the stroke or strokes responsible for the cognitive change are single versus multiple and large vessel versus small vessel. As mentioned above, a single large vessel stroke can cause a dementia syndrome. Such presentations are often obvious because they typically present within the context of an acute, clearly diagnosable large vessel stroke. Some patients will have multiple large vessel strokes. Greater amounts of stroke-related brain damage commonly associate with greater degrees of cognitive dysfunction.

Single small strokes can also alter cognition when they happen to damage specific areas that are critical to cognitive performance. The thalamus, caudate head, and fornix constitute some examples in which a strategically placed small stroke can impact cognition. Cognitive decline severe enough to qualify for a syndromic dementia diagnosis also results from multiple small vessel strokes that, on neuroimaging, appear as multiple lacunar strokes. As is the case with large vessel multiinfarct dementias, this type of small vessel multiinfarct vascular dementia often presents within the context of a stepwise decline occurring in association with diagnosed acute strokes.

When it comes to diagnosing a vascular dementia, the most difficult cases are those in which the patient has developed a clinical dementia, there is no clinical history of a previously diagnosed acute stroke, but a neuroimaging study reveals extensive stroke-induced damage to the brain. In many such instances, the imaging shows extensive changes to the subcortical white matter. These changes may appear confluent or more anatomically restricted. The changes may coalesce around the lateral ventricles and may or may not also separately project into other white matter

areas in a patchy or punctuate pattern. When this white matter change is indeed driving the dementia, a diagnosis of subcortical ischemic vascular dementia should be considered, and a pathologic survey may reveal changes consistent with Binswanger disease. However, nondemented elderly individuals and patients with neurodegenerative dementias may also show similar patterns of subcortical white matter change. In the latter situation, the white matter change may represent a consequence of the true underlying disease as opposed to a cause of the dementia. When

considering such cases, the overall clinical picture, including the clinical history, general neurologic exam, and cognitive neurologic exam, needs to be synthesized and interpreted very cautiously. Sometimes these patients will ultimately receive a diagnosis of mixed vascular-degenerative dementia, or *Alzheimer disease plus cerebrovascular disease.* This point notwithstanding, clinical strokes do increase the risk of a patient developing AD, and the frequent association of AD with cerebrovascular pathology suggests that these conditions may be linked.

Plate 2.30

Cerebral Cortex and Neurocognitive Disorders

TREATABLE DEMENTIAS

Although in some ways cognitive performance abilities evolve throughout adulthood, many elderly people remain mentally sharp into their ninth and tenth decades. The emergence of uncharacteristic changes in an individual's cognition that impacts their usual activities should therefore trigger an evaluation for possible etiologies.

Because AD is the most common cause of intellectual decline in later life, symptoms or signs that are unusual in AD should alert the physician to a different diagnosis and the possibility of reversing the dementing process. Such features include early age at onset; prominent headache; disturbances of gait or incontinence early in the course of the illness; seizures; fever; precipitous decline over a period of weeks or months; alteration of consciousness, especially sleepiness, stupor, or delirium; history of head trauma; focal neurologic signs, such as lateralized visual, motor, or sensory abnormalities; accompanying dysfunction of peripheral nerves characterized by paresthesias and absent distal reflexes; and known systemic cancer, collagen vascular disease, or endocrinopathy. The presence of any of these features should dictate further evaluation and consideration of the following treatable dementias.

METABOLIC DISEASE WITH ENCEPHALOPATHY

When intellectual decline is caused by systemic metabolic disease, there are usually four associated features: diminished alertness; asterixis; a global decrease in mental function, often with a flight of ideas; and variability of intellectual function during the day. The metabolic dysfunction can be either *endogenous* or *exogenous*. An endogenous abnormality indicates that too much or too little of a substance or metabolite usually found in the body, such as calcium, sodium, thyroid hormone, sugar, and so forth, may be responsible.

Failure of the lungs, kidneys, or liver is also in this category. Exogenous metabolic dysfunction is caused by a deficiency of a dietary substance, such as vitamin B_{12} or nicotinic acid or by intoxication with a growing variety of agents, such as alcohol, barbiturates, or narcotics.

BRAIN TUMORS

Primary benign brain tumors, such as meningiomas, that affect the olfactory grooves and frontal lobes decrease mental function by pressing on brain tissue or by obstructing the ventricular system. Malignant primary metastatic tumors can also cause intellectual decline, usually with focal or multifocal signs and seizures.

HEAD TRAUMA

A history of head injury, sleepiness, and slight lateralized weakness are clues, particularly to a subdural hematoma. The physician should be aware of this possibility because many patients will have forgotten the inciting trauma by the time they seek medical attention. In elderly patients, patients with alcoholism, and those on anticoagulant or antiplatelet agents relatively minor head injury can manifest with intracranial hemorrhages.

NORMAL-PRESSURE HYDROCEPHALUS

In most patients, this occult condition is unrecognized until the pathologic state causes overt symptoms, which are further described below.

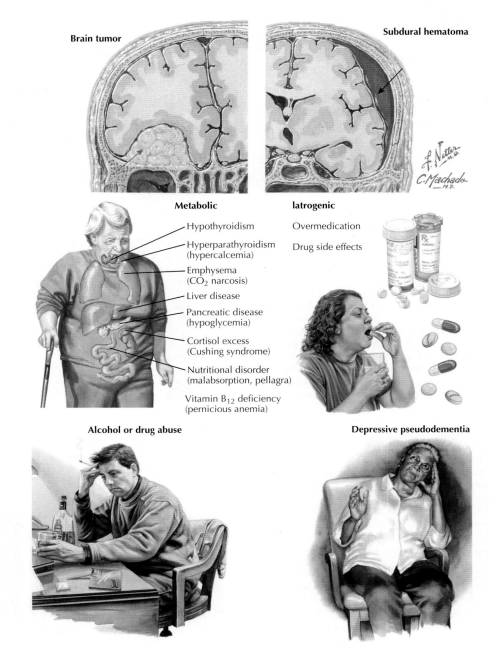

Brain tumor

Subdural hematoma

Metabolic
- Hypothyroidism
- Hyperparathyroidism (hypercalcemia)
- Emphysema (CO_2 narcosis)
- Liver disease
- Pancreatic disease (hypoglycemia)
- Cortisol excess (Cushing syndrome)
- Nutritional disorder (malabsorption, pellagra)
- Vitamin B_{12} deficiency (pernicious anemia)

Iatrogenic
- Overmedication
- Drug side effects

Alcohol or drug abuse

Depressive pseudodementia

INFECTION

An altered mental state, usually with headache and cerebrospinal fluid (CSF) pleocytosis, may be the first indication of CNS syphilis, tuberculosis, or fungal meningitis. Systemic infections, such as a urinary tract infection, frequently result in confusion and acute encephalopathy in elderly patients.

DEPRESSION

Depression is associated with measurable declines in some aspects of memory, and memory complaints are a frequent symptom of depression. Frequently patients will score poorly on many aspects of neuropsychological testing. *Depressive pseudodementia* is a concept that arose to characterize depression as a potential mimic of dementia and is likely a misnomer. Typically, patients with untreated or undertreated mood disorders will have relatively intact function; for example, still driving without difficulty. Depression should be considered in patients with dementia, although depression is often an

early manifestation of neurodegenerative disease. Depression in patients with AD contributes to greater functional decline and should be treated.

CEREBROVASCULAR DISEASE

Strokes can decimate the regions of the brain that govern thought processes. When this occurs, motor and reflex abnormalities usually parallel or exceed the degree of intellectual decline. Usually, the patient also has a history of an abrupt decline, as well as hypertension and coronary or peripheral vascular disease.

DIAGNOSTIC STUDIES

Screening of biochemical parameters, especially vitamin B_{12} level and thyroid, renal, liver, and lung function, can be important in evaluating potential causes of dementia. Neuroimaging, electroencephalography, and CSF analysis may also detect unsuspected causes of dementia.

Plate 2.31

Brain: PART I

NORMAL-PRESSURE HYDROCEPHALUS

The "plumbing system" of the CNS operates in a delicate balance. Fluid produced in the choroid plexus of the lateral ventricles circulates through the third ventricle, cerebral aqueduct (of Sylvius), and fourth ventricle. After exiting from the roof of the fourth ventricle, the CSF circulates around the brain within the subarachnoid cisterns and is ultimately absorbed by the arachnoid granulations into the circulation. If more CSF is produced than is absorbed, the ventricles and subarachnoid space distend with fluid. This imbalance leads to enlargement of the ventricles, which then encroaches on the normal cerebral white matter, especially frontally.

Conditions known to cause scarring of the pia-arachnoid membranes, such as meningeal infection, subarachnoid hemorrhage, or bleeding from past trauma, can cause hydrocephalus by decreasing the effectiveness of CSF absorption. In most elderly patients, communicating hydrocephalus has no easily identifiable cause. Although it could possibly result from degeneration of the arachnoid granulations and membranes, there has been little detailed study of the morphologic structure of the arachnoid in either normal persons or patients with hydrocephalus. Because the CSF pressure is usually high in obstructive hydrocephalus due to tumor and, for uncertain reasons, is within normal range in communicating hydrocephalus, the latter disorder has been called normal-pressure hydrocephalus (NPH).

NPH usually develops over a period of 6 to 12 months but at times progresses insidiously for a few years. Neuroimaging shows markedly enlarged ventricles, often with little or no cortical atrophy. Disproportionately enlarged subarachnoid space hydrocephalus is likely a more specific finding of NPH.

CLINICAL MANIFESTATIONS

Most symptoms relate to enlargement of the anterior (frontal) horns and loss of frontal lobe white matter. There is a classic triad of abnormality of gait dementia, and urinary incontinence. Not all components of the triad must be present to make the diagnosis.

1. *Abnormality of gait:* Patients with NPH have significant abnormalities in their gait, often described as "magnetic" with limited step height and difficulty with step initiation. It can appear that their feet are "stuck" to the floor. Other psychomotor slowing can be seen, and patients may be mistaken for having parkinsonism.
2. *Dementia:* Cognitive deficits reflect frontal network dysfunction, and some describe NPH as a "subcortical dementia." Patients typically exhibit deficits in working memory, psychomotor slowing, attention, and processing speed.
3. *Urinary incontinence:* The patient loses the ability to retain urine despite normal perception of the urge and need to urinate. Often incontinence is worsened by gait difficulties. A range of bladder findings has been reported in NPH, but the detrusor overactivity is most common.

TREATMENT

Spinal puncture with a high volume of CSF fluid drainage can lead to temporary improvement in gait and alertness. Acetazolamide has been trialed as a

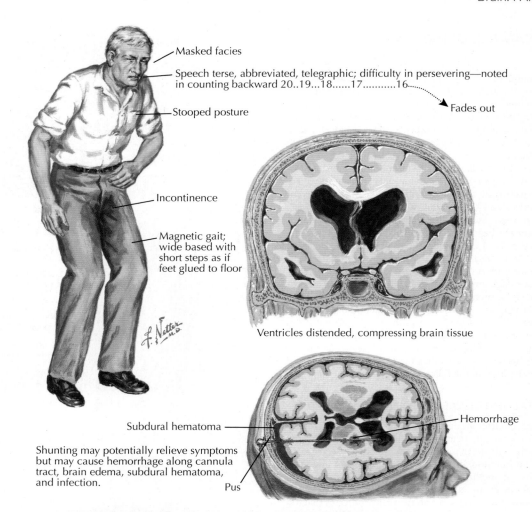

Masked facies

Speech terse, abbreviated, telegraphic; difficulty in persevering—noted in counting backward 20..19...18......17..........16........

Fades out

Stooped posture

Incontinence

Magnetic gait; wide based with short steps as if feet glued to floor

Ventricles distended, compressing brain tissue

Subdural hematoma

Hemorrhage

Shunting may potentially relieve symptoms but may cause hemorrhage along cannula tract, brain edema, subdural hematoma, and infection.

Pus

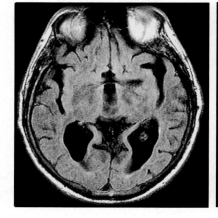

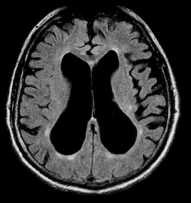

Axial FLAIR images demonstrate moderate enlargement of the third and lateral ventricles, more normal sulcal pattern, and patchy periventricular increased T2 changes.

treatment but without clear benefit. *Ventriculoperitoneal (VP) shunts* are the definitive treatment for NPH. *VP shunts* seem to be most effective in patients who have the classic triad of symptoms and in whom the course of the dementia has been short and a cause of the disorder, such as past subarachnoid hemorrhage, can be identified. Complications of ventriculoperitoneal shunts in adults include intracerebral or intraventricular hematoma during insertion of the tube; infection of the shunt and peritoneal space; oversiphoning of CSF, which causes subsequent brain swelling to take up the void; and collapse of the thin cerebral mantle, with tearing of bridging veins and formation of a subdural hematoma. The incidence of subsequent shunt infection is high.

DIAGNOSTIC STUDIES

Cisternography after introduction of a radionuclide by lumbar puncture may be of value in assessing abnormal CSF flow patterns. Impaired cerebral blood reactivity to acetazolamide with single-photon emission computed tomography imaging may help predict positive response to shunting. Fluorodeoxyglucose PET has been used with some success to determine the presence of other co-occurring neurodegenerative diseases, which may result in shunt failure. Unfortunately, there is no single definitive test that reliably predicts whether a patient will improve after surgical placement of a VP shunt. However, a positive response to large volume spinal puncture, multiple spinal punctures, or lumbar drain can suggest a higher probability for a positive response to VP shunt.

EPILEPSY

Plate 3.1

Brain: PART I

ELECTROENCEPHALOGRAPHY

The electroencephalogram (EEG) is a record of the electrical activity of the nerve cells in the brain. The EEG is based on the measurement of electrical fields generated by volume conduction of ionic currents from nerve cells through the extracellular space. Recorded EEG potentials arise from extracellular current flow from summated excitatory postsynaptic potentials (EPSPs) and inhibitory postsynaptic potentials (IPSPs). The EEG does not record activity from single neurons but is dependent on the summation of thousands to millions of postsynaptic potentials and therefore represents activity from large neuronal aggregations. Although nerve action potentials have higher voltage changes than EPSPs and IPSPs, due to the lack of summation and short duration of action potentials, they usually add little to EEG activity. During seizures, there is synchronous firing of large ensembles of action potentials from neurons, which may contribute to the EEG signal. The usual way to record an EEG is to attach small metal electrodes to the scalp in standardized positions. The signal from these electrodes is amplified, digitized, and electronically stored. The EEG is then read on a computer screen.

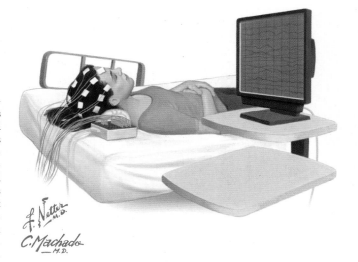

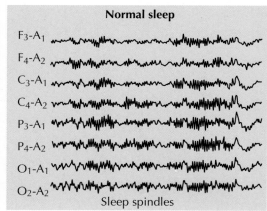

Electrode placement and lead identification

Odd numbers, left side;
even numbers, right side;
z locations, midline

BRAIN WAVE ACTIVITY

Brain activity consists of waveforms that vary in polarity, shape, and frequency and usually range in voltage from 20 to 60 microvolts. Scalp EEG activity shows oscillations at a variety of frequencies, representing synchronized activity over a network of neurons. EEG waveforms are labeled according to their frequency, measured in cycles per second or Hertz (Hz). Alpha activity ranges between 8 and 13 Hz. The alpha rhythm is predominantly over the posterior head region and is the characteristic background frequency of the normal awake person. It occurs when the eyes are closed and attenuates when the eyes are open. Beta activity is low-amplitude, fast activity with a frequency of 13 to 30 Hz and is usually present over the anterior head regions. Theta activity ranges from 4 to 7 Hz, and delta activity occurs at a frequency of less than 4 Hz. The EEG shows development maturation. For example, in the newborn infant, the EEG does not show continuous mixed-waveform activity, as would be expected in an adult. Instead, an infant has continuous amorphous delta activity. The other waveform frequencies progressively emerge as the infant's brain develops. EEG patterns change during different stages of sleep and contribute to the definition of sleep stages. The EEG patterns are very different for rapid eye movement (REM) stages compared with non-REM sleep. For stage II non-REM sleep, the EEG shows spindle activity (10–14 Hz sinusoidal activity) and vertex sharp waves. During stage III to IV non-REM sleep, high-voltage delta activity predominates. The EEG during REM sleep resembles the EEG during wakefulness, with a low-amplitude background consisting of a mix of frequencies.

The main types of abnormalities that may be seen in the EEG are slowing of background frequencies, epileptiform activity, and suppression of activity. Slowing of background activities can be either diffuse or focal. Diffuse slowing suggests widespread brain dysfunction, which can be caused by a variety of insults, such as global brain injury, toxins, inflammation, or degenerative processes. Focal slowing is often indicative of a

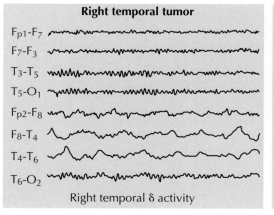

EEG in normal awake person, eyes closed

$F_{p1}-F_3$ β
F_3-C_3
C_3-P_3
P_3-O_1 α
$F_{p2}-F_4$ β
F_4-C_4
C_4-P_4
P_4-O_2 α

Right temporal tumor

$F_{p1}-F_7$
F_7-F_3
T_3-T_5
T_5-O_1
$F_{p2}-F_8$
F_8-T_4
T_4-T_6
T_6-O_2

Right temporal δ activity

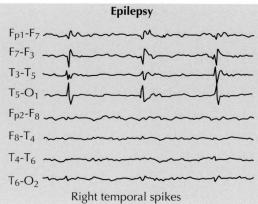

Normal sleep

F_3-A_1
F_4-A_2
C_3-A_1
C_4-A_2
P_3-A_1
P_4-A_2
O_1-A_1
O_2-A_2

Sleep spindles

Epilepsy

$F_{p1}-F_7$
F_7-F_3
T_3-T_5
T_5-O_1
$F_{p2}-F_8$
F_8-T_4
T_4-T_6
T_6-O_2

Right temporal spikes

structural lesion, such as a tumor or a stroke. Epileptiform activity indicates the patient is at risk for seizures. Suppression of activity can be either focal or diffuse, and it indicates a severe derangement of brain function.

INDICATIONS FOR EEG

The main indications for obtaining an EEG are to assess for seizure disorders, intracranial disease processes, coma, and brain death. The most common reason for an EEG is to characterize a seizure disorder. The EEG is useful in defining epilepsy syndromes and for localization of a seizure focus. Because seizures occur infrequently, EEG activity is usually measured between seizures to determine whether characteristic waveforms, such as sharp

waves or spikes, are present. These waveforms signify a predisposition to epilepsy. Capturing a seizure on EEG usually requires long-term monitoring with video. For some disease processes, the EEG shows specific diagnostic patterns, such as generalized periodic sharp waves in Creutzfeldt-Jakob disease. The EEG is also very useful in the evaluation of comatose patients. There may be distinctive patterns that can suggest a diagnosis of an underlying condition, such as triphasic waves in hepatic coma, spike discharges in nonconvulsive status epilepticus, and excessive beta activity associated with a benzodiazepine or barbiturate drug overdose. Finally, the EEG can be used to confirm brain death in patients in whom the EEG activity has ceased and the clinical criteria for brain death are present.

Plate 3.2

Epilepsy

SEIZURES AND EPILEPSY

Epilepsy is medically defined as a condition characterized by an individual having two or more unprovoked seizures. A seizure is a paroxysmal disorder characterized by an abnormal excessive, hypersynchronous discharge of neurons that results in an alteration of normal brain function. This alteration of function can be quite dramatic, such as during a generalized tonic-clonic (GTC) seizure, or much more subtle, such as during an absence seizure. If the seizures are consistently provoked, such as by fever or hypoglycemia, the term epilepsy should not be used. Epilepsy is not a single disorder but rather a symptom of an underlying brain disorder. Epilepsy is a chronic disorder, although many children will go into remission. Although many people with epilepsy are typical in all other respects, approximately 50% will also have additional cognitive or behavioral impairments.

The history and neurologic examination are the cornerstones of neurologic diagnosis. When assessing whether a patient may have had a seizure, it is important to obtain a description of a paroxysmal change in behavior, whether there was a loss of consciousness, the duration of the spell, and whether stimuli were encountered that might precipitate a seizure. A family history of epilepsy should always be ascertained. Of particular importance in the history is the description of the initial signs or symptoms. For example, the approach to a patient with an aura before a GTC seizure is quite different from the patient who has a GTC seizure without an aura. In the former, it is likely that the patient has a focal onset to the seizure, increasing the chances that there is a structural lesion responsible for the seizure, whereas in the latter instance, it is likely that the patient has a seizure-inducing stimulus, such as low blood sugar or perhaps an underlying genetic condition. Absence seizures of childhood are brief, typically lasting 30 seconds or less, and have a rapid offset, with the child quickly returning to normal mental status. Complex partial seizures are of longer duration, lasting 30 seconds to several minutes, and are typically associated with some degree of confusion and fatigue after the event.

Many episodic disorders resemble seizures. Episodes such as night terrors, breath-holding spells, or syncope may resemble epileptic seizures. The timing of the event is important. When nocturnal, epileptic seizures typically occur in the early morning hours, whereas sleep disorders such as night terrors typically occur several hours after the child falls asleep. A young child for whom the event always occurs in association with provoked crying likely has breath-holding spells. Individuals who feel lightheaded and clammy before losing conscious likely have syncope rather than epilepsy. If there is doubt about the diagnosis, it is usually better to wait before beginning therapy.

Seizures are classified into two major categories: focal and generalized. Focal seizures originate within a localized region of the brain and may evolve into generalized convulsions. Generalized seizures rapidly engage both hemispheres of the brain. Generalized seizures are further classified into tonic, clonic, tonic-clonic, absence, myoclonic, and atonic.

FOCAL (PARTIAL) SEIZURES

Focal seizures originate within networks of a limited region of the brain, often confined to one hemisphere.

FOCAL (PARTIAL) SEIZURES

Focal aware seizures

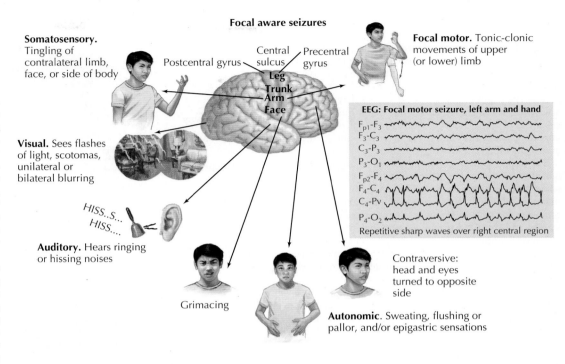

Somatosensory. Tingling of contralateral limb, face, or side of body

Central sulcus • Precentral gyrus • Postcentral gyrus

Leg Trunk Arm Face

Focal motor. Tonic-clonic movements of upper (or lower) limb

Visual. Sees flashes of light, scotomas, unilateral or bilateral blurring

EEG: Focal motor seizure, left arm and hand

F_{p1}-F_3
F_3-C_3
C_3-P_3
P_3-O_1
F_{p2}-F_4
F_4-C_4
C_4-P_V
P_4-O_2

Repetitive sharp waves over right central region

HISS..S.... HISS....

Auditory. Hears ringing or hissing noises

Grimacing

Contraversive: head and eyes turned to opposite side

Autonomic. Sweating, flushing or pallor, and/or epigastric sensations

Focal impaired awareness seizures

Impairment of consciousness: cognitive, affective symptoms

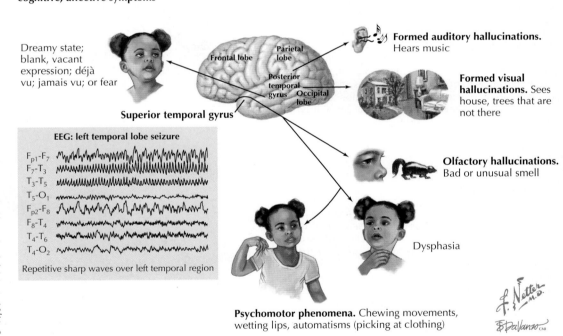

Dreamy state; blank, vacant expression; déjà vu; jamais vu; or fear

Frontal lobe • Parietal lobe • Posterior temporal gyrus • Occipital lobe

Superior temporal gyrus

Formed auditory hallucinations. Hears music

Formed visual hallucinations. Sees house, trees that are not there

Olfactory hallucinations. Bad or unusual smell

EEG: left temporal lobe seizure

F_{p1}-F_7
F_7-T_3
T_3-T_5
T_5-O_1
F_{p2}-F_8
F_8-T_4
T_4-T_6
T_4-O_2

Repetitive sharp waves over left temporal region

Dysphasia

Psychomotor phenomena. Chewing movements, wetting lips, automatisms (picking at clothing)

They can occur at any age. Focal seizures may be classified further into those without impairment of consciousness or awareness (formerly termed simple partial seizures) and those with impairment of consciousness or awareness (formerly termed complex partial seizures). Seizures without impairment of consciousness or awareness can be further subdivided into seizures with (1) observable motor or autonomic components or (2) subjective sensory or psychic phenomenon. The signs or symptoms of focal seizures depend on the location of the focus within the brain. Seizures involving the motor cortex most commonly consist of rhythmic or semirhythmic clonic movements of the face, arm, or leg. There is usually no difficulty in diagnosing this type of seizure. Seizures with somatosensory or autonomic and psychic symptoms (hallucinations, illusions, déjà vu) may be more difficult to diagnose.

Most commonly, psychic symptoms occur as a component of a focal seizure with impaired consciousness

Plate 3.3

Brain: PART I

SEIZURES AND EPILEPSY
(Continued)

or responsiveness. Focal seizures with impairment of consciousness or awareness, formerly termed temporal lobe or psychomotor seizures, are one of the most common seizure types encountered in both children and adults. The beginning of the focal seizure may serve as a warning to the patient (i.e., aura) that a more severe seizure is pending. It is important to recognize that the aura may enable the clinician to determine the cortical area from which the seizure is beginning.

The impairment of consciousness or awareness may be subtle. For example, the patient may either not respond to commands or respond in an abnormally slow manner. Although focal seizures with altered consciousness or awareness may be characterized by simple staring and impaired responsiveness, behavior is usually more complex during the seizure. Automatisms, semipurposeful behaviors of which the patient is unaware and subsequently cannot recall, are common during the period of impaired consciousness. Types of automatism behaviors are quite variable and may consist of activities such as facial grimacing, gestures, chewing, lip smacking, snapping fingers, and repeating phrases. The patient does not fully recall this activity after the seizure. Most patients have some degree of postictal impairment, such as fatigue or confusion after the seizure.

The EEG in focal seizures is characterized by focal spikes or sharp waves. There is often a relationship between the location of the spikes and the seizure type; that is, occipital lobe spikes are associated with occipital lobe seizures, whereas frontal lobe spikes are associated with frontal lobe seizures.

Different types of seizures may evolve in temporal succession in the same patient. For example, a focal seizure starting with normal consciousness and awareness may become associated with alteration in consciousness and subsequently evolve to a generalized convulsive seizure as the seizure starts within a local neural circuit and then spreads to involve an increasing proportion of the brain and ultimately both hemispheres.

GENERALIZED SEIZURES: TONIC-CLONIC SEIZURE

A GTC, or grand mal, seizure is the most severe type of seizure. It starts with a sudden loss of consciousness and generalized tonic stiffening and extension of the body secondary to a widespread contraction of the muscles. The patient may utter a piercing cry resulting from forced expiration of air from the lungs through closed vocal cords. Cessation of respirations with associated cyanosis is secondary to the tonic muscle contractions that prevent normal respiratory movements. The patient often bites their tongue during this phase of the seizure. Salivation occurs because the patient cannot swallow during the seizure. In addition, urinary incontinence is often present.

The initial *tonic phase* of the seizure is followed by the *clonic phase*, in which generalized bilaterally synchronous clonic jerks of the body alternate with brief periods of relaxation. As the periods of relaxation become more prolonged, the clonic movements gradually decrease and finally cease.

During the *postictal phase* after the seizure, the patient is limp, obtunded, and unresponsive. The actual seizure may last about 1 to 2 minutes, and the postictal phase may last from 5 to 20 minutes. Afterward, the patient may arouse but remains confused and, if left undisturbed, may sleep for an hour or so and awaken with a headache and generalized muscle soreness.

GTC seizures may occur at any age. They may be primary generalized seizures, which are generalized from onset, or secondary generalized seizures, which start as focal seizures and then become generalized as the seizure activity progresses to involve widespread areas of the brain.

The EEG of a GTC seizure shows various types of seizure activity that correspond to the different phases of the seizure. During the tonic phase, the EEG shows fast, repetitive, generalized spike discharges. During the clonic phase, the EEG shows spike-and-wave discharges, with the spike corresponding to the clonic jerks and the slow wave to the period of relaxation.

GENERALIZED TONIC-CLONIC SEIZURES

A. Tonic phase

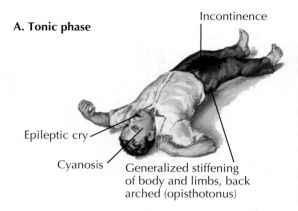

Incontinence

Epileptic cry

Cyanosis

Generalized stiffening of body and limbs, back arched (opisthotonus)

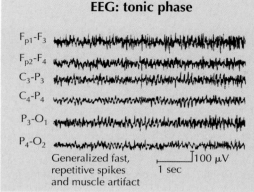

EEG: tonic phase

F_{p1}-F_3
F_{p2}-F_4
C_3-P_3
C_4-P_4
P_3-O_1
P_4-O_2

Generalized fast, repetitive spikes and muscle artifact

100 µV
1 sec

B. Clonic phase

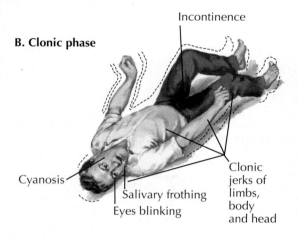

Incontinence

Cyanosis

Salivary frothing

Eyes blinking

Clonic jerks of limbs, body and head

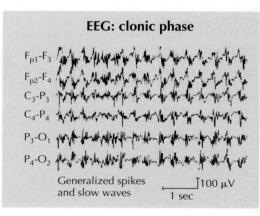

EEG: clonic phase

F_{p1}-F_3
F_{p2}-F_4
C_3-P_3
C_4-P_4
P_3-O_1
P_4-O_2

Generalized spikes and slow waves

100 µV
1 sec

C. Postictal phase

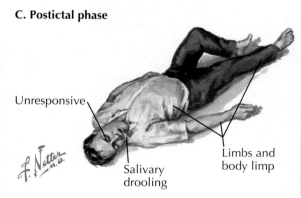

Unresponsive

f. Netter M.D.

Salivary drooling

Limbs and body limp

EEG: postictal phase

F_{p1}-F_3
F_{p2}-F_4
C_3-P_3
C_4-P_4
P_3-O_1
P_4-O_2

Generalized attenuation

100 µV
1 sec

Plate 3.4

Epilepsy

SEIZURES AND EPILEPSY
(Continued)

Finally, during the postictal phase, the EEG shows generalized attenuation of background activity followed by slowing, which gradually decreases as the patient recovers from the seizure.

GENERALIZED SEIZURES: ABSENCE SEIZURES

Absence seizures typically begin and end in childhood, although they can be seen in adults. Absences start abruptly without an aura, lasting from a few seconds to half a minute and ending abruptly. Absence seizures are generalized seizures indicating bihemispheric initial involvement clinically and electroencephalographically. There is typically a sudden cessation of activities with a blank, distant look to the face. As the seizure continues, there are often automatisms and mild clonic motor activity, such as jerks of the arms and eye blinking. Patients are often unaware that they have had a seizure but usually recognize experiencing a "blank" period.

In the untreated patient, absence seizures can occur quite frequently during the day. They sometimes occur in clusters, particularly when the child is tired or drowsy. In a child not on antiseizure drugs, typical absence seizures can almost always be precipitated by hyperventilation.

There are four major syndromes in which typical absence seizures are a major component: childhood absence epilepsy (pyknolepsy), juvenile absence epilepsy, juvenile myoclonic epilepsy, and epilepsy with myoclonic absences. The absence epilepsies appear to have a complex genetic basis. Atypical absence seizures, a form of absence seizures, usually occur in cognitively impaired children who have other seizure types. Unlike typical absence seizures, atypical absence seizures are often longer and have a less distinct onset.

The EEG reveals a bilateral, synchronous symmetric, three cycles per second, spike-and-wave discharge with normal interictal background activity. The interictal EEG in this disorder is distinctive and easily distinguished from other forms of generalized epilepsies. In atypical absence, the spike-and-wave discharges are irregular in frequency and shape and occur at a frequency that is less than three cycles per second.

OTHER GENERALIZED SEIZURES

Myoclonic Seizures

Myoclonic seizures are characterized by sudden, brief (<350 msec), shocklike contractions that may be generalized or confined to the face and trunk or to one or more extremities or even to individual muscles or groups of muscles. Myoclonic seizures result in short bursts of synchronized electromyographic activity. The contractions of muscles are quicker than the contractions with clonic seizures. Any group of muscles can be involved in the jerk. Myoclonic seizures may be dramatic, causing the patient to fall to the ground, or be quite subtle, resembling tremors. Because of the brevity of the seizures, it is not possible to determine whether consciousness is impaired. Myoclonus may occur as a component of an absence seizure or at the beginning of a GTC seizure. The interictal EEG pattern seen in patients with myoclonic seizures typically consists of generalized spike-and-wave discharges.

Tonic Seizures

Tonic seizures are brief seizures (usually <60 seconds) consisting of the sudden onset of increased

tone in the extensor muscles. If standing, the child usually falls to the ground. The seizures are longer than myoclonic seizures. Electromyographic activity is dramatically increased in tonic seizures. There is impairment of consciousness during the seizure, although in short seizures this may be difficult to assess. The EEG ictal manifestations of tonic seizures usually consist of bilateral synchronous spikes of 10 to 25 Hz of medium to high voltage with a frontal accentuation.

Atonic Seizures

Atonic (astatic) seizures, or drop attacks, are characterized by a sudden loss of muscle tone. They begin suddenly and without warning and cause the patient, if standing, to fall quickly to the ground. Because there may be total lack of tone, the child has no protective response, and injuries occur. The attack may be fragmentary and lead to dropping of the head with slackening of the jaw or dropping of a limb. In atonic seizures, there is a loss of electromyographic activity.

ABSENCE SEIZURES

Absence seizures represent abnormal interactions between cortical and thalamic transmissions

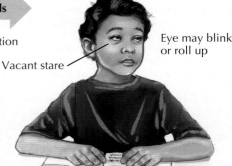

Cortex

Thalamus

Generalized bilateral seizure activity

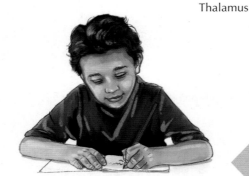

Child alert and attentive before and after seizure

Sudden onset

2–15 seconds

Sudden cessation

Loss of attention

Vacant stare

Eye may blink or roll up

Typical absence seizure. Impaired awareness and responsiveness for 2–15 seconds.

F_{p1}-F_3
F_3-C_3
F_{p1}-P_3
F_{p2}-F_4
F_4-C_4
C_4-P_4

EEG, atypical absence pattern. Atypical absence seizures may be associated with intellectual disability and tonic or atonic seizures.

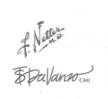

F_7-T_3
F_3-C_3
C_3-P_3
F_3-T_4
F_4-C_4
C_4-P_4

EEG, typical absence pattern

Plate 3.5

Brain: PART I

Infantile spasms (West syndrome)

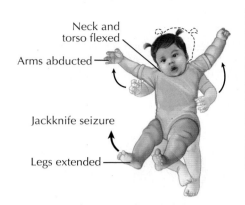

Neck and torso flexed

Arms abducted

Jackknife seizure

Legs extended

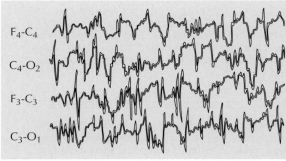

EEG. Hypsarrhythmia typical of interictal pattern in children with infantile spasms

EPILEPSY SYNDROMES

Once the seizure type has been identified, the clinician should try to determine the epileptic syndrome. An epilepsy syndrome is a cluster of clinical and EEG features that occur together more commonly than would be expected by chance. Epilepsy syndrome identification aids in identifying etiology and provides the clinician with guidance regarding long-term prognosis. A large proportion of epilepsy syndromes have a genetic basis.

An example of an epilepsy syndrome with generalized seizures is *juvenile myoclonic epilepsy* (JME). The seizure types are GTC, absence, or myoclonic, which often occur upon awakening. The seizures begin in adolescence or early adulthood in an otherwise healthy individual. The interictal EEG reveals spike-and-wave activity at a frequency of 3.5 to 6.0 Hz, and neuroimaging is normal. Although the seizures are usually controlled with antiseizure drugs, the condition is lifelong. A single-gene mutation has not been identified, and many investigators feel the condition likely involves multiple genes. Once diagnosed with JME, the patient can be provided specific information regarding prognosis and treatment.

Benign rolandic epilepsy, also called benign childhood epilepsy with central-temporal spikes, is a genetic disorder confined to children. It is characterized by nocturnal generalized seizures of probable focal onset, diurnal simple partial seizures arising from the lower rolandic area, and an EEG pattern consisting of midtemporal-central spike foci. The characteristic features of daytime seizures include (1) somatosensory stimulation of the oral-buccal cavity, (2) speech arrest, (3) preservation of consciousness, (4) drooling, and (5) tonic or tonic-clonic activity of the face. Less often, the somatosensory sensation spreads to the face or arm. Most attacks involve the face, and arrest of speech may initiate the attack or occur during its course. Consciousness is rarely impaired during the daytime attacks, although the child cannot speak because of the motor involvement. Often the child's gestures will indicate to the parents that the child is totally aware during the event. The characteristic interictal EEG abnormality is a high-amplitude, usually diphasic spike, with a prominent following slow wave. The spikes or sharp waves appear singly or in groups in the midtemporal and central (rolandic) region (C3, C4).

Infantile spasms are brief episodes of tonic flexor or extensor movements, or both, of the body and limbs. These spasms are seen in infants and young children

Juvenile myoclonic epilepsy

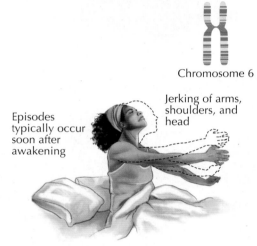

Chromosome 6

Episodes typically occur soon after awakening

Jerking of arms, shoulders, and head

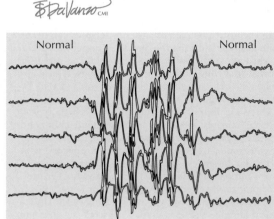

Normal   Normal

EEG. 3–6 Hz spikes and polyspikes and slow waves

Benign rolandic epilepsy

Heterozygous affected

Normal

Dominant inheritance pattern

Motor, sensory, or autonomic seizures involving face or oropharynx

Seizures often occur during sleep

$F_{p2}-F_8$
F_8-T_4
T_4-T_6
C_3-C_z
C_z-C_4
C_4-T_4

EEG. Pattern typical of benign rolandic epilepsy

up to 4 years of age and usually result from a severe cerebral insult before, at, or shortly after birth or from an insult or disease process occurring within the first few months to 1 year after birth. One of the most common types of infantile spasm is characterized by forward flexion of the head and body, with the arms flung forward or outward. The EEG in infantile spasms shows a characteristic pattern called hypsarrhythmia, consisting of high-amplitude multifocal spikes and slow waves. During the spasm, the EEG shows an abrupt generalized decrement in the amplitude of the ongoing activity.

Infantile spasms are often treated with adrenocorticotropic hormone, corticosteroids, or vigabatrin.

Lennox-Gastaut syndrome is a severe seizure syndrome that typically begins between the ages of 3 and 5 years. Children have different types of seizures, most commonly tonic, GTC, atonic, and atypical absence seizures. The EEG shows high-amplitude, slow (<2.5 Hz) spike-and-wave activity. Cognitive impairment is a common feature of the disorder. The syndrome can be very difficult to treat with antiseizure medications, and most children need a combination of different drugs or nondrug treatments such as the ketogenic diet or vagus nerve stimulation.

Plate 3.6

Epilepsy

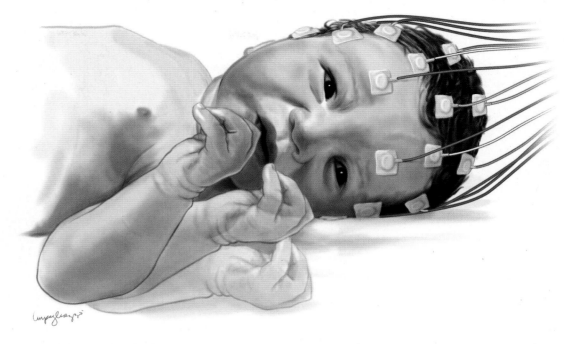

The most common seizure type in neonates is focal. In this example, the newborn is having focal clonic activity of the left arm with eye deviation to the left. The EEG shows electrographic seizures with rhythmic spikes coming from the right hemisphere. The seizure in the right hemisphere is responsible for both the left arm jerking and eye deviation.

NEONATAL SEIZURES

Neonatal seizures are one of the most common, yet most ominous, neurologic signs in newborns. Because seizures may be the first and only sign of a central nervous system disorder, their recognition is extremely important. A considerable difference is apparent in the behavior observed during seizures in neonates and the behaviors seen in older children and adults. Infants are unable to sustain organized generalized epileptiform discharges, and GTC and absence seizures do not occur. The age-dependent clinical and EEG features of seizures in neonates are a result of the immaturity of cortical organization and myelination.

Neonatal seizures are classified as clonic, tonic, and myoclonic. Clonic seizures consist of rhythmic jerking of groups of muscles and occur in either a focal or multifocal pattern. In multifocal clonic seizures, movements may migrate from one part of the body to another. Although focal seizures may be seen with localized brain insults, such as neonatal strokes, they may also be seen in disorders that diffusely affect the brain, such as asphyxia, subarachnoid hemorrhage, hypoglycemia, and infection. In tonic seizures, the infant develops asymmetric posturing of the trunk or deviation of the eyes to one side. Myoclonic seizures are similar to those seen in older children, consisting of rapid jerks of muscles. The myoclonic seizures can consist of bilateral jerks, although occasionally unilateral or focal myoclonus can occur.

Sick neonates often display repetitive, stereotyped behavior that may be confused with seizures. These

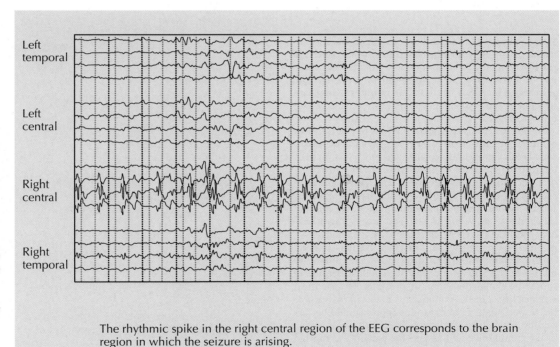

The rhythmic spike in the right central region of the EEG corresponds to the brain region in which the seizure is arising.

behaviors include repetitive sucking and other oral-buccal-lingual movements, assumption of an abnormal posture, pedaling movements of the legs or paddling movements of the arms, blinking, momentary fixation of gaze with or without eye deviation, nystagmus, and apnea. However, when these behaviors are observed during EEG recordings, epileptiform activity is usually not recorded. Likewise, when tonic posturing involves all four extremities and the trunk, an associated EEG

epileptiform discharge rarely appears. Myoclonus not associated with epileptiform discharges can also be seen in sick neonates.

Although the diagnosis of seizures relies primarily on clinical observation, the EEG may be extremely valuable in confirming the presence of epileptic seizures. In addition, the EEG is very useful in the detection of electrographic seizures in paralyzed infants or in assessing response to antiseizure medications.

Plate 3.7

Brain: PART I

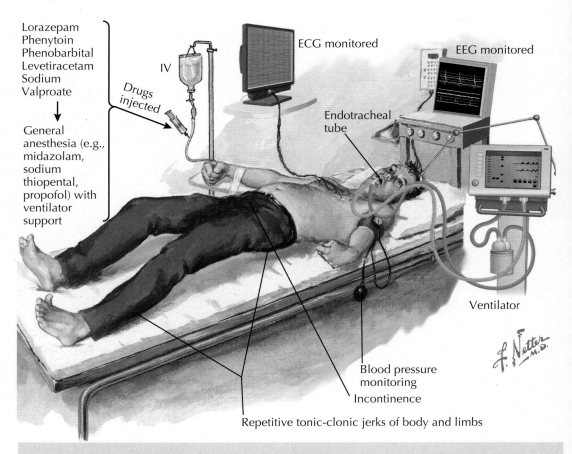

Lorazepam
Phenytoin
Phenobarbital
Levetiracetam
Sodium
Valproate

↓

General
anesthesia (e.g.,
midazolam,
sodium
thiopental,
propofol) with
ventilator
support

Drugs
injected

IV

ECG monitored

EEG monitored

Endotracheal
tube

Ventilator

Blood pressure
monitoring

Incontinence

Repetitive tonic-clonic jerks of body and limbs

STATUS EPILEPTICUS

Status epilepticus is a condition in which the mechanisms that usually terminate seizures have failed. It is usually defined as a seizure or series of seizures without full recovery of consciousness between the seizures, which last at least 30 minutes. There are two major types of status epilepticus: convulsive and nonconvulsive.

Convulsive status epilepticus (CSE) is one of the most common medical neurologic emergencies and is associated with significant mortality and morbidity. In people with epilepsy, CSE is often provoked by withdrawal or reduction of antiseizure drugs. However, more than 50% of people with CSE have never had an epileptic seizure before. The most common causes in children are febrile seizures, meningitis, and preexisting neurologic disorders such as cerebral palsy. In adults, CSE is often caused by cerebrovascular insults, cerebral anoxia, alcohol withdrawal, drug abuse, and tumors. To minimize the risk of an adverse outcome, treatment should be initiated as soon as possible. Because most seizures begin in the community, medications such as rectal, buccal, or nasal benzodiazepines should be carried by emergency medical technicians, administered in the community setting, and the patient transported urgently to the nearest emergency department. In the hospital setting, an airway should be immediately provided and maintained. Cardiorespiratory status and other vital functions should be assessed and support given if necessary. Blood samples should be drawn for analysis, and an infusion of normal saline should be started. The initial in-hospital treatment is usually a benzodiazepine, such as lorazepam, administered intravenously. If benzodiazepines fail to terminate the seizure, levetiracetam, sodium valproate, phenytoin, or phenobarbitone may be administered. If seizures remain uncontrolled, general anesthesia and artificial ventilation may be required.

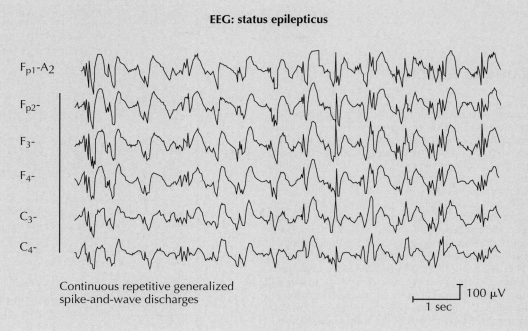

EEG: status epilepticus

F_{p1}-A_2

F_{p2}-

F_3-

F_4-

C_3-

C_4-

Continuous repetitive generalized
spike-and-wave discharges

100 µV

1 sec

Nonconvulsive status epilepticus (NCSE) refers to the condition in which there is EEG evidence of continuous epileptiform abnormalities in the absence of obvious clinical motor manifestations. NCSE in patients with epilepsy often occurs in the context of absence epilepsy and focal seizures, particularly those arising in the temporal lobe. Patients with confusion may have NCSE, and patients admitted to an intensive care unit may also develop NCSE. Because NCSE may worsen the prognosis of the underlying disorder, treatment of the status epilepticus is recommended. However, there is debate on whether aggressive therapy with anesthetic agents is warranted. Epilepsia partialis continua refers to continuous focal motor activity that may last months to years. The most common cause is Rasmussen encephalitis.

Plate 3.8

Epilepsy

Primary

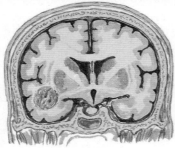

?　?

Unknown (genetic or
biochemical predisposition)

Extracranial

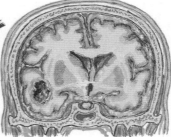

Metabolic

Electrolyte

Biochemical

Inborn errors
of metabolism

Anoxia

Hypoglycemia

Drugs

Drug withdrawal

Alcohol
withdrawal

CAUSES OF SEIZURES

The etiology of epilepsy is classified into three broad categories: genetic and neurometabolic, structural, and systemic.

GENETIC AND NEUROMETABOLIC CAUSES

Many genetic and neurometabolic causes lead to seizures, typically beginning in childhood. Genetic disorders include severe myoclonic epilepsy of childhood, tuberous sclerosis, Rett syndrome, Angelman syndrome, and fragile X syndrome. Neurometabolic disorders, which may also have a genetic cause, result in disturbances of metabolism and can lead to seizures. Disorders such as urea cycle defects, pyridoxine dependency, biotinidase deficiency, and glucose transporter deficiencies can cause severe seizures.

STRUCTURAL CAUSES

The most common types of brain lesions causing seizures are tumors, vascular lesions, head trauma, infectious diseases, congenital malformation of the brain, and biochemical or degenerative disease processes affecting the brain.

Brain tumor is an important cause of seizures, particularly in the adult patient, and becomes an increasingly likely cause after the second decade of life and one of the main causes in the fourth and fifth decades. A brain tumor should be suspected in any person who has onset of seizures, especially focal seizures, after age 20 years.

Head trauma is a major cause of seizures, which may occur shortly after the head injury or, more often, several months to several years later. Factors that increase the chance of development of posttraumatic seizures are a penetrating head injury, severe damage to the brain, prolonged periods of unconsciousness, posttraumatic amnesia, complications of wound healing, and a persistent neurologic deficit.

Vascular disease is one of the most common causes of seizures in older persons, particularly after age 50 years. Seizures can occur transiently after an acute stroke (thrombotic, embolic, or hemorrhagic) or may develop later as a sequela of cerebrovascular disease. Although uncommon, arteriovenous malformations are frequently associated with seizures. Other vascular causes include subdural hematomas, venous thrombosis, and hypertensive encephalopathy.

Seizures may occur with any *acute infection* of the nervous system or as a complication of damage to the

Intracranial

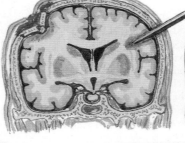

Tumor

Vascular (infarct or hemorrhage)

Lissencephaly

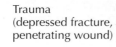

Trauma
(depressed fracture,
penetrating wound)

Infection
(abscess,
encephalitis)

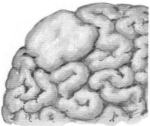

Congenital and
hereditary diseases
(tuberous sclerosis)

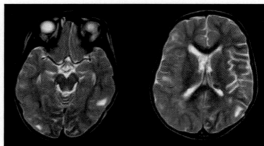

Tuberous sclerosis complex

nervous system by the inflammatory process. Patients with *cerebral abscesses* have a high incidence of seizures, and *encephalitis* and *meningoencephalitis* may be associated with either focal or generalized seizures.

Congenital brain malformations are a common cause of childhood seizures. With improved neuroimaging, many patients who were thought to have idiopathic epilepsy have now been found to have brain malformations. The severity of the seizures is related to the type and extent of the malformation.

SYSTEMIC CAUSES

Disease processes or disorders that can cause seizures include various types of metabolic, electrolyte, and biochemical disturbances; hypoxia; hypoglycemia; toxic processes; drugs; or abrupt withdrawal from drugs or alcohol. Various conditions, such as fever, fatigue, sleep deprivation, flashing lights, sound, or emotional factors, may also precipitate seizures in susceptible individuals. In young children, fever is a common cause of seizures.

Plate 3.9

Brain: PART I

Neurobiology of Epilepsy

The core feature of brain electrochemical signals is the neuron membrane. Like all cell membranes, the neuron membrane is a phospholipid bilayer. This lipid bilayer prevents the exchange of ionized substrates between the cell and its environment, which is critical for electrical signaling. The inside of the cell at rest is negatively charged compared with the outside of the cell due to concentration differences in ions. Sodium (Na$^+$), calcium (Ca^{2+}), and chloride (Cl$^-$) are predominantly found extracellularly, whereas potassium (K$^+$) and organic ions are concentrated intracellularly. These concentration differences are due to specific ion transporters that use the cell's energy supply to continuously move ions in and out of the cell. These pumps create concentration differences (between the inside and outside of the neuron) by transporting ions against their concentration gradients (from regions of low concentration to regions of high concentration). This concentration gradient across the membrane provides the electrochemical energy to drive signaling. These ions will flow through the membrane through protein channels. Most channels are ion selective and will allow the passage of a specific ion. Unlike the continuous transport by the ion pumps, transport by the ion channels is noncontinuous. Ion channels open or close in response to signals from their environment. Voltage-gated channels open or close in response to changes in electrical potential across the cell membrane, whereas ligand-gated channels require a binding of a particular signaling molecule to open or close.

The two most important ions in the transmission of action potentials are Na$^+$ and K$^+$. Voltage-gated Na$^+$ channels have three types of states: deactivated (closed), activated (open), and inactivated (closed). During excitation of the cell, Na$^+$ channels are activated through removal of an intracellular "activation gate," and Na$^+$ begins flowing into the cell. Once some Na$^+$ ion channels begin opening, the voltage drops further, causing more channels to open until the membrane depolarizes. Na$^+$ channels are more sensitive to voltage change than K$^+$ channels are and open more rapidly. Thus, in a depolarization, the Na$^+$ ions will rush into the cell faster than the K$^+$ ions move outward. This sudden depolarization, called an action potential, will briefly result in a +30 millivolt potential difference. Once the slowly opening voltage-gated K$^+$ ion channels have opened and allowed K$^+$ to flow out, the action potential is ended. Once Na$^+$ channels are activated, they quickly are inactivated because of an "inactivation gate" that blocks the inside of the channel shortly after it has been activated. During an action potential, the channel remains inactivated for a few milliseconds after depolarization. The inactivation is removed when the membrane potential of the cell repolarizes after the falling phase of the action potential. This allows the channels to be activated again during the next action potential. Thus the Na$^+$ ion channels initiate the action potential and the K$^+$ ion channels terminate it. The channels then close, and the sodium pump can restore the resting potential of −70 millivolts.

Membrane polarity is also affected by ligand-gated channels that open when neurotransmitters, the ligands of synaptic transmission, bind to specific receptors connected to the channels. Glutamate is the primary excitatory neurotransmitter and γ-aminobutyric acid

ION CHANNELS IN EPILEPSY

A. The movement of ions across the cell membrane is dependent upon both concentration and electrostatic forces. Ions flow from high concentrations to lower concentrations as depicted by the flow of K$^+$ ions from inside the cell, where the concentration is high, to outside the cell, where the concentration is lower.

B. Ions are attracted to charges of the opposite polarity. In this example, K$^+$ ions flow from the extracellular environment, which is positive in relationship to the intracellular space, which is negative. Both concentration and electrostatic forces determine flow of ions. The equilibrium potential for the ion is the membrane potential at which a particular ion does not diffuse through the membrane in either direction.

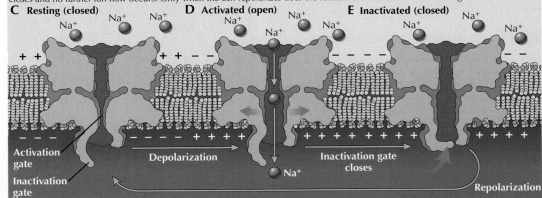

Concentration gradient moves K$^+$ out of cell

Electrical potential difference moves K$^+$ into cell

Extracellular

Intracellular

Three states of the sodium channel. C. In the resting state, no ion flow occurs due to closure of the activation gate. **D.** When the membrane begins to depolarize, the activation channel opens and ion flow occurs. **E.** As the cell becomes depolarized, the inactivation gate closes and no further ion flow occurs. Only when the cell repolarizes does the sodium channel return to the resting state.

C Resting (closed)

D Activated (open)

E Inactivated (closed)

Activation gate

Inactivation gate

Depolarization

Inactivation gate closes

Repolarization

F. An action potential is a short-lasting event in which the electrical membrane potential of a cell rapidly rises and falls. Action potentials begin with an inward flow of Na$^+$ ions, which changes the electrochemical gradient, which in turn produces a further change in the membrane potential. This then causes more channels to open, producing a greater electric current. The process proceeds until most of the available ion channels open, resulting in a large upswing in the membrane potential. The rapid influx of Na$^+$ ions causes the polarity of the plasma membrane to reverse, and the ion channels then rapidly inactivate. Potassium channels are then activated, and there is an outward current of K$^+$ ions, returning the electrochemical gradient to the resting state. After an action potential has occurred, there is a transient negative shift, called the afterhyperpolarization, or refractory period, due to additional potassium currents.

G. The release of a neurotransmitter is triggered by the arrival of a nerve impulse (or action potential) and occurs through a process called exocytosis. Within the presynaptic nerve terminal, vesicles containing neurotransmitter sit "docked" and ready at the synaptic membrane. The arriving action potential produces an influx of Ca^{2+} ions through voltage-dependent, Ca^{2+}-selective ion channels. Ca^{2+} ions then bind with the proteins found within the membranes of the synaptic vesicles, allowing the vesicles to "dock" with the presynaptic membrane, resulting in the creation of a fusion pore. The vesicles then release their contents to the synaptic cleft.

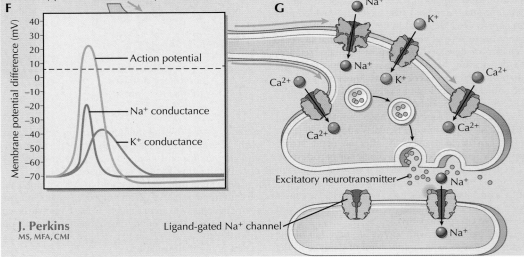

F — Membrane potential difference (mV): 40, 30, 20, 10, 0, −10, −20, −30, −40, −50, −60, −70

Action potential

Na$^+$ conductance

K$^+$ conductance

G — Excitatory neurotransmitter

Ligand-gated Na$^+$ channel

J. Perkins
MS, MFA, CMI

Plate 3.10

Epilepsy

SYNAPTIC RECEPTORS IN EPILEPSY

NEUROBIOLOGY OF EPILEPSY (Continued)

(GABA), the principal inhibitory transmitter. Synaptic transmission is mediated by glutamate that is released from the pyramidal neurons and depolarizes and excites the target neurons via ionotropic receptors (NMDA, α-amino-3-hydroxy-5-methylisoxazole-4-proprionic acid [AMPA], and kainic acid). Glutamate channel opening allows Na^+ and Ca^{2+} to enter the cell, resulting in depolarization, whereas with GABA channel opening, Cl^- enters the cell, resulting in hyperpolarization.

Once the action potential is generated, it propagates to the synapse. Depending on the type of cell, an excitatory or inhibitory neurotransmitter is released. The effect of the neurotransmitter on the postsynaptic membrane will determine current flow into or out of the postsynaptic cell, thus determining whether the postsynaptic cell will generate action potentials.

Epilepsy is a paroxysmal disorder characterized by abnormal neuronal discharges. Although epilepsy has many causes, the fundamental disorder is secondary to abnormal synchronous discharges of a network of neurons. Epilepsy is secondary to an imbalance between excitatory and inhibitory input to cells.

The hallmark of epileptic neurons in experimental models of epilepsy is membrane depolarization, which results in an interictal spike recorded by EEG. During an interictal discharge, the cell membrane near the soma undergoes a relatively high-voltage (approximately 10–15 mV) and relatively long (100–200 μsec) depolarization. The long depolarization has the effect of generating a train of action potentials that are conducted away from the soma along the axon of the neuron. This large depolarization is called the paroxysmal depolarization shift (PDS). The PDS is caused by an imbalance of excitation over inhibition. This enhanced excitation, or reduced inhibition, can be secondary to a variety of abnormalities, including disturbances in the intrinsic properties of neuronal membranes, excess excitation through NMDA and AMPA receptors, reduced inhibition through GABA channels, and abnormalities of potassium and calcium channels. The net effect is an imbalance of excitation over inhibition. The interictal PDS is followed by a large hyperpolarization, which serves to limit the duration of interictal paroxysms. It is important to remember that an epileptic area is made up of numerous abnormal neurons that discharge in an abnormal synchronous manner. The PDS may occur because of intrinsic membrane abnormalities in a group of neurons or because of excessive excitatory input (or reduced inhibitory input) to a group of neurons.

With time, a progressive loss of hyperpolarization after the PDS may occur in the epileptic focus. During seizures, the epileptic neurons undergo prolonged depolarization with waves of action potentials during the tonic phase of the seizure and oscillations of membrane potentials with bursts of action potentials, separated by quiet periods during the clonic phase. An EEG recorded at the scalp at this time shows continuous spikes, which generally coincide with the tonic stage of a GTC seizure. During the next stage, large inhibitory potentials occur (with slowing or flattening on surface EEG) and alternate with recurrent, rhythmic PDSs (with spikes on surface EEG). This pattern generally coincides with the clonic stage of the seizure.

Focal seizures may spread along the cortex and propagate to distant regions via white matter tracts.

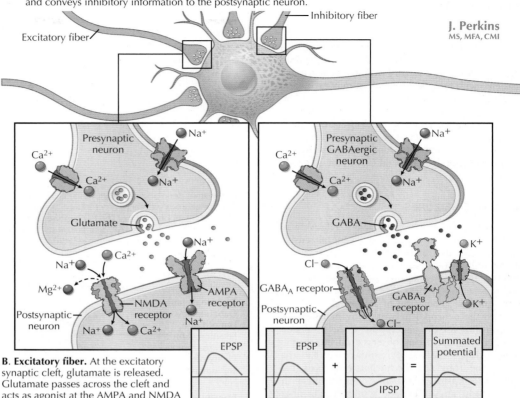

A. Postsynaptic neuron at which several presynaptic afferent fibers terminate. Fibers colored in pink convey excitatory information across the synaptic cleft to the postsynaptic neuron, whereas the inhibitory fiber is blue and conveys inhibitory information to the postsynaptic neuron.

J. Perkins
MS, MFA, CMI

B. Excitatory fiber. At the excitatory synaptic cleft, glutamate is released. Glutamate passes across the cleft and acts as agonist at the AMPA and NMDA ionotropic receptor. The excitatory neurotransmitters signal the AMPA channel to open, permitting the inflow of Na^+. This results in depolarization in the membrane potential so that the difference in potential across the membrane is shifted toward the positive (i.e., depolarization). With depolarization, there is a release of Mg^{2+} from the NMDA receptor, permitting Na^+ and Ca^{2+} ions to enter the postsynaptic neuron. An excitatory postsynaptic potential (EPSP) is generated.

C. Inhibitory fiber. The inhibitory neurotransmitters, principally GABA, act on GABA receptors in the postsynaptic neuron membrane, permitting the entry of Cl^- ions, shifting the membrane potential to a more negative potential (i.e., hyperpolarization). An inhibitory postsynaptic potential (IPSP) is generated. In normal synaptic transmission, there is a balance between excitatory and inhibitory neurotransmitters so that the summation of EPSP and IPSP maintains the polarization of the membrane at a level below the threshold at which bursts of firing occur, termed the resting potential.

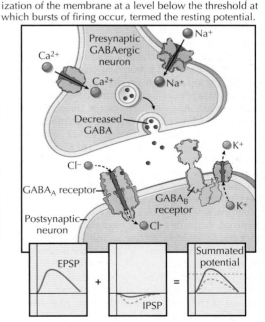

D. Increase in glutamate EPSP. With an increase in excitatory neurotransmitters, the postsynaptic neuron membrane becomes more positive, producing an increase in EPSP. The summation of the excitatory and inhibitory signals moves across the threshold value, and an action potential occurs.

E. Decrease in IPSP. When there is a decrease in inhibitory neurotransmitters, the IPSP decreases, and the postsynaptic neuron membrane becomes more positive. The summation of the excitatory and inhibitory signals moves across the threshold value, and an action potential is fired.

Plate 3.11

Brain: PART I

NEUROBIOLOGY OF EPILEPSY
(Continued)

Many patients with focal seizures will have an aura at the onset. The type of aura depends on the region of the brain in which the seizure originated. For example, patients with temporal lobe onset may experience déjà vu (the experience of feeling sure that one has already witnessed or experienced a current situation), whereas a patient with parietal lobe onset may experience a sensation of numbness or tingling. With propagation, more and more neurons are recruited into synchronous firing, which could culminate in a GTC seizure.

GENERALIZED SEIZURES

Unlike focal seizures, which involve a relatively restricted group of neurons at onset, generalized seizures result from dysfunction of networks of neurons involving multiple brain regions. The basic underlying mechanism in absence seizures, and possibly other generalized seizure types, involves thalamocortical circuitry and the generation of abnormal oscillatory rhythms in the neuronal network. The neuronal circuit responsible for the generation of the oscillatory thalamocortical burst firing observed during absence seizures includes cortical pyramidal neurons, thalamic relay neurons, and the nucleus reticularis thalami (NRT). The principal synaptic connections of the thalamocortical circuit include glutamatergic fibers between neocortical pyramidal cells and the NRT; GABAergic connections between cells of the NRT, which activate $GABA_A$ receptors; and GABAergic fibers from NRT neurons, which activate $GABA_A$ and $GABA_B$ receptors on thalamic relay neurons.

The cellular events that underlie the ability of NRT neurons to shift between an oscillatory and tonic firing mode are the low-threshold (T) Ca^{2+} spikes that are present in thalamocortical and NRT neurons. These T-type Ca^{2+} channels are a key membrane property involved in burst firing excitation and are associated with the change from oscillatory to burst firing in thalamocortical cells. Mild depolarization of these neurons is sufficient to activate these channels and to allow the influx of extracellular Ca^{2+}. Further depolarization produced by Ca^{2+} inflow will exceed the threshold for firing a burst of action potentials. After T-channels are activated, they become inactivated rather quickly; hence the name *transient*. Deinactivation of T-channels requires a relatively lengthy hyperpolarization. $GABA_B$ receptor–mediated hyperpolarization is a primary factor in the deinactivation of T-channels.

Recurrent collateral GABAergic fibers from the NRT neurons activate $GABA_A$ receptors on adjacent NRT neurons. Activating $GABA_A$ receptors in the NRT therefore results in an inhibition of inhibitory output to the thalamic relay neurons. Because of the decreased $GABA_B$ activation, there would be a reduced likelihood that Ca^{2+} deinactivation would occur. This would result in decreased oscillatory firing. However, direct $GABA_A$ and $GABA_B$ activation of thalamic relay neurons would be expected to have detrimental effects, increasing hyperpolarization and therefore increasing the likelihood of deinactivation of the T-channels. The abnormal oscillatory rhythms in absence seizures can be caused by abnormalities of the T-type Ca^{2+} channels or enhanced $GABA_B$ function.

ANTISEIZURE DRUG TARGETS

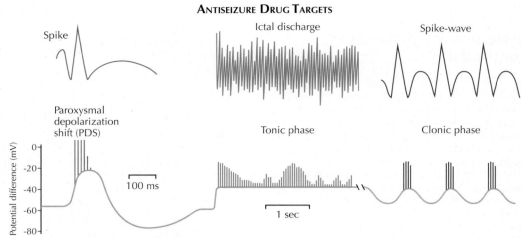

A. Paroxysmal depolarization shift (PDS) is a cellular marker of epilepsy and consists of a large depolarization of a group of neurons with action potentials, as indicated by the vertical lines on the large depolarization. The PDS is followed by repolarization. The PDS and repolarization correspond to a spike and wave on the EEG. A seizure occurs when there is a massive depolarization of cells without intervening periods of repolarization. This would correspond to the tonic phase of the seizure. As inhibition increases during the seizure, there is a cycle of PDS followed by repolarization. This corresponds to the clonic phase of the seizure

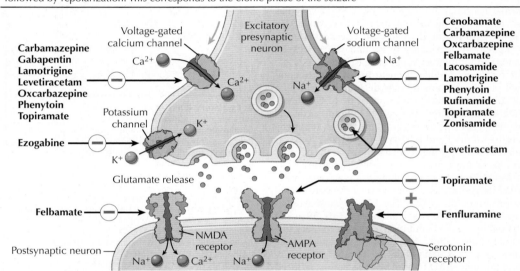

B. Examples of molecular targets of antiepileptic drugs that reduce excitability. This may occur through blockage of calcium, sodium, and potassium channels or through reducing ion flow through NMDA and AMPA receptors. Levetiracetam binds to synaptic vesicles, which may lead to reduced neurotransmitter release.

J. Perkins

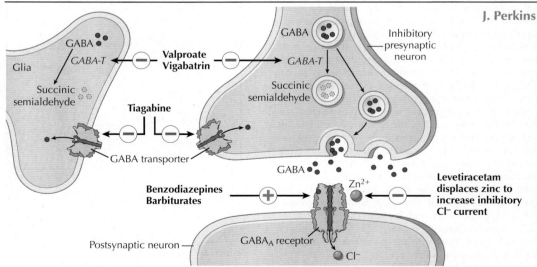

C. Examples of molecular targets of antiepileptic drugs that enhance inhibition. Drugs may increase amount of GABA postsynaptically by blocking GABA uptake or increase intracellular GABA by reducing degradation of GABA. Enhancing chloride flow through the GABA receptor is a common mechanism of inhibitory drugs, such as barbiturates and benzodiazepines. Levetiracetam displaces zinc from the GABA receptor, which results in increased chloride currents.

Plate 3.12

Epilepsy

PREOPERATIVE EVALUATION

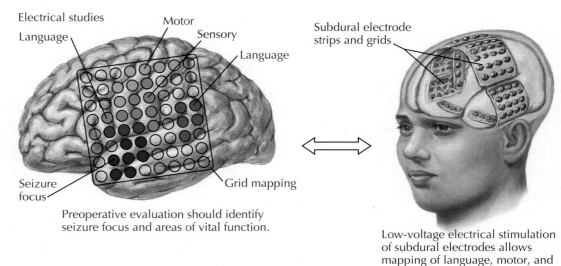

Electrical studies
Motor
Sensory
Language
Language

Seizure focus
Grid mapping

Preoperative evaluation should identify seizure focus and areas of vital function.

Subdural electrode strips and grids

Low-voltage electrical stimulation of subdural electrodes allows mapping of language, motor, and other vital areas.

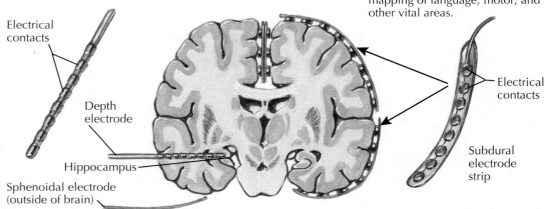

Electrical contacts

Depth electrode

Hippocampus

Sphenoidal electrode (outside of brain)

Electrical contacts

Subdural electrode strip

TREATMENT OF EPILEPSY

Although there are a variety of treatment options for seizures, the three main approaches are antiseizure drugs, dietary therapy, and surgery.

The vast majority of patients are treated with antiseizure drugs that work on a variety of targets that alter the excitatory/inhibitory balance of the brain: (1) blocking sodium and calcium channels or opening potassium channels, (2) reducing excitation by blocking glutamate receptors, (3) increasing inhibition by enhancing GABA currents or increasing extracellular or intracellular GABA concentrations, (4) increasing inhibition through increased serotonin release, and (5) reducing excitability via activating endocannabinoid receptors.

Drugs targeting the Na^+ channel reduce the likelihood of a seizure by either increasing the amount of time the channel stays in the inactive state or by altering the shape of the Na^+ channel. In both cases, the drugs prevent sustained repetitive firing of the cells. Likewise, Ca^{2+} channel blockers are used to block T-type Ca^{2+} channels or high-voltage activated channels, resulting in decreased excitability of the cells. Ca^{2+} is also critical in the release of a neurotransmitter from synaptic vesicles. Reducing release of glutamate would reduce the likelihood of a seizure. Levetiracetam binds to synaptic vesicles and appears to reduce seizure frequency by altering the release of neurotransmitters from synaptic vesicles.

Blocking excitation through the NMDA, AMPA, and kainate receptors can reduce excitation by reducing the inward flow of Na^+ and Ca^{2+} ions. Likewise, drugs

Multiple depth electrodes (stereoencephalography) placed around the probable seizure onset zone to identify an area of brain to be resected.

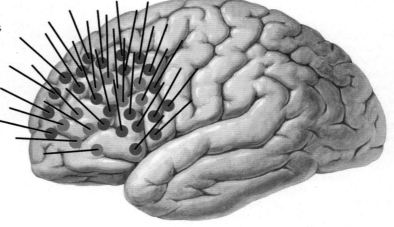

acting on $GABA_A$ receptors facilitate the passage of Cl^- into cells. Their passage into the cell makes the resting membrane potential more negative inside the cell and makes it more difficult for the cell to depolarize. The $GABA_A$ receptor has benzodiazepine and barbiturate receptor sites. Activation of the benzodiazepine receptor enhances the frequency of openings of the $GABA_A$

receptor. Activation of the barbiturate receptor increases the duration of openings of the $GABA_A$ receptor. The GABA effect can also be increased by blocking reuptake of GABA by neurons and glia, increasing the concentration of GABA at postsynaptic receptors, or reducing GABA breakdown in the neurons through inhibition of GABA transaminase.

Plate 3.13

Brain: PART I

RESECTIVE SURGERY

Temporal lobectomy

Amygdaloid body

Hippocampus

Temporal lobe

Insula

Amygdaloid body remnant

Temporal lobe remnant

Hippocampus

Lateral ventricle

Area of resection

Temporal lobe containing seizure focus resected. Amygdaloid body and distal hippocampus usually included in resection.

Hemispherectomy

Cingulate gyrus

Corpus callosum

3rd ventricle

Frontal lobe remnant

Insula and basal ganglia preserved

Parieto-occipital remnant

Basal ganglia

JOHN A. CRAIG—AD

Temporal lobe and central suprasylvian cortex are resected, preserving basal ganglia. All connections of frontal and parieto-occipital remnants to corpus callosum are severed.

Area of resection

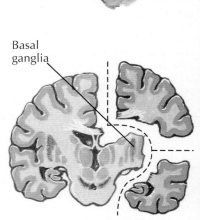

TREATMENT OF EPILEPSY
(Continued)

The ketogenic diet is typically used to treat children with severe epilepsy who do not respond to antiseizure drugs. The ketogenic diet consists of a high proportion of fats and small amounts of carbohydrate and protein. The basis of the therapeutic effectiveness of the ketogenic diet is thought to be the ketosis that develops when the brain is relatively deprived of glucose as an energy source and must shift to use of ketone bodies as the primary fuel.

Patients who do not respond to antiseizure drugs or dietary therapy may benefit from surgery. In patients with well-localized seizures focus, resection of the epileptic tissue may be possible. If the epileptic focus is coming from a brain area where resection would result in a significant neurologic deficit, such as weakness, aphasia, or memory impairment, focal surgery is not recommended. The most common surgery for focal seizure is a temporal lobe resection. In rare individuals with a severely damaged hemisphere who have unilateral weakness and seizures arising from that hemisphere, a hemispherectomy can be curative. Patients with severe focal seizures with secondary generalization may be helped by cutting the corpus callosum (corpus callosotomy). This reduces the likelihood that a focal seizure will become generalized.

Vagus nerve stimulation (VNS) is an adjunctive treatment for certain types of intractable epilepsy and treatment-resistant depression. VNS uses an implanted stimulator that sends electric impulses to the left vagus nerve in the neck via a lead wire implanted under the skin. The tenth cranial nerve arises from the medulla and carries both afferent and efferent fibers. The afferent vagal fibers connect to the nucleus of the solitary tract, which in turn projects connections to other locations in the central nervous system. Little is understood about exactly how vagal nerve stimulation improves seizure control, but proposed mechanisms include alteration of norepinephrine release by projections of solitary tract to the locus coeruleus, elevated levels of inhibitory GABA related to vagal stimulation, and inhibition of aberrant cortical activity by reticular system activation.

PSYCHIATRY

Plate 4.1

Brain: PART I

LIMBIC SYSTEM

Initially identified by Broca, the limbic system comprises interconnected structures whose functions include memory, drive, affect, autonomic tone, endocrine control, and immunoregulation. Major limbic structures include the amygdala, piriform cortex (parahippocampal gyrus, uncus, and amygdala), hippocampus, substantia innominata, and septal area.

The amygdala connects extensively to the hypothalamus and other limbic structures. It receives input from widespread sensory cortical regions and paralimbic structures (piriform cortex, entorhinal cortex, and parahippocampal cortex on the temporal lobe medial surface and the cingulate cortex just above the corpus callosum). It is critical for channeling drive and affect. In lesion studies of monkeys, visual information from one eye was restricted to an intact amygdala while visual information from the other eye was directed toward a lesioned amygdala. The monkey's typical aggressive behavior when visually provoked was intact only when stimulated through the intact visual pathway. When provoked via the lesioned pathway, the monkey remained passive.

A similar phenomenon in humans is observed in Klüver-Bucy syndrome, which arises when the amygdala is disconnected from cortical sensory input. The typical features of Klüver-Bucy syndrome include (1) indiscriminate sexual behavior toward objects in the immediate extrapersonal space, (2) absence of fight-or-flight reaction toward threat, and (3) inability to visually distinguish edible from inedible objects except by orally inspecting objects.

In addition, the amygdala of the right hemisphere plays the dominant role in channeling appropriate emotional response toward sensory targets while also having an important role in the interpretation and display of affective gestures, including vocalization. The amygdala also plays an integral role in the experience of strong emotions, including fear, rage, and experiences of familiarity. It imparts the affective coloring of personal experience that reflects a person's history, present internal state, and characteristics of their present mental experience. Certain disease states engender disruptions of this balance. Thus the affective color of a particular mental process may be distorted, amplified, or diminished, thereby changing the very meaning of the entire experience. This occurs in panic attacks, dissociative states, depression, and schizophreniform conditions. In humans, the amygdala does not appear to play a direct role in memory formation, although amnesia resulting from hippocampal damage seems more severe if there is involvement of the amygdala, suggesting that it may link affect to memorization. Additional amygdala roles include regulation of autonomic, endocrine, and immunologic function.

The piriform cortex is a relay area for cortical and olfactory information, much the way the thalamus is the relay area for every other sensory modality. This area also has numerous connections with the hypothalamus and other limbic regions. Animal studies suggest a role in regulation of the direction of drive within extrapersonal space, such as attack or sexual behaviors.

The hippocampus receives almost all its input from paralimbic areas, which in turn receive inputs from cortical sensory areas, the hypothalamus, amygdala, and septal area. The hippocampus's major role is memory and learning. These structures are necessary for the formation of new memories (recording experience)

rather than storage of memories. In addition, they rekindle memories during retrieval. The motivational relevance of experience makes it more likely to be memorized and recalled. Storage and retrieval are affected with relative preservation of memory banks (long-term memory) in diseases affecting these structures. Isolated hippocampal damage is relatively rare, but combined lesions of hippocampal and parahippocampal areas in infarcts lead to severe amnestic states, even when the amygdala is spared.

The septal nuclei and substantia innominata contain the major cholinergic cells of the brain, located in the medial septal nucleus, the vertical and horizontal limb nuclei of Broca's diagonal band, and the nucleus basalis of Meynert. These areas project to the hippocampus,

olfactory region, widespread cortical regions, and the amygdala. The hypothalamus and various limbic and paralimbic structures give rise to most of the inputs to these structures. This cholinergic network is essential for intact memory function. Patients with anterior communicating artery aneurysms or with septal tumors may develop amnestic states. In Alzheimer disease, where memory loss is the major clinical feature, there is a profound loss of cholinergic neurons in the nucleus basalis and widespread cortical regions. Septal lesions may also produce exaggerated emotional reactions to novel or threatening stimuli, hyperdipsia, hyperphagia, and altered taste preference. There is evidence suggesting a role in attaching motivational value to extrapersonal objects.

Anterior nucleus of thalamus
Interthalamic adhesion
Interventricular foramen
Fornix
Anterior commissure
Stria terminalis
Precommissural fornix
Stria medullaris
Septum pellucidum
Habenula
Cingulate gyrus
Indusium griseum
Corpus callosum
Septal nuclei
Subcallosal area
Hypothalamus
Paraterminal gyrus
Lamina terminalis
Olfactory { bulb / tract / medial stria / lateral stria }
Anterior perforated substance
Optic chiasm
Postcommissural fornix
Mammillary body and mammillothalamic tract
Medial forebrain bundle
Amygdaloid body (nuclei)
Interpeduncular nucleus
Uncus
Fasciculus retroflexus
Calcarine sulcus (fissure)
Gyrus fasciolaris
Dentate gyrus
Fimbria of hippocampus
Hippocampus
Parahippocampal gyrus
Descending connections to reticular and tegmental nuclei of brainstem (dorsal longitudinal fasciculus)

Plate 4.2

Psychiatry

MAJOR DEPRESSIVE DISORDER

Major depressive disorder (MDD) is a mood disorder characterized by the occurrence of one or more major depressive episodes during one's lifetime. To diagnose MDD, five (or more) of the following nine symptoms must been present every day or almost every day during the same 2-week period and represent a change from previous level of functioning. At least one symptom must be either (1) depressed mood, or (2) anhedonia (markedly diminished interest or pleasure in all, or almost all, activities), along with (3) significant decrease or increase in appetite or weight, (4) insomnia or hypersomnia, (5) psychomotor retardation or agitation, (6) fatigue or loss of energy, (7) feelings of worthlessness or excessive or inappropriate guilt, (8) poor concentration or difficulty making decisions, and (9) recurrent thoughts of death, suicidal ideation, or a suicide attempt. The symptoms must cause clinically significant distress or impairment in social, occupational, or other important areas of functioning and must not be due to the direct physiologic effects of a substance (e.g., drug of abuse, medication) or a general medical condition (e.g., hypothyroidism). Subtypes of depression may be defined by the presence of psychotic features (delusions, hallucinations), catatonic features (motor disturbances such as immobility or agitation, stereotyped movements, mutism), melancholic features (weight loss, insomnia, morning worsening) or atypical features (hypersomnia, hyperphagia), or by onset of depression during the postpartum period. Longitudinal course specifiers are with or without interepisode recovery and with seasonal pattern.

Dysthymia is a distinct form of depression that usually has fewer or less severe symptoms compared with major depression, but much longer duration (at least 2 years, during which there has been no interval free of symptoms of 2 months in duration). Dysthymia is characterized by depressed mood for most of the day, more days than not, and is accompanied by at least two of the following symptoms: lack of appetite or overeating, insomnia or hypersomnia, low energy or fatigue, low self-esteem, poor concentration, difficulty making decisions, and feelings of hopelessness. Approximately 75% of people with dysthymia will develop at least one major depressive episode during their lifetime. Differentiating dysthymia from MDD may be challenging; for example, in major depression with a partial response to treatment.

MDD is a common psychiatric disorder that affects about 280 million people worldwide, or 3.8% of the general population. According to the World Health Organization, the prevalence seems to be largely unrelated to ethnicity or geography (region of the country or urbanicity). In a recent epidemiologic study in the United States, the 12-month and lifetime prevalences of MDD were 10.4% and 20.6%, respectively. Although MDD can develop at any age, the mean age of onset is in the early 30s. The incidence of MDD is relatively low in childhood, increases sharply between ages 12 and 16 years, and continues to increase, albeit more gradually, up to the early 40s. The diagnosis of MDD is associated with the presence of one or more psychiatric disorders during one's lifetime in nearly 75% of cases, including anxiety disorders (ADs) (60%), substance use disorders (25%), and impulse control disorders (30%).

Despite intensive research during the past several decades, the neurobiologic basis and pathophysiology of MDD still remain unknown. MDD is heterogeneous and may not be a single disorder but a group in which various genetic and environmental factors play a role.

The Face of Depression

"Doctor, what's wrong with me?"

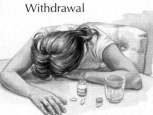

5-HT, NE

Depression is a biochemically mediated state most likely based on abnormalities in metabolism of 5-HT and norepinephrine.

Clinical syndrome characterized by withdrawal, anger, frustration, and loss of pleasure

Associated Symptoms and Comorbidities

Depressed mood with feelings of worthlessness and guilt

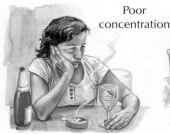

Poor concentration

Fatigue

Withdrawal

Substance abuse

Weight loss from poor nutritional habits

Sleep disturbance

Increased suicide risk

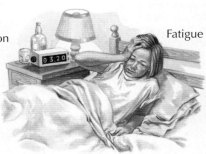

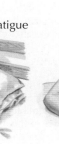

Specific neurotransmitters (serotonin, norepinephrine, dopamine, and more recently glutamate), neuroendocrine and neuroimmune responses to stress, or neurotrophic factors regulating plasticity in the brain may be relevant. Neural circuits are implicated from postmortem and imaging studies that show subtle alterations of complex neural networks involving the prefrontal cortex, subgenual cingulate cortex, amygdala, and hippocampus in patients with MDD.

The genetics of MDD are complex. MDD frequently runs in families and has an estimated heritability of approximately 40%. Genetic linkage and genome-wide association studies have identified several candidate genes and regions of the genome that may contribute to MDD, but findings have been inconsistent. Each individual gene likely contributes only a small percentage of the variance and interacts with environmental factors.

The choice of the initial treatment modality in MDD is influenced by several factors such as severity of symptoms, co-occurring psychiatric or medical conditions, psychosocial stressors, and the patient's preference. Different classes of antidepressant medications are available. Selective serotonin reuptake inhibitors (SSRIs) are typically used as a first-choice treatment option. Serotonin-norepinephrine reuptake inhibitors (SNRIs), tricyclic antidepressants (TCAs), monoamine oxidase inhibitors (MAOIs), and others (including bupropion, trazodone, and mirtazapine) are also approved for use. The choice of an antidepressant is based on side effect profile, tolerability, safety, and history of prior response to treatment. After an initial phase of pharmacologic treatment of 2 to 3 months, aiming at achieving full remission of symptoms, it is strongly recommended to continue pharmacotherapy for approximately 6 to 9 months to prevent early relapse. Psychotherapy, as monotherapy or combined with medications, may also be considered as initial treatment for patients with mild to moderate MDD. Electroconvulsive therapy (ECT) should be considered as a potential treatment option for patients who are severely ill or acutely suicidal or who present psychotic features or catatonia.

Plate 4.3

Brain: PART I

Postpartum Depression

The postpartum period has been clearly defined as a time of increased vulnerability to psychiatric illness in women; up to 85% of women experience some type of mood disturbance after childbirth. Most of these women experience transient and relatively mild mood symptoms ("the blues"); however, about 10% to 15% of women experience a more disabling and persistent form of mood disturbance: either postpartum depression (PPD) or postpartum psychosis. Although postpartum psychiatric illness was initially conceptualized as a group of disorders specifically related to childbirth, more recent evidence suggests that affective illness emerging during the postpartum period is clinically indistinguishable from affective illness occurring at other times during a woman's life. In fact, most women with postpartum illness have mood episodes that are not related to either pregnancy or childbirth.

The American Psychiatric Association's *Diagnostic and Statistical Manual of Mental Disorders (DSM-5)* defines postpartum psychiatric disorders using a "With Peripartum Onset" specifier to indicate an episode that has its onset during pregnancy or during the first 4 weeks after delivery. Although risk of postpartum psychiatric illness is the highest in the first 4 weeks after childbirth, several studies indicate that women remain at very high risk for affective illness during the first 3 months after delivery. In fact, women remain at heightened risk up to 1 year after childbirth. Thus many experts define *postpartum psychiatric illness* as any episode occurring within the first year after childbirth.

POSTPARTUM BLUES

During the first week after the birth of a child, many women experience a brief period of affective instability, commonly referred to as postpartum blues or the "baby blues." Given the high prevalence of this type of mood disturbance, it may be more accurate to consider the *blues* as a normal experience associated with childbirth rather than a psychiatric disorder. Women with postpartum blues report a variety of symptoms, including a rapidly fluctuating mood, tearfulness, irritability, and anxiety. These symptoms typically peak on the fourth or fifth day after delivery and may last for a few days, remitting spontaneously within 2 weeks of delivery.

POSTPARTUM DEPRESSION

Ten percent to 15% of women will present with more significant depressive symptoms or PPD after childbirth. Unlike the blues, PPD is more pervasive and may significantly interfere with a mother's ability to function and care for her child. Clinically, an episode of PPD is indistinguishable from other types of major depressive episodes, with symptoms of depressed mood, irritability, loss of interest in their usual activities, sleep disturbance, and fatigue. Women often express ambivalent or negative feelings toward their infant and may express doubts about their ability to care for their child. Anxiety symptoms may be prominent in this population, and women may present with comorbid generalized anxiety, panic disorder, or obsessive-compulsive disorder (OCD).

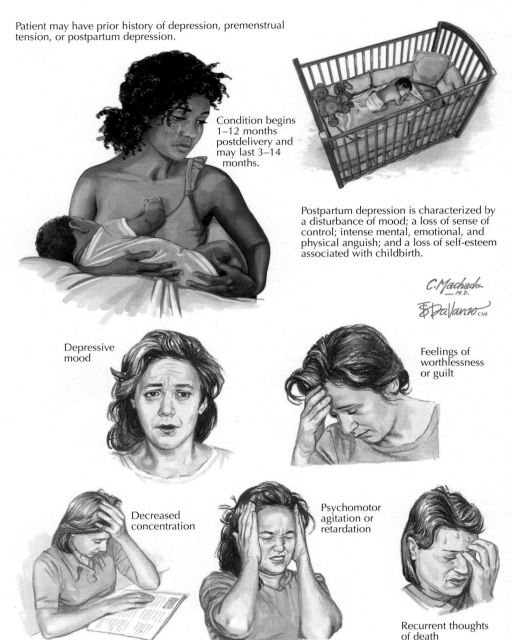

Patient may have prior history of depression, premenstrual tension, or postpartum depression.

Condition begins 1–12 months postdelivery and may last 3–14 months.

Postpartum depression is characterized by a disturbance of mood; a loss of sense of control; intense mental, emotional, and physical anguish; and a loss of self-esteem associated with childbirth.

Depressive mood

Feelings of worthlessness or guilt

Decreased concentration

Psychomotor agitation or retardation

Recurrent thoughts of death

POSTPARTUM PSYCHOSIS

This is the most severe form of postpartum psychiatric illness. It is a rare event that occurs in approximately 1 to 2 per 1000 women after childbirth. Its presentation is often dramatic, with onset of symptoms early, typically within the first 2 postpartum weeks. Longitudinal studies indicate that most women with postpartum psychosis have bipolar disorder, and the symptoms of postpartum psychosis most closely resemble those of a rapidly evolving manic or mixed episode. The earliest signs are restlessness, irritability, and insomnia, followed by a rapidly shifting depressed or elated mood, disorientation or confusion, and disorganized behavior. Delusional beliefs are common and often center on the infant.

TREATMENT

Because the blues are typically mild and resolve on their own, no specific treatment is required. The treatment of PPD depends on its severity. Milder cases may respond to psychotherapy, whereas more severe depressive symptoms are best treated with a combination of psychotherapy and medication. In this setting, SSRI antidepressants are preferred because they are effective for both depression and anxiety and are compatible with breastfeeding. Postpartum psychosis is a psychiatric emergency and typically requires hospitalization. Symptoms are treated with a combination of antipsychotic medications, benzodiazepines, and mood stabilizers, most commonly lithium. ECT may be helpful for treating psychosis or severe PPD.

In addition, a new class of medications may be helpful for the treatment of PPD. Brexanolone is a positive allosteric modulator of the γ-aminobutyric acid (GABA) A receptor, and in 2019 it was approved by the US Food and Drug Administration (FDA) for the treatment of PPD. In contrast to conventional antidepressants, which typically take weeks to improve symptoms, brexanolone's effects are evident within a few days of intravenous administration. Orally available medications with a similar mode of action are currently under investigation.

Plate 4.4

Psychiatry

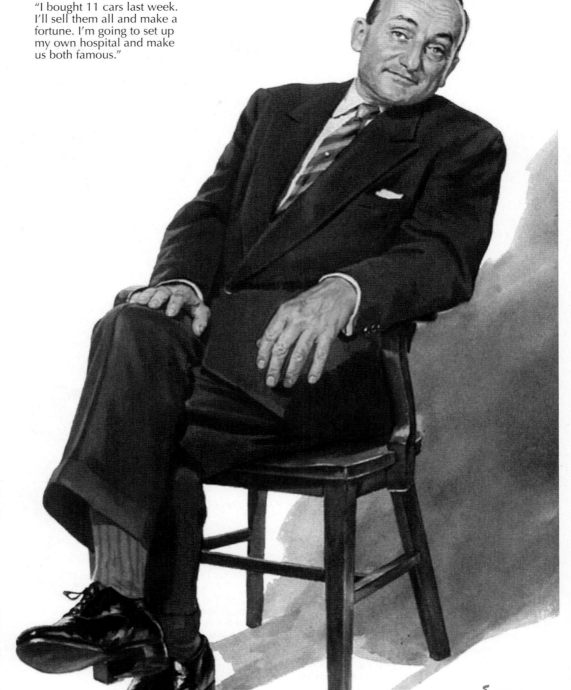

"I bought 11 cars last week. I'll sell them all and make a fortune. I'm going to set up my own hospital and make us both famous."

BIPOLAR DISORDER

Bipolar disorder is a severe and chronic mood disorder characterized by episodes of mania or hypomania and depression. *Bipolar I disorder* is characterized by one or more manic episodes. *Bipolar II disorder* is defined by one or more hypomanic episodes plus one or more depressive episodes. Cyclothymic disorder (milder illness in which mood swings do not meet severity or duration of hypomanic and major depressive episodes) and other specified bipolar disorder are related disorders within the bipolar spectrum.

Manic episodes, the defining feature of bipolar I disorder, consist of a week or more of abnormally and persistently elevated, expansive, or irritable mood, abnormally and persistently increased energy, and three or more of the following associated symptoms (four if mood is only irritable): distractibility; engagement in risky activities without regard for negative consequences (e.g., spending sprees, reckless driving, sexual indiscretions); grandiosity; flight of ideas; increase in goal-directed activity or agitation; decreased need for sleep; and loud, excessive, or pressured speech. Manic episodes are discrete periods that are uncharacteristic of the individual, cause impairment in functioning, and often require hospitalization. Psychotic symptoms (e.g., delusions, hallucinations) may also occur in the setting of mania and resolve when the mood disturbance is ameliorated (otherwise consider primary psychotic disorders such as schizoaffective disorder). The criteria for hypomania are the same as for mania, except the disturbance may last only 4 days and is not severe enough to cause marked impairment in functioning, be associated with psychotic symptoms, or necessitate hospitalization.

Depressive episodes, which represent the other polarity in bipolar disorder, consist of depressed mood; anhedonia (loss of interest or pleasure); sleep disturbance (insomnia or hypersomnia); appetite changes; fatigue; psychomotor retardation or agitation; feelings of excessive guilt or worthlessness; poor concentration and/or indecisiveness; and/or recurrent thoughts of death, suicidal ideation, or a suicide attempt. To meet criteria for a major depressive episode, an individual must experience five or more of these symptoms (one of which is either depressed mood or anhedonia) most of the day nearly every day during the same 2-week period. A depressive episode is not required to make a diagnosis of bipolar I disorder. However, most patients with bipolar I disorder experience both manic and depressive episodes, and depressive episodes typically account for a greater proportion of illness duration in both types of bipolar disorder. Moreover, patients can present with mixed features (i.e., presence of ≥3 depressive symptoms during a manic episode or ≥3 manic symptoms during a depressive episode).

The estimated global lifetime prevalence of bipolar I disorder is 0.6% to 1.0% and that of bipolar II disorder is 0.4% to 1.1%. The disorder affects men and women at

Plate 4.5

Brain: PART I

Emotion processing and emotion regulation circuitry

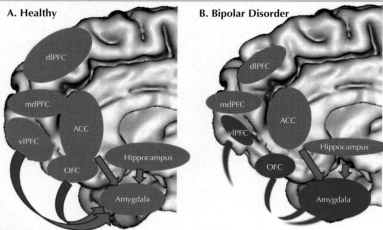

A, Schematic diagram highlighting key nodes in emotion processing and emotion regulation neural circuitry in healthy individuals. *Arrows* represent key regulatory connections between prefrontal cortical regions and the amygdala. **B,** Key functional abnormalities in individuals with bipolar disorder are highlighted in red (in regions and connections between regions); these include abnormally increased amygdala activity during emotion processing, emotion regulation, and performance of nonemotional tasks; abnormally decreased activity in the ventrolateral prefrontal cortex and orbitofrontal cortex during emotion regulation; and decreased functional connectivity between these prefrontal cortical regions and the amygdala during emotion regulation. In parallel, there are widespread abnormal decreases in gray matter volume and cortical thickness in prefrontal cortical regions, decreased gray matter volume in the amygdala and hippocampus, and abnormally decreased fractional anisotropy in white matter tracts connecting the ventral prefrontal cortex and anterior temporal regions. These changes are indicated by smaller sizes of ovals representing these regions. *ACC,* anterior cingulate cortex; *dlPFC,* dorsolateral prefrontal cortex; *mdPFC,* mediodorsal prefrontal cortex; *OFC,* orbitofrontal cortex; *vlPFC,* ventrolateral prefrontal cortex.

Reward processing neural circuitry

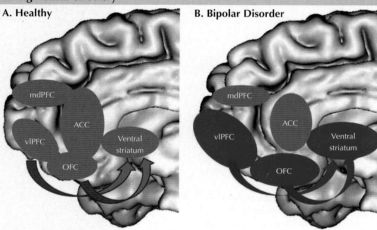

A. Schematic diagram highlighting key nodes in reward processing circuitry in healthy individuals. **B,** Key functional abnormalities in individuals with bipolar disorder are highlighted in red; these include abnormally increased activity in the ventral striatum, ventrolateral prefrontal cortex, and orbitofrontal cortex during reward processing, especially during reward anticipation. While not yet reported in the literature, it is likely that patterns of aberrant functional connectivity among these regions are exhibited by individuals with bipolar disorder during reward processing. In parallel, there are widespread decreases in gray matter volume and cortical thickness in prefrontal cortical regions and striatal regions in individuals with bipolar disorder. *ACC,* anterior cingulate cortex; *mdPFC,* mediodorsal prefrontal cortex; *OFC,* orbitofrontal cortex; *vlPFC,* ventrolateral prefrontal cortex. *From Phillips ML, Swartz HA. A critical appraisal of neuroimaging studies of bipolar disorder: toward a new conceptualization of underlying neural circuitry and a road map for future research. Am J Psychiatry. 2014;171(8):829-43. Copyright © 2014, American Psychiatric Association.*

BIPOLAR DISORDER
(Continued)

equal rates. Onset is usually in late adolescence/early adulthood. However, delays in accurate diagnosis often result in bipolar disorder being diagnosed and treated 6 to 10 years after age at onset; this may be due, in part, because depression is often the index presentation for many people. Mood episodes are often recurrent; the risk of relapse is 40% to 60% within 1 to 2 years after recovery from a first episode of mania.

Bipolar disorder is a complex disease with multiple genetic and environmental contributions. Twin studies demonstrate that bipolar disorder is strongly (60%–80%) heritable, with concordance rates of 40% to 45% in monozygotic twins and 4% to 6% in dizygotic twins. Bipolar I disorder shares overlapping risk with schizophrenia, whereas bipolar II disorder is highly genetically correlated with MDD. Genome-wide association studies have identified approximately 30 loci associated with bipolar disorder, including genes encoding ion channels and proteins involved in signal transduction, synaptic plasticity, or neurotransmitter reuptake. Though the pathophysiology remains unclear, research suggests possible mitochondrial dysfunction in addition to excessive inflammation, which may be activated, in part, by lifestyle and environmental stressors that are more common in people with bipolar disorder (e.g., childhood adversities, substance use including higher rates of tobacco use, poor diet). Neuroimaging studies point to alterations in emotion processing and emotion regulation neural circuitry, with abnormally increased amygdala activity, decreased activity in prefrontal cortical areas (i.e., ventrolateral prefrontal cortex [VLPFC], orbitofrontal cortex [OFC]) during emotion regulation, and decreased prefrontal-amygdala structural and functional connectivity. Imaging studies also implicate alterations in reward processing neural circuitry, with abnormally increased activity in the

ventral striatum, VLPFC, and OFC, especially during reward anticipation.

Mood stabilization is the goal of treatment for bipolar disorder. Lithium is the gold standard for mood stabilization, and evidence suggests that early initiation of lithium (i.e., after a first episode of mania) may alter the neurobiologic progression of bipolar disorder. Other pharmacologic therapies include anticonvulsant (e.g., carbamazepine, valproic acid, lamotrigine,

oxcarbazepine) and second-generation antipsychotic medications. Psychosocial interventions, such as cognitive-behavioral therapy (CBT) and lifestyle modifications (e.g., sleep hygiene), are also useful in illness management. The use of antidepressants to treat bipolar depression is controversial; though frequently prescribed, they are associated with induction of mania and mood destabilization, especially in the absence of adjunctive mood-stabilizing medications.

Plate 4.6

Psychiatry

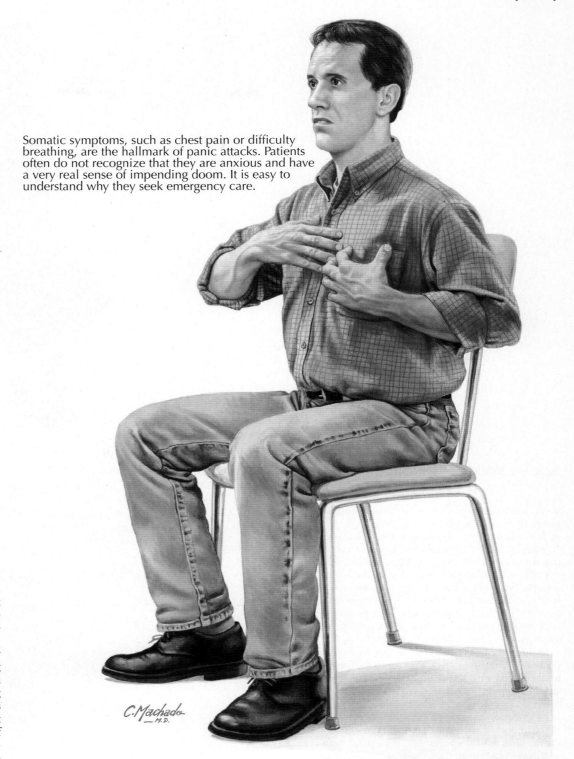

Somatic symptoms, such as chest pain or difficulty breathing, are the hallmark of panic attacks. Patients often do not recognize that they are anxious and have a very real sense of impending doom. It is easy to understand why they seek emergency care.

GENERALIZED ANXIETY DISORDER

Generalized anxiety disorder (GAD) is an AD characterized by excessive, uncontrollable, and often irrational worry about everyday things that is disproportionate to the actual source of worry. To diagnose GAD, excessive worry must be present most days for at least 6 months. The person finds it difficult to control the worry, and anxiety and worry are associated with three (or more) of the following six symptoms: (1) restlessness or feeling keyed up or on edge, (2) being easily fatigued, (3) difficulty concentrating or mind going blank, (4) irritability, (5) muscle aches or tension, and (6) sleep disturbances (difficulty falling or staying asleep or restless, unsatisfying sleep). The symptoms must cause clinically significant distress or impairment in social, occupational, or other important areas of functioning and must not be due to the direct physiologic effects of a substance (e.g., drug of abuse, medication) or a general medical condition (e.g., hyperthyroidism) and do not occur exclusively during worsening of a mood or psychotic disorder.

The lifetime prevalence of GAD is 3.7% and 12-month prevalence is 1.8%, with higher prevalence in women (2:1 female/male ratio). The age of onset is variable, ranging from childhood to late adulthood, with the median age of onset being approximately 31 years. There is significant comorbidity with other psychiatric disorders, most frequently major depression, alcohol abuse/dependence, other ADs (e.g., social phobia, agoraphobia, panic), and posttraumatic stress disorder (PTSD). The presence of comorbid disorders is associated with worse prognosis.

Some research suggests that GAD may run in families, and twin studies suggest genetic predisposition, but there is good evidence favoring an environmental component as well. Few studies have examined the long-term course of GAD; however, available data suggest that GAD has a chronic course, with significant long-term morbidity.

The treatment of GAD should incorporate both psychological and psychopharmacologic approaches. The choice of the initial treatment modality in GAD is influenced by factors such as severity of symptoms, co-occurring psychiatric or medical conditions, psychosocial stressors, and the patient's preference. Different classes of antidepressant medications have shown efficacy in GAD, including SSRIs (typically used as first choice), SNRIs, TCAs, MAOIs, and others (including buspirone and mirtazapine). Often other medications are used in combination with antidepressants, such as benzodiazepines and atypical antipsychotics. The choice of an antidepressant is based on side effect profile, tolerability, safety, and history of prior response to treatment. Psychotherapy, alone or combined with medications, may also be considered as initial treatment for patients with mild to moderate symptoms.

Plate 4.7

Brain: PART I

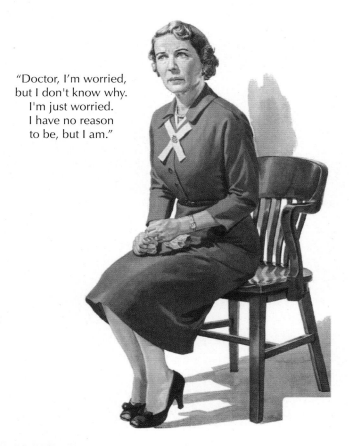

"Doctor, I'm worried, but I don't know why. I'm just worried. I have no reason to be, but I am."

Brain Regions Associated With Panic and Anxiety Disorders

Cerebral cortex

Thalamus

Bed nucleus of the stria terminalis

Hypothalamus

Amygdala

Locus coeruleus

Hippocampus

J. Perkins
MS, MFA

SOCIAL ANXIETY DISORDER

Social anxiety disorder (SAD), or social phobia, is characterized by persistent fear of social situations in which an individual will face exposure to unfamiliar people or scrutiny by others. The individual typically fears behaving in an embarrassing or humiliating fashion or revealing symptoms of anxiety. Exposure to these situations almost always provokes anxiety or panic symptoms, leading the individual to avoid such situations whenever possible. Physical symptoms may include diaphoresis, tachycardia, trembling, nausea, flushing, and difficulty speaking.

In addition to the presence of fear or anxiety, per *DSM-5* criteria, the anxiety should be out of proportion to the actual threat and the individual would avoid those situations or endure them with intense fear. Finally, this anxiety must cause significant functional impairment or distress (e.g., in social, occupational, or other important areas of functioning). Social anxiety can be often misinterpreted as a personality trait such as shyness rather than a disorder; however, it is critical to consider the functional impairment criterion.

Epidemiology. The lifetime prevalence of SAD is approximately 12%, with 12-month prevalence of roughly 7%, and is more common in women than in men. SAD often has early onset in the childhood or teenage years. Comorbid disorders are highly prevalent, occurring in as many as 90% of cases, particularly with other ADs, MDD, and alcohol use disorder (AUD).

Pathophysiology. SAD has been noted to be familial and data suggest SAD is approximately 20% to 40% heritable, with environmental factors accounting for the remaining variability. Although candidate gene studies have implicated multiple genes, no single association has been convincingly demonstrated. The

potential role of neuropeptides involved in social cognition, such as oxytocin and arginine vasopressin, is also under active investigation. Functional magnetic resonance imaging implicated the connectivity between amygdala, insula, and parietal regions in SAD, for example, on tasks requiring processing of emotional faces.

Treatment. CBT, exposure therapy, and antidepressant medications are effective treatments for SAD. Standard medication treatment includes SSRIs, although

other antidepressants, including SNRIs and MAOIs, have also demonstrated efficacy. Anxiolytic medications, such as benzodiazepines, are sometimes used in addition to adjunct therapy. β-Blockers can help control some of the physical symptoms of SAD, such as tachycardia and tremors. Short-acting β-blockers are commonly used for social anxiety related to public speaking or performance. Scales such as the Liebowitz Social Anxiety Scale may be used to assess severity over time.

Plate 4.8

Psychiatry

PANIC DISORDER

Patients complaining of panic often describe a dramatic presentation, including the sudden, unexpected onset of extreme fearfulness or alarm, quickly rising to a crescendo within minutes of commencement, and accompanied by a spectrum of physical, behavioral, and cognitive symptoms. These may include the bodily sensations of choking, chest pain, trembling, heat sensation, and rapid heart rate, which mimic a sympathetic, fight-or-flight response. The urge to escape, to find shelter, or to seek help can be overwhelming. Panic victims may believe they are dying, losing control, or going crazy and will often seek urgent medical care. The indelible, negative impression left by a panic attack often results in persistent fear of having another attack or in marked behavioral changes. Although isolated panic attacks are relatively common, it is these persistent sequelae that define the diagnosis of panic disorder. By *DSM-5* criteria, this disorder may also be accompanied by agoraphobia, characterized by the phobic avoidance of situations that may be difficult or embarrassing to escape if a panic attack recurs.

Panic disorder is common, with a lifetime prevalence in the United States of up to 5%. The disorder occurs nearly twice as often in women and tends to manifest in early adulthood. Comorbid substance use disorders and psychiatric illness are very common; MDD occurs in nearly two-thirds of patients with panic disorder. These comorbid conditions, if left untreated, may exacerbate the symptoms of panic or make treatment more difficult. Of particular concern, panic disorder is associated with higher risk for suicide. Of interest, the onset of panic disorder is often related to a stressful life event. Although most patients experience some remission of symptoms over time, the course of panic disorder is chronic for most affected individuals. Complications can include persistent anxiety symptoms, mood disorders, phobic avoidance, drug and alcohol use disorders, and significant impairments in functioning and quality of life.

The differential diagnosis of panic disorder includes a broad list of cardiac, respiratory, endocrine, metabolic, and drug-related causes, as well as other psychiatric conditions that may include panic attacks. An individual experiencing a panic attack often presents for treatment initially at emergency departments or in primary care settings, and although the classic presentation of panic attack may be familiar to most practitioners, a careful consideration of possible organic causes must be undertaken. A personal or family history of anxiety and recent stressful life events may suggest a primary AD.

Early family studies of panic disorder have demonstrated a higher risk in first-degree relatives of probands; twin studies estimate the heritability of ADs to be 20% to 40%. Although these studies suggest that genetic factors play a role, the investigation of particular genetic risk factors is complicated by the high level of comorbidity with other anxiety and depressive disorders. Explanatory neurobiologic models emphasize the role of an extended neural fear circuit, including the amygdala and related structures, hypothalamus, anterior and midcingulate cortex, insula, and prefrontal cortex. Hypothesized abnormalities in the serotonergic, noradrenergic, and GABAergic neurotransmitter systems are supported by the efficacy of pharmacologic treatments aimed at these systems (e.g., SSRIs, SNRIs, and benzodiazepines).

During the early stages of presentation, before phobic avoidance or recurrent attacks begin, a patient may

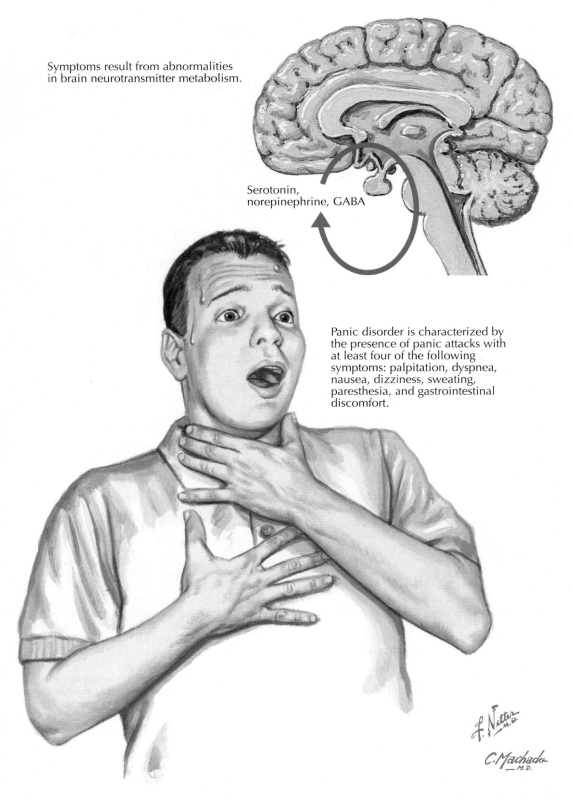

Symptoms result from abnormalities in brain neurotransmitter metabolism.

Serotonin, norepinephrine, GABA

Panic disorder is characterized by the presence of panic attacks with at least four of the following symptoms: palpitation, dyspnea, nausea, dizziness, sweating, paresthesia, and gastrointestinal discomfort.

respond well to reassurance, education, and supportive psychotherapy. Once phobic avoidance or recurrent attacks begin, the aims of treatment are to prevent further panic attacks and to eliminate the associated avoidance and anticipatory anxiety. Pharmacologic treatment for panic includes antidepressants; placebo-controlled trials support the efficacy of SSRIs, the SNRI venlafaxine, and the TCAs imipramine and clomipramine. Benzodiazepines provide rapid symptomatic relief and may be prescribed alone or together with antidepressants. CBT for panic disorder is validated and studied widely, proving effective whether delivered in individual or group therapy settings. CBT conceptualizes *panic* as the acquired fear of the bodily sensations associated with autonomic arousal, and *agoraphobia* as the behavioral response to the anticipation of such sensations. Therapists teach cognitive and somatic coping skills that are then used to manage anxiety during exposure to feared situations and bodily sensations. Multiple studies and meta-analyses show that the combination of medication and psychotherapy is more effective in treating panic than either therapy alone.

Plate 4.9

Brain: PART I

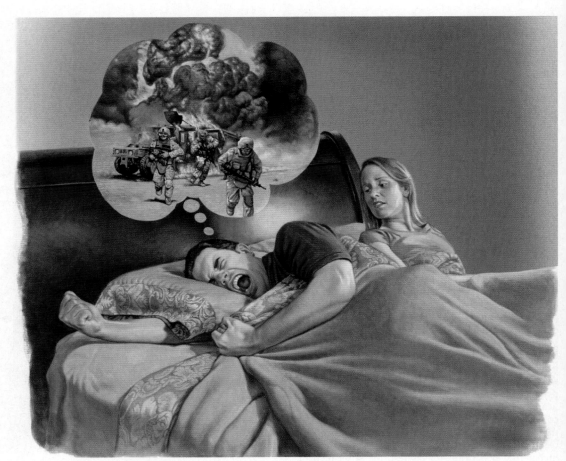

Individuals with PTSD may have flashbacks of traumatic events during the day and/or nightmares related to the event during sleep.

C. Machado
M.D.

Posttraumatic Stress Disorder

Posttraumatic stress disorder (PTSD) is a mental health condition that develops in response to a traumatic event: experiencing real or threatened death, serious injury, or sexual violation. PTSD is characterized by four clusters of symptoms: (1) *reexperiencing symptoms,* wherein the patient relives the trauma through thoughts and dreams and cannot get it out of their mind; (2) *avoidance symptoms,* wherein the patient avoids people, places, and anything that reminds them of the trauma and shuts off their emotional responses; (3) *negative alterations in cognitions and mood,* wherein the patient might have distorted thoughts related to the causes and consequences of the event, leading to blaming oneself or others, in addition to possible decreased interest in preferred activities, withdrawal, and depressed mood; and (4) *hyperarousal symptoms* that involve difficulty concentrating, constantly feeling on edge and in danger, difficulty sleeping, and irritability. To be diagnosed with PTSD, these symptoms must occur for at least 1 month, and there must be significant distress or impairment in various areas of daily functioning, such as in social or work-related settings. When these symptoms occur for less than 1 month and/or have an incomplete representation of all four cluster symptoms, it may be an acute stress reaction or an other-specified trauma and stressor-related disorder. In young children, their PTSD cluster symptoms may present with angry and irritable behaviors instead of negative self-image and blame.

PTSD is distinct from other mental health disorders in that trauma exposure is a prerequisite for diagnosis. Threatening events initiate the body's fight-or-flight response via the hypothalamic-pituitary-adrenal axis, the locus coeruleus, and the noradrenergic system. These systems have important reciprocal interconnections with the amygdala and hippocampus, limbic structures involved in fear conditioning and memory consolidation, and with prefrontal brain structures necessary for extinction of fear memories and reward motivation. Initially, this neurobiologic stress response is considered adaptive, as it mobilizes energy, increases vigilance and focus, facilitates memory formation, and depresses the immune response. When the acute threat has passed, an elaborate negative feedback system will return the body to homeostasis. However, in some individuals, this acute adaptive response to threat becomes persistent and pathologic.

Although most adults will experience at least one traumatic event in their lifetime, only a minority develop PTSD. The lifetime prevalence of PTSD in the United States has been estimated to be between 3.5 and 6%. The disorder is diagnosed twice as often in women. Although many individuals will experience some PTSD symptoms in the immediate days and weeks after a trauma, only a minority of individuals show the persistent symptoms required for the PTSD diagnosis. Uncontrollable and threatening events, such as sexual violence, childhood abuse/repeated exposure to abuse, near-death experiences, and military combat, are consistently associated with the highest risk for developing PTSD. Although the risk for developing clinical PTSD is low, it is very serious and can affect individuals from any racial/ethnic group with various intersecting identities (e.g., gender, sexual orientation, socioeconomic status). There continue to be efforts to identify protective factors to help lower the risk of developing PTS and to promote factors of resiliency after exposure to a traumatic event. Extant research suggests pretrauma characteristics, such as family and personal history of psychopathology, childhood adversity, and low cognitive ability; trauma-related factors, such as type of event experienced, perceived life threat, and peritraumatic psychologic response; and posttrauma factors, such as less social support, all contribute to increased vulnerability of developing PTSD. There are multiple studies that suggest PTSD is moderately heritable and that genetic factors can influence development of the disorder.

Some individuals recover from PTSD within 6 months, whereas for others it can become chronic (i.e., lasting for more than 3 months). Treatment can benefit those with both short-lived and chronic symptoms. Trauma-focused CBT (TF-CBT) is an evidence-based treatment for PTS. The core strategies of TF-CBT include (1) exposure and (2) cognitive restructuring. Both use the conceptualization that PTSD is reinforced through avoidance of traumatic event triggers, such as thoughts, feelings, places, and people associated with the memory. Exposure therapy targets the avoidance by having the patient slowly and gradually reexperience the memory and reminders of the traumatic event both in and outside the therapy session. Cognitive restructuring targets the avoidance by addressing irrational or inaccurate beliefs about the causes and consequences of the traumatic event. A primary focus of cognitive restructuring is to use cognitive techniques to help patients gain their own understanding of the event and subsequently to modify the meaning attributed to the traumatic event. Together, exposure and cognitive restructuring can be effective for treatment of PTSD. In some cases, pharmacotherapy can also be helpful in treating certain symptoms of PTSD. The only FDA-approved pharmacologic agents for the treatment of PTSD symptoms are the SSRIs sertraline and paroxetine. More research is needed to better understand their effectiveness in the treatment of PTS. Pharmacologic augmentation of TF-CBT is also the focus of ongoing research.

Plate 4.10

Psychiatry

Obsessive-Compulsive Disorder

Obsessive-comupulsive disorder (OCD) is diagnosed based on recurrent and intrusive thoughts, referred to as obsessions, and/or compulsive behaviors or rituals. The obsessions or compulsions are recognized by the patient, at least at some point, as excessive and unreasonable, leading to marked distress or functional impairment; they may be extremely time consuming. These symptoms are experienced as intrusive and inappropriate and are not simply excessive worries about real-world concerns.

Multiple subtypes of OCD are identified primarily based on factor analysis. Typical obsessions may include fears of contamination, sexual/religious or other moral transgression, harming others, or unrecognized illness. Compulsions may include checking, cleaning, repeating, and ordering. Of these, the most common symptom is checking behavior, seen in nearly 80% of cases. Patients may, for example, check repeatedly that the stove is turned off, reread paragraphs for typographic errors, or contact family members to confirm that they are healthy. Of importance, such behavior does not occur once but may persist for hours at a time. Of note, compulsions may be mental rituals as well; for example, needing to count to a certain number or recite a prayer to prevent a catastrophic event. OCD is highly comorbid with other psychiatric disorders, particularly ADs, mood disorders, and substance use or impulse control disorders. OCD is sometimes observed in individuals with comorbid tic disorders such as Tourette syndrome.

Epidemiologic studies indicate a lifetime prevalence of approximately 2% among the general population, with 1% reporting symptoms in the past 12 months. Subthreshold symptoms may be far more common, with up to 25% of respondents reporting some lifetime obsessions or compulsions. Mean onset age is between 19 and 20 years, but up to 25% of males may have onset before age 10 years; female incidence increases in adolescence. New cases are rarely observed after age 35 years. Twin and family studies suggest that OCD, particularly childhood-onset OCD, is a heritable disorder, with between 45% and 65% of vulnerability attributed to inherited risk.

Clinical Presentation. OCD symptoms are generally chronic and contribute to substantial functional and social impairment, although their severity may fluctuate over time.

Pathophysiology. Functional neuroimaging studies implicate cortico-striato-thalamo-cortical circuit dysfunction in the pathophysiology of OCD symptoms with a particular focus on the OFC, anterior cingulate cortex, and caudate. However, recent investigation suggests a somewhat broader network including the temporal, parietal, and occipital lobes as well as other subcortical structures. Investigation of OCD is facilitated by the availability of mouse models with OCD-like symptoms, particularly excessive grooming behavior. Despite the efficacy of serotonergic antidepressants for OCD, the role of glutamatergic neurotransmission is receiving increasing focus based on animal studies and genetic data.

In rare cases, OCD symptoms may emerge in children after streptococcal infection, a phenomenon referred to as *pediatric autoimmune neuropsychiatric disorders associated with streptococcal infections* (PANDAS). This syndrome has focused attention on the role of basal ganglia and immune mechanisms in OCD.

Treatment. Treatment for OCD typically relies on either behavioral therapy, medication treatment, or both;

"I am embarrassed that my hands are so chapped. I never told you before about my fear of germs and constant washing because I was afraid you would think I was crazy."

the individual treatments have similar effect sizes. The gold standard behavioral therapy for OCD is exposure and response prevention therapy. SSRIs or the TCA clomipramine are prescribed most often; these medications may require greater dosages and longer treatment durations (i.e., 12 weeks or more) to achieve response compared with the treatment of other psychiatric disorders.

For those with only a partial response to serotonergic antidepressants, antipsychotic medications and transcranial magnetic stimulation may be used as augmentation treatments. For severe and refractory OCD, neurotherapeutic approaches, such as ablative neurosurgery and deep brain stimulation targeting neural circuits implicated in OCD (see below), are options.

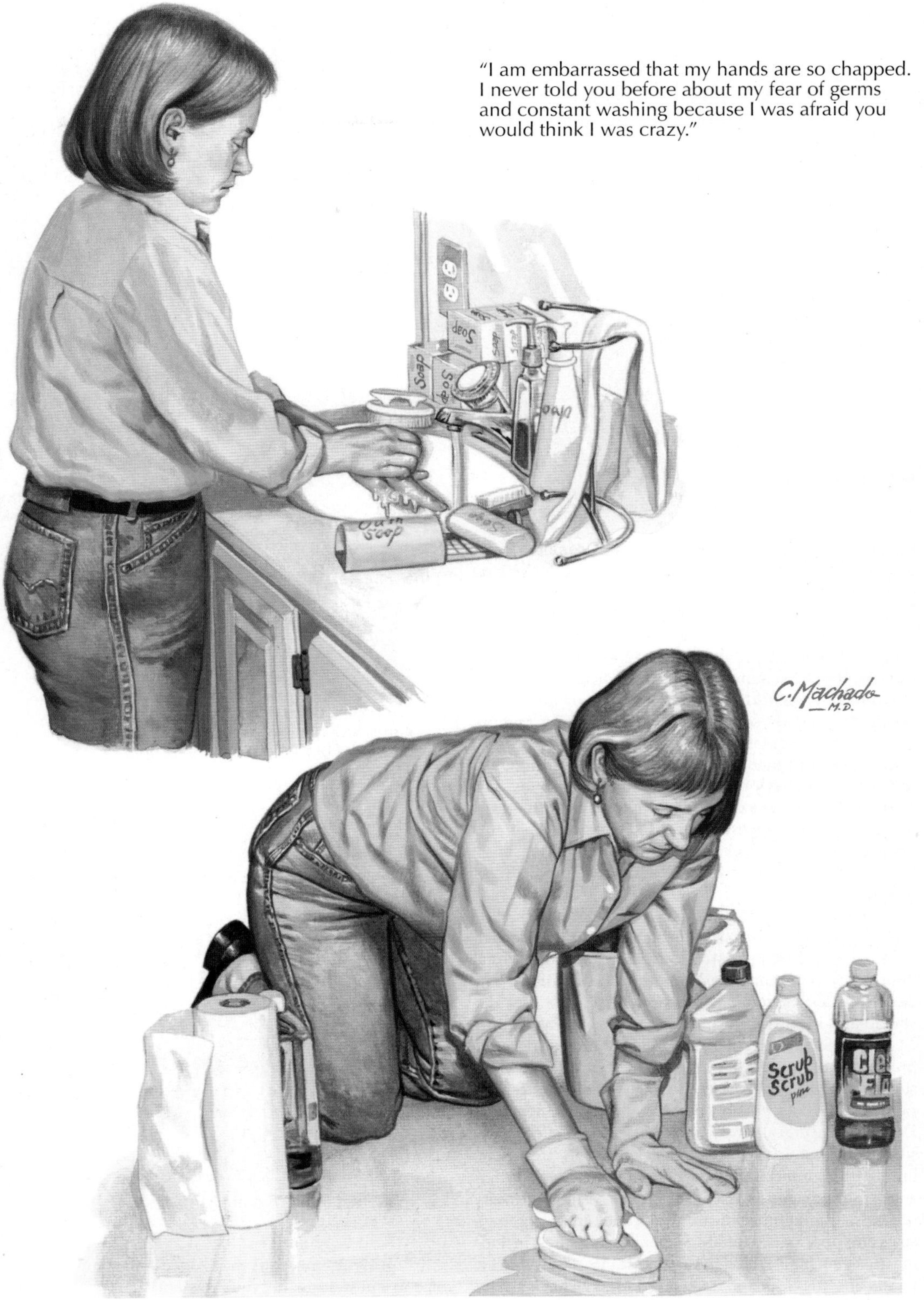

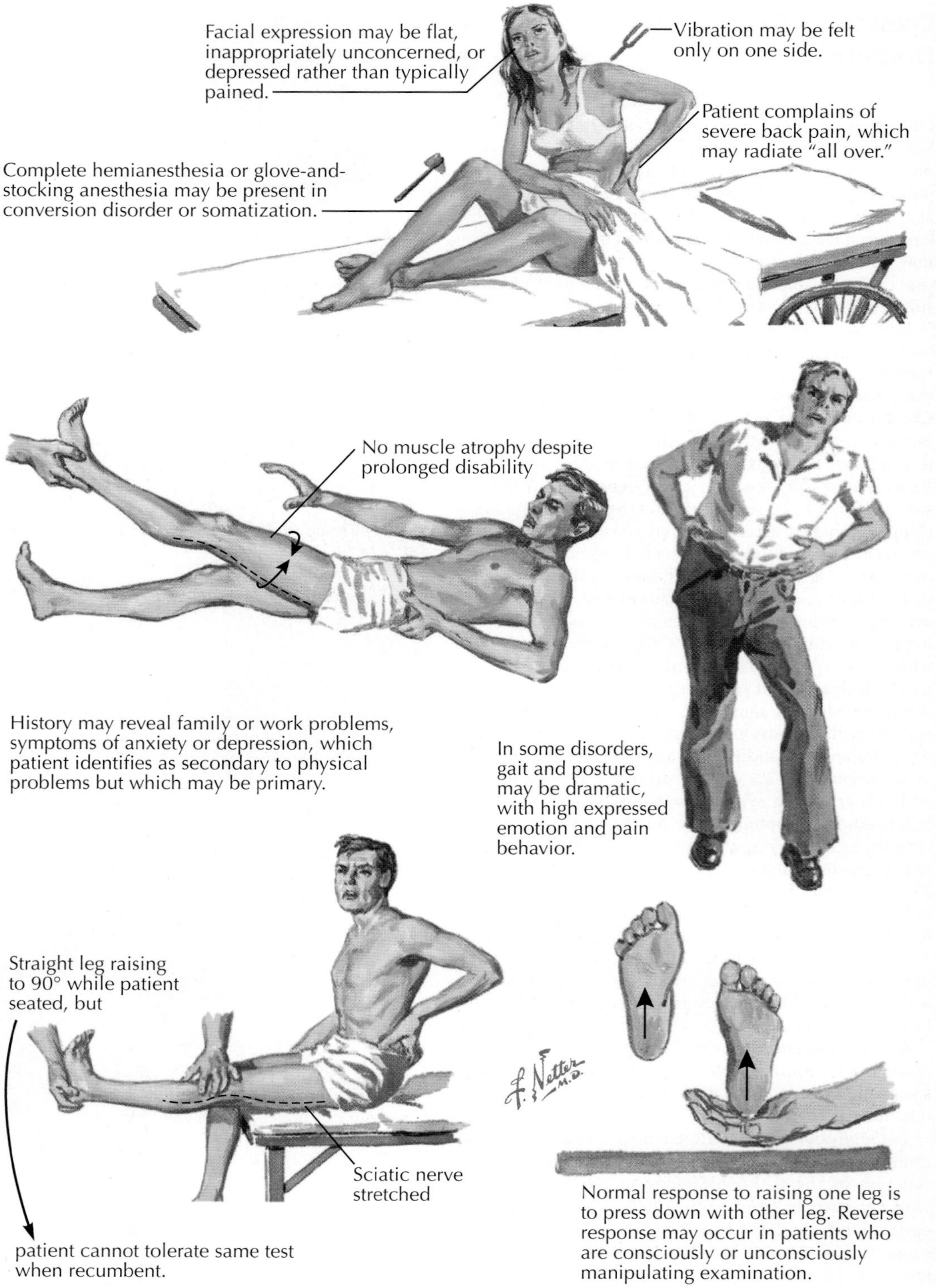

Plate 4.11

Brain: PART I

Facial expression may be flat, inappropriately unconcerned, or depressed rather than typically pained.

Vibration may be felt only on one side.

Patient complains of severe back pain, which may radiate "all over."

Complete hemianesthesia or glove-and-stocking anesthesia may be present in conversion disorder or somatization.

No muscle atrophy despite prolonged disability

History may reveal family or work problems, symptoms of anxiety or depression, which patient identifies as secondary to physical problems but which may be primary.

In some disorders, gait and posture may be dramatic, with high expressed emotion and pain behavior.

Straight leg raising to 90° while patient seated, but

Sciatic nerve stretched

patient cannot tolerate same test when recumbent.

Normal response to raising one leg is to press down with other leg. Reverse response may occur in patients who are consciously or unconsciously manipulating examination.

SOMATIZATION

Somatic symptom disorder is one of five somatic disorders identified by the *DSM-5*. Others include conversion disorder (or functional neurologic symptom disorder), illness AD, psychological factors affecting other medical conditions, factitious disorder, and other unspecified diagnoses. Fundamentally, somatization is a constellation of physical symptoms lacking medical explanation.

Clinical Presentation and Diagnosis. DSM-5 diagnostic criteria for somatic symptom disorder require one or more somatic symptoms causing distress or impairment in function, along with excessive thoughts, feelings, or behaviors related to the symptoms and associated health concerns. The symptoms range in severity and may be suggestive of disability. These patients disproportionately seek healthcare interventions; the total number of symptoms is a reliable predictor of healthcare use.

Patients with somatic symptom disorder have a variety of symptoms without a verifiable medical disorder. Pain, fatigue, gastrointestinal, urologic, and functional neurologic symptoms are all common. In patients undergoing sleep studies, paradoxical insomnia is widespread and minimally responsive to usual treatment.

Epidemiologic data suggest somatic symptom disorder prevalence of 5% to 7% in the general population. Twin studies suggest a genetic component. A female-to-male ratio of 10:1 exists, possibly because of ascertainment bias. Despite high prevalence rates, clinicians rarely diagnose somatic symptom disorder. Deficiencies in treatment, limited reassurance by medical practitioners, and avoidance of the diagnosis lead to excessive testing, specialty referrals, and high healthcare use overall, incurring high costs and poor quality of life. Screening measures, including the Patient Health Questionnaire–15, the Whiteley Index, and the Scale for Assessing Illness Behavior, have reasonable diagnostic utility compared with clinical interview alone.

Pathophysiology. The pathophysiology of somatic symptom disorders is not well understood. Connections have been made with experiences from childhood neglect and abuse, unpredictable living environment, substance use disorders, and personality disorders. Ability to switch attention from emotional content may be altered, especially in individuals with childhood trauma, dissociation, or depression. Alexithymia, habitual suppression or expression of anger, or belief that certain emotions are unacceptable may contribute.

Clinical presentations may suggest aberrant function of the autonomic nervous system or hypothalamic-pituitary-adrenal axis, or alterations in central processing of sensory input. It has been hypothesized that activation of proinflammatory cytokines by internal and external stressors may sensitize the central nervous system (CNS) and afferent peripheral nerves to cause altered body perceptions. Postinfectious syndromes may be relevant, with previous bacterial or viral infection a frequent precursor to irritable bowel syndrome, possibly by disruption of the brain-gut-microbiota axis.

Treatment and Prognosis. Despite their high prevalence, somatic symptom disorders are understudied and have limited evidence-based therapies. Purely "ruling out" general medical disorders leads to serial negative tests and ineffective interventions. Most treatments targeting specific symptoms are minimally effective. The most beneficial treatment uses a combination of exercise and minimal pharmacotherapy. Behavioral therapies such as CBT can improve symptoms and function and reduce comorbid depressive symptoms. Treatment outcome studies suggest TCAs have a slight advantage over other centrally acting agents such as SSRIs for treating pain. Providers suspecting a somatic symptom disorder diagnosis should schedule frequent time-limited visits to offer reassurance and address patient concerns.

Plate 4.12

Psychiatry

CONVERSION DISORDER

Conversion disorder, or functional neurologic symptom disorder (previously called hysteria), is defined by the *DSM-5* as a somatic symptom disorder with one or more losses or distortions of a neurologic function (1) not explained by a recognized organic neurologic lesion or medical disease, (2) not better explained by another medical or mental disorder, and with symptoms or deficits (3) not consciously produced or intentionally feigned. The diagnosis requires appropriate neurologic assessment and test results confirming the physical symptoms as incompatible with neurologic pathophysiology and/or inconsistent with recognized conditions.

Clinical Presentation and Diagnosis. Conversion disorder can affect any body system. Examples include functional limb weakness, paralysis, tremors, deafness, dysphonia, amnesia, and abnormal movements; anesthesia that does not follow nerve distributions or dermatomes; vision deficits incongruent with anatomically possible visual field deficits; and nonepileptic seizures with normal electroencephalogram (EEG) findings during events. A further complication is that 10% to 30% of individuals with nonepileptic seizures have a history of confirmed epileptic seizures. Patients with astasia-abasia exhibit an unusual, dramatic gait disturbance and falls. Focused physical examination can elicit findings suggesting conversion disorder. Functional leg weakness is demonstrated with the Hoover test (Plate 4.12), where weakness of hip extension resolves during contralateral hip flexion against resistance. Functional tremor may be suspected when it resolves or matches the frequency of voluntary rhythmic movement of the unaffected leg (entrainment). Overall, conversion symptoms typically become worse with attention and can lessen or disappear with distraction.

Conversion disorder is more prominent in developing nations, rural areas, in females, and in individuals with lower socioeconomic status with less access to education. Like other somatic symptom disorders, patients with conversion disorder have significant impairment and high use of healthcare. Some providers stigmatize these patients because of difficulty distinguishing conversion disorder from malingering and other factitious disorders. Given widespread lack of effective approaches to manage conversion disorder, patients may become dissatisfied and seek multiple providers.

Pathophysiology. The term "conversion" implies an etiology whereby psychologic stress is unconsciously converted into body symptoms. However, the actual mechanism is largely unknown and poorly understood. Historic hypotheses focused on anosognosia from an altered state of self-consciousness or altered awareness of body state. Functional brain imaging studies in which participants with conversion disorder and matched controls were asked to feign a deficit or symptom have been unrevealing. Inhibition of motor, sensory, or special sensory networks by increased prefrontal and cingulate cortex activity has been suggested. Involvement of the pathways from and to limbic structures and the temporoparietal junction, dorsolateral prefrontal cortex, and ventromedial prefrontal cortex may explain alterations in self-referential and autobiographical information processing. Preexisting vulnerabilities in emotional regulation may be activated, such as in a diathesis-stress model.

Management. Conversion disorder highlights relationships between the body and the mind, but additional research is needed to understand the underlying cause and potential treatments. Emphasis should be placed on confirming the diagnosis clinically. Body-based approaches such as massage, acupuncture, or rehabilitation may be more beneficial in some instances than talk therapies.

Treatment and Prognosis. Most conversion symptoms spontaneously remit. CBT is considered more effective than pharmacologic approaches, although antidepressants may have a role. Young age, sensory rather than motor symptoms, acuteness of presentation, association with a stressful event, high socioeconomic status, and absence of psychiatric or medical comorbidities are associated with a favorable prognosis. Concurrent depression and/or personality disorder is associated with a more chronic course.

Tests for Paralysis of Upper Extremity

1. Patient lies supine; examiner raises paralyzed arm to position over patient's face

2. Arm is suddenly released; examiner notes manner in which it falls

(Test may also be used for functional unconsciousness)

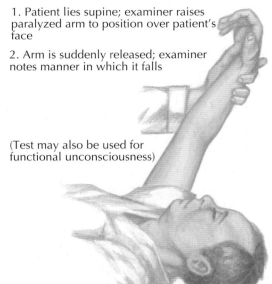

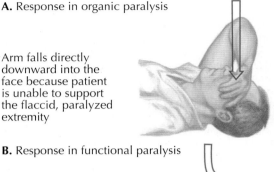

A. Response in organic paralysis

Arm falls directly downward into the face because patient is unable to support the flaccid, paralyzed extremity

B. Response in functional paralysis

Arm does not hit the face but follows, a slow or circuitous course downward, landing safely to the side of the head

JOHN A.CRAIG—AD

Tests for Weakness in Lower Extremity

Thigh adduction test

1. Patient is instructed to adduct unaffected leg against resistance by examiner

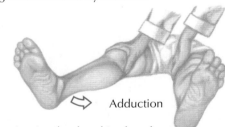

Adduction

2. Examiner's other hand is placed against affected thigh to detect contraction

 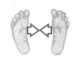

A. Response in organic paralysis

Patient can accomplish adduction with no contralateral adduction palpable in affected leg

B. Response in functional paralysis

In adduction of unaffected leg, patient involuntarily adducts affected leg

Hoover test

1. Patient is instructed to elevate unaffected leg against resistance by examiner

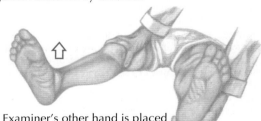

2. Examiner's other hand is placed beneath heel of affected leg to detect reciprocal downward thrust used by patient for leverage

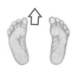

A. Response in organic paralysis

Patient is able to elevate unaffected leg without concomitant downward thrust of affected leg

B. Response in functional paralysis

Elevation of unaffected leg is accompanied by downward thrust of affected leg

Plate 4.13

Brain: PART I

SCHIZOPHRENIA

Schizophrenia is the prototype of a psychotic disorder, with the core symptoms of delusions and hallucinations as well as disorganized speech. Some patients also display prominent psychomotor disturbances, including catatonia. Together, these florid and often dramatic symptoms are referred to as *positive symptoms*. They contrast with negative and cognitive symptoms that are responsible for much of the disability that characterizes schizophrenia. *Negative symptoms* are categorized into a reduced emotional expressivity cluster (blunted or flat affect) and an avolition/asociality/anhedonia cluster. Many patients with schizophrenia struggle with cognitive impairment in the realms of working memory, attention/vigilance, verbal learning and memory, visual learning and memory, reasoning and problem solving, speed of processing, and social cognition. These patients can often have prominent mood symptoms, which are not inconsistent with a diagnosis of schizophrenia. However, if mood symptoms dominate the overall course of a psychotic illness, a diagnosis of *schizoaffective disorder* can be given. *Schizophrenia is a diagnosis of exclusion;* various street drug usage, medications, and medical causes of psychosis must initially be excluded before diagnosis because these can mimic the core symptoms of schizophrenia.

Many patients with schizophrenia experience symptoms that in hindsight are recognized as a prodrome before the onset of their florid psychosis. Unspecific prodromal symptoms (anxiety, depression, social withdrawal) eventually give rise to attenuated psychotic symptoms before schizophrenia declares itself by the onset of frank psychosis. Because schizophrenia is a syndrome, not all patients experience symptoms from all domains. Schizophrenia is also characterized by a fluctuating illness course, where periods of exacerbation with prominent psychosis alternate with periods of remission.

Schizophrenia has a prevalence of approximately 1.5%, with large public health implications because of its onset during young adulthood and persistence throughout life. The typical age at onset is between 15 and 30 years, with onset after age 45 years being rare. Males are 40% more likely to develop schizophrenia than females (ratio of 1.4:1) and have an earlier onset. Only about 20% of patients have a good overall prognosis. Patients with schizophrenia often die decades earlier than people in the general population. The excess medical mortality is partly preventable because modifiable risk factors (i.e., nicotine dependence and metabolic syndrome) contribute to death from cardiovascular disease. Suicide is responsible for 5% of deaths.

Schizophrenia is highly heritable. Other important risk factors for schizophrenia include in utero insults during brain development, such as exposure to infections; obstetric complications; advanced paternal age; social factors, such as urbanicity or immigration status; and early heavy cannabis use.

The neuropathology and pathophysiology of the network dysfunction in schizophrenia remain to be resolved. Critical brain regions involved include frontal cortical areas, particularly dorsolateral prefrontal cortex, the thalamus, and various limbic and dopaminergic midbrain areas. Although varied developmental pathways can eventually lead to schizophrenia, psychosis emerges as the result of dopamine (DA) dysregulation as a final common pathway. Other neurotransmitters such as glutamate may play a key role in the pathophysiology of schizophrenia.

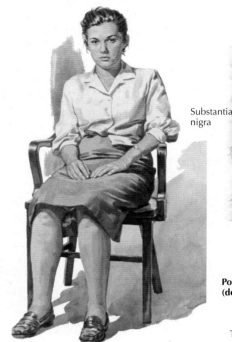

This patient exhibits flat affect that is common to schizophrenia. She appears to be responding to internal stimuli. Alternatively, she may have parkinsonism secondary to antipsychotic medications, which mimics negative symptoms. Finally, she may have parkinsonism secondary to antipsychotic medication.

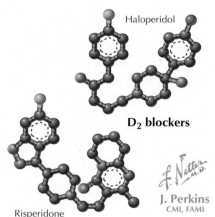

Haloperidol

D_2 blockers

Risperidone

J. Perkins
CMI, FAMI

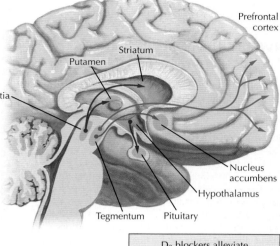

Neural Pathways Involved in Schizophrenia

Prefrontal cortex

Striatum

Putamen

Substantia nigra

Nucleus accumbens

Hypothalamus

Tegmentum   Pituitary

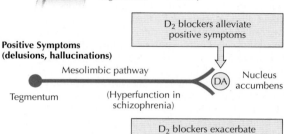

D_2 blockers alleviate positive symptoms

Positive Symptoms (delusions, hallucinations)

Mesolimbic pathway

Nucleus accumbens

Tegmentum   (Hyperfunction in schizophrenia)

DA

D_2 blockers exacerbate mesocortical dysfunction

Negative and Cognitive Symptoms (e.g., lack of motivation, executive dysfunction)

Mesocortical pathway

Prefrontal cortex

Tegmentum   (Hypofunction in schizophrenia)

DA

D_2 blockers cause extrapyramidal side effects

Adverse Effects (e.g., parkinsonism)

Nigrostriatal pathway

Corpus striatum

Substantia nigra

DA

D_2 blockers cause prolactin elevation

Adverse Effects (prolactin elevation)

Tuberoinfundibular pathway

Pituitary gland

Hypothalamus

DA

Schizophrenia can be viewed as a neurodevelopmental disorder that affects brain circuits and develops in stages. A prodromal stage is characterized by initial subtle symptoms and role failure; eventually, this results in an active psychosis stage and subsequently gives rise to a stage of chronic disability. According to this model, psychosis is a late symptom. Therefore prevention of this severe outcome requires treatment of target patients at earlier stages.

Antipsychotic medications are the treatment of choice for acute psychosis. After resolution of the initial psychosis, most patients require maintenance treatment with an antipsychotic medication to reduce the likelihood of a psychotic relapse. Antipsychotics are antagonists of dopamine 2 (D_2) receptors, and many antipsychotics combine D_2 with 5-hydroxytryptamine 2a receptor blockade as their basic receptor profile. Despite great differences in individual receptor pharmacologic sites of activity, currently available antipsychotics are equally effective and differ mostly in their propensity toward side effects. Only clozapine is shown to be more effective in treatment-refractory patients with schizophrenia. Problematic long-term side effects of all antipsychotics include tardive dyskinesia and metabolic syndrome.

Antipsychotics are not effective against all aspects of schizophrenia. In particular, negative and cognitive symptoms show little improvement with antipsychotics alone. Instead, the comprehensive treatment of schizophrenia requires integration of pharmacologic treatment with psychological therapies and concomitant psychosocial rehabilitation. Psychological treatments such as CBT and cognitive remediation are critical for treating persistent symptoms and cognitive deficits. Newer antipsychotics with nondopaminergic mechanisms of action and broader clinical efficacy beyond psychosis are under development.

Plate 4.14

Psychiatry

ALCOHOL USE DISORDER

The World Health Organization estimates 3 million alcohol-related deaths worldwide annually. Yet many who drink alcohol do not experience negative health or social consequences, and some healthcare studies suggest health benefits may be associated with alcohol consumption. How can we distinguish between risky drinking and safe drinking? The National Institute on Alcohol Abuse and Alcoholism (NIAAA), dedicated to providing scientific leadership in the assessment of alcohol use and its health and social consequences, has established sex-specific guidelines based on current evidence for "low-risk" drinking. To normalize these guidelines, a "standard drink" is defined as an ethanol alcohol content of 14 g (equivalent to 12 oz of beer, 5 oz of table wine, or 1.5 oz of liquor). It is considered low risk for healthy adult males younger than 65 years to consume no more than 14 standard drinks per week, with up to 4 drinks per day, and for healthy adult nonpregnant females younger than 65 years and healthy males and females age 65 years and older to consume no more than 7 standard drinks per week and up to 3 standard drinks per day.

The following risk factors may increase the potential negative health consequences of drinking even with low-risk patterns of consumption: (1) first-degree relative with alcohol or drug use disorder (i.e., heritable risk for developing AUD), (2) history of mental illness, (3) history or family history of cancer, and (4) history of adverse reaction to consumption. Conditions in which no amount of alcohol is established as safe, or any amount of alcohol is established as potentially harmful, include (1) pregnancy, (2) age younger than 21 years, (3) operation of a vehicle or other machinery, (4) consumption of medications that interact with alcohol, and (5) acute physical or mental health symptoms.

AUD is defined by *DSM-5* criteria and scaled from mild to severe. The cardinal aspect of AUD is *loss of control or self-regulation* over alcohol intake, resulting in negative consequences to health, safety, occupational performance, and social/family roles. NIAAA research in the United States has defined at least five phenotypic subtypes of AUD based on data from large national community survey studies. These subtypes are briefly described below and represent nongeriatric patient presentations. Geriatric AUD typically involves a prominence of alcohol-related health consequences, cognitive deficits, and loss of independent self-care and functioning.

Young Adult (31.5%). Comprising the largest group with AUD nationally, young adults tend to lack common risk factors for AUD (family history of AUD, co-occurring drug use, or mental illness). This subtype is a priority for medical screening because they rarely seek treatment.

Young Antisocial (21%). This group includes individuals in their mid-20s with high rates of co-occurring drug use (>75% smoke cigarettes and cannabis) and strong AUD family histories. Drinking begins in youth, which may in part account for early severity of AUD. Co-occurring mental illnesses are common (depression, anxiety, and personality disorders). One-third actively seek treatment. This group is of particular importance for pediatrician- and school-based screenings for substance use.

Functional (19.5%). Typically, this group encompasses well-educated, middle-aged individuals with stable jobs and relationships, colloquially referred to as "high-functioning alcoholics." A lack of prominent negative consequences to drinking creates a strong

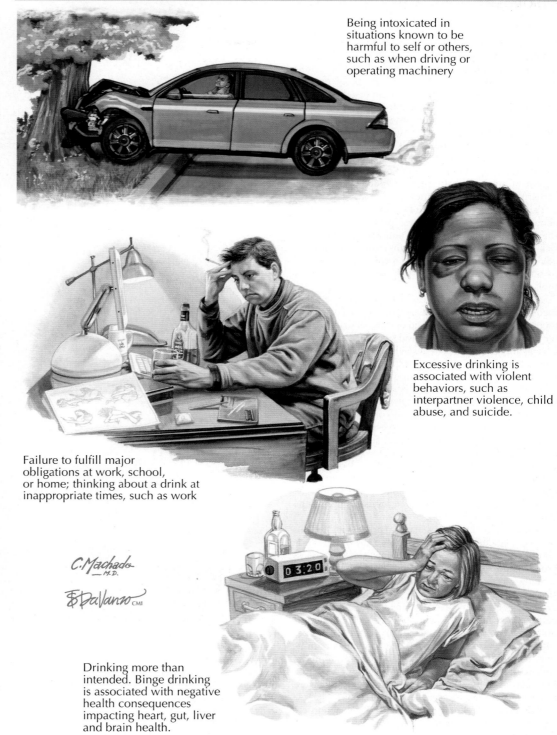

Meeting two or more of 11 *DSM-5* criteria in a 12-month period having to do with loss of control over consumption, craving/preoccupation, and negative health or social consequences

Being intoxicated in situations known to be harmful to self or others, such as when driving or operating machinery

Excessive drinking is associated with violent behaviors, such as interpartner violence, child abuse, and suicide.

Failure to fulfill major obligations at work, school, or home; thinking about a drink at inappropriate times, such as work

C. Machado
—M.D.

B. DaVanzo CMI

Drinking more than intended. Binge drinking is associated with negative health consequences impacting heart, gut, liver and brain health.

vulnerability to denial of illness and lack of incentive for seeking treatment; thus medical screening for alcohol-related problems is important to engage them in treatment. About half smoke cigarettes, one-third have strong AUD family histories, and one-quarter have a lifetime history of depression.

Intermediate Family (19%). This group of middle-aged individuals, half of whom have a lifetime history of depression and strong AUD family histories, has high rates of co-occurring mental illness and drug use, and the majority smoke cigarettes. Despite overt problems

with functioning, only 25% actively seek treatment for alcohol-related reasons. This group frequently presents for psychiatric care, making screening for substance use critical to diagnosing AUD.

Chronic Severe (9%). This group of middle-aged individuals has early-age onset of drinking, high rates of co-occurring mental illness and drug use, and high rates of antisocial personality disorder (ASPD) and criminal behavior with legal consequences. Two-thirds will actively seek treatment because of prominent negative consequences of alcohol use.

Plate 4.15

Brain: PART I

TREATMENT FOR ALCOHOL USE DISORDER

In the United States the prevalence of past-year AUD among persons aged 12 years and older was 10.2% in 2020. Past-month binge drinking (>5 drinks per drinking day for males, >4 drinks per drinking day for females) occurred in 22.2% of those surveyed, and 6.4% reported heavy drinking (binge drinking on ≥5 days per month), yet only 6.5% of those with AUD received any past-year treatment.

Screening identifies individuals at risk for developing alcohol-related problems and those with AUD. Evidence-based screening, brief intervention, and referral to treatment are universally recommended and result in earlier therapeutic interventions.

Treatment for at-risk drinkers involves education about AUD and alcohol-related problems, review of the NIAAA guidelines to sex- and age-specific "low-risk" drinking, a brief intervention consisting of clear advice to reduce or abstain from drinking, and referral to online and in-person self-help or mutual-support tools.

Treatment for AUD begins with assessing whether medically managed withdrawal (i.e., detoxification) is required for people with physiologic dependence at risk for dangerous alcohol withdrawal syndromes; this is especially important for patients with co-occurring hypertension, diabetes, seizure disorder, autonomic instability, and history of suicidality. Withdrawal management may be monitored on an outpatient basis, but many patients will require inpatient withdrawal management to prevent recurrent drinking. Medically stabilized patients with AUD may be referred to professional counseling and/or mutual-help groups (e.g., participation in Alcoholics Anonymous doubles the efficacy of professional counseling). For individuals dependent on alcohol, abstinence is most effective at maintaining recovery gains; however, meaningful health improvements may be achieved by lowering drinking risk levels defined by the World Health Organization.

Primary care physicians have a prominent role in treating AUD using medical management (MM) models of care. MM consists of (1) frequent visits to assess progress and health, (2) education about AUD, (3) prescribing and monitoring tolerance and adherence to an alcohol treatment medication, (4) facilitating weekly drinking goals and recovery behaviors, (5) encouraging participation in mutual-help or specialty counseling if indicated, and (6) screening and treating disorders that commonly co-occur with AUD (e.g., medical condition, mental illness, other substance misuse, domestic violence). There are three FDA-approved and two non–FDA-approved medications to treat moderate to severe AUD. Medications are reviewed briefly below.

Naltrexone. An antagonist at central mu-opioid receptors, naltrexone attenuates opioid-mediated reward of drinking and clinically reduces alcohol cravings and drinking days; it also increases the probability of containing recurrent drinking to a lower-consumption episode. Naltrexone is available in daily oral dosage and in an extended-release monthly intramuscular formulation that improves adherence. It poses hepatotoxicity risk and is contraindicated in those with severe hepatic disease and those requiring narcotic analgesia. Oral naltrexone is currently the only evidence-based medication to treat geriatric AUD.

Acamprosate (N-Acetylhomotaurine). A glutamate neuromodulator, acamprosate is an abstinence-promoting medication appropriate for patients who have achieved

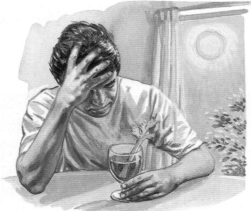

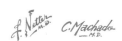

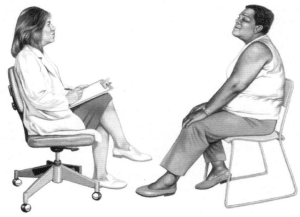

Alcohol use disorder is common and treatable. All patients should be routinely screened with evidence-based assessments, such as the 3-item AUDIT-C, and offered medical assistance for positive screening.

Brief counseling assists patients with alcohol use disorder to create and maintain effective treatment plans to reduce or quit drinking. Lifestyle changes and reducing drinking are associated with improved health outcomes.

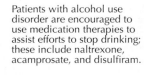

Patients with alcohol use disorder are encouraged to use medication therapies to assist efforts to stop drinking; these include naltrexone, acamprosate, and disulfiram.

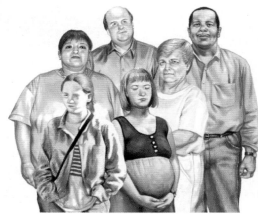

Patients who actively use mutual support groups (Alcoholics Anonymous or SMART Recovery) in addition to professional help improve their chances of achieving and sustaining recovery from alcohol use disorder.

early abstinence. It increases time to first drinking recurrence. It is metabolized within the kidney, providing a good choice for those with severe hepatic disease. It has poor bioavailability, and the dosing (three times daily) requires adherence.

Disulfiram. This aldehyde dehydrogenase inhibitor prevents the final metabolic conversion of ethanol to water. Usage results in accumulation of toxic acetaldehyde metabolites, leading to flushing, headache, hypertension, sweating, and nausea/vomiting. Disulfiram is most effective at reducing anticipated rewards of alcohol and thus reducing drinking days. Adherence is problematic, and the estimated incidence of acute liver injury is 1 per 10,000 to 30,000 patient-years of disulfiram treatment; thus careful hepatic monitoring is required. It is contraindicated in those with autonomic instability and generally considered too risky for use in adults older than 65 years. It may offer advantages as a contingency treatment for

impaired professionals and parents at risk of losing child custody.

Topiramate. Topiramate is a non–FDA-approved but evidence-based medication that reduces drinking in patients with AUD who seek treatment.

This GABAergic potentiator can be administered to patients who are actively drinking but want to reduce and are willing to commit to drinking-reduction goals and medication adherence. Topiramate reduces heavy drinking days and promotes abstinence. Because of its renal metabolism, it is contraindicated with renal calculi or glaucoma.

Gabapentin. Gabapentin is a non–FDA-approved but evidence-based medication that reduces drinking in patients with AUD who seek treatment. It is a GABAergic potentiator. The evidence base for its efficacy in treating AUD is less robust compared with topiramate, but it has greater tolerability and may be an appropriate alternative for those who do not respond to other FDA-approved medications.

Plate 4.16   Psychiatry

Alcohol Withdrawal

Alcohol withdrawal syndrome (AWS) occurs when an individual who has AUD with physiologic dependence experiences a period of reduced dosage or abstinence from drinking. *AWS may be life-threatening* as it poses a risk for seizures, hypertensive crisis, and autonomic instability (especially in patients with comorbid hypertension or diabetes) as well as delirium tremens, leading to death if not rapidly treated. AWS must be medically managed with close monitoring in either an outpatient or inpatient setting, depending on the patient risk profile.

Pathophysiology. Alcohol tolerance occurs with neuroadaptations to chronic alcohol exposure. Alcohol is a sedative; chronic exposure leads to compensatory changes with reduced neurotransmission at GABA$_A$ receptors and enhanced neurotransmission at excitatory *N*-methyl-D-aspartate (NMDA) glutamatergic receptors. During abrupt abstinence episodes, the unopposed activity of these compensatory changes results in central hyperexcitability responsible for objective and subjective AWS symptoms.

Presentation. AWS onset typically peaks within 48 to 72 hours of the last ethyl alcohol intake. Clinical signs of AWS include diaphoresis, tachycardia, hypertension, fever, vomiting, insomnia, anxiety, tremor, hyperreflexia, delirium, and grand mal seizures. Delirium tremens ("DTs") is a severe withdrawal syndrome with fatal potential if not recognized or if undertreated. It involves autonomic instability, agitation, altered mental state, hallucinations, and tremor. Risk factors include advanced age, advanced alcohol dependence, prior episodes of delirium tremens, and medical illness. Clinical symptoms of AWS include anxiety, irritability, dysphoria, nausea, anorexia, alcohol craving, headache, fatigue, and auditory and visual and/or tactile hallucinations. AWS is measured using a standardized instrument, the Clinical Institute Withdrawal Assessment for Alcohol (CIWA). This tool measures 10 AWS symptom categories with a 0-to-7 scoring range for each. Moderate scores (8–15) reflect autonomic hyperactivity, and high scores (>15) predict seizures and delirium; high scores warrant immediate initiation of medical treatment.

Persistent AWS may endure for 1 to 6 months and consists of anxiety or dysphoria, insomnia, and restlessness as well as frequent cravings for alcohol. Some medical treatments assisting recovery and promoting abstinence are hypothesized to address persistent central hyperexcitability. These include acamprosate, gabapentin, and topiramate. Medications must be combined with a comprehensive alcohol reduction or abstinence plan to effectively reduce symptoms that commonly lead to alcohol relapse.

Treatment. Benzodiazepines are the gold standard AWS treatment because of their cross-reactivity with alcohol at GABA$_A$ receptors. Symptom-triggered detoxification protocols are used because they prevent medical morbidity and death while minimizing dosing requirements for benzodiazepines and thus adverse effects. Typical protocols initiate treatment with either short-acting (lorazepam) or longer-acting (diazepam, chlordiazepoxide) benzodiazepines once autonomic arousal is recognized, and therapeutic selection is dependent on the treatment setting (whether benzodiazepine administration route must be oral or may be administered intravenously) and access to specific medication supplies. Alternatively, phenobarbital dosing protocols may be preferred in cases at high risk for delirium tremens. Benzodiazepine dosing is repeated as needed to control AWS

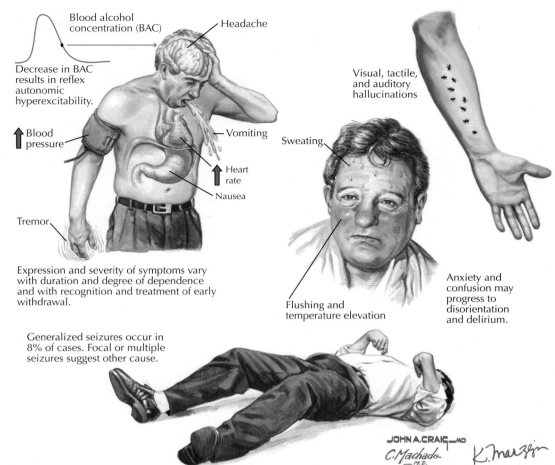

Expression and severity of symptoms vary with duration and degree of dependence and with recognition and treatment of early withdrawal.

Generalized seizures occur in 8% of cases. Focal or multiple seizures suggest other cause.

Stages of alcohol withdrawal			
	Stage 1	**Stage 2**	**Stage 3**
Hours after alcohol consumption	24 36 48 (peak)	48–72	72–105
Symptoms	Mild to moderate anxiety, tremor, nausea, vomiting, sweating, elevation of heart rate and blood pressure, sleep disturbance, hallucinations, illusions, seizures	Aggravated forms of stage 1 symptoms with severe tremors, agitation, and hallucinations	Acute organic psychosis (delirium), confusion, and disorientation with severe autonomic symptoms

Stage 1 withdrawal is usually self-limited. Only a small percentage of cases progress to stages 2 and 3. Progression is prevented by prompt and adequate treatment.

during the initial 24 hours and then tapered over the following days at a rate of not more than 25% per day. These protocols are guidelines because ongoing clinical assessment is required for safety; doses should be held if increasing sedation or gait instability develops. Treatment must include nutritional repletion of thiamine, folate, and multivitamins.

Carbamazepine and valproate are anticonvulsants that may be useful AWS therapeutic adjuncts; however, the comparatively favorable efficacy and tolerability of benzodiazepines generally render these treatments as second-line options.

Medical stabilization of acute AWS must always be paired with appropriate referral to maintenance treatment that supports drinking reduction. This includes medication management per Plate 4.15, treatment of co-occurring psychiatric and medical illnesses, and referral to ongoing care for substance use disorder. Level of care determinations may be assisted by the evidence-based Patient Placement Criteria developed by clinical researchers from the American Society of Addiction Medicine. Six domains influencing probability of good outcome are assessed to help determine the appropriate level of care: (1) severity of intoxication and withdrawal, (2) medical comorbidity, (3) psychiatric illness and psychosocial stability, (4) patient readiness to participate actively in treatment, (5) history of past treatment outcomes, and (6) recovery environment. Levels of care range from least restrictive outpatient to increasing medical and psychiatric outpatient supervision (intensive outpatient, partial hospitalization) to residential treatment. The highest level of care is inpatient hospitalization with both intensive medical and psychiatric stabilization of life-threatening symptoms.

Plate 4.17

Brain: PART I

BRAIN SUBSTRATES OF ADDICTIVE BEHAVIORS

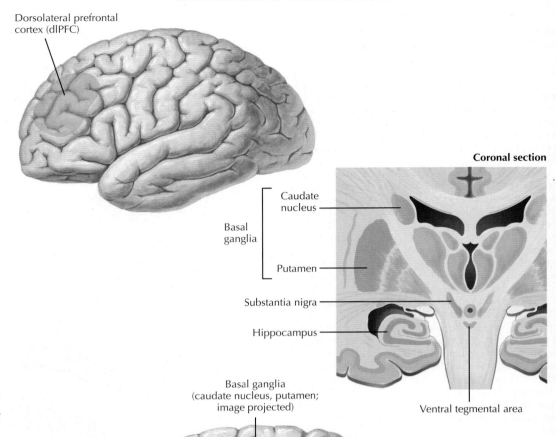

Dorsolateral prefrontal cortex (dlPFC)

Coronal section

Basal ganglia
- Caudate nucleus
- Putamen

Substantia nigra

Hippocampus

Basal ganglia (caudate nucleus, putamen; image projected)

Ventral tegmental area

Anterior cingulate cortex

dlPFC (image projected from lateral surface)

Subcallosal gyrus

Ventromedial prefrontal cortex (vmPFC)

Nucleus accumbens

Amygdala

Hippocampus

Substantia nigra

Ventral tegmental area

J. Netter

J. Perkins
CMI, FAMI

OPIOID USE DISORDERS

Opioid misuse and opioid use disorder refer to the pathologic self-administration of substances that activate central mu-opiate receptors for the purpose of experiencing an altered mental state (euphoria or relaxation), or in the opioid-dependent individual for the purpose of avoiding opioid withdrawal. Naturally occurring opiates (morphine, codeine) are found in *Papaver somniferum* poppy pods as a latex sap (opium); heroin is a semisynthetic opioid derived from opium. Prescription analgesics include semisynthetic (e.g., hydrocodone, oxycodone) and synthetic (e.g., methadone, fentanyl) opioids. Both heroin and opioid analgesics may be insufflated or injected to get "high"; other routes include smoking heroin and swallowing/chewing opioid analgesics. Routine toxicology detects only opiates (e.g., the heroin metabolites codeine and morphine); special gas chromatograph/mass spectrometry detection is required for semisynthetic and synthetic opioid analgesics.

According to the 2020 National Survey on Drug Use and Health, 513,000 US residents age 12 years and older acknowledge past-month heroin use, and 2.5 million endorse past-month prescription opioid misuse. Opioid-related drug poisoning deaths have increased sixfold since 1999 and continue to rise despite public health efforts aimed at reducing opioid supply in communities. Opioids, especially potent synthetic opioids such as illicitly manufactured fentanyl analogs, are implicated in most drug-associated poisoning deaths, in both intentional and unintentional drug poisoning categories.

Opioid intoxication may be recognized by miosis, dysarthria, altered mental state and sedation, constipation, impaired judgment, and slowed reaction time. Recurrent opioid use results in tolerance to the central effects and progression to physiologic dependence on opioid-taking to avoid opioid withdrawal. Physiologic dependence alone is not an opioid use disorder; however, use becomes a disorder when the individual also experiences preoccupation with obtaining, using, and recovering from opioid use such

that normal social and occupational functioning is reduced or impaired. Symptoms of opioid withdrawal include mydriasis, diaphoresis and fever, increased heart rate, abdominal cramps, nausea/vomiting and diarrhea, lacrimation, rhinorrhea, piloerection, leg cramping, yawning, insomnia, and anxiety. Although physiologic dependence alone is not sufficient to define an opioid use disorder, it poses a risk for developing an opioid use disorder, particularly in vulnerable populations, such as those with a history of substance

use disorder, mental illness, or genetic loading for addiction disorders.

Medical consequences of opioid misuse are many, and risk is proportionate to the quantity and type of opioid self-administration, the route of administration (with injection use carrying the highest probability of overdose death and high rates of blood-borne infectious disease transmission, especially hepatitis C virus and human immunodeficiency virus [HIV]), and the duration of use (females being more rapidly susceptible to

Plate 4.18

Psychiatry

Pinpoint pupils

Opioid overdose reversal with naloxone

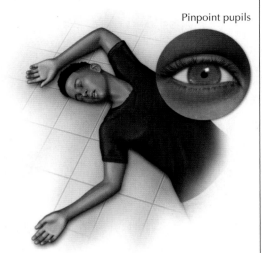

Unresponsive, cyanosis of lips and fingers

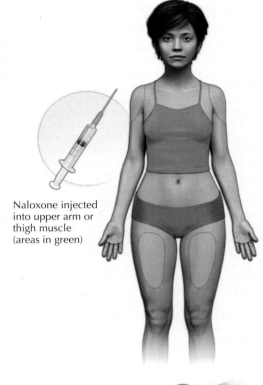

Naloxone injected into upper arm or thigh muscle (areas in green)

Opioid Use Disorders
(Continued)

both medical and social consequences, often referred to as a "telescoping course"). Opioid poisoning mortality is associated with high-dose prescription opioid use, illicitly manufactured fentanyl and fentanyl analog use, co-occurring use of alcohol and other sedatives, and injection drug use. Injection use is commonly associated with cellulitis and staphylococcal infection, phlebitis, and endocarditis. Pain is frequently comorbid among youth and adults dependent on opioids. Social and legal consequences include loss of employment, domestic violence, and arrest for drug-related criminal behaviors.

FDA-approved medications for opioid use disorder (MOUD) includes the mu-opiate receptor antagonist naltrexone, the mu-opiate receptor partial agonist buprenorphine, or the mu-opiate receptor full agonist methadone. Behavioral therapies without medication maintenance have high failure rates (recurrent opioid use) in both youth and adults. Optimal treatment combines medication management with behavioral therapy and participation in self-help programs. Naltrexone therapy has been limited by poor patient adherence to oral naltrexone; the development of an extended-release injection formulation that endures 4 weeks has superior outcomes. Buprenorphine has a favorable safety and tolerability profile compared with methadone and offers office-based access for patients as opposed to daily monitored dosing at federally regulated methadone maintenance clinics, also known as opioid treatment programs. Patients needing close medical monitoring and more intensive social service supports may benefit more from the structure of opioid treatment programs, which may administer either methadone or buprenorphine treatments. Although much of buprenorphine therapy is provided by daily transmucosal formulations, the development of depot formulations of buprenorphine may confer optimal treatment effects because of improved adherence, particularly during early recovery phases of care.

Safe opioid prescribing will prevent diversion of opioid analgesics. Prescribers screen patients for vulnerability

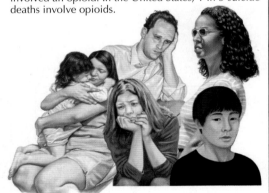

Opioid use disorder can affect anyone. Over 70% of the nearly 71,000 drug overdose deaths in 2019 involved an opioid. In the United States, 1 in 5 suicide deaths involve opioids.

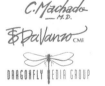

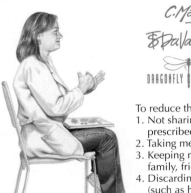

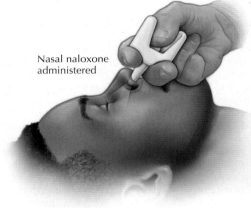

Nasal naloxone administered

To reduce the risk of prescription opioid addiction, talk to your patient about:
1. Not sharing medication with others and only taking prescription medication that is prescribed to them.
2. Taking medication as prescribed (not in greater amounts or more often).
3. Keeping medication in a safe and secure place, preferably that is locked so children, family, friends, and visitors cannot access.
4. Discarding expired or unused prescription opioids properly (such as https://www.dea.gov/takebackday).
Visit https://www.cdc.gov/injury/features/manage-your-pain/ for more information.

to opioid misuse and discuss these risks with patients. Prevention strategies include limiting quantity; using state prescription monitoring databases, designated pharmacies and treatment contracts, toxicology, and pill counts; and monitoring aberrant behaviors (e.g., "doctor shopping," running out early, "lost" or stolen prescriptions). Functional improvement with opioid analgesics is monitored closely to prevent unnecessary chronic opioid treatment. Patient education on safe storage (lockbox use), safe dosing, and safe disposal are essential.

It is recommended that all patients prescribed MOUD receive training and access to intranasal naloxone rescue kits. Naloxone rapidly reverses respiratory depression and restores breathing in the event of an opioid overdose. Guidelines also suggest making naloxone available to patients on chronic opioid therapy for pain, particularly with high-dose therapy, which has been defined by the US American National Institutes of Health guideline as a daily morphine equivalent dose of 50 mg/d for general practitioners and 90 mg/d for specialists.

Plate 4.19

Brain: PART I

OPIOID WITHDRAWAL

Opioid withdrawal syndrome (OWS) occurs when an individual who is physiologically dependent on opioids (either because of chronic opioid analgesic treatment or opioid use disorder) experiences a period of reduced dosage or abstinence from opioid-taking. OWS is both physically aversive and powerfully anxiogenic; thus individuals with moderate to severe OWS are highly motivated to seek opioid sources for immediate relief.

Pathophysiology. Opioid tolerance and withdrawal occur as neuroadaptations to chronic opioid exposure. This neurobiology is complex, involving adaptations at all levels of opioid-sensitive brain signaling, including (1) mu-opiate receptor desensitization, (2) opioid-sensitive neuron cellular tolerance due to upregulation of adenylyl cyclase activity and changes to cyclic adenosine monophosphate response element-binding signaling, (3) system feedback adaptations of neuronal and glial networks interacting with opioid-sensitive neurons, and (4) opioid-sensitive neural circuit changes in synaptic plasticity. Clinically, opioid signaling is inhibitory in function (e.g., suppression of pain, respiratory drive, arousal, and anxiety); in contrast, OWS symptoms are mediated by rebound hyperactivity due to reduction or removal of chronic opioid agonism.

Presentation. OWS onset, duration, and severity vary according to type of opioid exposure (short acting vs. long acting, full agonist vs. partial agonist), exposure duration, dosing of exposure, and periodicity of withdrawal episodes. OWS is more severe with high-dose, full-agonist opioid exposure; more frequent OWS episodes worsen future withdrawal episodes. Individuals using short-acting opioids (heroin, oxycodone, or hydrocodone) experience mild to moderate OWS within 8 to 12 hours of last dosing, whereas persons using long-acting opioids (sustained-release oxycodone or methadone) experience mild to moderate OWS within 24 to 36 hours of last dosing. The duration of OWS is briefer (days) with shorter-acting opioids and may persist for weeks with longer-acting opioids. In both instances, protracted withdrawal may persist for weeks to months characterized by residual dysphoria with persistent physical discomfort often interfering with an individual's motivation and capacity for remaining abstinent from opioids. Craving and mental preoccupation associated with opioid addiction is nearly universal, persisting beyond the acute withdrawal episode and frequently leading to recurrent opioid use.

Clinical symptoms of OWS include anxiety, irritability, dysphoria, nausea, anorexia, chills, muscle aches and cramps, abdominal cramping, opioid craving, headache, and fatigue. Patients with OWS demonstrate mydriasis, lacrimation, diaphoresis, yawning, piloerection, rhinorrhea, tachycardia, hypertension, fever, diarrhea, vomiting, insomnia, and restlessness. Individuals vary in their presentation; some primarily experience gastrointestinal distress, whereas others demonstrate high anxiety with cardiovascular hyperexcitability. Of interest, each individual exhibits a consistent pattern of OWS symptoms from episode to episode. OWS may be measured using a standardized instrument such as the Clinical Opiate Withdrawal Scale (COWS), which is useful for medical documentation and opioid dosing needs assessment.

Treatment. Typically, OWS is not considered a medical emergency; however, special circumstances may constitute medical emergencies. These include pregnancy

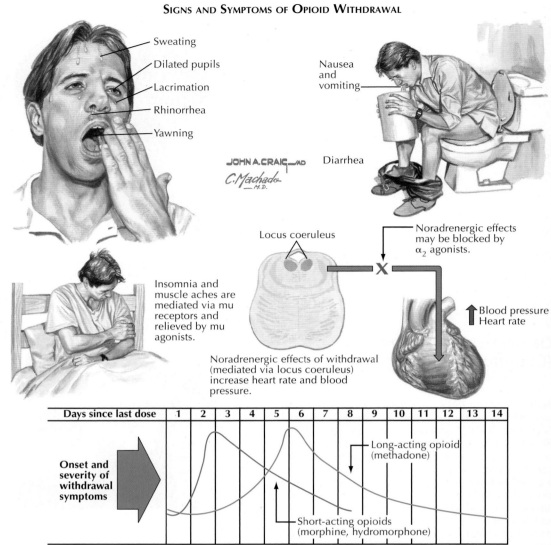

SIGNS AND SYMPTOMS OF OPIOID WITHDRAWAL

Sweating

Dilated pupils

Lacrimation

Rhinorrhea

Yawning

JOHN A. CRAIG—MD
C. Machado—M.D.

Nausea and vomiting

Diarrhea

Insomnia and muscle aches are mediated via mu receptors and relieved by mu agonists.

Locus coeruleus

Noradrenergic effects may be blocked by α₂ agonists.

Blood pressure
Heart rate

Noradrenergic effects of withdrawal (mediated via locus coeruleus) increase heart rate and blood pressure.

Days since last dose	1	2	3	4	5	6	7	8	9	10	11	12	13	14

Onset and severity of withdrawal symptoms

Long-acting opioid (methadone)

Short-acting opioids (morphine, hydromorphone)

Severity of opioid withdrawal varies with dose and duration of opioid use. Onset and duration of symptoms after last drug dose depend on half-life of particular drug.

(deleterious cardiovascular effects on the fetus and third trimester premature labor risk), cardiovascular disease, disorders involving autonomic instability, and vulnerability to dehydration. Optimal treatment includes rapid symptom stabilization to prevent opioid misuse and medical consequences of OWS.

Agonist replacement is the most rapidly effective treatment and is achieved by administering previously used opioids or an agonist substitution therapy, including the full agonist methadone or the partial agonist buprenorphine. Full agonists are administered to prevent OWS at any time; however, the partial agonist buprenorphine requires OWS be sufficiently moderate in severity (COWS score ≥9) before administration. This avoids inadvertently precipitating severe withdrawal (buprenorphine competes superiorly with full agonists at mu-opiate receptors and thereby has functional antagonist activity in this setting). New microdosing protocols are under investigation to improve the induction experience of those dependent on illicitly manufactured fentanyl, as routine buprenorphine induction protocols in fentanyl users frequently precipitate significant OWS.

Standard protocols for first-day dosing of opioid-dependent individuals are 5 to 10 mg oral methadone every 4 hours as needed, not exceeding 40 mg/24 hr, or 2 to 4 mg sublingual buprenorphine every 4 hours as needed, not exceeding 16 mg/24 hr. Dosing in pregnancy is generally similar, although requirements may be higher during the third trimester. Methadone peak and trough monitoring is recommended in pregnant women, concomitant with obstetric consultation. Although detoxification protocols may follow first-day dosing, opioid detoxification generally demonstrates poor outcomes in outpatient settings, with very high rates of recurrent opioid use occurring despite behavioral treatments for opioid use disorder. Agonist stabilization or maintenance is frequently preferred to improve long-term stability (antagonist maintenance has a higher dropout rate) and to reduce all-cause mortality. Although α₂ agonists, including clonidine, are widely used to treat OWS, they only ameliorate autonomic symptoms (hypertension and tachycardia) without providing efficacy for other symptoms. Patient comfort and treatment retention with clonidine are poor compared with opioid agonist treatments. During any treatment protocol, other symptom-specific medical adjuncts may be needed, including sedatives for insomnia, antiemetics for nausea, and dicyclomine for abdominal cramping.

Plate 4.20

Psychiatry

Develops in early childhood

Lack of control over anger

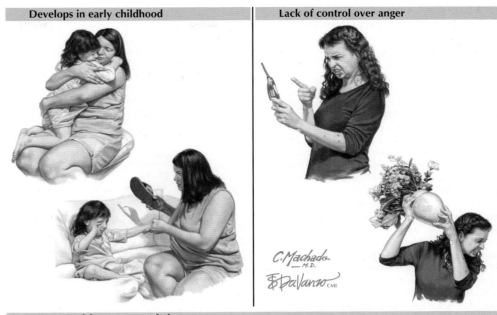

Intense and frequent mood changes

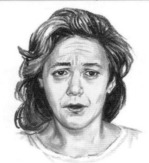
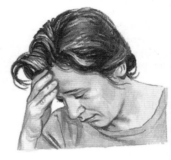
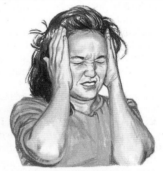

Impulsive behavior, including drug or alcohol abuse

Volatile interpersonal relationships

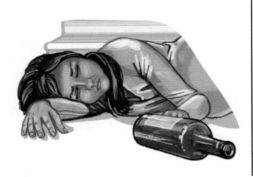
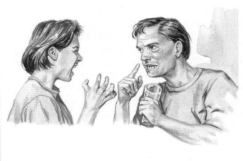

BORDERLINE PERSONALITY DISORDER

According to the *DSM-5,* the essential feature of borderline personality disorder (BPD) is a "pervasive pattern of instability of interpersonal relationships, self-image, and affects, and marked impulsivity that begins by early adulthood." Symptoms must occur in multiple contexts and include five or more of the following: frantic efforts to avoid real or imagined abandonment; a pattern of unstable, intense interpersonal relationships marked by alternating between idealization and devaluation; marked identity disturbance; impulsivity in at least two areas that are potentially self-damaging; recurrent suicidal behaviors, gestures, or threats; affective instability due to marked mood reactivity; chronic feelings of emptiness; inappropriate intense anger or difficulty controlling anger; transient, stress-related paranoid ideation; or severe dissociative symptoms.

BPD is common in both the general population and in clinical settings. The prevalence of BPD is estimated to be 1.6% but may be more common within specific groups. The prevalence of BPD has been found to be as high as 10% among individuals seen in outpatient and mental health clinics and about 20% among psychiatric inpatients. Impairment from symptoms and risk for suicide are greatest during young adulthood, especially in those with co-occurring depressive disorders or substance use disorders. The severity and prevalence of BPD decrease with age; approximately 75% of individuals with BPD regain close to normal functioning by age 40 years, and by age 50 years, almost 90% recover.

Both biologic and psychosocial factors contribute to the development of BPD. Neurobiologic research suggests (1) stress exerts demanding effects on the brain, specifically the hippocampus; (2) heightened activity in brain circuits involved in the experience of negative emotions; and (3) reduced activation that normally suppresses negative emotion once it is generated. BPD is about five times more common among first-degree biologic relatives of those with the disorder than in the general population. There is also an increased familial risk for substance use disorders, ASPD, and depressive or bipolar disorders. Contributing psychosocial factors include family dysfunction, frequent traumatic

childhood events, invalidating environments, history of sexual and/or physical abuse, and history of childhood neglect.

BPD historically has been thought to occur more frequently in females; however, two epidemiologic surveys of the US general population have found the lifetime prevalence of BPD does not differ significantly between males and females. Thus the apparent increased prevalence in women may represent selection and confirmation bias. BPD has been found to occur in all races and ethnicities.

Although pharmacotherapy can have a role in symptom management, psychosocial treatment is the primary treatment for BPD. Dialectical behavior therapy (DBT) is the most empirically supported treatment for BPD with the most consistent efficacy. DBT

focuses on the concepts of mindfulness (e.g., paying attention to the present emotion) and teaches skills to control intense emotions, reduce self-destructive behavior, manage distress, and improve relationships. DBT seeks a balance between acceptance and change-oriented behaviors, and treatment includes individual therapy sessions, skills training in a group setting, and phone coaching as needed. Psychodynamic treatments, such as mentalization-based therapy, have demonstrated encouraging results. Finally, medications can help treat other conditions that often accompany BPD, such as depression, impulsivity, and anxiety, but they do not treat or cure BPD itself. Often individuals with BPD are treated with several medications, but there is little evidence that this approach is necessary or effective.

Plate 4.21

Brain: PART I

ANTISOCIAL PERSONALITY DISORDER

Antisocial personality disorder (ASPD) is defined by the *DSM-5* as "a pervasive pattern of disregard for, and violation of, the rights of others" beginning in early childhood or adolescence and continuing into adulthood. To meet criteria for a diagnosis of ASPD, individuals must have a history of conduct disorder before the age of 15 years, characterized by aggression toward people and animals, destruction of property, deceitfulness or theft, or serious violation of rules or social norms. As adults, these persons may continue to ignore social rules, be manipulative and deceitful, be impulsive without considering the consequences, be irritable and aggressive, disregard their own or other's safety, behave irresponsibly, lack remorse for the consequences of their actions, and may be involved in criminal activity. Antisocial behavior has a negative effect on academic and professional achievement, material-life success, physical health, social relationships, and psychologic well-being and is linked to negative outcomes, such as legal problems, incarceration, and increased mortality due to reckless behavior. Although not all persons with ASPD are violent, ASPD is strongly associated with violence toward others compared with other psychiatric disorders.

The prevalence of ASPD is estimated to be 0.2% to 3% of the adult general population (3% of males and 1% of females) (APA, 2013). One potential explanation for the sex discrepancy is that females are more likely to be diagnosed with other personality disorders, such as BPD. The prevalence of ASPD is higher in males in substance abuse treatment and forensic settings and incarceration. This disorder is represented across all races, ethnicities, and cultures, but the prevalence is higher in individuals with lower socioeconomic status. Comorbid psychiatric disorders are common among individuals with ASPD. ASPD overlaps with psychopathy, which is not defined in the *DSM* but refers to individuals with features of ASPD plus manipulativeness, callousness, and shallow affect. ASPD is highly associated with substance use disorders, other personality disorders, and ADs. Symptoms of ASPD, like many personality disorders, appear to decline with age.

The exact etiology of ASPD is unknown, although several possible biologic and psychosocial factors are identified. Adoption studies suggest a genetic link, with higher rates of ASPD in the offspring of males with the disorder. The stability of antisocial behavior also appears to be related to genetic influences, whereas nonshared environmental influences account for change in antisocial behavior over time. Biologic theories suggest that the impulsive and sometimes violent behavior seen in ASPD may be linked to low levels of serotonin, low thresholds for limbic stimulation, or brain damage secondary to injury, disease, or substances; however, causal relationships have yet to be established. ASPD is also associated with deficits in neural networks that involve the dorsolateral prefrontal cortex. Individuals with ASPD demonstrate difficulties with executive function and memory, specifically with problems requiring higher-level planning ability.

Psychosocial factors are also associated with ASPD. Adults with ASPD often have experienced insufficient emotional attachment and nurturing during childhood. Childhood behavioral disorders also contribute to the development of ASPD in adulthood.

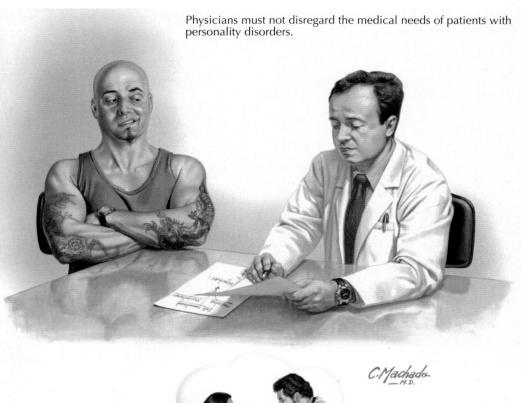

Physicians must not disregard the medical needs of patients with personality disorders.

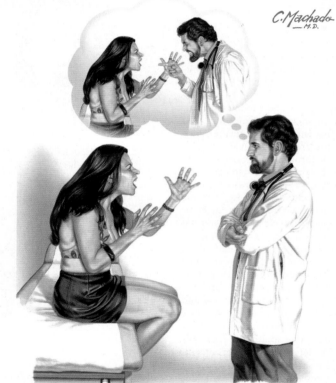

Patients with personality disorders often provoke intense and hostile feelings in their caregivers.

The consensus regarding treatment for ASPD is that it is difficult to treat. There are little to no efficacy data on pharmacologic interventions for ASPD, and presently there are no guidelines put forth by the APA for the treatment of ASPD. One of the challenges to identifying an effective treatment is the absence of research on this population, as they are frequently excluded from psychiatric care and studies. Patients with ASPD are characterized as having poor insight and minimal motivation to change behavior. When they do present for treatment, it may be because of legal mandate or the presence of a comorbid condition. Individual psychotherapy is not recommended for ASPD. Beyond the difficulty of establishing a therapeutic alliance, therapy itself provides yet another opportunity for deception and manipulation. The most promising treatment modality for ASPD is cognitive and behavioral interventions that focus on reducing offending behavior. A more productive target may be early intervention and prevention programs to reduce the likelihood that childhood conduct disorder will evolve into ASPD.

Plate 4.22   Psychiatry

INTIMATE PARTNER VIOLENCE

Intimate partner violence refers to physical, sexual, or psychological maltreatment by a current or prior partner or spouse. It can take place in the context of any intimate relationship and can consist of a single incident or recurrent, severe violence lasting many years. There are four major categories of intimate partner violence: (1) *physical abuse,* whereby physical force is used to kill, disable, injure, or otherwise hurt a partner; (2) *sexual abuse,* which involves coercing a partner to engage in a sex act or sexual behavior without consent; (3) *threats of violence,* in which verbal statements, gestures, or weapons convey a desire to kill, disable, injure, or otherwise hurt a partner; and (4) *psychologic or emotional abuse,* including insults, controlling behavior, deliberate damage to self-esteem, stalking, and preventing a partner from accessing family, friends, information, money, or other resources.

In the United States 1 in 3 females and 1 in 6 males experience some form of sexual violence during their lives. Perpetrators of attempted or completed rape are highly likely to be known to the survivor. One in four females and 1 in 9 males experience physical violence, sexual assault, or stalking behavior that causes them significant sequelae requiring treatment or a diagnosis of PTSD. One in seven females and 1 in 25 males have received physical injuries from an intimate partner; only 34% of individuals with injuries received any treatment.

Clinical Presentation and Diagnosis. Risk factors for committing intimate partner abuse include poor self-esteem, poverty, substance use disorders, minimal social supports, belief in strict gender roles, social isolation, past physical or psychologic abuse, BPD (Plate 4.20), ASPD (Plate 4.21), relationship instability, financial stressors, and community tolerance of intimate partner violence. Victims of intimate partner abuse can present with physical injuries, such as scratches, cuts, bruises, welts, broken bones, internal bleeding, and head trauma. The psychological trauma from intimate partner violence can manifest as depression, suicidal ideation and attempts, flashbacks, panic attacks, and difficulty sleeping.

The mnemonic *SAFE* (Sebastian, 1996) is often used to facilitate the discussion of intimate partner abuse by asking about (1) *stress* and *safety* in the relationship, (2) being *afraid* of or *abused* by one's partner, (3) having *friends* or *family* who can serve as social supports, and (4) having an *emergency* plan if in danger. The Danger Assessment originally developed by Campbell in 1986 (https://www.dangerassessment.org) and a short-form, five-item version assess whether violence has increased over the past year, the amount and extent of incidents involving weapons or strangulation, concern that the abuse could cause death, and extent of jealous motivation. Assessing specifically for experiences of being "choked" by a partner is particularly sensitive in predicting future violence and homicide.

Management. Clinicians must provide victims of intimate partner abuse with a safe environment. History taking and physical examination should be conducted in a trauma-informed manner, with detailed, sensitive, and confidential documentation in the medical record of all findings and interventions. All necessary steps must be taken to prevent discovery of the evaluation by the abusive partner or their associates. Intimate partner abuse must be acknowledged and the victim told that they are not at fault.

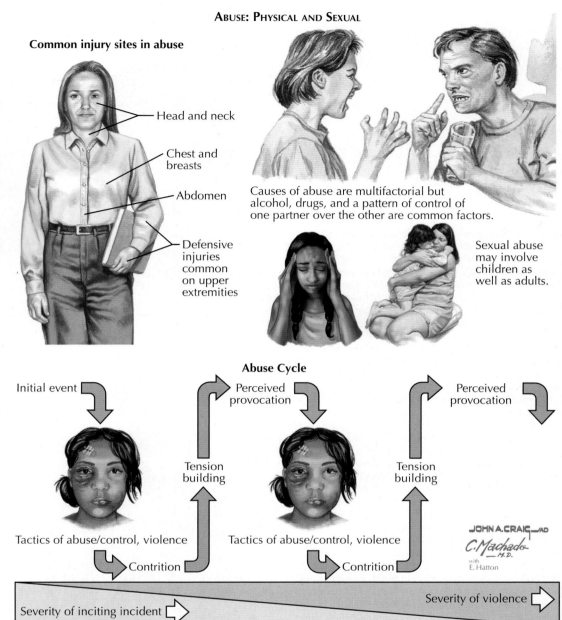

ABUSE: PHYSICAL AND SEXUAL

Common injury sites in abuse

- Head and neck
- Chest and breasts
- Abdomen
- Defensive injuries common on upper extremities

Causes of abuse are multifactorial but alcohol, drugs, and a pattern of control of one partner over the other are common factors.

Sexual abuse may involve children as well as adults.

Abuse Cycle

Initial event — Perceived provocation — Perceived provocation

Tension building — Tension building

Tactics of abuse/control, violence — Contrition — Tactics of abuse/control, violence — Contrition

JOHN A. CRAIG—MD
C. Machado—M.D.
with E. Hatton

Severity of inciting incident ⟶   Severity of violence ⟶

Cycle of abuse is characterized by progressively smaller incidents inciting progressively greater violence and interspersed with periods of remorse.

The patient must receive all needed medical and surgical treatment for sequelae of abuse as well as evaluation for signs and symptoms of psychological trauma. Those in abusive relationships need the information that violence often becomes more severe with time. Intimate partner abuse may be reported to legal authorities if appropriate. Clinicians need to formulate a safety plan with the patient, including identifying potential escape routes in a conflict, discussing feasibility of making copies of or keeping important documents in an offsite location that the partner cannot access, having a few days' worth of clothes and toiletries packed, and providing referrals for shelter, legal assistance, and mental health services.

Treatment and Prognosis. Lenore Walker classically described a cyclic pattern of abuse relationships in 1979. (1) The *tension-building phase* occurs before an abusive incident; (2) the *acting-out phase* involves violent or otherwise abusive acts; and (3) the *reconciliation/honeymoon phase,* which consists of statements of apology, displays of affection, or attempts to overlook the preceding abuse, followed by a *calm phase.*

In addition to risks of bodily harm and homicide, physical, mental, sexual, and reproductive health outcomes have been linked with intimate partner violence. These include adolescent pregnancy, unintended pregnancy, miscarriage, stillbirth, intrauterine hemorrhage, nutritional deficiency, gastrointestinal problems, neurologic disorders, chronic pain, disability, substance use disorders, anxiety and PTSD, and dissociative disorders, as well as noncommunicable diseases such as hypertension, cancer, and cardiovascular diseases. Around 1 in 15 children in the United States are exposed to intimate partner violence, and 90% of this group are eyewitnesses. Observing intimate partner abuse in the home can have an adverse effect on the emotional, social, behavioral, and cognitive development of a child that can include repeating the observed patterns in their future relationships.

Plate 4.23

Brain: PART I

ABUSE IN LATER LIFE

Abuse of an older adult refers to the maltreatment or neglect of adults age 60 years or older, usually by a caregiver or person on whom the older adult relies. It includes *physical abuse* (injury, physical threats, or inappropriate restraints), *sexual abuse* (sexual acts, contact, or exposure to sexual content without the older adult's consent), *psychologic or emotional abuse* (insults, name-calling, humiliation), *neglect or abandonment* (failure to meet the older adult's physical, emotional, and social needs or to provide protection), and *financial abuse* (inappropriate use of the older adult's resources for personal gain, including forgery, theft, manipulation of the elder to transfer money or belongings, and exploitation of guardianship or power of attorney).

Clinical Presentation and Diagnosis. A WHO-funded meta-analysis in 2017 estimated the worldwide prevalence of elder abuse in the community at approximately 1 in 6 older adults, and in all settings the most experienced were psychological abuse and financial abuse, followed by neglect, physical abuse, and sexual abuse. In the Americas, the total prevalence is estimated at 11.7%. Worldwide, 64.2% of staff in institutional care settings admitted to abusing an older adult in the past year. Individuals experiencing abuse are often reluctant to report it out of fear.

Risk factors for perpetrating abuse of an older adult include insufficient training for caregiving, emotional overwhelm, untreated or undertreated mental illness, alcohol abuse, personal history of physical or emotional abuse, significant emotional or financial dependence upon the older adult, inadequate social support, lack of formal support services, negative cultural beliefs about aging, and institutional settings with poor working conditions for staff and/or insufficient administrative monitoring. Risk factors for experiencing abuse as an older adult are being female, being 74 years or older, having a cognitive impairment or disability, and having worsening health and requiring more assistance.

The older adult reporting abuse must be listened to, and there may be observable, abrupt changes in the older adult's behavior. The caregiver may keep visitors from seeing the older adult alone. However, signs and symptoms of abuse of an older adult include bruises, welts, cuts, lacerations, rope marks or other signs of being restrained, broken bones, and internal bleeding. Additionally, the abused older adult patient may have injury to the breasts or genitals, unexplained sexually transmitted illnesses, dehydration, malnutrition, bed sores, poor hygiene, and unauthorized or unexplained banking transactions. Laboratory results may indicate medication overdose or inadequate dosing.

Prevention and Management. Caregivers can use a variety of strategies to reduce stress and decrease their likelihood of perpetrating abuse. Obtaining adequate training before assuming caregiving responsibilities can

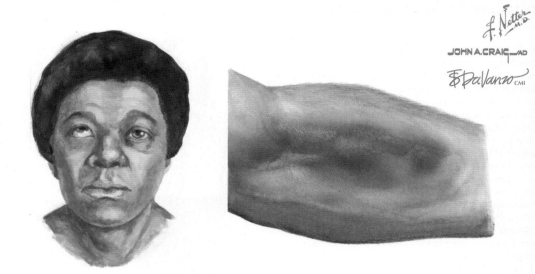

Physical abuse

Physical abuse demonstrated through assaults, rough handling, burns, and sexual abuse

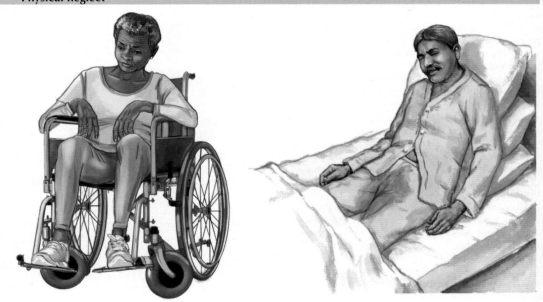

Physical neglect

Physical neglect demonstrated through poor hygiene, malnutrition, soiled clothing, receiving wrong medicines, not getting medical care when needed, or complete abandonment without supervision or care

markedly reduce overwhelm. Caregivers should also enlist the help of other community members, including family, friends, and local assistive services. Respite for caregivers, including adult day care programs and volunteer programs, can be beneficial. Independent financial planning services to manage an older adult's assets can decrease the risk of financial abuse. Finally, caregivers should never hesitate to seek mental health counseling for themselves.

At facilities for the care of older adults, appropriate staffing ratios, thorough employee training, availability of registered nurses, regular monitoring for abuse, clear policies and protocols outlining proper treatment of older adults with and without dementia, and regular visits to the facility by community members may all

decrease the risk of abuse. Suspected abuse of older adults must be reported to adult protective services. The patient may require hospital admission to ensure safety and provide medical or surgical treatment in the aftermath of abuse. A multidisciplinary team approach to abuse in later life is optimal, and referrals to appropriate supportive services are essential.

Treatment and Prognosis. Experiencing abuse in later life increases the risk of adverse health consequences, including physical injuries, malnutrition, dehydration, poor sleep, sexually transmitted illnesses, exacerbation of preexisting medical conditions, and premature death. Psychologic sequelae include increased rates of depression, ADs, symptoms of PTSD, and other forms of distress.

Plate 4.24

Psychiatry

DELIRIUM AND ACUTE PERSONALITY CHANGES

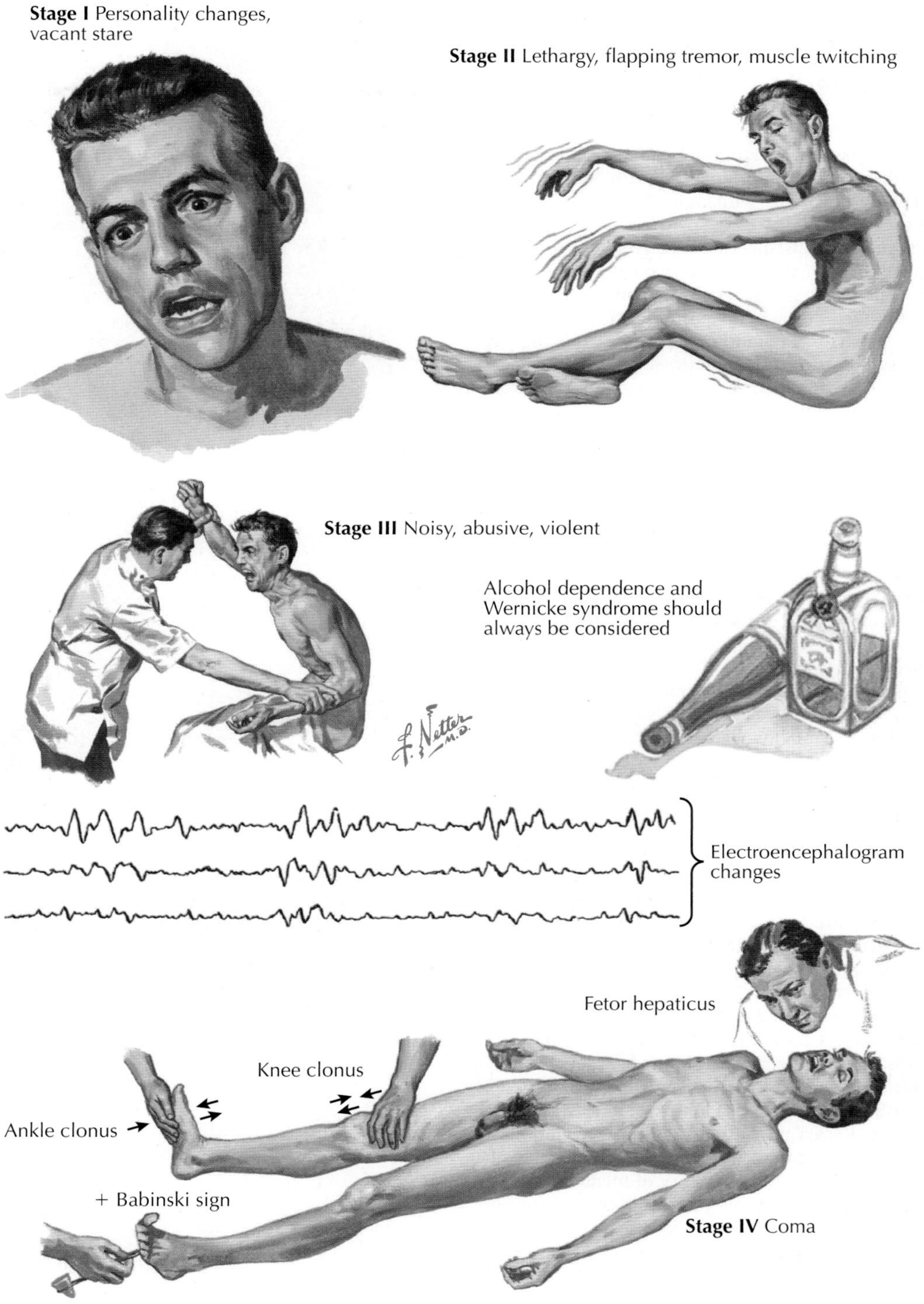

Delirium is an acute and fluctuating change of mental status commonly seen in medically ill patients. It is a medical emergency. Approximately 30% of elderly patients experience delirium during hospitalization. Its prevalence in the intensive care unit can reach up to 70%. Delirium encompasses four key clinical features: (1) a new-onset disturbance in attention and awareness, (2) acute development typically over hours to days, (3) symptom fluctuation in severity, and (4) disturbances in other cognitive domains (e.g., memory deficit, disorientation, language, visuospatial ability, perception). Other disorders that cause altered attention, awareness, or cognition should be excluded. Positive evidence should emerge that the cognitive disturbances are the direct physiologic consequence of a systemic medical condition, substance intoxication or withdrawal, or exposure to a toxin. Delirium can be due to multiple medical etiologies at once.

The three main subtypes of delirium are hyperactive, hypoactive, and mixed. Hyperactive delirium presents with symptoms of restlessness, agitation, emotional lability, auditory hallucinations, visual hallucinations, and delusions. Sometimes patients strike out at staff or aggressively pull at tubes or lining. Hyperactive delirium can be confused with agitated dementia, psychosis, mania, or excited catatonia. Hypoactive delirium presents with symptoms of apathy, blunted affect, withdrawal, and slowed cognition. Hypoactive delirium may be confused with dementia, depression, or akinetic catatonia. Mixed delirium presents with cycling between hyperactive and hypoactive states. Sleep dysregulation with "sundowning" can be an early sign of emerging delirium: patients may present as lethargic during the daytime yet be agitated and awake overnight.

Several evidence-based tools exist to facilitate screening for delirium. For adults, these include the Confusion Assessment Method (CAM), the Confusion Assessment Method—Intensive Care Unit (CAM-ICU), and the Delirium Rating Scale (DRS). Pediatric screening tools include the Cornell Assessment of Pediatric Delirium (CAPD) and the Pediatric Confusion Assessment Method—Intensive Care Unit (pCAM-ICU). Delirium screening tools are not diagnostic tools. Psychiatric examination remains the evidence-based standard for diagnosing delirium.

The neurobiologic basis of delirium remains poorly understood. Multiple pathophysiologic mechanisms are causative, and several neural pathways are involved. Affected areas of the brain include the subcortical ascending reticular activating system, which contributes to arousal, and the integrated cortical regions, which support proper orientation and higher-level processing.

One of the best-understood neurochemical pathogenic mechanisms associated with delirium is the cholinergic system. Conditions that may predispose to delirium secondary to acetylcholine depletion include hypoxia, hypoglycemia, thiamine deficiency, and Alzheimer disease. Additional neurotransmitter systems that may be involved in delirium include GABA, endorphins, neuropeptides, serotonin, and norepinephrine. Endogenous neurochemical precipitants include proinflammatory cytokines and tumor necrosis factor-α.

Hospitalized elderly patients with multiple medical comorbidities are at highest risk for delirium. Other vulnerable populations include patients on multiple

Stage I Personality changes, vacant stare

Stage II Lethargy, flapping tremor, muscle twitching

Stage III Noisy, abusive, violent

Alcohol dependence and Wernicke syndrome should always be considered

F. Netter M.D.

Electroencephalogram changes

Fetor hepaticus

Knee clonus

Ankle clonus

+ Babinski sign

Stage IV Coma

medications, terminally ill patients, young children, patients with sensory deprivation, and patients who are sleep deprived. In the hospital setting, patients with dementia, malnourishment, burns, Parkinson disease, HIV, AUD, sedative-hypnotic use disorder, dialysis, and poststroke or postsurgical status all carry additional risk for delirium.

Primary delirium management requires identifying and treating underlying physiologic disturbances. In hospitalized patients, emerging infection is among the most common causes of delirium. Other common causes include medications, substance intoxication or withdrawal (sometimes iatrogenic), metabolic derangement, hypoxia, dehydration, thyroid disease, and neurovascular disease. Delirium warrants comprehensive

review of a patient's medical history, physical exam, labs, medications (prescription and over the counter), and substance use history. Psychiatric consultation may be appropriate for diagnostic clarification and psychotropic management. Secondary management involves supporting and managing behavioral and neuropsychiatric disturbances.

Behavioral management is a universal intervention that involves environmental strategies that minimize excessive stimulation and refocus the patient. Strategies include frequent reorientation, environmental optimization to promote daytime wakefulness and nighttime sleep, early mobilization, access to hearing and visual aids, cognitive stimulation, and adequate hydration and

Plate 4.25

Brain: PART I

DELIRIUM AND ACUTE PERSONALITY CHANGES (Continued)

nutrition. Psychoeducation to patients and families about delirium is important. Delirium can be a very frightening experience with high rates of PTSD in caregivers.

Although nonpharmacologic interventions should remain the core of secondary management, short-duration antipsychotic use for hyperactive or mixed-type delirium may be indicated to ensure patient safety and control behavioral agitation related to distressing psychotic symptoms. Antipsychotics should be used with caution. They do not treat underlying physiologic disturbances causing delirium itself, and they are not a benign intervention, as they carry increased risk of mortality and stroke. The largest collection of data supports low-dose haloperidol as needed for severe agitation in delirium. Several studies show the second-generation antipsychotics risperidone, olanzapine, and quetiapine as largely comparable to haloperidol in management of hyperactive delirium. No evidence currently supports the use of antipsychotic agents or stimulant agents in the management of hypoactive delirium. No evidence currently supports the prophylactic use of medication in delirium.

Anticholinergic, sedative-hypnotic (e.g., benzodiazepines), and opiate medications should generally be avoided in delirium management because of the risk of exacerbating symptoms. For select cases, strategic use of sedative-hypnotics or opioid medications may be warranted (e.g., taper protocols for substance withdrawal syndromes or opioids for postoperative pain).

Delirium can be confused with primary psychiatric disorders, so understanding the neuropsychiatric baseline of the patient is critical. Cognitive decline that is chronic and progressive suggests a major neurocognitive disorder such as dementia. Primary psychoses classically present with psychotic symptoms in early adulthood. A first psychotic episode occurring in a middle age or older adult warrants medical evaluation for delirium. Characteristics of hallucinations may help distinguish primary psychotic disorders from delirium. Patients with hyperactive delirium can present with visual hallucinations alone, which is unusual for psychoses. Recurring episodes of odd behavior, indifferent attitude, amnesia, atypical presenting age, absence of patient or family history of mental illness, or abnormal signs on neurologic examination should indicate evaluation for neurologic disease. Seizures or focal signs on neurologic examination may warrant brain imaging or electroencephalography to assess for acute structural lesions, infection, or inflammation. It is important to rule out potentially treatable neurologic conditions that can cause permanent damage to the nervous system such as Wernicke encephalopathy, herpes encephalitis, paraneoplastic syndromes, or autoimmune encephalitides.

Anti–NMDA receptor (NMDA-R) encephalitis is a novel and significantly underdiagnosed autoimmune encephalitis. Clinically, anti-NDMA-R encephalitis presents with acute new-onset neuropsychiatric symptoms of psychosis, catatonia, abnormal involuntary movements, memory deficits, or seizures, sometimes after a nonspecific prodromal illness. Approximately 40% of cases occur in patients younger than 18 years. Females make up the majority of cases, and 58% are diagnosed with an underlying ovarian teratoma. Testing should include serum and cerebrospinal fluid studies for anti-NMDA-R

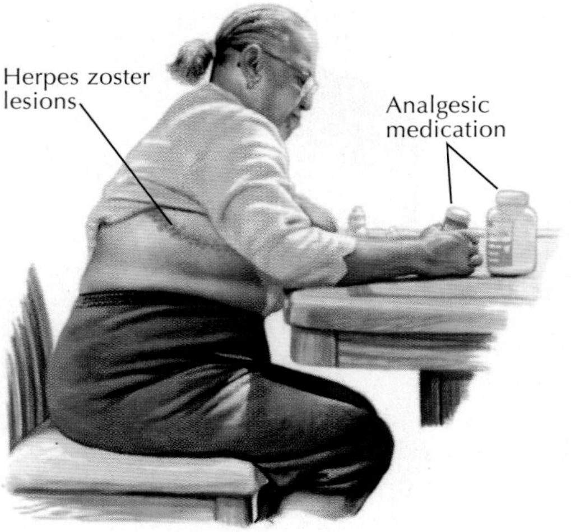

Use of analgesics and sedatives can precipitate delirium in patients with limited cognitive reserve, especially the elderly and those with dementia.

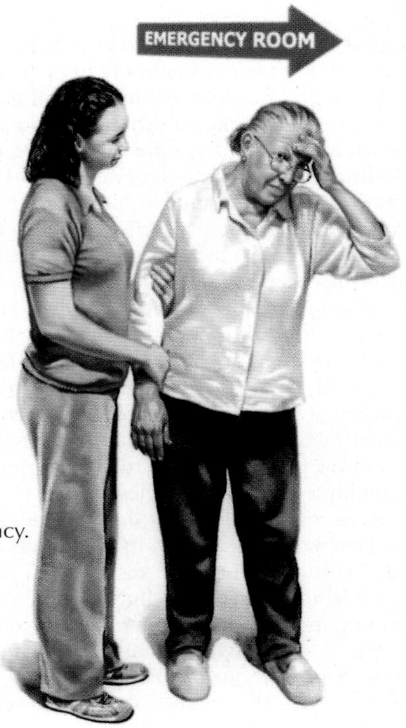

Delirium is a medical emergency.

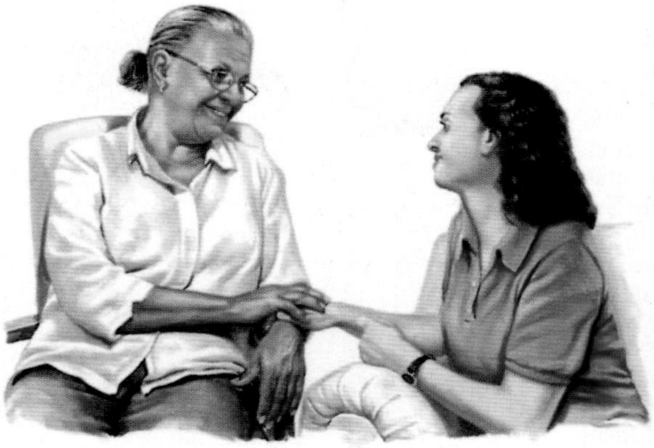

The mental state of delirious patients often changes from hour to hour.

C. Machado —M.D.

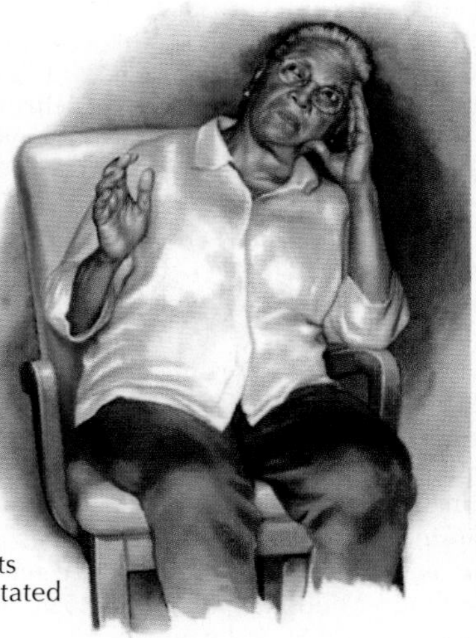

"Sundowning." Delirious patients are often more confused and agitated at night.

autoantibodies and abdominal/pelvic imaging. Prognosis depends on adequate immunotherapy and, in paraneoplastic cases, complete tumor removal.

In rare cases, psychiatric medications may cause emergent medical syndromes. Antipsychotic medications can precipitate neuroleptic malignant syndrome, a triad of acute confusion, muscle rigidity, and hyperthermia. Combinations of antidepressants, migraine medications, and some antibiotics can trigger serotonin syndrome, causing a triad of confusion, autonomic instability, and clonus. Lithium and other drugs that have a narrow therapeutic window, such as digitalis, can cause delirium even when levels are in the recommended therapeutic range. Lithium toxicity usually manifests with vomiting, diarrhea, severe tremors, and ataxia, whereas digitalis toxicity often causes paranoia and hallucinations. Drug

toxicity accounts for 30% of cases of delirium. Serum levels should be checked for all drugs the patient is taking, and all nonessential medications should be held.

Delirium is associated with significant morbidity and mortality. Negative outcomes include longer hospital stays, increased medical complications, and increased risk of death. Although most patients experience rapid resolution of delirium with correction of the underlying medical etiology, full recovery may take up to 12 months. Elderly individuals and those with baseline neurocognitive injury are less likely to achieve full recovery. Optimal delirium treatment requires prompt identification and correction of the underlying medical problem, judicious use of psychotropic or other medications to control unwanted symptoms, and maintenance of a peaceful environment.

Plate 4.26

Psychiatry

INSOMNIA

Most people experience occasional insomnia sometime in their lives. However, insomnia disorder, which is present in 10% to 15% of adults, is a more chronic problem with more substantial consequences. It requires a *symptom,* that is, difficulty with sleep onset, sleep maintenance, or nonrestorative sleep; a *frequency and duration* present at least 3 nights per week over a period of at least 3 months; and a *consequence* of associated distress or social or occupational dysfunction. Insomnia disorder can be diagnosed (and should be treated) even when it is in the context of an additional medical, psychiatric, or sleep disorder, as we now understand that sleeplessness can predispose to and can certainly aggravate those disorders.

Insomnia disorder is more common during increased social and familial stress and in females and those with poor physical health. Insomnia is often a chronic condition, with 60% of those with insomnia disorder continuing to meet criteria after 5 years, particularly in those with more severe symptoms. However, specific insomnia symptoms (initial insomnia, nocturnal awakenings) are often dynamic, shifting over the course of the disorder. Insomnia disorder is often a marker of greater medical, neurologic, and psychiatric illness severity. Insomnia disorder is an independent risk factor for incident major depressive episodes. It is not established whether insomnia treatment improves outcomes or prevents incidence in such disorders. People with insomnia have an increased risk of hypertension and diabetes.

The construct of hyperarousal helps understand much of the physiology of insomnia disorder, although it is unclear whether the hyperarousal is a cause or consequence (or both) of insomnia. Evening cortisol elevations, increased body temperature and basal metabolic rate, waking EEG patterns, elevated glucose metabolism (detected by positron emission tomography) during non–rapid eye movement sleep, and reductions in brain GABA during wakefulness all point to nervous and autonomic system hyperarousal in insomnia disorder. Insomnia disorder may not be primarily a nocturnal disorder but rather something that is present throughout the 24-hour day, with insomnia its primary expression.

Insomnia neurobiology is not fully defined, although advances in sleep biology provide guidance to potential CNS substrates. The brain contains multiple systems promoting sleep and others enhancing wakefulness. Pedunculopontine and laterodorsal tegmental nuclei cholinergic neurons innervate the thalamus and cortex, firing most actively during wakefulness. Similarly, noradrenergic, serotonergic, and histaminergic cells in the locus coeruleus, raphe nucleus, and tuberomammillary nucleus project to the lateral hypothalamus, thalamus, and frontal cortex, respectively, and fire most actively during the waking state. Orexin-containing cells in the lateral hypothalamus project widely to the cerebral cortex and fire actively during waking to support arousal. The latter receive afferents from monoaminergic brainstem arousal centers, also providing extensive input to these centers. The cortex itself aids the arousal centers with reciprocal innervations.

GABAergic-containing neurons in the ventrolateral preoptic nucleus (VLPO) promote sleep by inhibiting arousal centers. Thus the current simplified understanding of sleep physiology informs us that redundant and interactive neural systems control sleep. It is not surprising that despite a powerful sleep drive, there

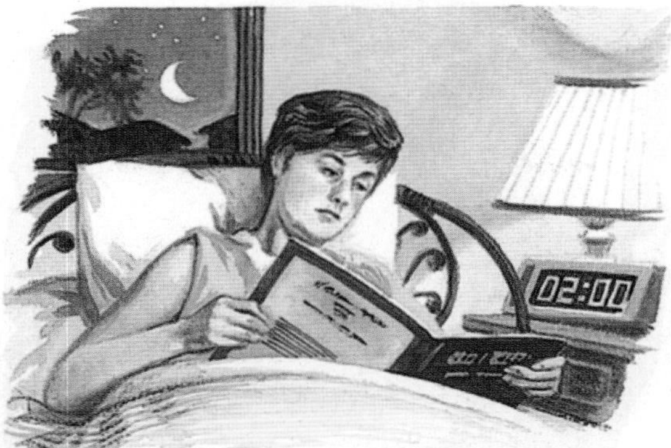

Reading in bed can assist those with insomnia relax, although watching the clock is not recommended.

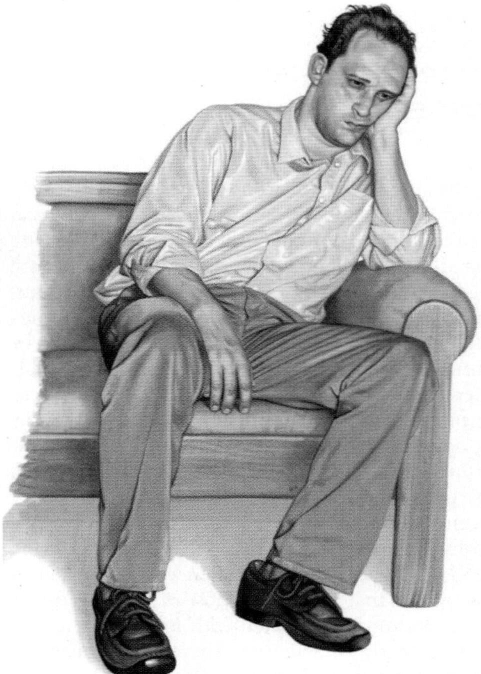

Symptoms of insomnia include fatigue, depressed mood, poor concentration, and worry.

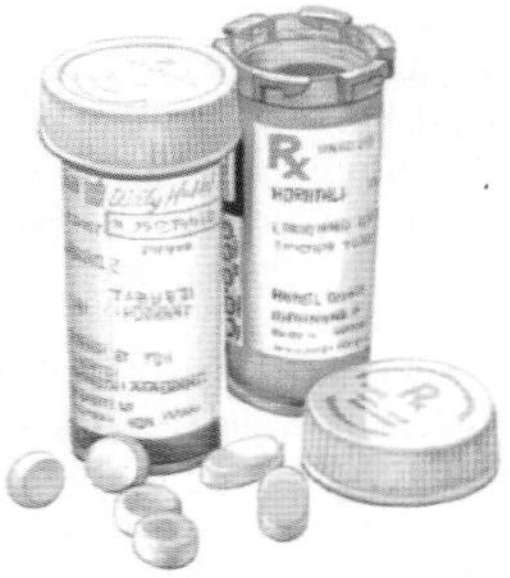

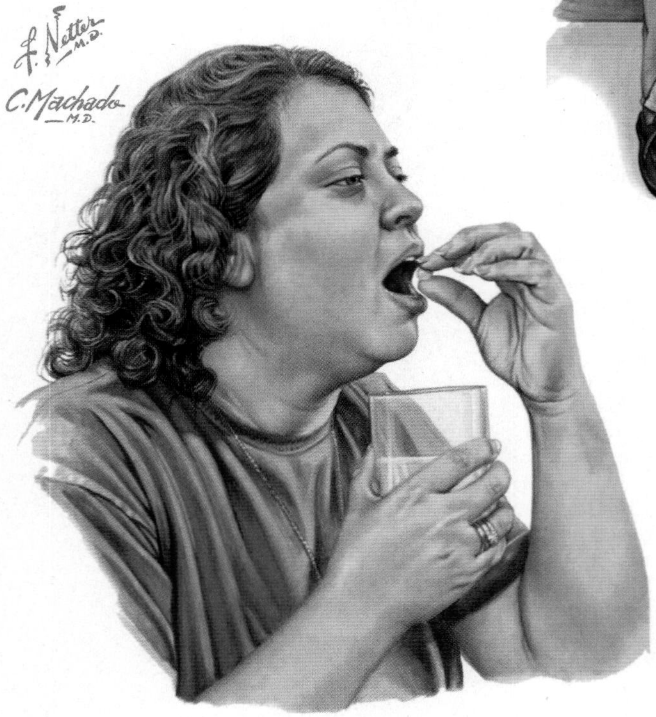

Hypnotic medications can be of great value for those who have not responded to cognitive-behavioral treatments.

are many neuroanatomic substrates for pathology to develop. Thus insomnia may be related to either inadequate inhibitory activity from VLPO sleep-promoting neurons or excess brainstem activation of arousal centers, or even simultaneous activation of both excitatory and inhibitory influences, leading to unstable sleep states.

The multiple neural systems controlling sleep provide diverse targets for behavioral and pharmacologic intervention for insomnia treatment. CBT for insomnia (CBT-I) is first-line therapy for insomnia disorder and includes education about productive sleep habits (sleep hygiene), reduction of time awake in bed (stimulus control), time in bed restriction to produce sleep deprivation and increase sleep drive, instruction in relaxation techniques such as meditation and progressive muscle relaxation, and substitution of realistic attitudes about the consequences of sleeplessness for prevailing catastrophic beliefs. CBT-I is effective for improving sleep satisfaction and reducing wake time before sleep and during the night, though it does not increase total sleep time during the night.

Marketed medications known to assist with sleep have existed for more than 50 years, although alcohol and opioids have been used for centuries. The commonly prescribed medications bind to benzodiazepine receptors, an allosteric site on the $GABA_A$ receptor, enhancing GABAergic (inhibitory) transmission throughout the CNS. Many benzodiazepine receptor agonists exist, and they differ from each other predominantly only in their half-life. These medications are also anticonvulsant, anxiolytic, and myorelaxant and may produce tolerance, physical and psychological dependence, and withdrawal symptoms upon rapid discontinuation. Therefore their use is controlled. Novel medications for insomnia disorder include the orexin antagonists, which bind to receptors regulating wakefulness. Other common medications used to promote sleep act at the monoaminergic receptors involved in CNS arousal. For instance, drugs with antihistaminergic properties are available for treatment of allergic reactions and as antidepressants and antipsychotics. Other insomnia medications bind to the melatonin receptor in the CNS, promoting sleep by uncertain mechanisms.

Plate 4.27

Brain: PART I

PEDIATRICS: DEPRESSIVE DISORDERS

Depressive disorders are a group of mental health problems in children and adolescents characterized by sad or irritable mood. In simple terms, these disorders are associated with differences in parts of the brain that are involved in the intensity of sad and irritable moods. Additionally, these disorders develop because of biologic vulnerabilities, such as a genetic predisposition or family history, and social vulnerabilities, such as maltreatment, bereavement, parent-child discord, and peer victimization. It is estimated that 4 to 5 of 100 youths have a depressive disorder. The three primary depressive disorders are MDD, persistent depressive disorder, and disruptive mood dysregulation disorder.

The most severe of these disorders, MDD, is characterized by a distinct period of at least 2 weeks during which the child/adolescent experiences a depressed or irritable mood that is present most of the day nearly every day and/or is associated with loss of interest or pleasure in nearly all activities. There are often severe problems with eating, sleeping, energy, concentration, feelings of worthlessness or extreme guilt, and/or loss of the desire to live. These symptoms may manifest as irritability, loss of interest in hanging out with friends, refusal to get out of bed for school in the morning, or preoccupation with death and dying. To meet this diagnosis, problems must cause distress and/or impair the youth's function at home, school, or with peers. After puberty, MDD is more common in females than in males regardless of gender identity. Furthermore, it is also more common in transgender youth than their cisgender peers.

The less severe but longer lasting of these disorders, *persistent depressive disorder,* is characterized by a depressed or irritable mood for most of the day, more days than not, *for at least 1 year.* As with MDD, the youth has problems with eating, sleeping, energy, concentration, feelings of hopelessness, and low self-esteem, and these problems must cause distress and/or impair the youth's function at home, school, or with peers. Children with this disorder are more likely to develop MDD in their teenage or early adult years.

Finally, disruptive mood dysregulation disorder is characterized by persistent irritability and behavioral difficulties in youth 12 years of age and younger. Frequent temper outbursts are present that are inconsistent with developmental level and occur consistently for 12 months or more. Disruptive mood dysregulation disorder is more common in males than in females, and children with this symptom pattern are more likely to develop another depressive disorder in their teenage or early adult years.

Diagnosis. Qualified health professionals experienced and trained in working with children and adolescents are most competent in accurately diagnosing these depressive disorders. The diagnostic evaluation is typically based upon information from interviews of parents/caregivers and the child or adolescent as well as a mental status examination. There are no imaging studies, blood tests, or other specific medical testing modalities to diagnose these disorders.

Treatment. Psychotherapy is an effective treatment for these disorders because it helps the youth understand and learn how to cope with sad feelings. These coping strategies include learning how to identify and talk about feelings, identify and change automatic negative

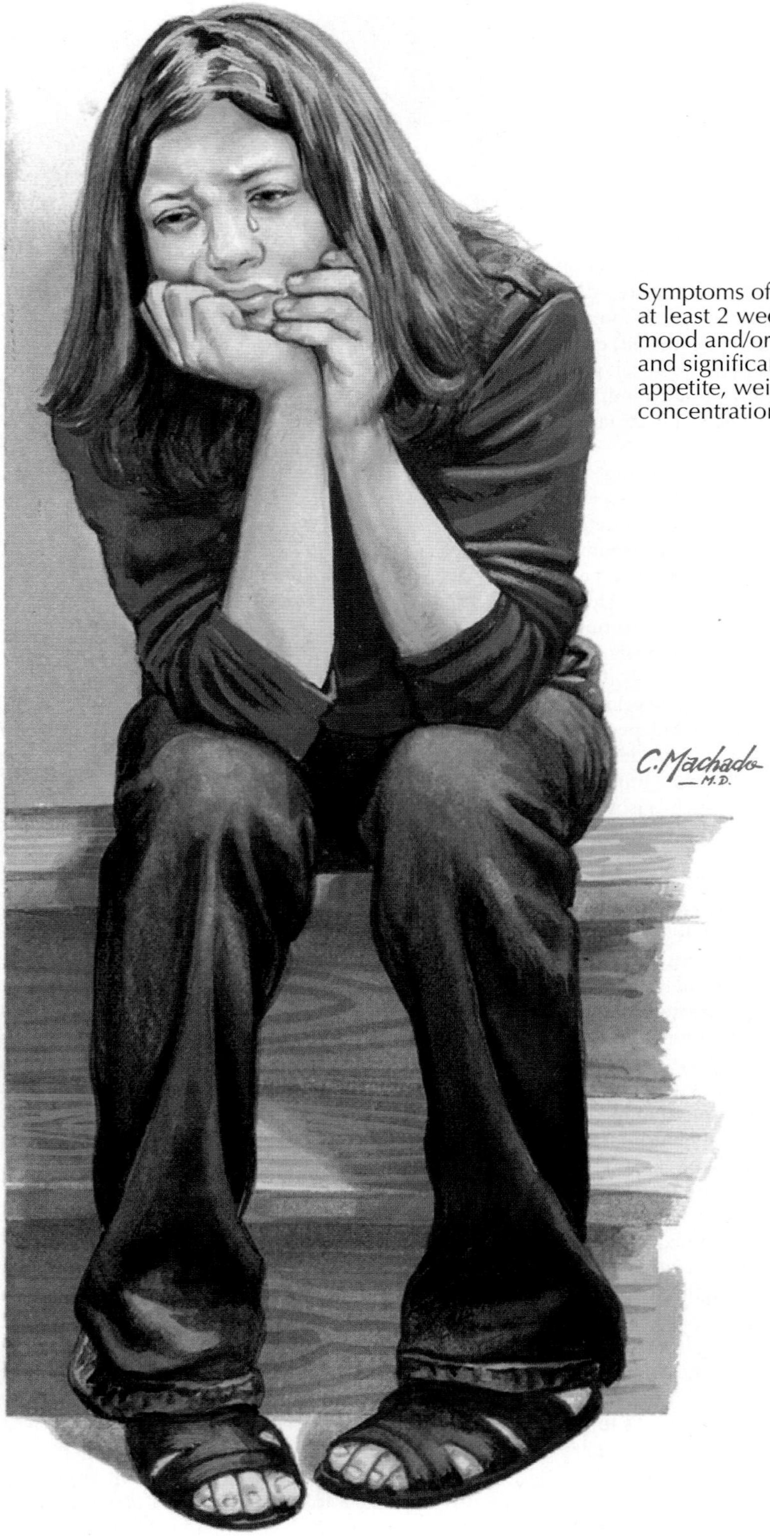

Symptoms of depressive disorder include at least 2 weeks of marked change in mood and/or loss of interest and pleasure, and significant changes in patterns of appetite, weight, sleep, activity, concentration, energy level, or motivation.

thoughts, engage in activities that are soothing and comforting, discover and appreciate good things about themselves, and build hope for the future. If the depressive disorder is severe, such that the youth is thinking about wanting to die or has lost most ability to function, or psychotherapy is not effective alone or not available, then antidepressant medication is indicated as a treatment. Antidepressant medication may help the youth feel more motivated to engage in therapy.

Treatment and Prognosis. The depressive disorders respond well to the above treatments when delivered by qualified mental health professionals. If left untreated, depressive disorders may lead to death through suicide. This very serious illness is also associated with failure in school and involvement in risky behaviors alongside subsequent difficulties with maintaining or establishing relationships and jobs in adulthood.

Plate 4.28

Psychiatry

PEDIATRICS: ANXIETY DISORDERS

Anxiety disorders (ADs) are mental health problems found in children and adolescents that are characterized by disabling worry or fear. These disorders are common, with 10 to 15 of 100 youths estimated to have one of these disorders. These occur more commonly in females. ADs are caused by a difference in the structure or function of the brain that controls worries and fears. Vulnerability to the development of ADs can be genetically transmitted. Parents who are overprotective or overcontrolling appear more likely to have anxious children, and children also can learn to be anxious from parents who are anxious. Sometimes environmental events can trigger an AD. For example, *separation anxiety disorder* can be caused by exposure to frightening events, such as intimate partner violence.

GENERALIZED ANXIETY DISORDER

GAD is characterized by excessive worry/angst occurring on more days than not about a variety of areas, such as schoolwork, friendships, family, health/safety, and world events. The worry is accompanied by feeling tired, tense, restless, or irritable; having difficulty focusing; and having trouble falling or staying asleep. There may be associated physical symptoms, including muscle aches, stomach cramps, or nausea. The youth finds it difficult to control the worry. To meet the diagnosis, the problems must be present for at least 6 months and must cause distress and/or impair the youth's function at home, at school, or with peers.

SEPARATION ANXIETY DISORDER

Separation anxiety disorder is characterized by excessive worry about separation from home or from parents. The child may feel very upset about leaving home to go to school, about being separated from the parent, about sleeping alone in their own bedroom, about something bad happening to the parent, or something bad happening to the child that will separate them from the parent. The child may refuse to go to school or may develop physical problems (e.g., headaches, nausea) before going to school or when at school. Some may experience bad dreams about being separated from the parent. To meet the diagnostic criteria, these problems must have persisted for at least 1 month, causing distress and/or impairing the youth's function at home, at school, or with peers.

SOCIAL ANXIETY DISORDER

SAD is characterized by excessive worry about social or performance situations where embarrassment may occur. This angst can arise when meeting new people or performing in front of others (e.g., speaking up in the classroom, performing musically or athletically). When worry becomes so severe that it causes panic, a pattern develops that leads to the youth avoiding social or performance situations. To meet the diagnosis, the problems must have been present for at least 6 months in addition to causing distress and/or impairing the youth's function at home, at school, or with peers.

Diagnosis. Qualified mental health professionals experienced with children (child and adolescent psychiatrists, child psychologists, child-trained social workers, counselors, and clinical nurse specialists) are best trained to accurately diagnose the various ADs. The evaluation for these diagnoses typically

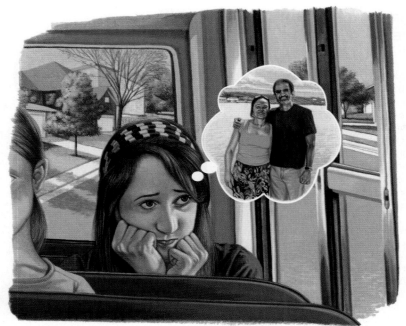

Generalized anxiety disorder (excessive worries and fears about various areas)

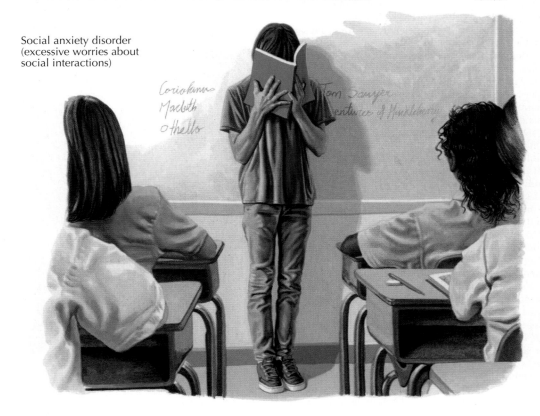

Social anxiety disorder (excessive worries about social interactions)

takes several hours and requires input from multiple people who know the child very well. The diagnosis is based upon the findings from parent and child interviews, questionnaires, and a mental status examination. In contrast to disruptive disorders, ADs often cause more distress in the child than the parents, and children tend to report their anxiety symptoms more accurately than their parents, who may not be aware of the child's symptoms. There are no imaging studies, blood tests, or other medical tests to diagnose these disorders.

Treatment. Psychotherapy to help the youth to learn how to cope with worry and fear is the best treatment. These coping strategies include learning how to confront and tolerate distress, how to identify and talk about feelings, how to reframe automatic negative thoughts, and how to relax the mind and body. When a child's AD does not respond to traditional therapy, antianxiety medication should be considered, as combination therapy of psychotherapy and medications has been shown to be superior to either therapy alone. Antianxiety medication may help the youth feel more relaxed when working on coping skills in therapy.

Prognosis. ADs respond well to the above treatments when delivered by qualified mental health professionals. If left untreated, ADs can cause long-standing distress and problems with social relationships and school performance.

Plate 4.29

Brain: PART I

PEDIATRICS: DISRUPTIVE BEHAVIOR DISORDERS

Disruptive behavior disorders (DBDs) are mental health problems occurring in children and adolescents, more commonly in males, characterized by out-of-control behavior. Prevalence rates vary from 1% to 16%. A cluster of factors, including the child's characteristics, parental interactions, and environmental factors contribute to their development.

A mismatch of parenting strategies and/or child-parent temperament and style often underly these disorders. Parents may have insufficient time and emotional energy for planning for the child's behavioral needs or may use methods inconsistently or for the wrong situation. *Authoritarian* parenting, in which the parent's style is low in warmth but high in firmness, and *permissive* parenting, with low firmness and high warmth, can result in behavioral challenges. *Authoritative* parenting, defined as having high levels of both warmth and firmness, is usually the most effective parenting strategy.

Children with DBDs may be strong willed because of genetically inherited personality characteristics, certain intrauterine exposures (e.g., nicotine, alcohol, or marijuana), lack of positive parent-child attachment, stress, or inconsistencies in the structure, routine, and safety of the home and community. Situational factors such as marital discord, low socioeconomic status, high crime rates, and systemic racism can exacerbate underlying mental health conditions in the parent or child, or both. These factors frequently result in reduced available resources for families and communities as well as less structure and consistency.

Diagnosis. DBDs are most accurately diagnosed by child and adolescent psychiatrists, child psychologists, child-trained social workers, and clinical nurse specialists. The evaluation requires input from multiple individuals from different environments. To confirm diagnosis of a DBD, symptoms must be present at least 6 months to 1 year, depending on the specific diagnosis, and the intensity and duration of outbursts must exceed that of a typical child and must affect functioning in the youth's home, school, and/or peer relationships. The diagnosis is based on findings from interviews and a mental status examination. There are no specific imaging studies, blood tests, or other medical tests that are diagnostic. One should always consider diagnoses that better capture the entire clinical picture, including oppositional behaviors. For example, ADs, PTSD, OCD, attention-deficit/hyperactivity disorder (ADHD), or autism could manifest with significant refusal of tasks and dysregulated behaviors.

Oppositional defiant disorder is characterized by a recurrent pattern of negativistic, defiant, disobedient, and hostile behavior, such as deliberately annoying others, frequent arguments, and angry outbursts directed toward authority figures, such as parents and teachers. Conduct disorder is characterized by a persistent pattern of serious rule-violating behavior, including instances that seriously harm or have the potential to seriously harm others. Physical aggression to people and animals, destruction of property, lying or stealing, running away from home, and truancy are typical examples. Intermittent explosive disorder is characterized by impulsive verbal or aggressive outbursts that are out of proportion for the context. Pyromania and kleptomania are also well-established DBDs.

Treatment. The best therapy for DBDs is to help the caregiver develop more effective strategies for managing behavioral concerns. Collaboration with a

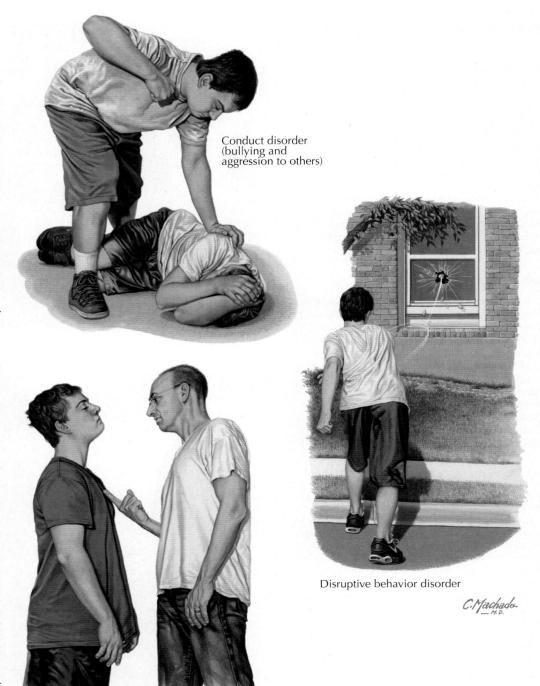

Conduct disorder (bullying and aggression to others)

Disruptive behavior disorder

Oppositional defiant disorder (defiant and disobedient)

psychotherapist can foster a systematic approach to managing behaviors in the home. Special parent-child time, even a few minutes a day, can help develop a warm, compassionate relationship between parent and child. Providing a predictable, structured environment and setting clear and simple household rules and consequences, while consistently praising and rewarding positive behaviors and ignoring disruptive behaviors, increases adaptive behaviors and diminishes maladaptive ones. CBT and social-emotional skills training help the child develop skills to identify and manage feelings, get along with others, and make good decisions based on thinking rather than feeling. Behavioral training is most effective when started early and can be challenging to begin in middle/late adolescence when the child is developing increasing autonomy.

Because conduct disorder is a more enduring condition, or when DBDs result in involvement of police, treatment must be more intensive and extensive, sometimes involving other child-serving agencies (e.g., juvenile justice, child welfare). Multisystemic therapy is a comprehensive approach to reduce recidivism and improve social, academic, and occupational outcomes.

Prognosis. DBDs respond well to the above treatments when delivered by qualified mental health professionals. Conduct disorder can be more enduring and necessitates more systemic treatment. If untreated, these DBDs can go on to cause significant problems, including difficult relationships with parents and other adults, failure at school and delinquency, and antisocial or criminal behavior in adulthood.

Plate 4.30

Psychiatry

PEDIATRICS: ATTENTION-DEFICIT/ HYPERACTIVITY DISORDERS

Attention-deficit/hyperactivity disorder ADHD is a group of childhood and adolescent neurodevelopmental problems characterized by difficulty controlling attention, motivation, and behavioral impulses. It is common, affecting about 5% of children worldwide and 9.4% of children in the United States. It is more common in males (12.9%) than in females (5.6%). A greater American prevalence may reflect different approaches to diagnosis. ADHD is associated with genetic and environmental risk factors, including maternal drinking or smoking during pregnancy, low birth weight, chemical injuries to the brain (e.g., lead poisoning), and severe child neglect.

Pathophysiology. ADHD occurs because of differences in the structure and function of the prefrontal cerebral cortex and reward circuit important for executive functioning. The neurotransmitters related to ADHD, dopamine and norepinephrine, are important for attention, behavioral regulation, impulse control, and delayed gratification.

Clinical Presentation and Diagnosis. ADHD is a neurodevelopmental disorder, and subtypes reflect predominant symptoms. The *predominantly inattentive type* is characterized by a persistent pattern of poor attention and lack of motivation, particularly when sustained mental effort is required (e.g., for schoolwork or homework). These children are often described as "daydreamers" or "spacey." The *predominantly hyperactive/ impulsive type* is characterized by a persistent pattern of overactive behavior (e.g., being fidgety or restless, walking around without permission in class, talking excessively when it is important to behave quietly) as well as impulsive behavior (e.g., difficulty waiting, not stopping to think before acting or blurting out answers). The *combined type* is characterized by both inattention and hyperactivity/impulsivity. To meet such diagnoses, these problems must be more frequent and severe than children normally exhibit, start before age 12 years, be present for at least 6 months, be noted in two or more settings, and impair the youth's function at home, at school, or with peers. A child with ADHD observed in a highly structured environment or engaged in a stimulating activity (e.g., playing video games) may not exhibit any symptoms. Unstructured, boring, and minimally supervised environments tend to enhance typical ADHD symptoms.

Evaluation. Child and adolescent psychiatrists and neurologists, pediatricians, child psychologists, child-trained social workers, counselors, and clinical nurse specialists are best trained to accurately diagnose ADHD. The evaluation typically takes several hours, requiring input in the form of interviews and/or questionnaires from parents/caregivers and teachers and careful examination. It is important to check other frequently associated comorbidities, such as AD, mood disorders, learning or language disorders, or DBD. There are no specific blood tests, imaging studies, or other medical tests to diagnose these disorders. Neuropsychological testing can aid but is not required for the diagnosis of ADHD.

Treatment. Treatment includes education about the disorder, appropriate school support, executive skills training, and medication. When needed, stimulant

Attention-deficit/hyperactivity disorder is a highly treatable neurodevelopmental disorder, common in school-age children, especially males. The core symptoms include inattention, hyperactivity, and/or impulsivity.

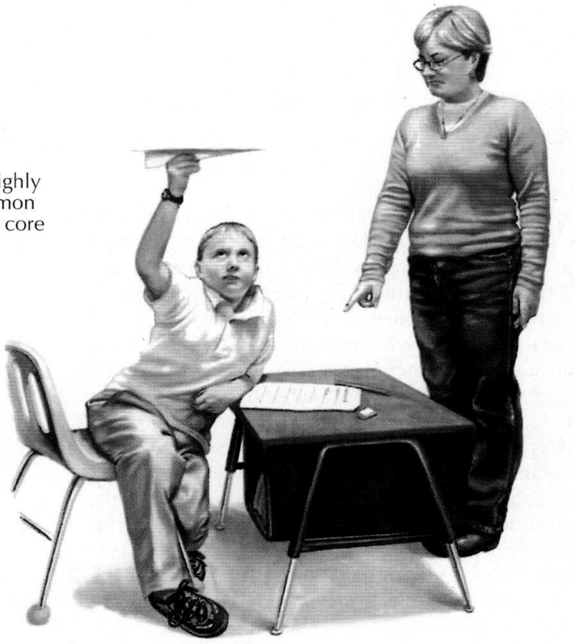

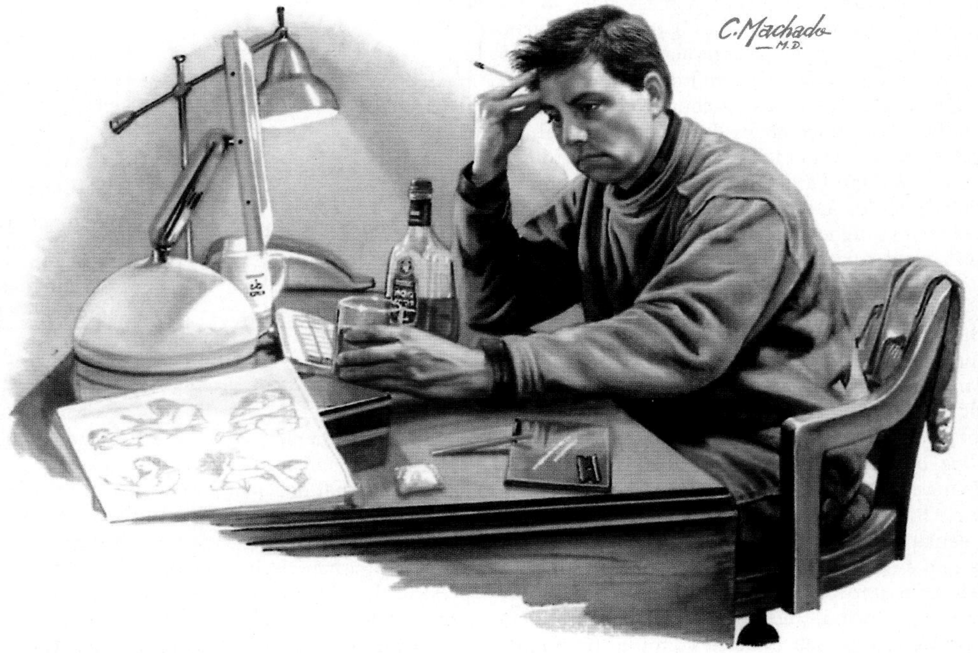

Hyperactivity improves or resolves spontaneously in adulthood, but symptoms persist in 50% of patients and may continue to require treatment. If untreated, it increases the risk of developing substance use or disruptive behavior disorders.

medications are the first line of treatment. Nonstimulant medications (such as atomoxetine) can also be considered in place of or in addition to stimulant medications.

Behavioral support at home and school is important, including a predictable, structured, and informed environment. Accommodations in school are identified through psychoeducational testing requested by teachers or caregivers under an individualized education plan. Other academic and behavioral strategies include frequent reminders to stay on task and complete assignments, reducing distractions, rewarding persistence, tutoring the child in effective study skills (e.g., setting goals, planning, self-rewarding), giving extra time to complete work, or providing a variety of interesting approaches to learning. It is helpful to provide opportunities for physical activity or "boredom breaks" during

the day and to give rewards for control of behavioral impulses or consequences for failure to control.

Prognosis. ADHD generally responds well to treatments. About one-third of children grow out of ADHD in the teen or early adult years. The remaining two-thirds may continue to need support as they grow into adulthood, including ongoing use of medication, and accommodations or supports at school, work, and home. If untreated, ADHD can cause significant problems, including failure at school, injuries and accidents, substance abuse, other risky behaviors, difficult relationships with parents and peers, and poor self-esteem. Contrary to many layperson concerns, studies show treatment with stimulants reduces incidence of future inappropriate substance use, not increasing substance use behaviors or disorders.

Plate 4.31

Brain: PART I

Pediatrics: Eating and Feeding Disorders

Eating and feeding disorders occur in adolescents who have intense preoccupation with body weight and shape and impaired eating habits. Patients have distorted thoughts and emotions concerning their appearance and have abnormal eating behaviors; these thoughts and behaviors lead to alterations in body composition and functioning. The etiology of eating and feeding disorders is multifactorial and includes a genetic component, sociocultural pressures to be thin, and the promotion of dieting. Performers and athletes, particularly those participating in activities that reward a lean body (e.g., gymnastics, running, wrestling, dance, modeling) are at particular risk. Girls with greater negative affect (e.g., guilt, fears, sadness), cultural idealization of thinness, and first-degree genetic relatives with an eating disorder may be at increased risk for the development of eating difficulties. Additionally, those who have a low body mass index (BMI) historically appear at greater risk for the development of anorexia nervosa (AN). The prevalence of eating and feeding disorders varies by condition from 0.8% to 14%. Their epidemiology has gradually changed concomitantly in the United States and worldwide, with an increasing prevalence in males and younger age groups. There is no significant difference between ethnic groups in United States for AN or binge eating disorder (BED), with somewhat higher rates of bulimia nervosa (BN) for Latinx and African American individuals. Acculturation to Western values is a risk factor for eating disorders in US immigrants.

Clinical Presentation. Eating disorders can be qualified into three major disorders: AN, BN, and BED. *Avoidant-restrictive food intake disorder* (ARFID) is a specific diagnosis of feeding disorder in the absence of evident body image distortion. *Other specified feeding or eating disorder* represents disorders not meeting criteria for a more specific eating or feeding disorder.

AN is characterized by fear of gaining weight, low BMI, denial of current low weight and its effect on health, and amenorrhea. Prevalence is highest in teenage girls; up to 0.8% may be affected. Behaviors used to reduce weight include restricting meals and calories, excessive exercising, self-induced vomiting (purging), and use of diet pills or laxatives. Binge eating episodes can occur within AN as well. Psychiatric disorders and personality characteristics, such as depression, ADs, OCD, and perfectionism, are common.

Patients with BN and BED have regular episodes of uncontrolled overeating (binge eating). BN is also associated with extreme measures to counteract the feared effects of the overeating, such as occur with AN. BED, on the other hand, is characterized by marked distress during the binge eating episode without compensatory behaviors such as marked dietary restriction or purging. Approximately 90% of BN patients are females who become symptomatic in late adolescence; their binge eating typically begins in the context of dieting. Because patients with BN and BED may have normal weight or be overweight, this diagnosis is more difficult to ascertain. Although patients with BN experience weight variations, they rarely approach the low weights of patients with AN. Higher obesity rates, mood disorder, sexual and physical abuse, parental obesity, and substance misuse exist in patients with BN.

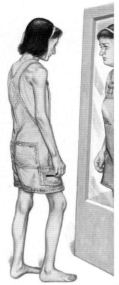

Refusal to maintain weight at or above a minimally normal weight or failure to gain weight during a period of expected growth; intense fear of gaining weight; disturbance in body image; and the absence of at least three spontaneous menstrual cycles in postmenarcheal females are symptoms/signs of an eating disorder.

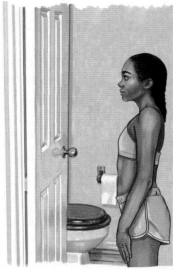

"No matter what anyone says, I am too fat!"

Anorexia Nervosa	Restrictive type or binge-eating/purging type
Common Findings	Body image distortion at ages 14–18; females > males Amenorrhea Weight loss >15% of ideal body weight Preserved secondary sex characteristics
Psychiatric Associated Disorders	Affective Anxiety Obsessive-compulsive disorder Personality Substance misuse
Differential Diagnosis	Adrenal insufficiency Inflammatory bowel and other gastrointestinal disease Recent-onset diabetes mellitus Central nervous system posterior fossa lesions Primary depression

ARFID is characterized by a persistent failure to meet nutritional needs, often with associated weight loss, nutritional deficiency, or dependence on supplemental nutrition. This condition is present in the absence of a fear of weight gain or disturbance in perceived body shape. When other medical conditions are present, the nutritional failure exceeds what would be expected for co-occurring medical illness. Prevalence for ARFID is as high as 14% in the pediatric population. Individuals with ARFID may restrict nutritional intake in the setting of sensory aversion to foods, lack of interest in eating, or concern for undesirable consequences of eating (e.g., nausea, fear of choking).

Short-term medical complications of ARFID and AN (and less so BN and BED) include electrolyte disturbances, esophageal tears, gastric disturbances, dehydration, orthostatic blood hypotension, and cardiac dysfunction; sometimes hospitalization is required. Long-term medical complications typically resulting from chronic malnutrition include growth hormone changes, hypothalamic hypogonadism, bone marrow hypoplasia, and brain structural abnormalities.

Diagnosis. Pediatricians, child and adolescent psychiatrists, child psychologists, child-trained social workers, counselors, and clinical nurse specialists are best trained to accurately diagnose eating disorders. Because these disorders can affect every organ system and the medical complications can be serious to life-threatening, a comprehensive history and physical examination are required.

Treatment. Treatment requires that individual, family, medical, and nutritional aspects be addressed. The initial therapeutic goal for patients with AN is the restoration of physical health. Family therapy provides the most promising results in adolescent AN and BN. CBT strategies are helpful in BN for behavioral changes; for example, for binge-purge reduction and to some extent in AN. Family therapy and CBT approaches have been helpful in the treatment of ARFID, particularly in supported graduated exposures to increasing amounts and/or variety of foods. No medications are approved by the FDA for AN treatment. Although pharmacotherapy is sometimes prescribed, it is typically targeted at comorbid depression and anxiety. SSRI antidepressants may reduce binge eating episodes and purging.

Prognosis. Although most individuals with an eating disorder recover completely or partially, 20% to 40% develop a chronic eating disorder. Even after recovery, there are high rates of residual psychiatric illness, predominantly depression and anxiety. There is less specific guidance available regarding long-term outcomes for ARFID, as this is a newer diagnosis. The potential for significant growth retardation, pubertal delay or interruption, and peak bone mass reduction are significant medical problems for adolescents in contrast to adults. Young females with AN have an increased risk of fractures later in life. Eating disorders in adolescents are identified as the psychiatric condition with the highest mortality rate (2%–5%). Mortality is most often attributable to the complications of starvation or to suicide.

Plate 4.32

Psychiatry

FRACTURES IN ABUSED CHILDREN

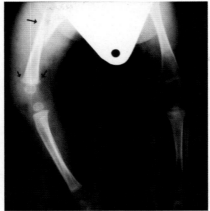

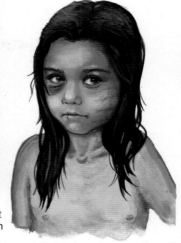

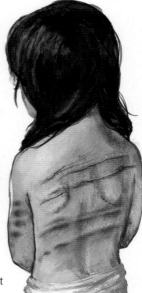

Radiograph shows fracture of proximal right femur for which patient was brought to the hospital. Healing fracture of growth plate of distal femur noted, arousing suspicion of child abuse.

Abused child characteristically sad or withdrawn. Signs such as poor skin and hair care or malnutrition should increase suspicion and should be understood within context of other important factors such as community and familial resources.

Further examination may reveal bruises, welts, or cigarette burns in various stages of healing on other parts of body.

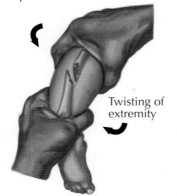

Twisting of extremity

Spiral fractures in young children may occur accidentally but often due to abuse.

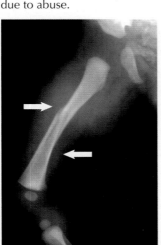

Spiral fracture in infant

Sudden jerk on extremity avulses metaphyseal tips.

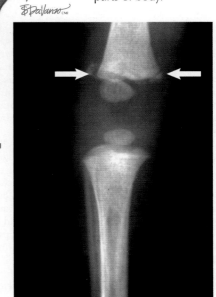

Avulsion fracture of metaphysis

CHILD ABUSE

Child abuse is defined by the Child Abuse Prevention and Treatment Act as "Any recent act or failure to act on the part of a parent or caretaker, which results in death, serious physical or emotional harm, sexual abuse or exploitation ... or an act or failure to act which presents an imminent risk of serious harm" (2010). There are multiple forms of child maltreatment, including medical neglect, neglect or deprivation of necessities, physical abuse, psychological or emotional maltreatment, sexual abuse, sex trafficking, and other forms of maltreatment included in state law.

In the National Child Abuse and Neglect System of the Administration of Children, Youth, and Families Annual Report 2019, there were 8.9 unique abuse victims per 1000 children in the United States. Youngest children were the most vulnerable to maltreatment, with 28.1% of victims between the ages of 0 and 2 years and an almost equal distribution of males and females. Neglect was most frequent (74.9%), followed by physical abuse (17.5%) and sexual abuse (9.3%). Children experiencing "other" types of maltreatment (e.g., threatened abuse or neglect, substance use, lack of supervision) constituted 6.8% of victims. Data show 15.5% of victims experienced multiple maltreatment types. The 2019 national fatality rate was 2.5 per 100,000 children, representing an estimate of 1840 children and an increase over the prior 5 years. Health professionals should remain vigilant about potential abuse every time they see a child.

Clinical Presentation. Presentations vary greatly depending on the type(s) of abuse as well as social and emotional developmental stages. Children diagnosed with disabilities, including intellectual disability, emotional disturbances, visual or hearing impairment, learning disability, physical disability, behavior problem, or other medical conditions are at an increased risk of being victims of abuse.

Physical abuse most often manifests with signs of bodily harm, including bruises, cuts, burns, restraint or gag marks, black eyes, and/or skeletal injury. Sexually abused children often present to physicians for evaluation of genital injury. Both physical abuse and sexual abuse are often associated with mental health challenges, including increased anger, aggression, anxiety, depression, PTSD, poor academic performance, sleep problems, substance use or misuse, and suicidality.

Psychologic abuse is often more difficult to detect and assess compared with physical abuse and sexual abuse. Psychological abuse of a child may have repeated occurrences but may also manifest as a single severe incident. Examples of psychologically abusive behaviors include spurning, ridiculing or humiliating, terrorizing or threatening violence, isolating or restricting social interactions, corrupting or exploiting by involving child in illicit activities, or withholding or denying emotional responsiveness such as

Plate 4.33

Brain: PART I

Staging of injuries

Bruises

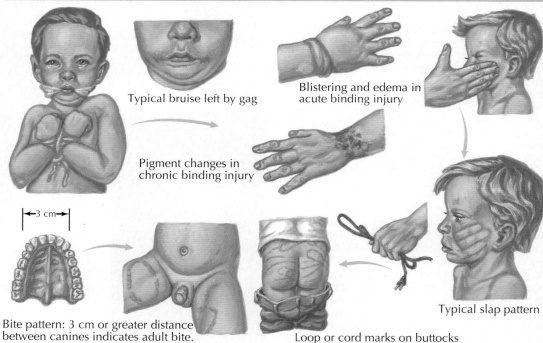

Acute bruise with marked swelling (1–3 days)

Purple (1–5 days)

Green (5–7 days)

Yellow (7–10 days)

Brown (>10 days)

Subdural hematomas

Organizing membranes

Organized clot mistaken for atrophic brain tissue on CT scan

Acute hemorrhage

Fluid

JOHN A. CRAIG_MD

Fresh subdural hematoma (acute)

Organized subdural hematoma (weeks)

Organized subdural hematoma (months)

Child abuse injury patterns

Typical bruise left by gag

Blistering and edema in acute binding injury

Pigment changes in chronic binding injury

|←3 cm→|

Bite pattern: 3 cm or greater distance between canines indicates adult bite.

Loop or cord marks on buttocks

Typical slap pattern

CHILD ABUSE
(Continued)

praise. Children experiencing psychologic abuse are more likely to present with depressive disorders, ADs, PTSD, and behavior problems compared with peers who were not psychologically abused. Often children are exposed to more than one type of abuse, so the consequences of abuse can be complex. In general, child abuse is associated with poor mental health outcomes and impairments in interpersonal relationships.

Diagnosis. Evaluations of child abuse should be carried out by qualified pediatric healthcare professionals. If there is a concern for physical abuse, physical and diagnostic examinations should be performed as soon as abuse is suspected. Concern for sexual abuse warrants evaluation for pregnancy or sexually transmitted infection. In all instances, information should be gathered from multiple people within the child's psychosocial sphere (e.g., parents/caregivers, family members, teachers, counselors).

Treatment. The first step after identification of suspected abuse is reporting to a child protective service (CPS) agency. The CPS will carry out a thorough investigation of the suspected person(s) abusing the child and their living situation. The CPS will engage a treatment team to support the child and the child's family. In instances where the child's safety has been compromised and/or future abuse is suspected without intervention, the child may be placed in a safe environment until the investigation is complete or sufficient supports are put in place for the child to return home. The primary treatment for child abuse is psychotherapy and can include CBT (change behavior by addressing distorted cognitions and modifying habitual responses to situations/stimuli), TF-CBT, family therapy (explore patterns of family interactions) such as parent-child interaction therapy or SafeCare, and developmental victimology (describes the processes involved in the

onset and maintenance of abusive behavior). Other options for treatment include family foster care and kinship care.

Prognosis. Child abuse is hypothesized to occur through response biases, resulting in impaired emotional and cognitive regulation. Adult victims of prior childhood abuse are found to have higher rates of sleep disorders, abdominal disorders, obesity, chronic pain (e.g., headache, backache, premenstrual syndrome), fatigue, and exaggerated startle responses. Longitudinal

studies indicate that adults continue to experience low self-esteem, maladaptive sexual behavior, and impaired interpersonal relationships (e.g., parenting, romantic/intimate). Despite these findings, not every child who experiences abuse develops significant mental health challenges, indicating a role for protective factors such as active coping, control beliefs, education, external attribution of blame, interpersonal and emotional competence, optimism, social attachment, and familial and social support.

HYPOTHALAMUS, PITUITARY, SLEEP, AND THALAMUS

Plate 5.1

Brain: PART I

ANATOMY AND RELATIONS OF THE HYPOTHALAMUS AND PITUITARY GLAND

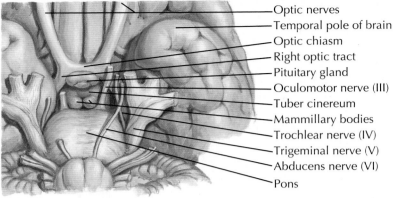

Optic nerves
Temporal pole of brain
Optic chiasm
Right optic tract
Pituitary gland
Oculomotor nerve (III)
Tuber cinereum
Mammillary bodies
Trochlear nerve (IV)
Trigeminal nerve (V)
Abducens nerve (VI)
Pons

Fornix
Interventricular foramen
Choroid plexus of 3rd ventricle
Thalamus
Pineal gland
Corpus callosum

Hypothalamic sulcus
Anterior commissure
Lamina terminalis
Tuber cinereum
Mammillary body
Chiasmatic cistern
Optic chiasm
Diaphragma sellae
Pituitary gland
Sphenoidal sinus
Nasal septum
Interpeduncular cistern
Nasopharynx
Pontine cistern

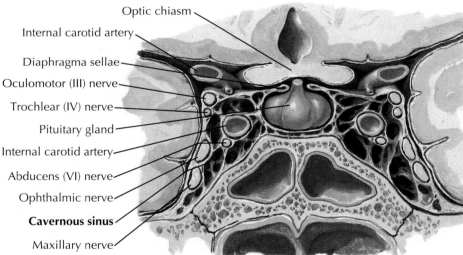

Optic chiasm
Internal carotid artery
Diaphragma sellae
Oculomotor (III) nerve
Trochlear (IV) nerve
Pituitary gland
Internal carotid artery
Abducens (VI) nerve
Ophthalmic nerve
Cavernous sinus
Maxillary nerve

ANATOMIC RELATIONSHIPS OF THE HYPOTHALAMUS

The hypothalamus is a small area, weighing about 4 g of the total 1400 g of adult brain weight, but it is the only 4 g of brain without which life itself is impossible. The hypothalamus is so critical for life because it contains the integrative circuitry that coordinates autonomic, endocrine, and behavioral responses that are necessary for basic life functions, such as thermoregulation, control of electrolyte and fluid balance, feeding and metabolism, responses to stress, and reproduction.

Perhaps for this reason, the hypothalamus is particularly well protected. It lies at the base of the skull, just above the pituitary gland, to which it is attached by the infundibulum, or pituitary stalk. In this position, it is shielded from trauma by the skull and the entire thickness of the cerebral hemispheres. It receives its blood supply directly from the circle of Willis (see Plate 5.3), so it is rarely compromised by stroke, and it is bilaterally reduplicated, with survival of either side being sufficient to sustain normal life.

On the other hand, the hypothalamus may be involved in several pathologic processes that arise from structures that surround it, and the signs and symptoms that first attract attention in those disorders are often due to the involvement of those neighboring structures. Examination of the ventral surface of the brain shows that the hypothalamus is framed by fiber tracts. The optic chiasm marks the rostral extent of the hypothalamus, and the optic tracts and cerebral peduncles identify its lateral borders. The pituitary stalk emerges from the midportion of the hypothalamus, sometimes called the tuber cinereum (gray swelling), just caudal to the optic chiasm. As a result, tumors of the pituitary gland, which are among the more common causes of hypothalamic dysfunction, typically involve the optic chiasm (producing bitemporal visual field defects) or the optic tracts as an early sign.

The posterior part of the hypothalamus is defined by the mammillary bodies, which are bordered caudally by the interpeduncular cistern, from which emerge the oculomotor nerves. These are joined in the cavernous sinus, which runs just below the hypothalamus and lateral to the pituitary gland, by the trochlear and abducens nerves. Hence pathologies such as aneurysms of the internal carotid artery or infection or thrombosis of the cavernous sinus, which may impinge on the hypothalamus, typically involve the nerves controlling eye movements at an early stage. If there is a mass of sufficient size, it may also involve the trigeminal nerve. The ophthalmic division, which traverses the cavernous sinus, is most involved, but if the mass is large

enough and posteriorly located, it can involve the maxillary or even the mandibular division of the trigeminal nerve as well. Just lateral to the cavernous sinus sits the medial temporal lobe. As a result, pathology in this area can also cause seizures, most commonly of the complex partial type, with loss of awareness for a brief period.

In the midline, the hypothalamus borders the ventral part of the third ventricle. The supraoptic recess of the

third ventricle, which surmounts the optic chiasm, ends at the lamina terminalis, the anterior wall of the ventricle. This is the most anterior part of the diencephalon in the developing brain. The infundibular recess defines the floor of the hypothalamus that overlies the pituitary stalk. This portion of the hypothalamus is called the median eminence and is the site at which hypothalamic-releasing hormones are secreted into the pituitary portal circulation (see Plate 5.3).

Plate 5.2   Hypothalamus, Pituitary, Sleep, and Thalamus

CYTOGENETIC DISEASE: PRADER-WILLI SYNDROME

Deleted segment 15q11-15q13

Interstitial deletion

Interstitial deletion in long arm of one chromosome 15

Skin lesions caused by scratching

Small genitalia and cryptorchidism

Obesity, small hands and feet

Abnormal glucose tolerance test

Dental caries

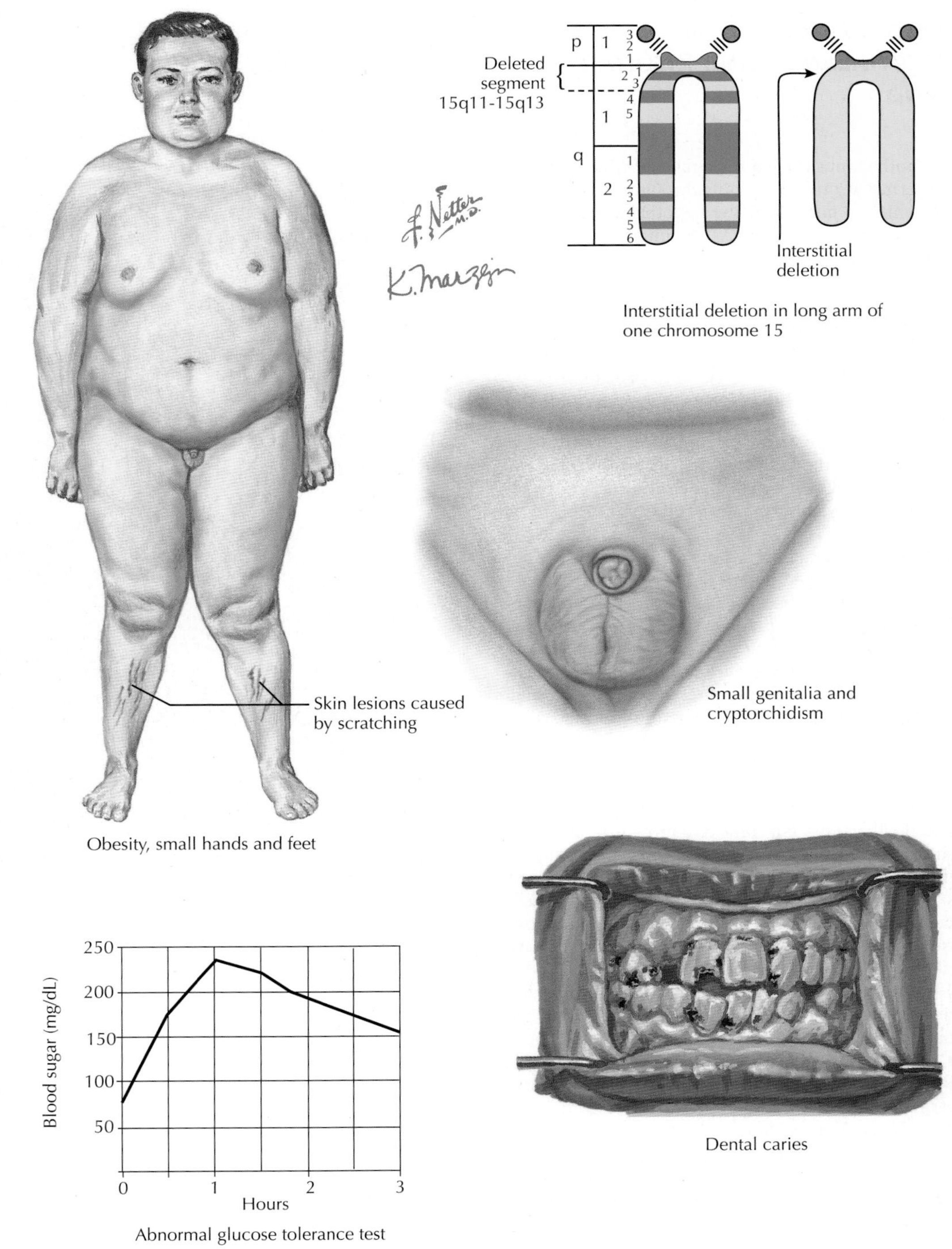

DEVELOPMENT AND DEVELOPMENTAL DISORDERS OF THE HYPOTHALAMUS

The hypothalamus in mammals arises as a part of the ventral diencephalon and the adjacent telencephalon, and its embryologic origins are intimately related to those of the optic chiasm and tracts and to the pituitary gland. Thus disorders that affect the hypothalamus frequently manifest with signs and symptoms resulting from dysfunction of neighboring, developmentally related structures. The developing neural tube is divided into three primary regions: forebrain, midbrain, and hindbrain. The forebrain is further subdivided into the telencephalon, which gives rise to the cerebral cortex and basal ganglia, and the diencephalon, from which the thalamus and hypothalamus are derived. The hypothalamus develops from the anterior portion of the diencephalon in a series of steps that involve the activation of suites of transcription factors, which determine the fates of the developing cell populations.

First, the prechordal mesoderm that underlies the developing neural tube secretes sonic hedgehog protein (Shh) that induces the normal patterning of the anterior midline of the brain, including the formation of the hypothalamus and the separation of the optic system. Abnormal mesodermal induction occurs with mutations that affect Shh signaling and can result in one of the most common human brain malformations, holoprosencephaly, which causes a spectrum of malformations due to failed division of the midline structures of the brain. In its most severe form, holoprosencephaly results in cyclopia and complete or partial loss of the hypothalamus, which is not compatible with life. In its milder forms, holoprosencephaly can result in endocrine abnormalities because of defective development of the hypothalamic-pituitary system. After initial patterning induced by Shh, hypothalamic precursor cells proliferate before exiting the cell cycle and undergo terminal differentiation into the many cell types that comprise the hypothalamus' compact yet complex structure. Finally, the developing neurons express unique combinations of transcription factors, such as Nkx and Lhx family members, Sim1, and Six3. Deletions of individual transcription factors have profound effects upon development of specific hypothalamic nuclei.

Terminal differentiation of the hypothalamic nuclei requires the combined action of "codes" of transcription factors that, when expressed with anatomically restricted and developmentally timed precision, give rise

to the regional complexity of the hypothalamus. Although still poorly understood, rare genetic mutations have been identified in humans and tested in animal models that demonstrate that dysfunction of specific genes results in loss of specific hypothalamic neurons and corresponding phenotypes. For example, Prader-Willi syndrome, which manifests as morbid obesity, hypersomnolence, hypogonadism, and intellectual disability, is caused by a deletion of the paternally inherited chromosome 15q11. This genomic region contains several genes implicated in the normal development of the paraventricular nucleus (PVN), a cell group with critical integrative functions in feeding and responses to stress.

The relationship of the hypothalamus and pituitary gland has its embryologic origins as an anatomic juxtaposition between the anterior diencephalon and the ectodermally derived Rathke's pouch, from which portions of the ventral pituitary are derived. Thus both the hypothalamus and pituitary are patterned by similar signaling pathways, and dysfunction in these systems may disrupt the development and function of both structures. Craniopharyngiomas are the most common nonneural intracranial tumors in childhood and derive from the remnants of Rathke's pouch. Clinical presentation includes optic, pituitary, and/or hypothalamic symptoms, including obesity, hypopituitarism, and sleep and circadian rhythm dysfunction.

Plate 5.3

Brain: PART I

BLOOD SUPPLY OF THE HYPOTHALAMUS AND PITUITARY GLAND

The hypothalamus is what the circle of Willis encircles. The internal carotid artery runs through the cavernous sinus, which is just below the hypothalamus, and the site of its venous drainage. As the internal carotid artery emerges from the cavernous sinus, it ends in the middle cerebral artery laterally, the posterior communicating artery caudally, and the anterior cerebral artery rostrally. The anterior cerebral artery runs above the optic nerve, crosses the olfactory tract, and meets the anterior communicating artery in the midline before turning upward and back to run above the corpus callosum. The posterior communicating artery runs back to meet the posterior cerebral artery shortly after it emerges from the basilar artery. As a result, the hypothalamus is fed by small penetrating arteries that originate directly from the vessels that form the circle of Willis.

The anterior part of the hypothalamus, above the optic chiasm, is supplied by arterial feeding vessels from the anterior cerebral artery. These vessels densely penetrate the basal forebrain (BF) just in front of the optic chiasm, giving it the name the *anterior perforated substance*. The tuberal, or midlevel of the hypothalamus, is fed mainly by small branches directly from the internal carotid artery and the posterior communicating artery. Posteriorly, small penetrating vessels from the posterior cerebral arteries running through the interpeduncular fossa give it the name *posterior perforated substance*. Many of these small blood vessels supply the posterior part of the thalamus, but some also provide blood to the posterior hypothalamus. The cell groups within the hypothalamus are not uniformly supplied with blood vessels. The paraventricular (PVN) and supraoptic (SON) nuclei, which contain neurons that make the vasoactive hormones oxytocin (OXY) and vasopressin (VP), have particularly rich capillary networks.

The superior hypophyseal artery is one of the branches derived from the internal carotid artery. It supplies the pituitary stalk, where it breaks up into a series of looplike capillaries in the median eminence and pituitary stalk. The hypothalamic neurons that make pituitary-releasing (and release-inhibiting) hormones send axons that terminate on these loops, which, unlike most brain capillaries, have fenestrations to permit easy penetration by these small peptide hormones (see Plate 5.6). These capillaries drain into the hypophyseal portal veins, which, along with some branches of the inferior hypophyseal artery, provide blood flow to the adenohypophysis or anterior pituitary gland. The posterior pituitary gland is supplied almost entirely by the inferior hypophyseal artery. Because most of the blood flow to the anterior pituitary gland is from the portal system, it is possible, on occasion, for the gland to outgrow its blood supply. This occurs mainly during pregnancy or can occur when a pituitary adenoma, an otherwise benign tumor, becomes larger than can be accommodated by the blood supply. At this point, there is infarction of the pituitary, often with bleeding, which may become life-threatening (pituitary apoplexy). The typical presentation is sudden onset of dysfunction of some combination of cranial nerves II, III, IV, or VI, with a severe headache that is generally localized between the eyes, and often impaired consciousness.

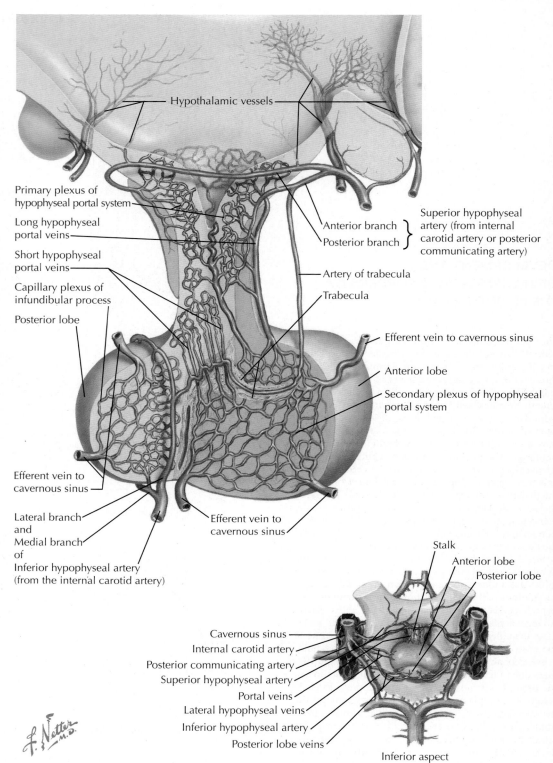

Hypothalamic vessels

Primary plexus of hypophyseal portal system

Long hypophyseal portal veins

Short hypophyseal portal veins

Capillary plexus of infundibular process

Posterior lobe

Efferent vein to cavernous sinus

Lateral branch and Medial branch of Inferior hypophyseal artery (from the internal carotid artery)

Anterior branch
Posterior branch
Superior hypophyseal artery (from internal carotid artery or posterior communicating artery)

Artery of trabecula

Trabecula

Efferent vein to cavernous sinus

Anterior lobe

Secondary plexus of hypophyseal portal system

Efferent vein to cavernous sinus

Cavernous sinus
Internal carotid artery
Posterior communicating artery
Superior hypophyseal artery
Portal veins
Lateral hypophyseal veins
Inferior hypophyseal artery
Posterior lobe veins

Stalk
Anterior lobe
Posterior lobe

Inferior aspect

Finally, the fenestrated capillary loops in the median eminence allow egress of hypothalamic-releasing hormones to the anterior pituitary gland and also permit blood-borne substances to enter the brain. The hormone leptin, which is made by white adipose tissue during times of plenty, is believed to enter the brain via the median eminence to signal satiety to cell groups in the basal medial hypothalamus. There is another area of fenestrated capillaries along the anterior wall of the third ventricle, called the *organum vasculosum of the lamina terminalis,* which may allow entry of other hormones, such as angiotensin, which may be involved in thirst and water balance, and perhaps some cytokines and prostaglandin E2 (PGE2), which play a role in the fever response. These regions are called *circumventricular organs* because they are around the edges of the ventricles. Another circumventricular organ, the area postrema, is found at the outflow of the fourth ventricle in the medulla and is probably involved in emetic reflexes based on blood-borne toxins or hormones, such as glucagon-like peptide 1.

Plate 5.4

Hypothalamus, Pituitary, Sleep, and Thalamus

GENERAL TOPOGRAPHY OF THE HYPOTHALAMUS

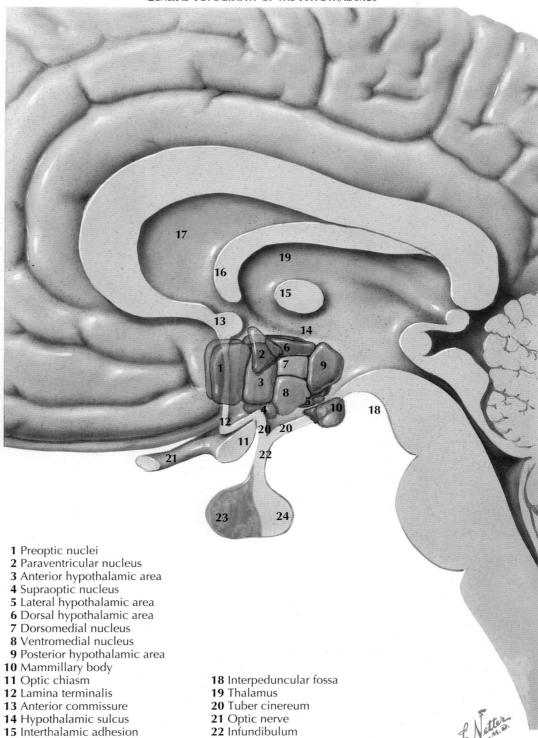

OVERVIEW OF HYPOTHALAMIC CELL GROUPS

The hypothalamus consists of a complex assemblage of cell groups. The borders of these cell groups often are not quite as distinct as those shown in Plates 5.4 and 5.5, but the different cell groups are also distinguished based upon their neurotransmitters, functions, and connections.

In general, the hypothalamus can be divided into three tiers of nuclei. Most medially, along the wall of the third ventricle, is the periventricular nucleus, shown in green on Plate 5.5. Along the base of the periventricular nucleus is an expansion laterally along the edge of the median eminence, known as the *arcuate* or *infundibular nucleus*. The periventricular stratum contains many neurons that make releasing or release-inhibiting hormones (see Plate 5.6) and whose axons end on the capillary loops of the hypophyseal portal vessels in the median eminence. Many axons from the brainstem run through the periaqueductal gray matter in the midbrain in the dorsal longitudinal fasciculus and into the periventricular region of the hypothalamus.

The next tier of nuclei is sometimes called the medial tier. These nuclei are generally involved in intrinsic connections within the hypothalamus that allow integration of various functions. The most rostral of the medial nuclei is the medial preoptic area (orange), which sits along the wall of the third ventricle as it opens. Along the anterior wall of the third ventricle is the median preoptic nucleus (not shown here). These two cell groups are involved in integrating control of body temperature with fluid and electrolyte balance, wake-sleep cycles, and reproductive function.

The next most caudal region is called the *anterior hypothalamic area* (pale purple). At the base of the anterior hypothalamic area, just above the optic chiasm, is the suprachiasmatic nucleus (Plate 5.5). The suprachiasmatic nucleus is the body's main biologic clock, and it sets the timing of rhythms of sleep, feeding, thirst, body temperature, reproduction, and social interaction. These functions are controlled by means of outputs to the portion of the anterior hypothalamic area between the suprachiasmatic nucleus and the PVN (blue) called

1 Preoptic nuclei
2 Paraventricular nucleus
3 Anterior hypothalamic area
4 Supraoptic nucleus
5 Lateral hypothalamic area
6 Dorsal hypothalamic area
7 Dorsomedial nucleus
8 Ventromedial nucleus
9 Posterior hypothalamic area
10 Mammillary body
11 Optic chiasm
12 Lamina terminalis
13 Anterior commissure
14 Hypothalamic sulcus
15 Interthalamic adhesion
16 Fornix
17 Septum pellucidum
18 Interpeduncular fossa
19 Thalamus
20 Tuber cinereum
21 Optic nerve
22 Infundibulum
23 Anterior lobe of pituitary
24 Posterior lobe of pituitary

the *subparaventricular zone*. The suprachiasmatic nucleus and subparaventricular zone provide circadian timing signals for autonomic, endocrine, and behavioral function to the rest of the hypothalamus.

The SON and PVN are also at this anterior level in the medial tier. Both nuclei contain large numbers of OXY and VP neurons, whose axons travel through the pituitary stalk in the tuberohypophyseal tract to the posterior pituitary gland, where they release their

hormones into the circulation. The PVN also contains neurons that make releasing hormones (including corticotropin-releasing hormone [CRH]) and project to the median eminence. A third population of neurons in the PVN sends axons through the medial forebrain bundle in the lateral hypothalamus to form a descending hypothalamic tract that runs through the brainstem and spinal cord, to control both the sympathetic and parasympathetic nervous systems. Many of these

Plate 5.5

Brain: PART I

OVERVIEW OF HYPOTHALAMIC NUCLEI

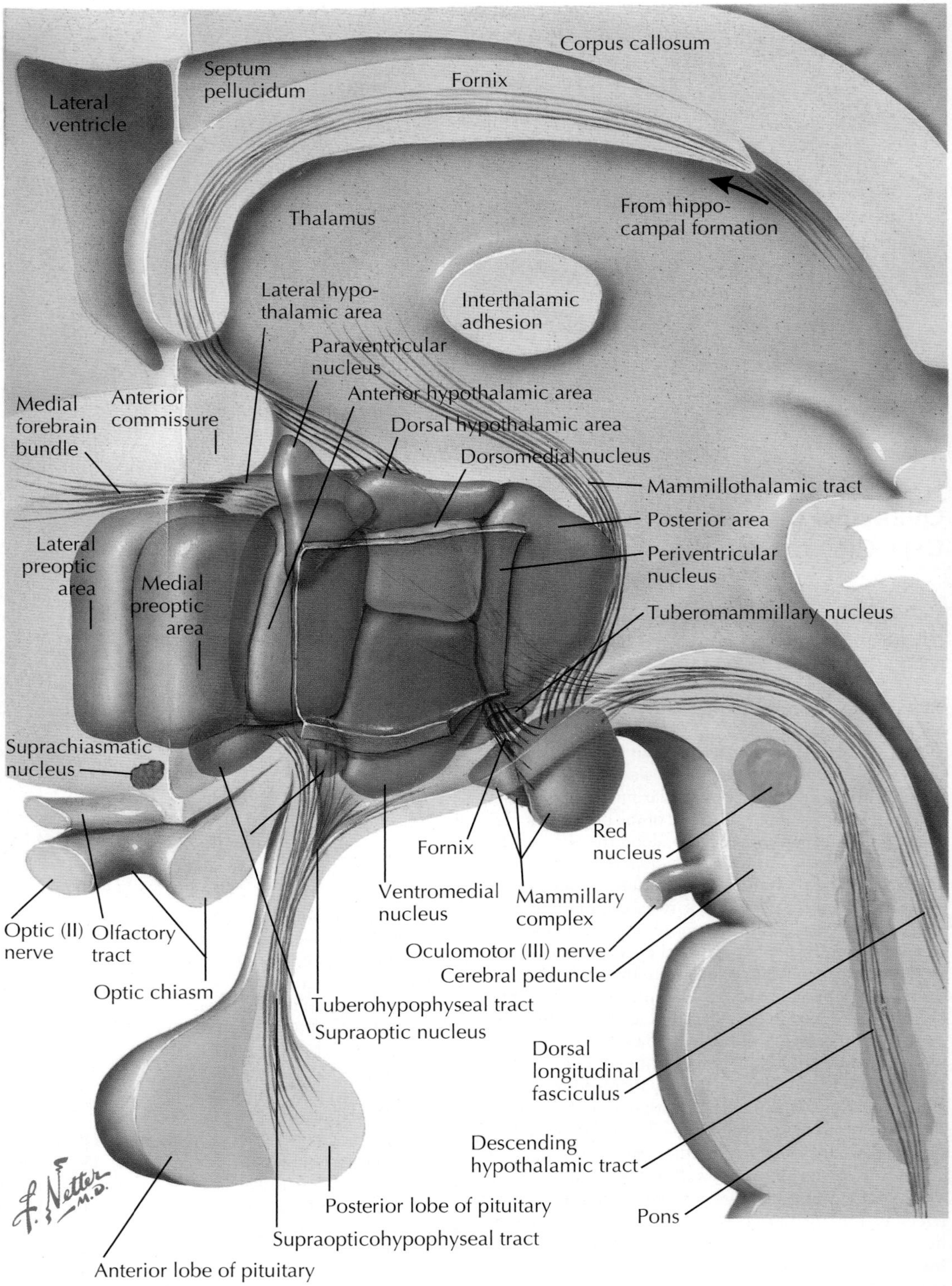

Corpus callosum
Septum pellucidum
Fornix
Lateral ventricle
Thalamus
From hippo-campal formation
Lateral hypo-thalamic area
Interthalamic adhesion
Paraventricular nucleus
Anterior hypothalamic area
Medial forebrain bundle
Anterior commissure
Dorsal hypothalamic area
Dorsomedial nucleus
Mammillothalamic tract
Posterior area
Lateral preoptic area
Medial preoptic area
Periventricular nucleus
Tuberomammillary nucleus
Suprachiasmatic nucleus
Red nucleus
Fornix
Ventromedial nucleus
Mammillary complex
Optic (II) nerve
Olfactory tract
Oculomotor (III) nerve
Cerebral peduncle
Optic chiasm
Tuberohypophyseal tract
Supraoptic nucleus
Dorsal longitudinal fasciculus
Descending hypothalamic tract
Posterior lobe of pituitary
Pons
Supraopticohypophyseal tract
Anterior lobe of pituitary

OVERVIEW OF HYPOTHALAMIC CELL GROUPS (Continued)

neurons use either OXY or VP as a central neurotransmitter in this autonomic pathway, but they are an entirely separate set of neurons from those that send axons to the posterior pituitary gland.

Just caudal to the anterior hypothalamic area, in the tuberal level of the hypothalamus, the medial tier contains three cell groups. The ventromedial nucleus (brown) sits just above the median eminence and is mainly involved in feeding, aggression, and sexual behavior. The dorsomedial nucleus (yellow), which is just dorsal to it, has extensive outputs to much of the rest of the hypothalamus. The subparaventricular zone sends circadian outputs to both the dorsomedial and ventromedial nuclei, and the dorsomedial nucleus uses this input to organize circadian cycles of wake-sleep, corticosteroid secretion, feeding, and other behaviors. The dorsal hypothalamic area, just above the dorsomedial nucleus, contains neurons that are involved in regulating body temperature.

At the most posterior end of the hypothalamus, the mammillary bodies form a prominent pair of protuberances along the base of the brain. Despite having very clear-cut, heavily myelinated connections, the function of the mammillary nuclei remains mysterious. They receive major brainstem input from the mammillary peduncle and a large bundle of efferents from the hippocampal formation through the fornix. The large fiber bundle that emerges from the mammillary body splits into a mammillotegmental tract to the brainstem and a mammillothalamic tract to the anterior thalamic nucleus. Neurons in the mammillary body and the supramammillary nucleus just above it appear to be concerned with head position in space and may be related to hippocampal circuits that remember the positions of objects in space (so-called place cells). However, lesions of the mammillary bodies in primates have relatively subtle effects on memory.

The lateral tier of the hypothalamus includes the lateral preoptic and lateral hypothalamic areas (LHAs). These regions are traversed by the medial forebrain bundle, which connects the brainstem below with the hypothalamus and the forebrain above. Many neurons

in the LHA project through the medial forebrain bundle, either to the BF or cerebral cortex, or to the brainstem or spinal cord. Among these are the neurons that contain the peptides orexins (ORXs) (also known as hypocretins) or melanin-concentrating hormone (MCH). These neurons are involved in regulating wake-sleep cycles, as well as metabolism, feeding, and other types of motivated behaviors. Loss of the ORX neurons causes the disorder known as narcolepsy (see Plate 5.22).

At the posterior hypothalamic level, there is also a cluster of histaminergic (His) neurons, called the tuberomammillary nucleus (TMN), in the lateral hypothalamus adjacent to the mammillary body. These neurons play a role in regulation of wakefulness and body temperature and have projections ranging from the cerebral cortex to the spinal cord. The posterior hypothalamic area sits just above the mammillary body. In humans, many of the ORX, MCH, and His neurons are found in this region.

Plate 5.6

Hypothalamus, Pituitary, Sleep, and Thalamus

HYPOTHALAMIC CONTROL OF THE ANTERIOR AND POSTERIOR PITUITARY GLAND

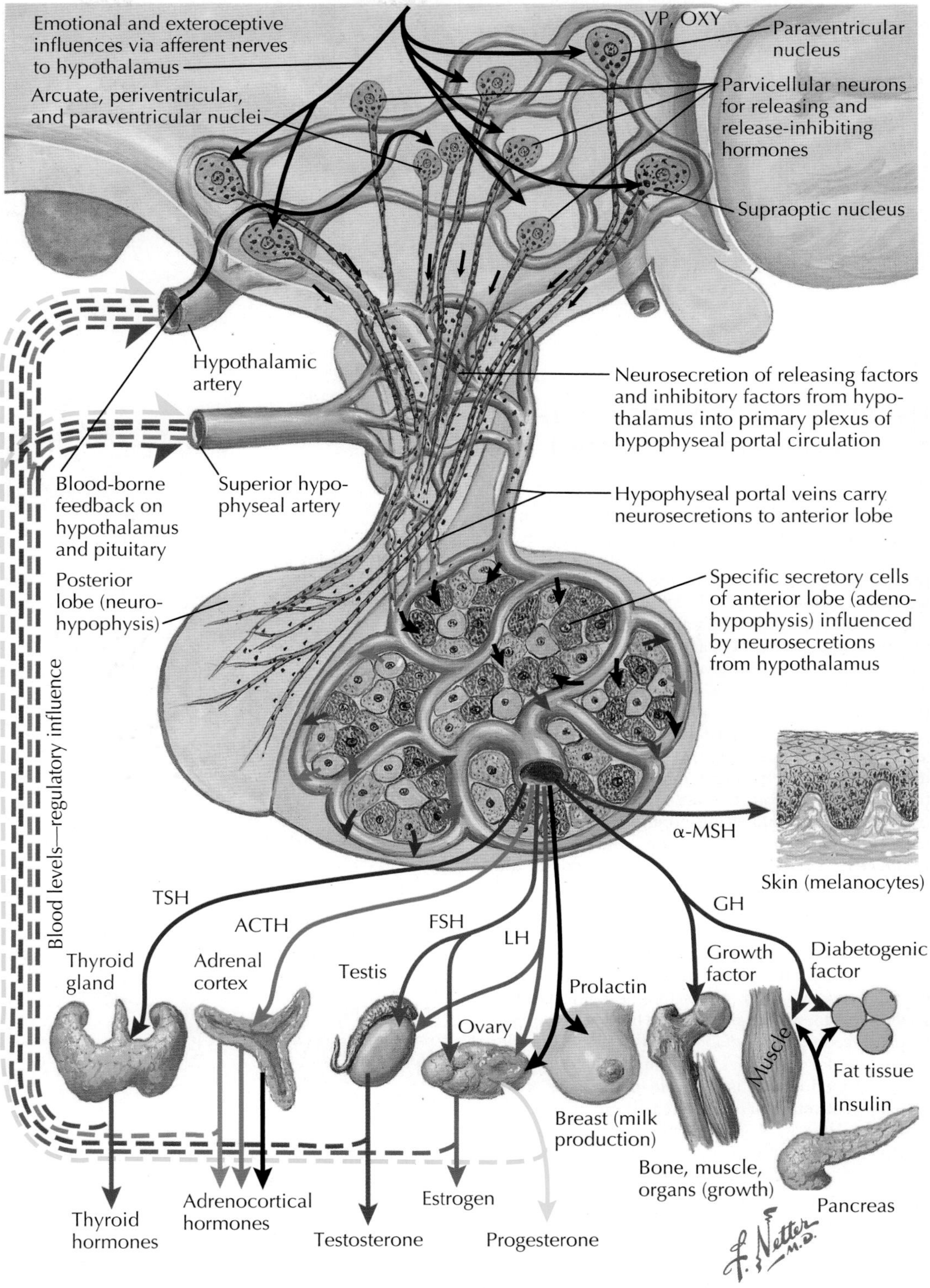

Emotional and exteroceptive influences via afferent nerves to hypothalamus

Arcuate, periventricular, and paraventricular nuclei

VP, OXY

Paraventricular nucleus

Parvicellular neurons for releasing and release-inhibiting hormones

Supraoptic nucleus

Hypothalamic artery

Neurosecretion of releasing factors and inhibitory factors from hypothalamus into primary plexus of hypophyseal portal circulation

Blood-borne feedback on hypothalamus and pituitary

Superior hypophyseal artery

Hypophyseal portal veins carry neurosecretions to anterior lobe

Posterior lobe (neurohypophysis)

Specific secretory cells of anterior lobe (adenohypophysis) influenced by neurosecretions from hypothalamus

Blood levels—regulatory influence

α-MSH

Skin (melanocytes)

TSH

ACTH

FSH

LH

GH

Growth factor

Diabetogenic factor

Thyroid gland

Adrenal cortex

Testis

Prolactin

Ovary

Muscle

Fat tissue

Insulin

Breast (milk production)

Bone, muscle, organs (growth)

Pancreas

Thyroid hormones

Adrenocortical hormones

Testosterone

Estrogen

Progesterone

HYPOTHALAMIC CONTROL OF THE PITUITARY GLAND

The hypothalamus contains two sets of neuroendocrine neurons: the magnocellular neurons, which send axons to the posterior pituitary gland, and the parvicellular neurons, which secrete releasing or release-inhibiting hormones into the pituitary portal circulation.

The magnocellular neurons consist of two clusters: the SON and PVN. Each cell group contains both OXY and VP neurons. These cells secrete the hormones from their terminals in the posterior pituitary gland into the general circulation. VP controls urinary water and sodium excretion and has direct vasoconstrictor effects on blood vessels. OXY has some vasoconstrictor properties and causes uterine contractions but also is involved in the milk let-down reflex during breastfeeding. Cutting the pituitary stalk causes loss of secretion of both hormones, but the predominant symptom is diabetes insipidus due to lack of VP. Such individuals have excess loss of water in the urine, requiring the ingestion of up to 20 L of water per day to maintain blood osmolality in the normal range unless the hormone is replaced.

The parvicellular neurons are located along the wall of the third ventricle in the periventricular, paraventricular, and arcuate nuclei. Different populations of parvicellular endocrine neurons, secreting specific pituitary releasing or release-inhibiting hormones, have characteristic locations within this region. The CRH neurons, which cause secretion of adrenocorticotrophic hormone (ACTH) and ultimately adrenal corticosteroids, are mainly located in the PVN. Many neurons that secrete thyrotropin-releasing hormone which causes secretion of thyroid-stimulating hormone (TSH), or somatostatin, which inhibits secretion of growth hormone (GH), are also in the PVN, but some are found rostral to it in the periventricular nucleus. Neurons that secrete gonadotropin-releasing hormone (which causes secretion of luteinizing hormone [LH] and follicle-stimulating hormone [FSH]) are found in the most rostral part of the periventricular nucleus and dorsal arcuate nucleus. The rostral part of the arcuate nucleus also contains GH–releasing hormone neurons. Neurons secreting dopamine (a prolactin release–inhibiting hormone) are found widely distributed along the wall of the third ventricle in the periventricular, paraventricular, and arcuate nuclei. The arcuate nucleus also contains neurons that express pro-opiomelanocortin (POMC), a precursor protein that can be differentially processed to produce ACTH (e.g., in the pituitary gland) but that is processed into α-melanocyte–stimulating hormone (α-MSH) and β-endorphin in the arcuate nucleus, which uses them as neurotransmitters.

The anterior pituitary gland contains a mixed population of pituitary cells, each of which secretes a different hormone: TSH, ACTH/α-MSH, FSH/LH, prolactin, or GH. These hormones and their releasing and release-inhibiting factors can feed back upon the parvicellular endocrine neurons, providing short loop feedback. Prolactin is the only pituitary hormone that is primarily under inhibitory tone from the hypothalamus. Hence when the pituitary stalk is damaged, the secretion of other anterior pituitary hormones is diminished but prolactin increases.

Endocrine disorders may ensue from either excess secretion or lack of secretion of either an anterior pituitary hormone or its hypothalamic-releasing or release-inhibiting hormones. Thus precocious puberty is sometimes seen with hypothalamic hamartomas that secrete gonadotropin-secreting factor. On the other hand, amenorrhea may occur from increased secretion of prolactin. Cushing syndrome, the oversecretion of adrenal corticosteroids, may result from a steroid-secreting adrenal tumor, a pituitary tumor (or sometimes a lung or other tumor) that secretes ACTH, or hypersecretion of CRH.

Plate 5.7

Brain: PART I

HYPOTHALAMIC CONTROL OF THE AUTONOMIC NERVOUS SYSTEM

Other than a relatively modest projection to the preganglionic neurons from the infralimbic cortex, the hypothalamus is the highest level of the neuraxis that provides substantial input to the autonomic nervous system. It regulates virtually all autonomic functions and coordinates them with each other and with ongoing behavioral, metabolic, and emotional activity. The hypothalamus contains several sets of neurons, using different neurotransmitters, that provide innervation to the sympathetic and parasympathetic preganglionic neurons, as well as brainstem areas that regulate the autonomic nervous system. Many of these neurons are in the PVN of the hypothalamus. These form populations of small neurons that are typically dorsal or ventral to the main endocrine groups, and most of the paraventricular-autonomic neurons contain messenger ribonucleic acid for either OXY or VP. The descending pathways also stain immunohistochemically for these peptides and are probably involved in stress responses.

A second set of hypothalamic-autonomic neurons is found in the LHA. These consist mainly of neurons containing ORX or MCH neurons, and sometimes the peptide cocaine- and amphetamine-regulated transcript (CART), which is thought to be involved in regulation of feeding and metabolism, as well as wake-sleep and locomotor activity. A third population of hypothalamic-autonomic cells is found in the arcuate nucleus and adjacent retrochiasmatic area. These neurons contain α-MSH and CART and may also be involved in feeding and metabolic regulation.

All three sets of neurons send axons to the brainstem, where they innervate the nucleus of the solitary tract (which receives visceral afferent input from the glossopharyngeal and vagus nerves), as well as the regions that coordinate autonomic and respiratory reflexes in the ventrolateral medulla. Other axons innervate the parasympathetic preganglionic neurons in the Edinger-Westphal nucleus (pupillary constriction), the superior salivatory nucleus (associated with the facial nerve, which supplies the submandibular and sublingual salivary glands and the cerebral vasculature), the inferior salivatory nucleus (associated with the rostral tip of the nucleus of the solitary tract, supplying the parotid gland), the dorsal motor vagal nucleus (which supplies the abdominal organs), and the nucleus ambiguus (which is the main source of vagal input to the thoracic organs, including the esophagus, heart, and lungs).

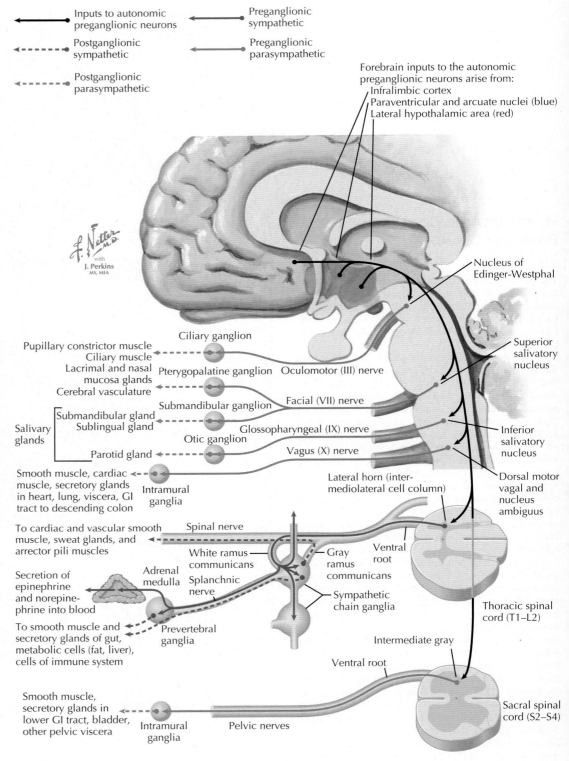

Inputs to autonomic preganglionic neurons

Postganglionic sympathetic

Postganglionic parasympathetic

Preganglionic sympathetic

Preganglionic parasympathetic

Forebrain inputs to the autonomic preganglionic neurons arise from:
Infralimbic cortex
Paraventricular and arcuate nuclei (blue)
Lateral hypothalamic area (red)

Nucleus of Edinger-Westphal

Superior salivatory nucleus

Ciliary ganglion

Pupillary constrictor muscle
Ciliary muscle
Lacrimal and nasal mucosa glands
Cerebral vasculature

Pterygopalatine ganglion

Oculomotor (III) nerve

Submandibular ganglion

Facial (VII) nerve

Submandibular gland
Sublingual gland

Glossopharyngeal (IX) nerve

Inferior salivatory nucleus

Salivary glands

Otic ganglion

Parotid gland

Vagus (X) nerve

Dorsal motor vagal and nucleus ambiguus

Smooth muscle, cardiac muscle, secretory glands in heart, lung, viscera, GI tract to descending colon

Intramural ganglia

Lateral horn (intermediolateral cell column)

To cardiac and vascular smooth muscle, sweat glands, and arrector pili muscles

Spinal nerve

White ramus communicans

Gray ramus communicans

Ventral root

Secretion of epinephrine and norepinephrine into blood

Adrenal medulla

Splanchnic nerve

Sympathetic chain ganglia

To smooth muscle and secretory glands of gut, metabolic cells (fat, liver), cells of immune system

Prevertebral ganglia

Thoracic spinal cord (T1–L2)

Intermediate gray

Ventral root

Smooth muscle, secretory glands in lower GI tract, bladder, other pelvic viscera

Intramural ganglia

Pelvic nerves

Sacral spinal cord (S2–S4)

Finally, descending axons from the hypothalamus innervate the sympathetic preganglionic neurons in the thoracic spinal cord. Different populations of hypothalamospinal neurons contact distinct targets. For example, the main projection from the ORX neurons is to the upper thoracic spinal cord, which may be important for control of pupilodilation and facial sweating. The OXY neurons innervate specific clusters of sympathetic preganglionic neurons at multiple spinal cord levels.

In addition, there is a major input to the medullary raphe nuclei from the preoptic area and dorsomedial nucleus of the hypothalamus. The medullary raphe nuclei contain both serotoninergic (5-HT) and glutamatergic neurons that innervate the sympathetic preganglionic column at multiple levels and regulate populations of neurons involved in thermoregulation. This pathway is thought to be a major mechanism for regulating body temperature and metabolic rate.

Damage to the descending hypothalamic-autonomic pathway, in the lateral medulla or spinal cord, causes ipsilateral central Horner syndrome. Such patients have a small pupil (miosis) and ptosis on that side as well as lack sweating (anhidrosis) on the affected side of the face and body.

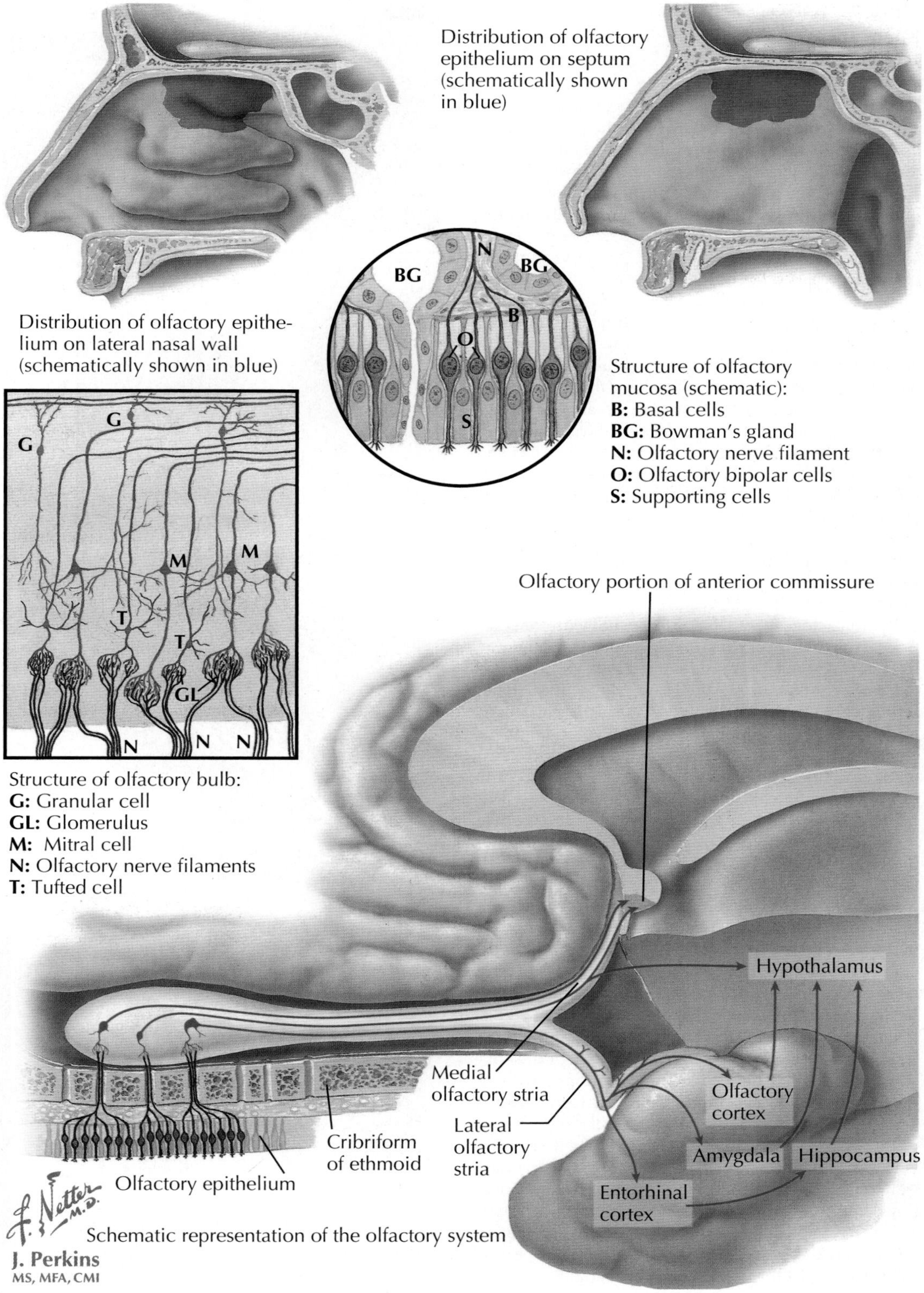

Plate 5.8

Hypothalamus, Pituitary, Sleep, and Thalamus

Distribution of olfactory epithelium on septum (schematically shown in blue)

Distribution of olfactory epithelium on lateral nasal wall (schematically shown in blue)

Structure of olfactory mucosa (schematic):
B: Basal cells
BG: Bowman's gland
N: Olfactory nerve filament
O: Olfactory bipolar cells
S: Supporting cells

Structure of olfactory bulb:
G: Granular cell
GL: Glomerulus
M: Mitral cell
N: Olfactory nerve filaments
T: Tufted cell

Olfactory portion of anterior commissure

Hypothalamus

Medial olfactory stria

Lateral olfactory stria

Olfactory cortex

Amygdala   Hippocampus

Entorhinal cortex

Cribriform of ethmoid

Olfactory epithelium

Schematic representation of the olfactory system

J. Perkins
MS, MFA, CMI

OLFACTORY INPUTS TO THE HYPOTHALAMUS

There are about 1000 olfactory receptor genes, each of which recognizes a different class of chemical olfactory stimulus. Each olfactory receptor cell expresses a single olfactory receptor type, and each gene is expressed in several hundred cells, spread across the olfactory mucosa. The axons from olfactory receptor cells then run through openings in the cribriform plate, which forms the base of the skull over the olfactory mucosa, and axons from individual cells, which express a single receptor gene, then converge in the olfactory bulb on one or a few individual olfactory glomeruli.

The glomeruli are on the surface of the olfactory bulb and are spherical areas, each about one-third millimeter across. The outside of the glomerulus is lined with tiny periglomerular interneurons. Just deep to the glomerular layer are mitral and tufted cells, which send their apical dendrites up into the glomeruli, where they receive olfactory sensory information. The mitral and tufted cells excite granule cells, which, in turn, inhibit the other mitral and tufted cells and receive centrifugal axons, which modulate the perception of the sensory stimulus. Only the mitral and tufted cells send their axons into the brain via the olfactory tract. In humans, this is a long white matter bundle that runs along the surface of the frontal lobe and is sometimes erroneously called the "olfactory nerve."

The olfactory tract supplies information about smell to a variety of targets in the brain. It bifurcates as it approaches the temporal lobe into one branch that runs medially into the BF and another that runs laterally to supply olfactory inputs to cortical structures.

The lateral olfactory branch provides inputs to the primary olfactory cortex, which appears to be necessary for processing the conscious appreciation of odors, and the entorhinal cortex, which is a point of convergence of information from multiple sensory systems and a major relay into the hippocampal formation. There is also input to the amygdala, which may be important for relaying olfactory signals related to food acquisition and sexual behavior to the hypothalamus.

In many mammals, there is an accessory olfactory system. A small pit in the nasal mucosa, called the vomeronasal organ, contains olfactory sensory neurons that are important for sensing pheromones. These olfactory neurons synapse in a specialized region called the accessory olfactory bulb and relay information concerned with social behaviors into the amygdala and hypothalamus. Such a system has never been clearly identified in humans, and its very existence remains controversial.

Plate 5.9

Brain: PART I

VISUAL INPUTS TO THE HYPOTHALAMUS

The hypothalamus is largely framed by the optic chiasm, which underlies its most rostral part (the preoptic area) and the optic tract, which provides the lateral boundary for its middle, tuberal part. Despite this close relationship, it remained a mystery for many years how the hypothalamus used visual input to synchronize its biologic clock with the external world. In 1972 two groups of scientists demonstrated that some axons leave the optic chiasm as it passes by the hypothalamus and provide an input that is now called the *retinohypothalamic tract*.

The retinohypothalamic tract originates from about 1000 scattered retinal ganglion cells in each retina. In 2001 it was discovered that these retinal ganglion cells have the peculiar property of making their own light-sensing pigment, called melanopsin. So although other retinal ganglion cells that are concerned with patterned vision are "blind" and depend on input from rods and cones to signal to them the presence of light in their receptive fields, the melanopsin-containing retinal ganglion cells are intrinsically photosensitive. These neurons act essentially as light level detectors and relay this information both to the hypothalamus and to the olivary pretectal nucleus, which is a critical relay in the pupillary light reflex pathway.

By replacing the melanopsin gene with one for β-galactosidase in mice, the melanopsin-containing retinal ganglion cells can be stained blue and their axons can be followed into the brain. The densest site of retinohypothalamic input is to the suprachiasmatic nucleus, although other axons, in smaller numbers, enter other parts of the hypothalamus. The suprachiasmatic nucleus is the brain's biologic clock; damage to this cell group causes animals and humans to lose their 24-hour patterns of activity in wake-sleep, feeding, body temperature, corticosteroid secretion, and other important physiologic and behavioral functions. Although the neurons in the suprachiasmatic nucleus maintain an approximately 24-hour rhythm of activity even when placed into tissue culture, retinal input is necessary to reset their clock rhythm to maintain synchrony with the external world. In the absence of light cues, circadian rhythms in both people and animals show a free-running cycle that is generally just a bit different from 24 hours and may vary among individuals (humans average about 24.1 hours). Although this may seem like a small difference from 24 hours, without a mechanism for synchronization, someone with a 24.1-hour cycle would be 3 hours off-cycle from the rest of the world by the end of 1 month. Some blind individuals, with total loss of retinal input to the brain, show this type of shift of their circadian rhythms over time (non-24 syndrome) so that they go through periods every few months where their cycles go out of phase with the rest of the world. Other blind people, such as those with rod and cone degeneration, who retain intrinsically photosensitive melanopsin-containing retinal ganglion cells, remain in synchrony with the world that they cannot see.

Melatonin is one of the hormones whose 24-hour cycle of secretion is driven by the suprachiasmatic nucleus. Suprachiasmatic axons directly contact neurons in the PVN, which, in turn, innervates the sympathetic preganglionic neurons in the upper thoracic spinal cord. The latter project to the superior cervical ganglion, which sends axons along the internal carotid artery intracranially to innervate the pineal gland, causing secretion of melatonin. The hormone is mainly

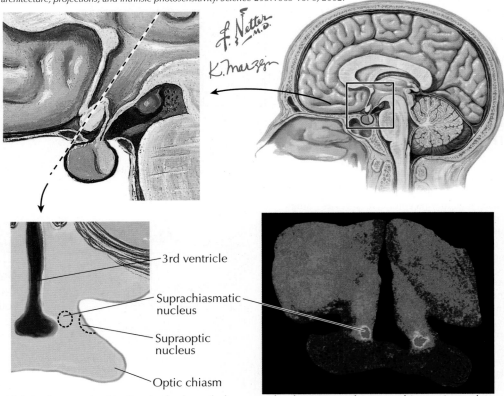

The axons bound for the suprachiasmatic nucleus have been stained blue, shown at higher magnifications.
Photographs reprinted with permission from Hattar S, Liao HW, Takao M, et al. Melanopsin-containing retinal ganglion cells: architecture, projections, and intrinsic photosensitivity. Science 295:1065-1070, 2002.

3rd ventricle

Suprachiasmatic nucleus

Supraoptic nucleus

Optic chiasm

Melatonin receptor binding in the hypothalamus with a hot spot at the suprachiasmatic nucleus.
Courtesy Dr. David Weaver, University of Massachusetts Medical School.

secreted at the onset of the dark period and in humans may promote sleepiness. One of the major targets in the brain for melatonin is the suprachiasmatic nucleus itself, which stands out when the brain is stained for melatonin receptors.

Other retinal axons to the hypothalamus may be important in providing visual inputs to neurons concerned with a variety of diverse functions. For example, retinal inputs to a sleep-promoting cell group,

the ventrolateral preoptic (VLPO) nucleus, may explain why people turn out the lights and close their eyes when falling asleep. Other inputs to the lateral hypothalamus may contact neurons involved in regulating arousal and feeding. In rodents, who might be recognized as potential prey when they venture into a lighted area, an important response to light is immobility. This reduced locomotion in light appears to be regulated by retinal inputs to the subparaventricular zone.

Plate 5.10

Hypothalamus, Pituitary, Sleep, and Thalamus

CONTROL OF HYPOTHALAMUS BY SENSORY INPUTS

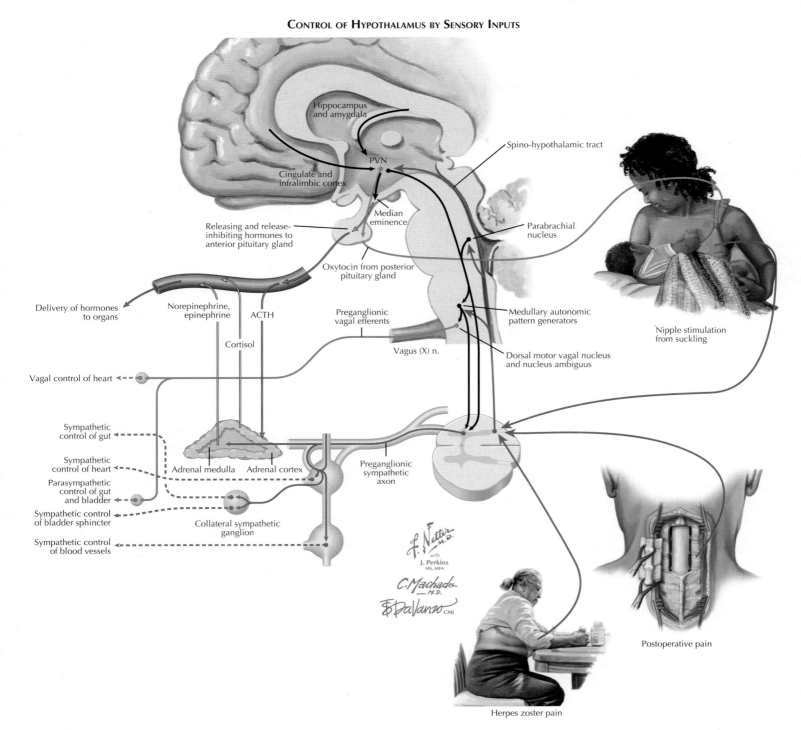

Hippocampus and amygdala

Spino-hypothalamic tract

PVN

Cingulate and infralimbic cortex

Median eminence

Parabrachial nucleus

Releasing and release-inhibiting hormones to anterior pituitary gland

Oxytocin from posterior pituitary gland

Delivery of hormones to organs

Norepinephrine, epinephrine

ACTH

Preganglionic vagal efferents

Medullary autonomic pattern generators

Nipple stimulation from suckling

Cortisol

Vagus (X) n.

Dorsal motor vagal nucleus and nucleus ambiguus

Vagal control of heart

Sympathetic control of gut

Sympathetic control of heart

Parasympathetic control of gut and bladder

Adrenal medulla

Adrenal cortex

Preganglionic sympathetic axon

Sympathetic control of bladder sphincter

Sympathetic control of blood vessels

Collateral sympathetic ganglion

Postoperative pain

Herpes zoster pain

SOMATOSENSORY INPUTS TO THE HYPOTHALAMUS

The somatosensory system provides a major source of direct inputs to the hypothalamus. For many years it was thought that the somatosensory system primarily fed through the thalamus to the cerebral cortex and that sensory inputs to the hypothalamus must be relayed from the cortex. However, in 1980 it was discovered that some axons from the ascending somatosensory pathways directly reach the hypothalamus. These inputs originate from somatosensory neurons in the spinal and trigeminal dorsal horn. Many of these neurons are concerned with painful stimuli. These may

play a role in orchestrating emotional responses, such as anger, fight, or flight in response to a physical injury. They may also be important stimuli for triggering the autonomic and endocrine responses associated with pain, such as elevation of blood pressure and heart rate, or secretion of cortisol.

Somatosensory inputs are also important in sexual behavior. Neurons in the preoptic area promote erection in males, and nerve cells in the ventromedial nucleus of the hypothalamus can potently drive sexual behaviors, including mounting postures in males and receptive postures in females. The neurons that produce these responses are, in turn, driven by a range of visual, olfactory, and tactile stimuli. In some species, ovulation is also triggered by sexual somatosensory stimuli (e.g., vaginal stimulation).

Another hypothalamically mediated response that is dependent on somatosensory input is the milk letdown reflex during breastfeeding. Breast milk production is stimulated by prolactin, but the release of the milk requires somatosensory stimulation as well. The infant suckling at the breast causes sensory input that reaches the OXY neurons in the PVN and SON in the hypothalamus. These neurons fire in bursts, which causes them to release OXY into the circulation from their axon terminals in the posterior pituitary gland. The OXY, in turn, causes milk to flow from the breast.

In each of these examples, autonomic, endocrine, and behavioral responses must be coordinated, the hallmark of a hypothalamically mediated behavior. The integration of these responses in each case depends on somatosensory input that is delivered directly to the hypothalamus.

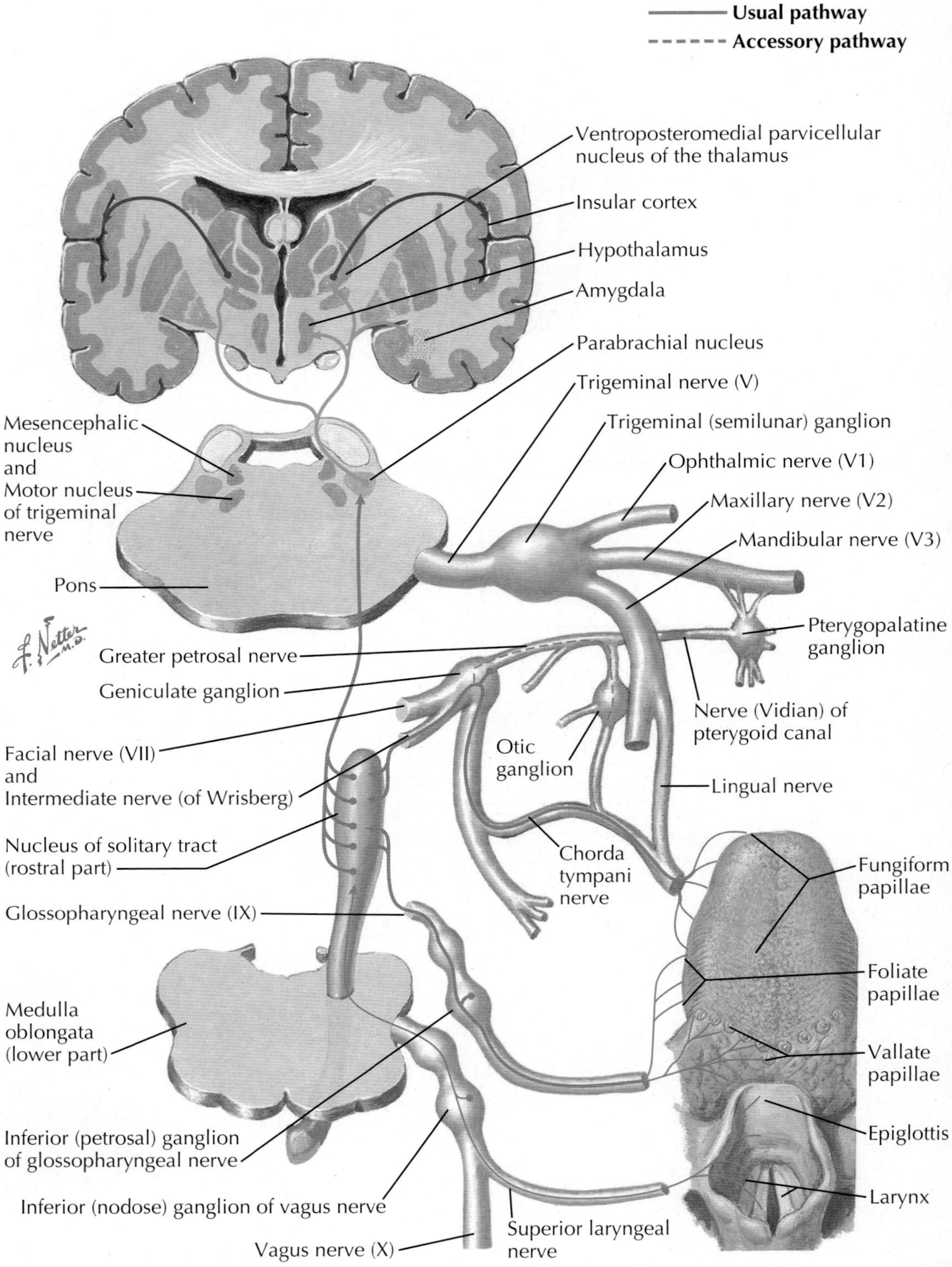

Plate 5.11

Brain: PART I

Usual pathway
------ Accessory pathway

Ventroposteromedial parvicellular nucleus of the thalamus

Insular cortex

Hypothalamus

Amygdala

Parabrachial nucleus

Trigeminal nerve (V)

Trigeminal (semilunar) ganglion

Ophthalmic nerve (V1)

Maxillary nerve (V2)

Mandibular nerve (V3)

Mesencephalic nucleus and Motor nucleus of trigeminal nerve

Pterygopalatine ganglion

Pons

Greater petrosal nerve

Geniculate ganglion

Nerve (Vidian) of pterygoid canal

Facial nerve (VII) and Intermediate nerve (of Wrisberg)

Otic ganglion

Lingual nerve

Nucleus of solitary tract (rostral part)

Chorda tympani nerve

Fungiform papillae

Glossopharyngeal nerve (IX)

Foliate papillae

Medulla oblongata (lower part)

Vallate papillae

Inferior (petrosal) ganglion of glossopharyngeal nerve

Epiglottis

Inferior (nodose) ganglion of vagus nerve

Larynx

Vagus nerve (X)

Superior laryngeal nerve

TASTE AND OTHER VISCERAL SENSORY INPUTS TO THE HYPOTHALAMUS

A special class of visceral sensory pathway provides taste information to the hypothalamus and other areas of the brain. Taste receptor cells are found in taste buds, located in clusters along the surface of the tongue. Different classes of taste receptors respond to different classes of chemicals in food, including acids (sour), sugars (sweet), sodium (salty), glutamate (an important amino acid component of proteins, whose taste is said to be "savory," or "umami" in Japanese), and complex plant alkaloids that often warn of poisonous compounds (bitter). The taste receptor cells are innervated by sensory neurons from the facial (VII nerve, to the anterior two-thirds of the tongue), glossopharyngeal (IX nerve, to the posterior tongue and tonsillar arches), and vagus (X nerve, to the posterior tongue and oropharynx) cranial nerves. Much like other somatosensory systems, the gustatory sensory neurons are located in ganglia (geniculate for the facial nerve, petrosal for the glossopharyngeal nerve, and nodose for the vagus nerve) and consist of pseudounipolar cells, with a single axon that bifurcates in the ganglion into a central and a peripheral branch. The central branches terminate in the rostral third of the nucleus of the solitary tract in the medulla. The axons end in a roughly topographic order with respect to the surface of the tongue (axons from the anterior two-thirds of the tongue ending most rostrally). The nucleus of the solitary tract gives off local connections in the brainstem to reflex pathways for salivation and for regulation of biting, chewing, and swallowing activity.

Ascending axons from the nucleus of the solitary tract travel through the brainstem, and a large proportion of them synapse in the parabrachial nucleus. From there, axons continue to the thalamus (for conscious appreciation of taste), amygdala (for taste associations), and hypothalamus (presumably for regulation of feeding). The inputs to the hypothalamus and amygdala are augmented by a smaller number of axons that reach these sites directly from the nucleus of the solitary tract. In primates, there is evidence that some axons from the taste portion of the nucleus of the solitary tract may reach the thalamus directly, without requiring a relay in the parabrachial nucleus. Taste neurons in the thalamus are located adjacent to the tongue somatosensory area, and they innervate the insular cortex, which contains the primary taste cortex.

The posterior two-thirds of the nucleus of the solitary tract receives inputs from other internal organs via the glossopharyngeal and vagus nerves. These terminate in a roughly topographic order, with gastrointestinal inputs in the middle part of the nucleus and cardiorespiratory in the caudal part. The nucleus of the solitary tract provides local inputs to cell groups in the medulla that control gastrointestinal functions, including gastric acid secretion and gut motility, as well as cardiovascular and respiratory reflexes (e.g., the baroreceptor reflex that stabilizes blood pressure when moving from a lying to a standing position, and the increase in both respiratory rate and blood pressure when there is a high level of carbon dioxide in the blood).

Other axons from the posterior two-thirds of the nucleus of the solitary tract terminate in the parabrachial nucleus. Parabrachial neurons then contact the visceral sensory thalamus, which, in turn, projects to the insular cortex, where sensations such as gastric fullness or air hunger reach conscious appreciation. Other parabrachial outputs are joined by smaller numbers of axons from the nucleus of the solitary tract itself in projecting to the amygdala, where they may be involved in visceral conditioned reflexes. Parabrachial inputs to the hypothalamus may play a role in a wide range of functions, from regulation of behaviors such as feeding and drinking to control of secretion of hormones such as VP (during hypovolemia) and OXY (during emesis).

Plate 5.12

Hypothalamus, Pituitary, Sleep, and Thalamus

LIMBIC AND CORTICAL INPUTS TO THE HYPOTHALAMUS

In addition to having direct sensory inputs, the hypothalamus receives highly processed information from the cerebral cortex, which is relayed via the limbic system. The limbic lobe of the brain was first defined by Paul Broca, in 1878, as the cortex surrounding the medial edge of the cerebral hemisphere, as shown in orange in the upper figure of Plate 5.12. Broca's limbic lobe includes the cingulate gyrus (the infralimbic, prelimbic, anterior cingulate, and retrosplenial areas), the hippocampal formation (including the entorhinal area, subiculum, hippocampal cornu ammonis [CA] fields, and dentate gyrus), and the amygdala. These limbic regions all receive highly processed sensory information from the association regions of the cerebral cortex, process that information for its emotional content, and then project back to the association cortical areas to provide emotional coloring to cognition.

Each of the limbic areas also sends descending inputs to the hypothalamus. The inputs from the cingulate gyrus mainly originate in the infralimbic and prelimbic regions (around and just beneath the splenium of the corpus callosum). These areas mainly send axons to the lateral hypothalamus, as well as to components of the autonomic system in the brainstem and the spinal cord, and are believed to provide much of the autonomic component of emotional response.

Neurons in the hippocampal formation, particularly the CA1 field and the subiculum, send axons to the hypothalamus through the fornix. This long looping pathway, shown in yellow in the upper figure, curves just under the corpus callosum and then dives into the diencephalon at the foramen of Monro. Many axons leave the fornix in the hypothalamus and provide inputs to the ventromedial nucleus. However, a dense column of fornix axons reaches the mammillary body, where they terminate. These structures are shown in blue in the upper figure and red in the lower one. Although the hippocampus appears to be very important in memory consolidation, isolated damage to the fornix or mammillary bodies has more limited and inconsistent effects on memory, so the function of this pathway remains enigmatic.

The mammillary nuclei provide another salient bundle of axons to the anterior nucleus of the thalamus. This mammillothalamic tract is heavily myelinated and easily seen, but its contribution to memory formation is more subtle, like that of the mammillary body itself. Lesions of the mammillothalamic tract have been reported to prevent the generalization of limbic seizures, however, and this pathway has been targeted for deep brain stimulation to prevent generalization of seizures. The anterior thalamic nucleus projects to the cingulate gyrus, and in 1937 James Papez hypothesized that

perhaps the momentum of emotions could be explained by a "reverberating circuit," completed by a projection from the cingulate cortex back to the hippocampus, to neurons that contribute to the fornix. Although there is no credible evidence for this last link in the "circuit" actually existing or for the proposed "Papez circuit" playing a role in emotion, the theory has achieved great attention.

The amygdala provides the hypothalamus with inputs via two pathways. Some axons leave the amygdala in

parallel to the fornix, running along the lateral edge of the lateral ventricle just below the tail and body of the caudate nucleus in the stria terminalis, shown in blue in the lower figure. Other amygdaloid inputs to the hypothalamus take a much more direct anterior route, running over the optic tract into the lateral hypothalamus. Many hypothalamic cell groups receive inputs from the amygdala, which are thought to be important for the visceral components of conditioned emotional responses.

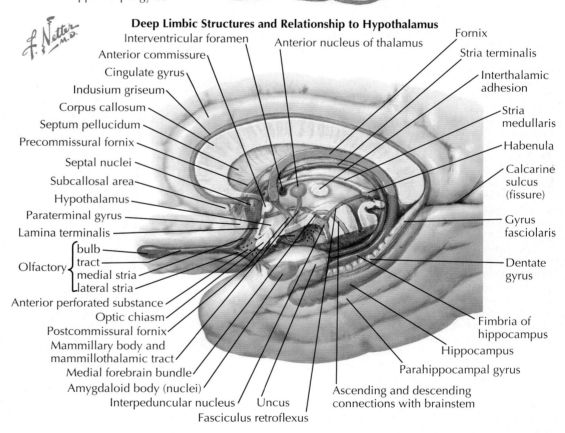

Limbic Cortex and Relationship to Hypothalamus

Supplementary motor (premotor) area
Cingulate gyrus
Fornix
Thalamus
Prefrontal area
Motor area
Somatosensory area
Corpus callosum
Visual area
Olfactory bulb
Orbital cortex
Hypothalamus
Amygdala
Hippocampal formation
Parahippocampal gyrus

Deep Limbic Structures and Relationship to Hypothalamus

Interventricular foramen
Anterior commissure
Cingulate gyrus
Indusium griseum
Corpus callosum
Septum pellucidum
Precommissural fornix
Septal nuclei
Subcallosal area
Hypothalamus
Paraterminal gyrus
Lamina terminalis
Olfactory { bulb, tract, medial stria, lateral stria }
Anterior perforated substance
Optic chiasm
Postcommissural fornix
Mammillary body and mammillothalamic tract
Medial forebrain bundle
Amygdaloid body (nuclei)
Interpeduncular nucleus
Fasciculus retroflexus
Uncus
Anterior nucleus of thalamus
Fornix
Stria terminalis
Interthalamic adhesion
Stria medullaris
Habenula
Calcarine sulcus (fissure)
Gyrus fasciolaris
Dentate gyrus
Fimbria of hippocampus
Hippocampus
Parahippocampal gyrus
Ascending and descending connections with brainstem

Plate 5.13

Brain: PART I

OVERVIEW OF HYPOTHALAMIC FUNCTION AND DYSFUNCTION

The hypothalamus works to integrate autonomic, endocrine, and behavioral functions of the brain that subserve basic life functions, such as maintaining fluid and electrolyte balance, feeding and metabolism, body temperature and energy expenditure, cycles of sleep and wakefulness, and a wide range of emergency responses. As a result, the range of disorders that occur when the hypothalamus malfunctions is also very great.

Because the hypothalamus is very small, injuries often involve multiple systems. Hence a patient with a pituitary tumor or craniopharyngioma impinging on the hypothalamus may have disorders extending into many functions. Such patients are often quite somnolent because an important branch of the ascending arousal system runs through the LHA. There may also be loss of circadian (24-hour) rhythms of behavior so that the relatively limited waking time may occur during the night rather than in the day.

Alfred Froehlich in 1901 described the patients with such lesions as having an "adiposogenital syndrome" because they became obese and had failure of sexual maturation. Research has identified the reason for this association. Feeding in humans (and other animals) is controlled in part by the hormone leptin, which is made by white adipose tissue during times of plenty. In the absence of leptin or its receptors, both humans and animals are ravenous and become quite obese. Leptin is now known to act on the hypothalamus in the region just above the pituitary stalk to decrease activity in circuits that promote eating. When tumors in the region of the pituitary gland damage this part of the hypothalamus, feeding circuits become disinhibited and the patient becomes obese. An adequate nutritional state is also required for the brain to trigger the hormonal changes that accompany puberty. These circuits are also dependent on leptin to provide a signal that there are sufficient energy stores to make reproduction possible. Patients whose pituitary tumors develop before puberty may fail to go through the transition. Adults who are severely underweight may have regression of sexual organs, accompanied by amenorrhea in females.

The hypothalamic-releasing hormones, in general, are required by the anterior pituitary gland to secrete adequate amounts of growth, thyroid, corticotropic, and gonadal hormones. In the presence of a pituitary tumor that damages the hypophyseal portal bed in the pituitary stalk, secretion of all these hormones is diminished. On the other hand, prolactin is mainly under inhibitory control by the hypothalamus, primarily through release of dopamine into the portal circulation. Damage to the pituitary stalk thus causes hyperprolactinemia, with galactorrhea (breast milk production) and amenorrhea in women.

Pituitary stalk lesions also sever the axons from the PVN and SON, which release the hormones OXY and VP from the posterior pituitary gland. Such patients have diabetes insipidus, with excessive urination, requiring compensatory drinking to avoid volume depletion.

Smaller, focal hypothalamic lesions can sometimes have different results. For example, bilateral lateral hypothalamic lesions, such as multiple sclerosis plaques, have been reported to cause emaciation. Lesions of the preoptic area can cause loss of thirst and loss of ability to increase VP secretion during dehydration. On hot days, such patients may have substantial volume depletion without becoming thirsty.

Hypothalamic lesions in children may also have somewhat different clinical presentations than in adults.

Hypothalamic hamartomas can cause gelastic epilepsy, in which the child laughs uncontrollably but mirthlessly, and sometimes precocious puberty (if the hamartoma includes gonadotropic-releasing hormone neurons). On the other hand, a large hypothalamic lesion in an infant is more likely to present with wasting and emaciation than with obesity, but such children may be quite happy and playful, rather than somnolent.

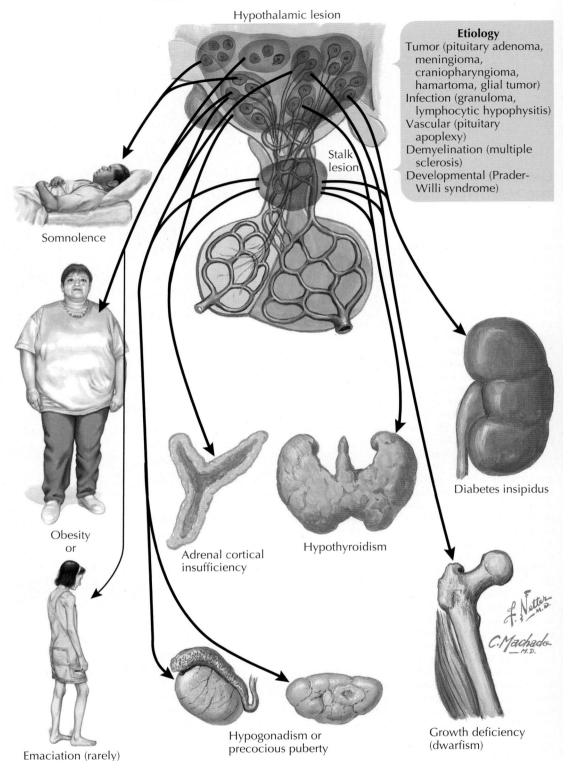

OVERVIEW OF HYPOTHALAMIC AND PITUITARY DISEASE

Hypothalamic lesion

Stalk lesion

Etiology
Tumor (pituitary adenoma, meningioma, craniopharyngioma, hamartoma, glial tumor)
Infection (granuloma, lymphocytic hypophysitis)
Vascular (pituitary apoplexy)
Demyelination (multiple sclerosis)
Developmental (Prader-Willi syndrome)

Somnolence

Obesity or

Emaciation (rarely)

Adrenal cortical insufficiency

Hypothyroidism

Hypogonadism or precocious puberty

Diabetes insipidus

Growth deficiency (dwarfism)

Plate 5.14

Hypothalamus, Pituitary, Sleep, and Thalamus

REGULATION OF OSMOLALITY AND WATER BALANCE

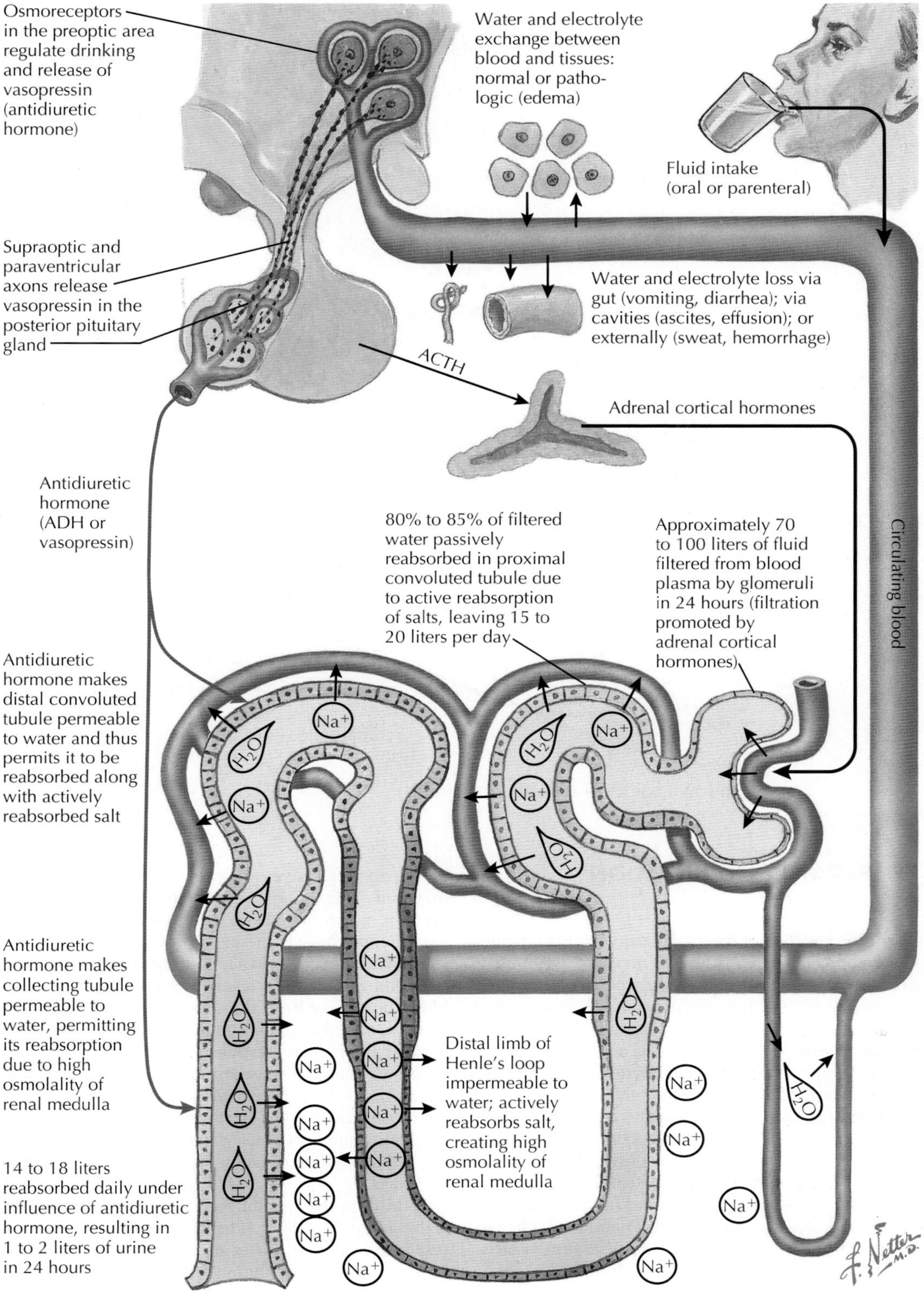

Osmoreceptors in the preoptic area regulate drinking and release of vasopressin (antidiuretic hormone)

Water and electrolyte exchange between blood and tissues: normal or pathologic (edema)

Fluid intake (oral or parenteral)

Supraoptic and paraventricular axons release vasopressin in the posterior pituitary gland

Water and electrolyte loss via gut (vomiting, diarrhea); via cavities (ascites, effusion); or externally (sweat, hemorrhage)

ACTH

Adrenal cortical hormones

Antidiuretic hormone (ADH or vasopressin)

80% to 85% of filtered water passively reabsorbed in proximal convoluted tubule due to active reabsorption of salts, leaving 15 to 20 liters per day

Approximately 70 to 100 liters of fluid filtered from blood plasma by glomeruli in 24 hours (filtration promoted by adrenal cortical hormones)

Circulating blood

Antidiuretic hormone makes distal convoluted tubule permeable to water and thus permits it to be reabsorbed along with actively reabsorbed salt

Antidiuretic hormone makes collecting tubule permeable to water, permitting its reabsorption due to high osmolality of renal medulla

Distal limb of Henle's loop impermeable to water; actively reabsorbs salt, creating high osmolality of renal medulla

14 to 18 liters reabsorbed daily under influence of antidiuretic hormone, resulting in 1 to 2 liters of urine in 24 hours

REGULATION OF WATER BALANCE

The anterior part of the preoptic area, just above the optic chiasm, contains the neurons of the median preoptic (MnPO) nucleus, which play an important role in sensing blood osmolality, sodium levels, and fluid volume. The individual neurons in this region appear to be sodium and osmolality sensors, and they also receive sensory inputs concerning fluid volume from atrial stretch receptors (through the vagus nerve and nucleus of the solitary tract). There are also mineralocorticoid sensor neurons in the nucleus of the solitary tract, which provide inputs that regulate salt appetite to the hypothalamus via a relay in the parabrachial nucleus. In addition, VP neurons in the suprachiasmatic nucleus provide circadian input to the preoptic neurons that control drinking behavior.

Fluid and electrolyte balance is maintained by autonomic, endocrine, and behavioral means. The renal blood flow is under autonomic control, as is the juxtaglomerular apparatus, which releases renin, an enzyme that acts on angiotensinogen to produce a range of angiotensin hormones. After conversion to angiotensin, this hormone increases both vasoconstriction (thus supporting blood pressure) and aldosterone secretion, and it causes drinking by direct action on the brain. The drinking behavior appears to be mediated by angiotensin II leaking across the blood-brain barrier to activate neurons expressing angiotensin II receptors at the anterior end of the third ventricle. These neurons then project into the hypothalamus to promote drinking via effects on salivary secretion (dry mouth, a signal to drink) and general arousal (foraging for water) and specific motor systems (that increase licking and swallowing responses) associated with drinking.

The endocrine response to dehydration includes both anterior and posterior pituitary limbs. The release of VP by the posterior pituitary causes active resorption of salt and water in the distal limb of the renal tubules and in the collecting ducts. At the same time, VP has a direct vasoconstrictor effect that supports blood pressure. The anterior pituitary gland releases more ACTH, under control of both CRH and VP secreted into the pituitary portal circulation from the hypothalamus. Cortisol itself has some mineralocorticoid effects, but

ACTH also primes the adrenal cortex to make aldosterone, the major mineralocorticoid. Aldosterone secretion is also stimulated by the presence of angiotensin III.

Individuals with lesions in the preoptic area are sometimes unable to appreciate thirst. Some of these individuals also have deficits in VP secretion in response to dehydration. Such patients must be reminded to drink, especially on hot days, to avoid dehydration.

Plate 5.15

Brain: PART I

HYPOTHALAMIC REGULATION OF BODY TEMPERATURE

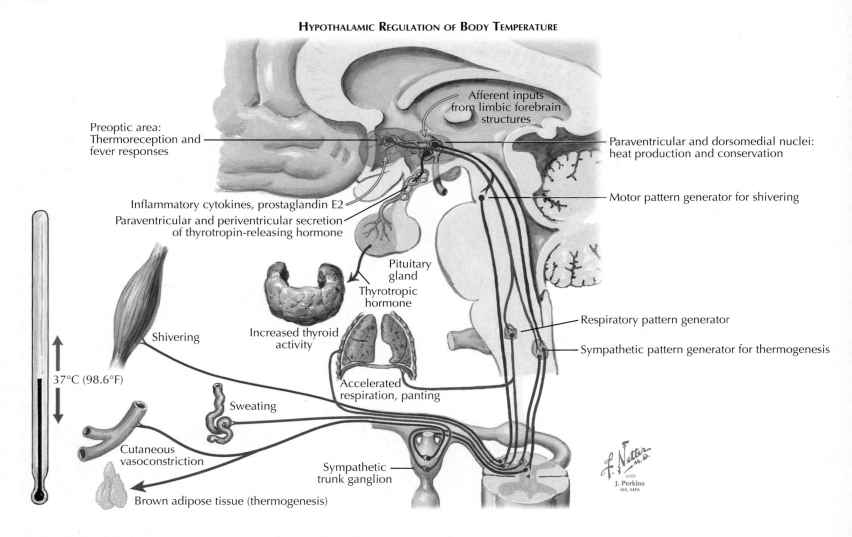

Preoptic area:
Thermoreception and
fever responses

Afferent inputs
from limbic forebrain
structures

Paraventricular and dorsomedial nuclei:
heat production and conservation

Inflammatory cytokines, prostaglandin E2

Motor pattern generator for shivering

Paraventricular and periventricular secretion
of thyrotropin-releasing hormone

Pituitary
gland

Thyrotropic
hormone

Shivering

Increased thyroid
activity

Respiratory pattern generator

Sympathetic pattern generator for thermogenesis

37°C (98.6°F)

Sweating

Accelerated
respiration, panting

Cutaneous
vasoconstriction

Sympathetic
trunk ganglion

Brown adipose tissue (thermogenesis)

TEMPERATURE REGULATION

One of the key roles of the hypothalamus is maintaining an even body temperature. This is necessary for optimal function of neurons, metabolic enzymes, and actions of the immune system. The preoptic area contains neurons that are specialized for thermoregulation. These are located in the preoptic area close to the neurons that detect osmolality and control fluid and electrolyte balance, and some neurons may have roles in both systems. (For example, on a hot day it is necessary to conserve fluid for use by sweat glands to maintain cooling.) The preoptic thermoregulatory neurons are responsive both to the local brain temperature and to skin temperature, relayed by warm- and cold-receptive neurons in the dorsal horn of the spinal cord to the parabrachial nucleus and then to the preoptic area. The preoptic warm-responsive neurons excite inhibitory neurons in the dorsomedial hypothalamus and medullary raphe. The latter neurons cause a rise in body temperature when they are stimulated, so inhibition by the preoptic warm-responsive neurons causes body temperature to fall. The preoptic warm-responsive neurons also have receptors for PGE2, which is made by blood vessels in the preoptic area during inflammatory conditions. Inhibitory E-type prostaglandin (EP) receptor (EP3) prostaglandin receptors reduce activity of the warm-responsive neurons, causing a rise in body temperature (fever).

This circuit controls body temperature in three ways. First it regulates metabolic rate. Increased firing by warm-responsive preoptic neurons can reduce metabolic rate by up to 80%. Second, activation of preoptic warm-responsive neurons causes cutaneous vasodilation, which increases heat loss through the skin. When this pathway is shut down (e.g., in a cold environment, during a fever), vasoconstriction shunts blood flow away from the skin to deep vascular beds to conserve heat. In animals with fur, piloerection, another sympathetic response, increases the thickness of the fur coat and thus conserves heat. Humans also have piloerection called gooseflesh, but this is not nearly as effective in heat conservation. The heat-producing and heat-conserving mechanisms are coordinated by medullary raphe neurons that activate both pathways.

A third mechanism for regulating body temperature is by motor activity. Activation of preoptic warm-responsive neurons causes animals to seek a cool environment, whereas inhibition by EP3 receptors during a fever promotes seeking a warm environment. In addition, heat may be generated by increased muscle activity or shivering. Little is known about the pathways by which preoptic neurons regulate motor activities.

Anterior pituitary hormones do not seem to play much of a role in the regulation of body temperature over a period of minutes or even hours, although in the absence of thyroid hormone, body temperature falls. Body temperature also rises (during the active cycle) and falls (during the sleep cycle) daily, and these adjustments typically occur before the onset of motor activity or rest and so are not due to a simple change in muscle activity. There are also changes in body temperature during the menstrual cycle, which may reflect the fact that the preoptic area is also involved in reproductive function.

In addition to inhibiting the heat production and conservation systems, warm-sensitive neurons in the preoptic area also increase blood flow to the skin, resulting in sweating to permit heat loss, and they increase VP secretion, which permits conservation of fluids that are necessary to support increased sweating. Sweating in humans is mediated by two sets of sympathetic nerves, one of which is noradrenergic (NE) and the other cholinergic. The cholinergic sympathetic input appears to be of primary importance for thermoregulatory sweating, whereas the NE axons may be more important for emotional sweating.

Paroxysmal hypothermia is a rare neurologic disorder, most often seen in individuals who have agenesis of the corpus callosum (due to a failure of the anterior wall of the third ventricle to develop properly) or a congenital tumor or other lesion affecting the preoptic area. Such individuals have periods of several days at a time during which their body temperature drops to about 30°C, and they lapse into a stuporous state. The mechanism for paroxysmal hypothermia is not known, although similar regulated reductions in body temperature for periods of hours (torpor) or weeks (hibernation) occur in many other species. In mice, preoptic warm-responsive neurons have been found to cause torpor during periods of inadequate energy supply.

Plate 5.16

Hypothalamus, Pituitary, Sleep, and Thalamus

CYTOKINES AND PROSTAGLANDINS CAUSE THE SICKNESS RESPONSE

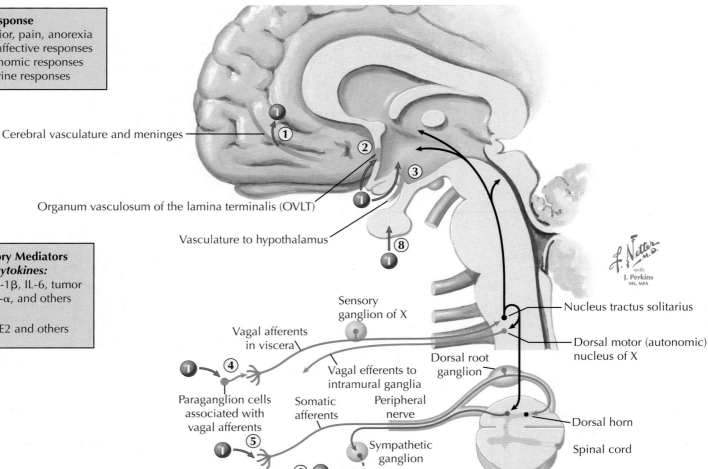

The Sickness Response
Sickness behavior, pain, anorexia
Cognitive and affective responses
Fever and autonomic responses
Cortisol/endocrine responses

Cerebral vasculature and meninges

Organum vasculosum of the lamina terminalis (OVLT)

Vasculature to hypothalamus

I = Inflammatory Mediators
Inflammatory cytokines:
  Interleukin (IL)-1β, IL-6, tumor
  necrosis factor-α, and others
Prostaglandins:
  Prostaglandin E2 and others

Sensory ganglion of X

Nucleus tractus solitarius

Vagal afferents in viscera

Dorsal motor (autonomic) nucleus of X

Vagal efferents to intramural ganglia

Dorsal root ganglion

Paraganglion cells associated with vagal afferents

Somatic afferents

Peripheral nerve

Dorsal horn

Spinal cord

Sympathetic ganglion

Target

① Prostaglandins crossing blood-brain barrier (BBB) or released from meninges can alter cognitive function.

② Cytokines and prostaglandins can enter brain at circumventricular organs, such as OVLT, that lack BBB.

③ Cytokines act on cerebral blood vessels to release prostaglandin E2, which directly crosses BBB into brain.

④ Cytokines and prostaglandins act on vagal afferents and associated paraganglion cells, activating visceral sensory pathways from the nucleus of the solitary tract that influence autonomic, endocrine, and behavioral responses.

⑤ Cytokines and prostaglandins act on sensory neurons, modulating pain.

⑥ Cytokine modulation of norepinephrine release from sympathetic nerve terminals.

⑦ Cytokine modulation of neurotransmitter intercellular signaling in target cells.

⑧ Cytokine modulation of pituitary hormone release.

FEVER AND THE HYPOTHALAMIC SICKNESS RESPONSE TO SYSTEMIC INFLAMMATION

During systemic infections, there is a characteristic, hypothalamically mediated "sickness response" that includes an array of adaptive adjustments. Among these are a feeling of malaise, achiness, and sleepiness (which reinforces rest); increased secretion of adrenocorticosteroids (to mobilize adipose energy stores); and anorexia (to keep blood sugar low because many microorganisms prefer sugars as fuel, whereas the human body can adapt to using fat stores such as ketone bodies). A prominent symptom of the "sickness response" is an elevation of body temperature called a fever. Experimental studies show that white blood cells are more active at 39°C than 37°C, whereas many microorganisms are less able to defend themselves at this temperature, so fever is an adaptive mechanism to augment immune response.

There are several processes by which invading infectious organisms can set off the sickness response. One is that they can act locally on white blood cells that then produce circulating hormones called cytokines. The cytokines can have direct actions on certain types of neurons, but most of the "sickness response" is due to the cytokines (or certain components of invading bacteria themselves) inducing white blood cells and vascular endothelial cells to make prostaglandins. The primary role of prostaglandins in the sickness responses is demonstrated by the fact that inhibitors of cyclooxygenase, the enzyme that produces prostaglandins, is sufficient to prevent most of these symptoms.

Prostaglandins can act on receptors on peripheral nerves, but they also can cross the blood-brain barrier and act directly on brain neurons that express prostaglandin receptors. The prostaglandin that is probably most important for causing sickness responses is PGE2, which has a series of four different EP receptors that are found on different classes of cells in the central nervous system (CNS). For example, EP3 receptors in the MnPO nucleus recognize PGE2 during an inflammatory response and are critical for causing a fever response. Activation of corticosteroid secretion during a sickness response requires EP3 receptors in the preoptic area and the ventrolateral medulla, as well as EP1 receptors, which may be in the PVN or the central nucleus of the amygdala. Increased sensitivity to pain during fever is likely to be due to EP3 receptors, but the exact locus of those receptors is not yet known.

Plate 5.17

Brain: PART I

HYPOTHALAMIC RESPONSES DURING INFLAMMATION MODULATE IMMUNE RESPONSE

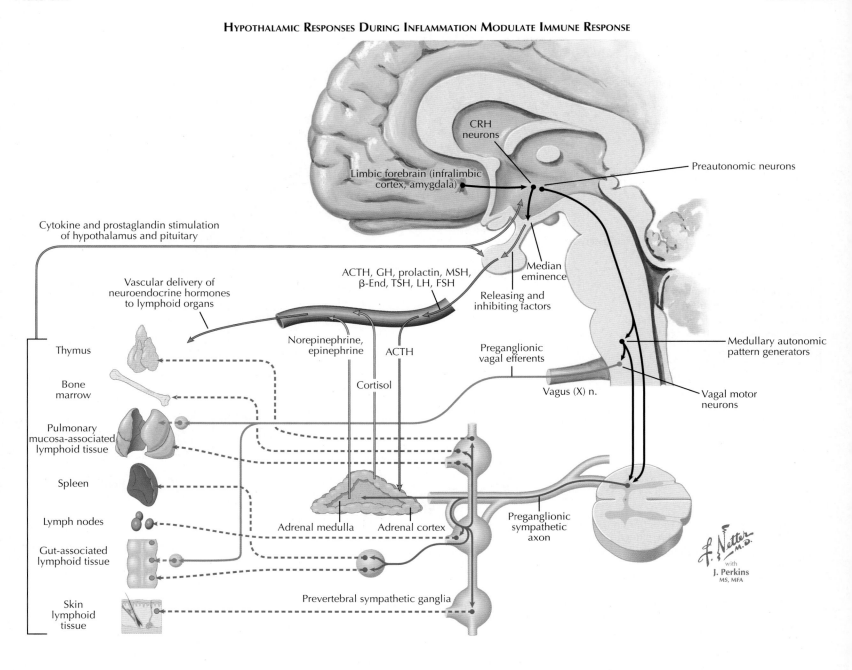

CRH neurons

Preautonomic neurons

Limbic forebrain (infralimbic cortex, amygdala)

Cytokine and prostaglandin stimulation of hypothalamus and pituitary

Median eminence

ACTH, GH, prolactin, MSH, β-End, TSH, LH, FSH

Releasing and inhibiting factors

Vascular delivery of neuroendocrine hormones to lymphoid organs

Medullary autonomic pattern generators

Thymus

Norepinephrine, epinephrine

ACTH

Preganglionic vagal efferents

Bone marrow

Cortisol

Vagus (X) n.

Vagal motor neurons

Pulmonary mucosa-associated lymphoid tissue

Spleen

Lymph nodes

Gut-associated lymphoid tissue

Adrenal medulla

Adrenal cortex

Preganglionic sympathetic axon

Skin lymphoid tissue

Prevertebral sympathetic ganglia

FEVER AND THE HYPOTHALAMIC SICKNESS RESPONSE TO SYSTEMIC INFLAMMATION (Continued)

The fever response during sickness appears to be due to EP3 receptor-mediated inhibition of preoptic warm-responsive neurons that tonically inhibit neurons in the dorsomedial hypothalamus and the medullary raphe that produce elevated body temperature. Disinhibition of the latter neurons allows body temperature to rise by about 2°C to 3°C. Fever in the range of 39°C to 40°C is uncomfortable but may be an adaptive response to help fight off invading organisms.

Changes in cognitive capacity and sleepiness during a sickness response are less well understood. EP1 and EP3 receptors are found on hypothalamic preoptic neurons that cause sleepiness, and EP4 receptors are found on His neurons in the posterior hypothalamus, which may cause arousal. However, prostaglandins are also made by the leptomeninges and may have direct effects on cortical neurons. PGE2 may also exacerbate meningeal and vascular pain perception (causing headache, particularly during coughing or straining, which increase intracranial pressure).

HYPOTHALAMIC CONTROL OF LYMPHOID TISSUE IN IMMUNE RESPONSE

A critical part of fighting off any infection is the activation of an appropriate immune response. During a sickness response, PGE2 acts on neurons in the medulla, amygdala, and hypothalamus, which results in an increase in the secretion of CRH into the pituitary portal circulation, elevated ACTH secretion by the pituitary gland, and increased levels of circulating adrenal corticosteroids. Cortisol then causes demargination of white blood cells that are adherent to the endothelium of blood vessels, elevating the circulating white blood cell count. Lymphocytes in a variety of tissues also respond directly to ACTH and to several other circulating hormones.

There is also direct sympathetic innervation of the lymphoid tissues. This input, which is also under hypothalamic control, may control the production and trafficking of specific lymphocyte subsets.

Plate 5.18

Hypothalamus, Pituitary, Sleep, and Thalamus

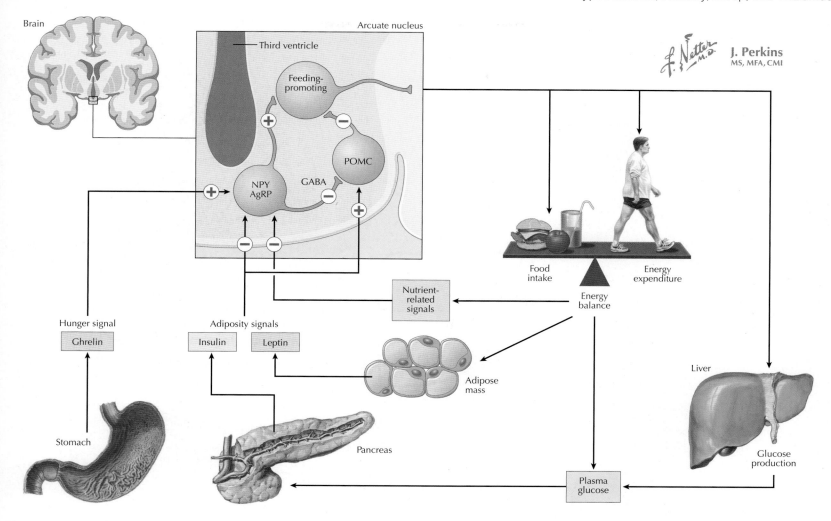

REGULATION OF FOOD INTAKE, BODY WEIGHT, AND METABOLISM

A key function of the hypothalamus is the control of feeding, body weight, and metabolism. Two systemic hormones are known to act on the hypothalamus to ensure that animals ingest sufficient food for their metabolic needs. Ghrelin, a hormone made by the gastric mucosa when the stomach is empty, causes increased eating. Similarly, low levels of leptin, a hormone made by white adipose tissue during times of metabolic plenty, also drive feeding. Hence a starving animal that has low leptin and high ghrelin levels will eat voraciously. Of interest, the opposite does not occur: in the presence of high leptin levels, animals are not inhibited from eating. Throughout evolution, starvation has been a constant problem for animals, but the prospect of obesity due to having too much available food was never a problem until humans recently learned to produce such an overabundance. Hence humans never evolved ways to deal with this modern situation, and obesity has become rampant in modern human societies.

The actions of leptin and ghrelin appear to involve neurons in the arcuate nucleus, a part of the hypothalamus that is just above the pituitary stalk. These hormones can enter the brain through the hypophyseal portal vessels, which lack a blood-brain barrier. Here they encounter neurons that have receptors for the hormones and form a key circuit in controlling eating. Neurons in the arcuate nucleus that contain the peptide neurotransmitters neuropeptide Y (NPY) and agouti-related protein (AgRP) form a positive part of the circuit. They contact cells in the paraventricular, ventromedial, and dorsomedial nuclei of the hypothalamus, as well as the LHA and parabrachial nucleus, and drive feeding responses. By contrast, a different set of arcuate neurons contains the peptides derived from the POMC precursor, including α-MSH, β-endorphin, and others. These POMC neurons contact many of the same targets as the NPY/AgRP neurons but use α-MSH and the melanocortin 3 and 4 receptors to inhibit the pathways that promote feeding. NPY neurons also contain γ-aminobutyric acid (GABA) and appear to inhibit the POMC neurons directly as well, whereas AgRP blocks melanocortin 3 and 4 receptors.

The feeding system also receives other CNS inputs. For example, there is a strong circadian input to feeding,

which is mediated by the pathway from the suprachiasmatic nucleus to the subparaventricular zone and then the dorsomedial nucleus. Dorsomedial hypothalamic neurons, in turn, send outputs to the LHA and the paraventricular, ventromedial, and arcuate nuclei, which may drive circadian cycles of feeding.

The mechanisms by which hypothalamic neurons promote feeding are not well understood. Although activation of AgRP neurons rapidly produces intense feeding behavior, the mechanism by which they do this is not understood. They appear to activate different populations of neurons controlling autonomic and behavioral responses that promote feeding. Some of the lateral hypothalamic neurons that are activated during starvation contain the peptide neurotransmitter ORX, and these neurons appear to cause arousal and to drive active exploration of the environment, which is necessary for most animals to acquire food. Other descending pathways may potentiate motor responses, such as sniffing, licking, chewing, and swallowing, which are a part of ingestive behavior. Other descending pathways that control the autonomic nervous system may increase gastric motility and acid production, which may be perceived by the individual as "hunger pangs."

Plate 5.19

Brain: PART I

AUTONOMIC, ENDOCRINE, AND BEHAVIORAL COMPONENTS OF STRESS RESPONSES

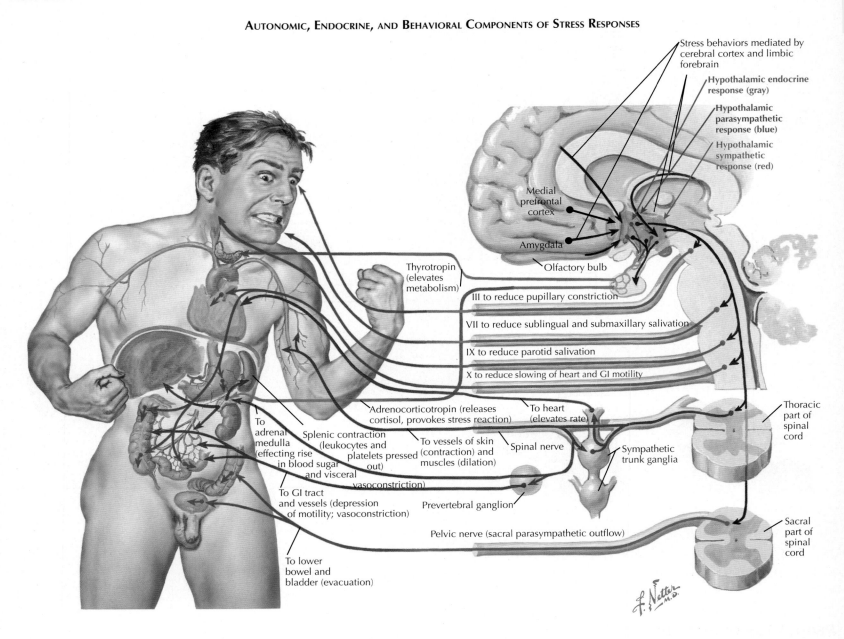

Stress behaviors mediated by cerebral cortex and limbic forebrain

Hypothalamic endocrine response (gray)

Hypothalamic parasympathetic response (blue)

Hypothalamic sympathetic response (red)

Medial prefrontal cortex

Amygdala

Olfactory bulb

Thyrotropin (elevates metabolism)

III to reduce pupillary constriction

VII to reduce sublingual and submaxillary salivation

IX to reduce parotid salivation

X to reduce slowing of heart and GI motility

Adrenocorticotropin (releases cortisol, provokes stress reaction)

To heart (elevates rate)

To adrenal medulla (effecting rise in blood sugar and visceral vasoconstriction)

Splenic contraction (leukocytes and platelets pressed out)

To vessels of skin (contraction) and muscles (dilation)

Spinal nerve

Sympathetic trunk ganglia

Thoracic part of spinal cord

To GI tract and vessels (depression of motility; vasoconstriction)

Prevertebral ganglion

Pelvic nerve (sacral parasympathetic outflow)

Sacral part of spinal cord

To lower bowel and bladder (evacuation)

STRESS RESPONSE

Stress was defined by the Nobel laureate Hans Selye as whatever increased the blood levels of corticosteroids. He was aware that the stimuli for elevated cortisol could include a very wide range of behavioral and physiologic stressors. However, as shown in Plate 5.19, stress involves much more than just corticosteroid secretion and includes other endocrine and autonomic and behavioral components.

Behavioral stress may come from many different sources, but the areas that most frequently show increased activity under stressful conditions include the medial prefrontal cortex (particularly the cingulate gyrus) and parts of the amygdala (particularly the central nucleus and the closely related bed nucleus of the stria terminalis). These regions also have direct inputs to the hypothalamus. The PVN of the hypothalamus is particularly important in producing stress responses. It contains separate populations of neurons that regulate anterior and posterior pituitary responses, as well as autonomic outputs. Most of the CRH neurons that regulate secretion of ACTH are found in the medial part of the PVN. These neurons are activated by virtually all stressful stimuli, and they secrete CRH and thus drive the systemic secretion of cortisol. The lateral part of the PVN contains neurons that release VP through the posterior pituitary gland. This response permits fluid conservation in case there is hemorrhage (e.g., associated with fighting). The dorsal and ventral parts of the PVN contain nerve cells that innervate the sympathetic and parasympathetic preganglionic neurons in the medulla and the spinal cord. These inputs reduce fluid loss through salivation (dry mouth), ready the cardiovascular system for fight or flight (elevated heart rate and blood pressure), and direct blood flow to muscular vascular beds to prepare for action.

However, the behavioral responses to stress are probably most familiar and distressing. The most prominent symptom of stress is hyperarousal, in which the individual reacts excessively to daily stimuli. This can include a tendency to become angry or aggressive more easily. At night, individuals who are under stress often have difficulty sleeping. Positron emission tomography studies on patients with insomnia show activation of the same brain regions (medial prefrontal cortex, amygdala, hypothalamus) that are activated in animals under experimental stress.

Plate 5.20

Hypothalamus, Pituitary, Sleep, and Thalamus

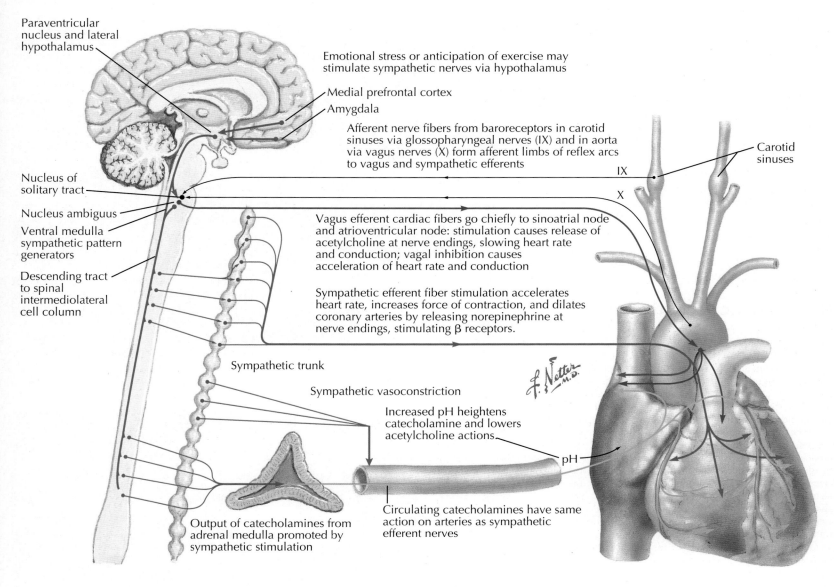

Paraventricular nucleus and lateral hypothalamus

Emotional stress or anticipation of exercise may stimulate sympathetic nerves via hypothalamus

Medial prefrontal cortex

Amygdala

Afferent nerve fibers from baroreceptors in carotid sinuses via glossopharyngeal nerves (IX) and in aorta via vagus nerves (X) form afferent limbs of reflex arcs to vagus and sympathetic efferents

Carotid sinuses

IX

X

Nucleus of solitary tract

Nucleus ambiguus

Ventral medulla sympathetic pattern generators

Descending tract to spinal intermediolateral cell column

Vagus efferent cardiac fibers go chiefly to sinoatrial node and atrioventricular node: stimulation causes release of acetylcholine at nerve endings, slowing heart rate and conduction; vagal inhibition causes acceleration of heart rate and conduction

Sympathetic efferent fiber stimulation accelerates heart rate, increases force of contraction, and dilates coronary arteries by releasing norepinephrine at nerve endings, stimulating β receptors.

Sympathetic trunk

Sympathetic vasoconstriction

Increased pH heightens catecholamine and lowers acetylcholine actions.

pH

Output of catecholamines from adrenal medulla promoted by sympathetic stimulation

Circulating catecholamines have same action on arteries as sympathetic efferent nerves

Hypothalamic Regulation of Cardiovascular Function

The hypothalamus is a key component of a CNS network that governs the heart and circulation. Different behaviors, ranging from emotional responses to motor activities, require activation of different components of the cardiovascular control network. Neurons in the cerebral cortex send inputs to the medial prefrontal cortex, particularly the infralimbic cortex, and the amygdala. These send axons to the hypothalamic neurons that govern cardiovascular response, including the PVN and LHA. The descending hypothalamic axons innervate brainstem sites involved in producing patterns of cardiovascular response, such as the parabrachial nucleus and both ventromedial and ventrolateral medullary reticular formation.

The parabrachial nucleus receives visceral sensory and pain inputs and organizes patterns of cardiovascular response seen during arousal due to pain, respiratory distress, or gastrointestinal discomfort (increased blood pressure and heart rate). It does this by direct projections

to sympathetic and parasympathetic preganglionic neurons, as well as to medullary pattern generators.

In the medulla, there are distinct pattern generators in the ventromedial and ventrolateral areas. The ventromedial medulla receives inputs from hypothalamic cell groups involved in thermoregulation, and it organizes patterns of sympathetic response necessary for thermogenesis (increased heart rate and activation of brown adipose tissue), as well as shifting of blood flow from cutaneous to deep vascular beds. This also requires elevation of heart rate to deal with the increased cardiac demand of hyperthermia. The ventrolateral medulla, by contrast, produces patterns of cardiovascular response necessary for maintaining blood pressure during erect posture, called baroreceptor reflexes.

Other descending hypothalamic axons go directly to the nucleus of the solitary tract, as well as the preganglionic neurons in the nucleus ambiguus in the medulla, which control heart rate through the vagus nerve and the intermediolateral column of the spinal cord, which controls vasoconstriction. These may produce patterns of autonomic activation that are organized at a hypothalamic level, such as stress or starvation responses.

The brainstem targets of this descending system coordinate cardiovascular reflexes. For example, the carotid sinus nerve (a branch of the glossopharyngeal nerve) and the aortic depressor nerve (a branch of the vagus nerve) bring information to the nucleus of the solitary tract about aortic and carotid stretch. When blood pressure is high, neurons in the nucleus of the solitary tract activate cardiovagal neurons in the nucleus ambiguus to slow the heart and inhibit neurons in the ventrolateral medulla that maintain tonic blood pressure by means of activating sympathetic preganglionic vasoconstrictor neurons. This baroreceptor reflex can be modified by descending hypothalamic input so that during times of stress, for example, there can be a simultaneous increase in blood pressure and heart rate without activating the baroreceptor reflex.

Projections from the hypothalamus to the intermediolateral column can directly activate sympathetic ganglion cells concerned with cardioacceleration and the strength of contraction to increase cardiac output. Other descending hypothalamic axons can contact adrenal preganglionic neurons, resulting in increased circulating adrenalin, which also increases vasoconstriction and cardiac output.

Plate 5.21

Brain: PART I

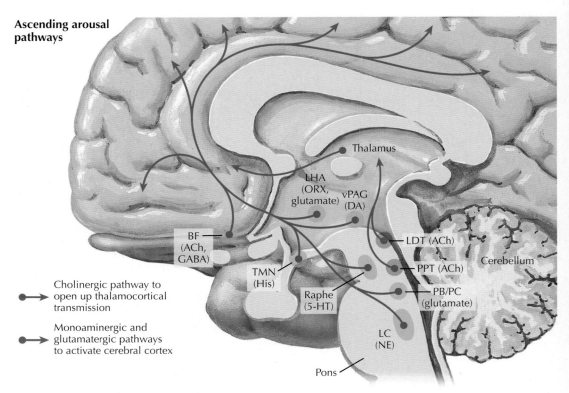

Ascending arousal
pathways

Thalamus

LHA
(ORX,
glutamate)

vPAG
(DA)

BF
(ACh,
GABA)

LDT (ACh)

PPT (ACh)

Cerebellum

TMN
(His)

Raphe
(5-HT)

PB/PC
(glutamate)

Cholinergic pathway to
open up thalamocortical
transmission

Monoaminergic and
glutamatergic pathways
to activate cerebral cortex

LC
(NE)

Pons

HYPOTHALAMIC REGULATION OF SLEEP

The brain is kept awake by an ascending arousal system that takes origin in the rostral pons and caudal midbrain. The neurons that activate forebrain arousal mainly consist of specific populations of cells that contain monoamine neurotransmitters, acetylcholine, and the excitatory transmitter glutamate. The cholinergic neurons in the pedunculopontine tegmental and laterodorsal tegmental nuclei provide the major input to the thalamic relay nuclei and the thalamic reticular nucleus. The latter is a sheet of inhibitory GABAergic interneurons that sit on the surface of the thalamus. The cholinergic input inhibits the reticular nucleus and activates the relay nuclei, thus enhancing thalamocortical transmission of sensory information.

At the same time, a series of monoaminergic cell groups in the upper brainstem provides an ascending pathway that largely bypasses the thalamus and goes directly to the cerebral cortex. These include noradrenergic (NE) neurons in the locus coeruleus (LC), serotoninergic (5-HT) neurons in the dorsal raphe and median raphe nuclei, dopaminergic (DA) neurons in the ventral periaqueductal gray matter (vPAG) and histaminergic (His) neurons in the tuberomammillary nucleus (TMN) in the hypothalamus. These are joined by glutamatergic neurons in the parabrachial and precoeruleus (PB/PC) nuclei. All of these cell groups send axons through the LHA, where they are joined by ascending axons from the ORX neurons and from glutamatergic neurons in the supramammillary nucleus and the LHA. The pathway then passes through the basal forebrain (BF), where additional cholinergic neurons (which innervate cortical pyramidal cells) and GABAergic neurons (which innervate cortical inhibitory interneurons) join in. These inputs are thought to excite cerebral cortical neurons and to enhance their capacity for information processing.

During wakefulness, both pathways are active at a maximal rate. As the brain falls asleep, the electroencephalogram (EEG) slows, the individual enters slow-wave (non–rapid eye movement [NREM] sleep), and the firing of all these cell groups is diminished. However, intermittently during the sleep cycle, when the individual enters REM, or active dreaming sleep, the cholinergic neurons and some of the glutamatergic neurons in the parabrachial nucleus begin firing again

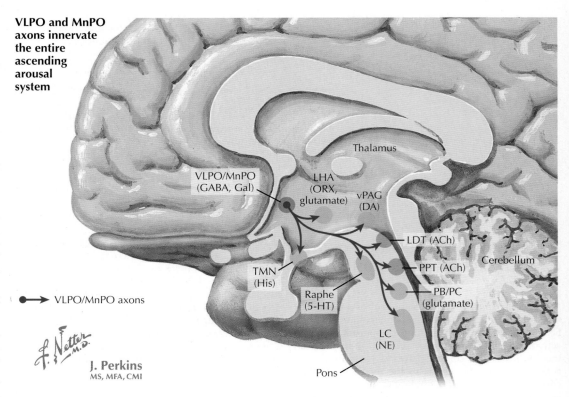

VLPO and MnPO
axons innervate
the entire
ascending
arousal
system

Thalamus

VLPO/MnPO
(GABA, Gal)

LHA
(ORX,
glutamate)

vPAG
(DA)

LDT (ACh)

PPT (ACh)

Cerebellum

TMN
(His)

Raphe
(5-HT)

PB/PC
(glutamate)

VLPO/MnPO axons

LC
(NE)

Pons

J. Perkins
MS, MFA, CMI

at a high rate, whereas the monoamine systems stop firing altogether. This disparity in activity is thought to cause the dreaming state.

Sleep is regulated at least in part by two populations of neurons in the preoptic area. MnPO neurons appear to fire in response to prolonged wakefulness and accumulate homeostatic drive for sleep. Neurons in the VLPO nucleus begin firing at the onset of sleep, and the two both continue to fire during sleep states. The VLPO

nucleus projects to the components of the ascending arousal system, and its neurons contain both the inhibitory neurotransmitter GABA and the inhibitory neuropeptide galanin (Gal), which appear to be important in turning off arousal and permitting sleep to occur. GABAergic neurons in the MnPO neurons also contact some of these same targets. Animals with VLPO lesions may lose a third or more of their total sleep.

Plate 5.22

Hypothalamus, Pituitary, Sleep, and Thalamus

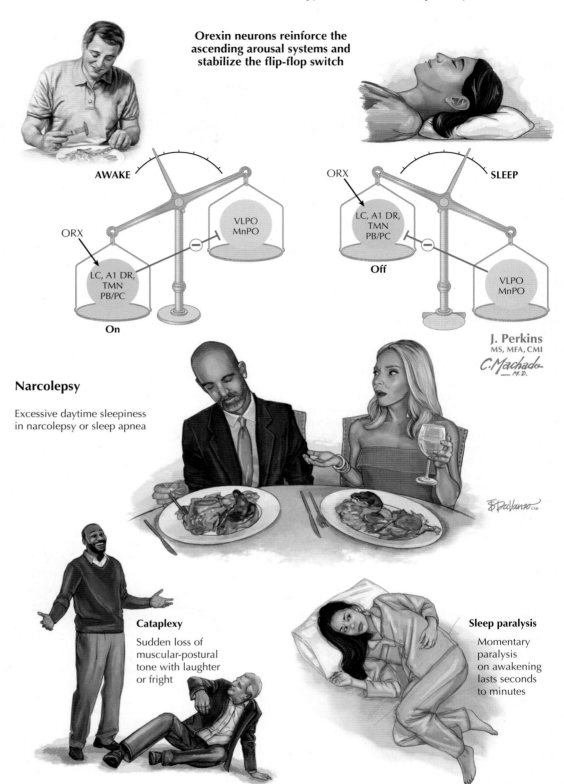

Orexin neurons reinforce the ascending arousal systems and stabilize the flip-flop switch

J. Perkins
MS, MFA, CMI

C. Machado
M.D.

Narcolepsy

Excessive daytime sleepiness in narcolepsy or sleep apnea

Cataplexy

Sudden loss of muscular-postural tone with laughter or fright

Sleep paralysis

Momentary paralysis on awakening lasts seconds to minutes

NARCOLEPSY: A HYPOTHALAMIC SLEEP DISORDER

Narcolepsy is a puzzling disorder that was first described in the late 1800s. Patients usually have onset of symptoms in their teens or 20s, when they become unusually sleepy during the day and may fall asleep if unstimulated even for a brief time. When a friend tells a joke, they may suddenly lose muscle strength and gradually slide to the floor, unable to stand or even sit, a condition called cataplexy. Narcoleptic patients also may have sleep paralysis when they are conscious but unable to move when just falling asleep or just waking up, or they may have dreams intrude into their waking state as they fall asleep (hypnagogic hallucinations) or wake up (hypnopompic hallucinations). All these phenomena represent a weakening of the boundaries between different wake-sleep states, particularly with components of REM sleep (muscle atonia, dreaming) intruding on wakefulness.

The cause of narcolepsy was mysterious until the neurotransmitter ORX (also called hypocretin) was discovered in 1998. ORX neurons are found in the LHA. They target the main components of the ascending arousal system, and both of the ORX receptors are excitatory. ORX neurons fire most rapidly during wakefulness, particularly during wakeful exploration of the environment. Thus the ORX neurons appear to play a key role in maintaining and stabilizing a wakeful state.

Soon after their discovery, it became apparent that gene defects that cause loss of signaling by the ORX neurons could cause narcolepsy in experimental animals. In humans, however, genetic mutations are a rare cause of narcolepsy, which is thought to be due to loss of the ORX neurons from an autoimmune attack. For example, waves of increased incidence of narcolepsy after H1N1 influenza epidemics or after immunization with a particular H1N1 vaccine suggested that the immune response to H1N1 may cause some cases of narcolepsy.

The ORX neurons stabilize the behavioral state by reinforcing wakefulness and blocking individuals from falling directly from wakefulness into REM sleep. In the absence of the ORX neurons, the waking state is less stable, and individuals fall asleep too easily. They also enter REM sleep very quickly after sleep onset and can have fragments of REM sleep (dreaming, muscle atonia) occurring even while they are awake, accounting for the episodes of hypnagogic hallucinations, sleep paralysis, and cataplexy.

Plate 5.23

Brain: PART I

SLEEP-DISORDERED BREATHING

Sleep-disordered breathing includes a spectrum of disorders, ranging from snoring to frank cessation of air flow, or apnea, during sleep. *Obstructive sleep apnea* occurs when relaxation of the tongue and airway muscles during sleep causes collapse of the airway, resulting in snoring, reduction in air flow (hypopnea), or even total blockage of air flow (apnea). Patients with *central sleep apnea* have reduced drive to breathe during sleep. Central sleep apnea may occur as a congenital problem in children, where it may be caused by a mutation in the *PHOX2B* gene, which is necessary for development of CO_2 chemosensory neurons in the medulla. However, it can also be caused by damage to the medulla or spinal cord causing failure of automatic breathing during sleep (Ondine's curse). Central sleep apnea also is seen in older adults with congestive heart failure or respiratory disease causing waxing and waning Cheyne-Stokes respiration during sleep. In older adult patients, a combination of central and obstructive sleep apnea may be seen, called *complex sleep-disordered breathing*. The typical patient with obstructive sleep apnea arouses after a brief interval of struggling to breathe, the airway opens, and breathing resumes. This cycle may repeat all night. The patient often is unaware that arousals occur but typically feels sleepy during the day. Sometimes the patient complains of impaired memory or cognitive function, which can be increased by sleep loss. Generally, the bed partner will first realize that something is wrong when snoring sounds become intolerable or notices the periodic loss of breathing. Episodes of apnea are often increased in frequency when the patient drinks alcoholic beverages or sleeps supine. Obstructive sleep apnea is most prevalent among older individuals, men, and those with obesity and large shirt collar sizes, but it is also seen in older women and in children and young adults who have enlarged tonsils or adenoids, anomalies of craniofacial structure that compromise airway diameter, or neuromuscular disorders that cause laxity of the airway muscles.

Clinical Presentation. Pronounced snoring, a classic indicator of potential sleep apnea, is related to vibration of upper airway tissue. Apnea occurs when upper airway obstruction becomes complete. There may be decreased blood oxygen saturation leading to arousal from sleep. The patient is usually unaware of these events; however, the bed partner is aroused and understandably frightened by the patient's respiratory status. Paradoxically, most patients with obstructive sleep apnea do not report choking or gasping for breath and are unaware of their apneas. Although patients may feel that they have slept well, they exhibit excessive daytime sleepiness, which results in lapses in attention and inappropriately falling asleep. Impairment of cognitive function may mimic depression or dementia, and children with sleep-disordered breathing show problems with attention and behavioral dyscontrol potentially disrupting their schoolwork. Severe cases (≥30 episodes per hour) and possibly those with moderate degrees of apnea (15–29 episodes per hour) are at significantly increased risk for cardiovascular disorders, including hypertension, myocardial infarction, cardiac arrhythmias, and stroke. Hypertension may develop from elevated catecholamine levels caused by the apneas. In addition, the negative intrathoracic pressure caused by struggling to breathe may lead to increased secretion of

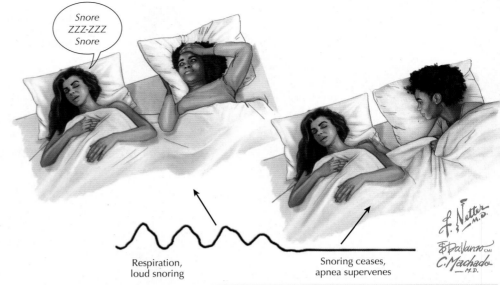

Respiration, loud snoring

Snoring ceases, apnea supervenes

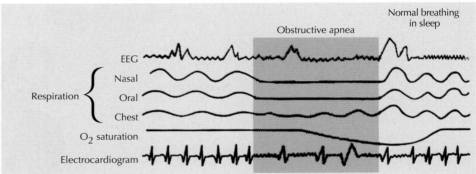

Normal breathing in sleep

Obstructive apnea

EEG

Nasal

Respiration { Oral

Chest

O_2 saturation

Electrocardiogram

Recordings from patient with obstructive sleep apnea

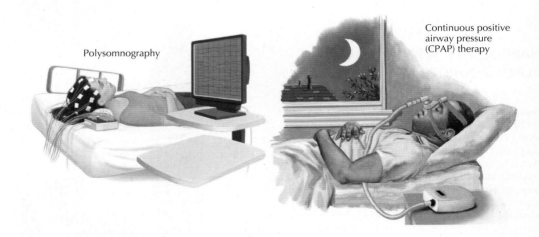

Polysomnography

Continuous positive airway pressure (CPAP) therapy

aldosterone, promoting increased intravascular fluid volume. Elevated central venous pressure paired with increased intrathoracic negative pressure increases transmural forces affecting the heart, which may cause cardiovascular remodeling and alteration of cardiopulmonary physiology. Sleep loss also causes insulin resistance, which can predispose to diabetes and increased body mass, which further worsens the sleep apnea and hypertension.

Diagnosis and Treatment. An all-night polysomnogram is the best means to detect and quantify apneic events. Healthy adults may experience fewer than five apneas per hour of sleep at night; in children younger than 12 years, more than one event per hour is

considered abnormal. Continuous positive airway pressure (CPAP), which uses air pressure to splint open the airway during sleep, prevents apneas and reduces daytime sleepiness and cardiovascular risk. Patients with severe and moderate sleep apnea significantly benefit from CPAP use, which improves daytime alertness and reduces cardiovascular risk. Often the treated patient may be unaware of their degree of sleepiness before experiencing the results of treatment. Treatment of obstructive sleep apnea may require correction of abnormalities of the airway, including removal of enlarged adenoids and tonsils in children. Reduction of risk factors, such as obesity and drinking alcohol in the evening, may help.

Plate 5.24

Hypothalamus, Pituitary, Sleep, and Thalamus

PARASOMNIAS

Parasomnias are characterized by certain unusual or unwanted movements or behaviors that occur during sleep.

PERIODIC LIMB MOVEMENTS OF SLEEP

Periodic limb movements of sleep (PLMS) are very brief episodic leg movements ranging from simple great toe dorsiflexion to violent flexion of the entire lower extremity. This may recur at regular intervals, up to several times per minute during sleep. If the movements are mild, neither the individual patient nor the bed partner may recognize the PLMS. On the other hand, if more violent, the movements may awaken the patient, bed partner, or both. Although mild PLMS may not be associated with arousals and are of no clinical significance, in some patients the more pronounced PLMS may cause repeated arousals. As a result, the patient may develop daytime sleepiness. PLMS can often be treated successfully with dopamine agonists, such as ropinirole or pramipexole, or with benzodiazepines, such as clonazepam.

RESTLESS LEG SYNDROME

Restless leg syndrome (RLS) often occurs in patients who have PLMS, although there are some RLS patients who do not get PLMS. The patient with RLS perceives an irresistible urge to move the legs, especially while sitting or lying down; these feelings are relieved when the patient stands or walks. The patient often describes the feeling as an uncomfortable sensation in the legs that is only relieved by leg movement. Many RLS patients demonstrate iron deficiency or low ferritin levels, and treatment with iron may help. Additionally, the symptoms of RLS may be successfully treated with dopamine agonists, benzodiazepines, or opioid drugs. Antidepressants and stimulants may exacerbate RLS and PLMS. Two genome-wide screening studies have identified a genetic polymorphism that correlates RLS with PLMS, suggesting that many cases may have a heritable cause.

REM SLEEP BEHAVIOR DISORDER

Patients with REM sleep behavior disorder (RBD) exhibit complex motor activity during REM sleep. During REM sleep, when active dreaming occurs, there is activation of reticulospinal pathways that result in profound inhibition of motor neurons, resulting in paralysis of voluntary muscles in intact individuals. In patients with RBD, this paralysis breaks down, and there are intermittent jerky movements and sometimes complex behaviors during REM sleep. In many respects, RBD is the opposite of the cataplexy attacks seen in patients with narcolepsy, who have activation of the REM sleep paralysis system while awake. RBD patients typically appear to be fighting off attackers and report dreams that match their actions. However, as with PLMS, patients with RBD are unaware of these occurrences, unless they are reported by a bed partner or the patient falls out of bed and is injured during episodes. RBD is usually treatable with either clonazepam or melatonin. However, in severe cases, the bed partner may have to sleep in a different room, and the mattress must be placed on the floor, the furniture removed, and windows boarded over to prevent

REM SLEEP BEHAVIOR DISORDER

Patients who lose their ability to be paralyzed during REM sleep begin to act out their dreams and are usually unaware of these occurrences because the episodes occur during sleep. Often the first episodes are observed by the spouses of the patients.

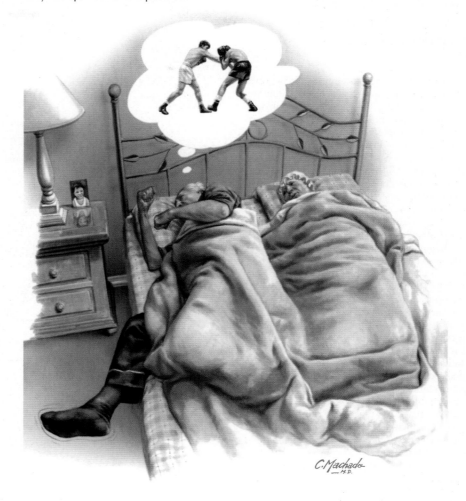

C. Machado
—M.D.

patients from injuring themselves or their bed partner during an attack. Some patients use large straps across the bed to avoid such excursions. Most patients with idiopathic RBD are men, and the peak onset is in the 50s or 60s. Studies show that most patients with idiopathic RBD subsequently develop a synucleinopathy, usually Parkinson disease or diffuse Lewy body dementia, and occasionally multiple-system atrophy. However, the time to diagnosis of these neurodegenerative disorders may be prolonged, with about half the patients with RBD developing a synucleinopathy within 12 years, and almost 80% by 20 years. In one case report a patient's wife noted that, although the patient had RBD on his wedding night at age 21, the patient did not develop Parkinson disease until age 71 years. Other risk factors include the use of antidepressants that prevent reuptake of serotonin or norepinephrine. Again, this situation represents the opposite of cataplexy (the development of REM atonia during waking in narcoleptic patients), where these antidepressants suppress the attacks.

NIGHT TERRORS, SLEEP WALKING, AND BED WETTING

These disorders commonly occur in children and rarely persist into adult life. As a group, these childhood parasomnias tend to occur during the deepest stage of slow-wave sleep and tend to become more brief and less profound during adulthood. Typically, the patient with night terrors suddenly sits up in bed and has dilated pupils, a frightened expression, and a rapid pulse. Occasionally, the individual may suddenly dash from the bed with such vigor that they may sustain an injury. Often, the child returns to sleep without any memory of the event. If awakened during the night terror, the child describes a frightened feeling or image but not a complex dream. Although there are no known adverse outcomes to night terrors, they can be quite frightening to parents, and it is important to distinguish them from other, more rare nocturnal events, such as seizures.

Sleep walking, or *somnambulism,* also tends to occur in children during deep slow-wave sleep. The child may walk and talk, but the speech is typically mumbled and incoherent. Patients can generally be led back to bed and will not remember the incident the next day. Often, an explanation of the problem to the family is sufficient.

Enuresis, or *bed wetting,* typically occurs in this same age range and during the deepest part of slow-wave sleep. In general the patient is not aware of the event, awakening in damp bedclothes.

Childhood parasomnias frequently do not require any treatment, although drugs that reduce the tendency for deep slow-wave sleep, such as tricyclic antidepressants or benzodiazepines, can be considered in adult patients.

Plate 5.25

Brain: PART I

DIVISIONS OF THE PITUITARY GLAND AND ITS RELATIONSHIPS TO THE HYPOTHALAMUS

The *pituitary gland (hypophysis)* is a midline structure at the base of the hypothalamus, to which it is connected through the pituitary stalk. The gland is approximately bean shaped, measures 6 mm (superior-inferior dimension) by 9 mm (anterior-posterior dimension) by 13 mm (transverse dimension) and weighs 500 to 600 mg.

The gland is composed of the adenohypophysis and the neurohypophysis, which are embryologically, anatomically, and functionally distinct. The former derives from *Rathke's pouch,* an ectodermal outgrowth of the primordial stomodeum, whereas the latter derives from the neural ectoderm and can be considered an extension of the hypothalamus.

The adenohypophysis is composed of the *pars distalis,* the *pars intermedia,* and the *pars tuberalis* (a small portion of the adenohypophysis wrapped around the neurohypophysis in the stalk). The *pars distalis* is also known as the *anterior lobe* (or pars glandularis), whereas the pars intermedia is poorly developed in humans. The pars intermedia contains connective tissue trabecula separating the anterior and posterior lobe as well as a narrow cleft or several small cysts at the site of the embryonic Rathke's pouch. During development, populations of stem cells differentiate into distinct groups of adenohypophyseal secretory cells under the influence of specific transcription factors.

Several differentiated cell types arise from a common stem cell precursor, including somatotrophs, lactotrophs, mammosomatotrophs, and thyrotrophs. *Somatotrophs* secrete GH, constitute about 50% of the cell population in the adenohypophysis, and are mainly present in the lateral wings of the anterior lobe.

Lactotrophs secrete *prolactin,* account for approximately 9% of adenohypophyseal cells, and are concentrated in the posterolateral areas of the anterior lobe. Mammosomatotrophs secrete both GH and prolactin.

Thyrotrophs secrete thyrotropin, constitute about 5% of adenohypophyseal cells, and are concentrated in the anteromedial areas of the pars distalis.

Corticotrophs synthesize POMC, which is cleaved into several proteolytic fragments, including corticotropin. Corticotrophs account for approximately 20% of cells in the adenohypophysis and are chiefly present in the midportion of the anterior lobe as well as the pars intermedia. In older individuals, some corticotrophs are also present in the adjacent neurohypophysis.

Gonadotrophs constitute approximately 10% of cells in the adenohypophysis, are distributed throughout the anterior lobe and pars tuberalis, and secrete both FSH and LH. Other nonsecretory cell populations in the adenohypophysis include follicular and folliculostellate cells.

The *neurohypophysis* is composed of the neural stalk, itself subdivided into the median eminence and the infundibular stem (also known as infundibulum), and the infundibular process (posterior lobe, pars nervosa, or neural lobe). The neurohypophysis contains neuronal axons whose cell bodies are present in the SON and PVN. Most of these axons terminate in the posterior lobe, with a minority of the axon terminals located in the median eminence and the infundibulum. VP (antidiuretic hormone) and OXY are synthesized in cell bodies of neurons in the SON and PVN, are transported down the axons, and are secreted by exocytosis from axon terminals in response to nerve impulses. Pituicytes are glial cells supporting the axon terminals in the neurohypophysis.

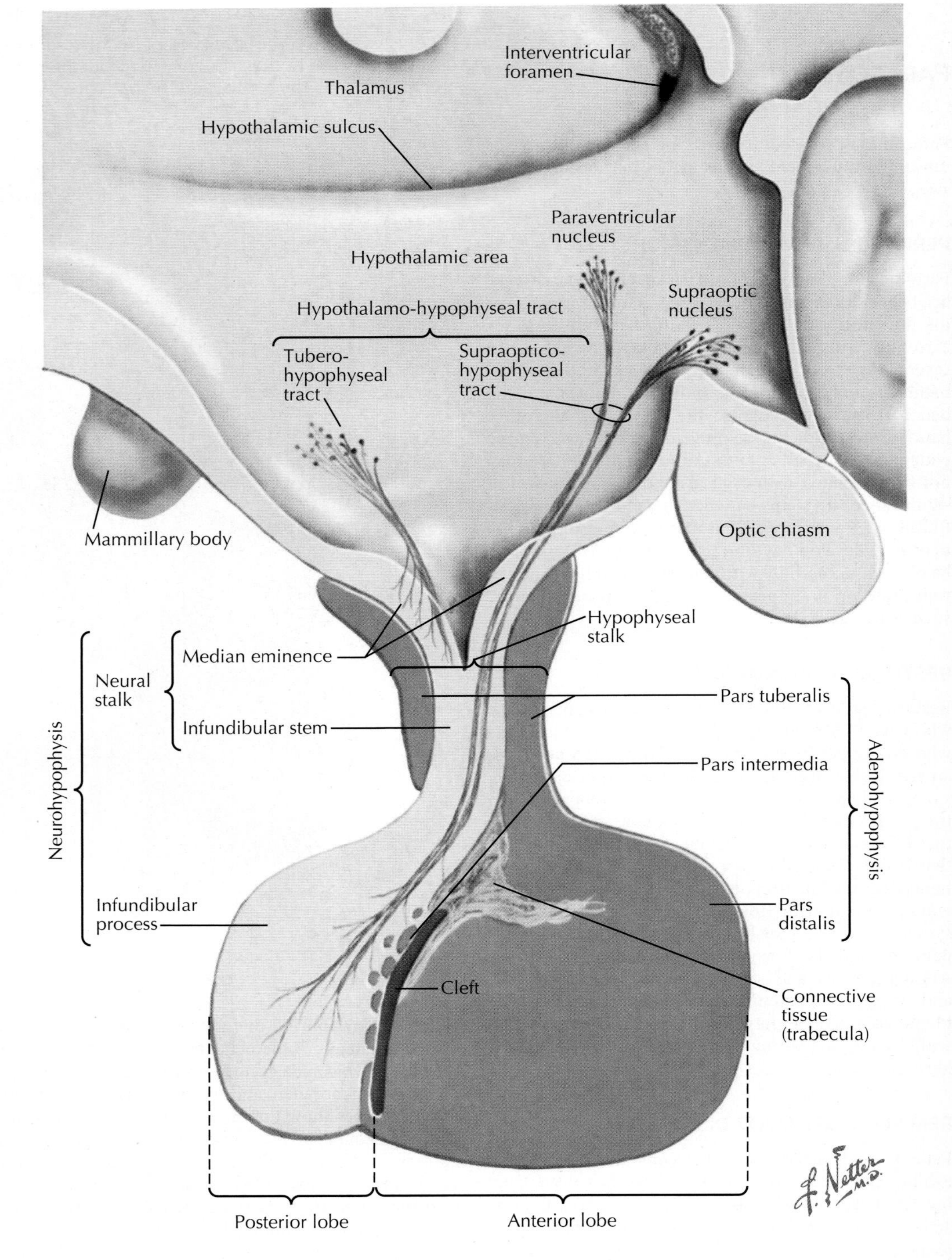

The pituitary gland receives a rich blood supply, commensurate with its role as an endocrine organ. Its blood supply derives from paired branches of the superior and inferior hypophyseal arteries, which are branches of the internal carotid arteries. Branches of the superior hypophyseal arteries form the primary plexus of the *hypophyseal portal capillary system* in the median eminence and infundibulum, where they are apposed to numerous terminals of nerve axons originating in the hypothalamus. Upon excitation, these neurons secrete several distinct releasing and inhibitory hormones into the portal system, which travel down the pituitary stalk in portal veins to reach the secondary plexus of the hypophyseal portal capillary system present in the adenohypophysis and either stimulate or inhibit hormone secretion in a cell-specific manner. Branches of the inferior hypophyseal arteries directly supply the posterior lobe and anastomose with branches of the superior hypophyseal vessels. Blood from the adenohypophysis and neurohypophysis leaves the pituitary through several hypophyseal veins that drain into the cavernous sinuses, which, in turn, drain into the superior and inferior petrosal sinuses, and from there into the sigmoid sinuses and the internal jugular veins.

Plate 5.26

Hypothalamus, Pituitary, Sleep, and Thalamus

POSTERIOR PITUITARY GLAND

The *neurohypophysis*, including the neural stalk and the posterior pituitary lobe, is an extension of the hypothalamus. It is embryologically derived from neural ectoderm. During development, magnocellular neurons of the SON and PVN send their axons inferiorly to form the neurohypophysis. These axons terminate in the posterior lobe of the pituitary. In addition, a smaller number of parvocellular neurons from the same nuclei send off shorter axons, which end in the median eminence or infundibular stem. *Pituicytes*, which are glial cells, support these axon terminals. Two *nonapeptide hormones* are secreted from distinct axon terminals in the neurohypophysis, including VP (antidiuretic hormone) and OXY. After secretion, these hormones enter neurohypophyseal capillaries and are carried via the inferior hypophyseal veins into the systemic circulation.

OXY and VP are made by distinct populations of large (magnocellular) neurons in both the PVN and SON nuclei, which release the hormones from their axons in the neurohypophysis. The PVN also contains populations of smaller (parvicellular) neuroendocrine neurons that produce CRH, thyrotropin-releasing hormone, or somatostatin, which is released into the hypothalamo-hypophyseal portal circulation. Some parvicellular neurons in the PVN also make either OXY or VP, which are used as central neurotransmitters to control the autonomic nervous system. OXY and VP are coded by distinct genes that code for precursor proteins that undergo posttranslational cleavage into the hormone, a neurophysin protein, and a carboxyterminal peptide called a copeptin. These are transported within secretory granules (vesicles), traveling along neuronal axons until they reach their respective axon terminals, where they are stored until secreted.

The presence of secretory granules within the posterior pituitary lobe gives rise to a bright signal on sagittal views of the pituitary on unenhanced, T1-weighted magnetic resonance imaging (MRI), termed the *posterior bright spot*. This is present in 80% to 90% of healthy individuals. An ectopic posterior pituitary may be present at the base of the hypothalamus or the pituitary stalk in some individuals, who usually have intact posterior pituitary function. However, anterior pituitary hypoplasia and variable anterior pituitary hormone deficiencies are often present in these patients.

Release of VP or OXY occurs via exocytosis in response to action potentials propagating along the respective axons. The release of VP and OXY is regulated by specific neural inputs to the hypothalamic nuclei synthesizing these hormones, with glutamate representing a major stimulatory neurotransmitter and GABA being inhibitory. Both osmotic (increase in plasma osmolality, sensed by hypothalamic osmoreceptors) and nonosmotic (significant decrease in effective arterial blood volume, pain, nausea, certain medications) stimuli mediate VP release. Once secreted, VP leads to increased water permeability in the collecting ducts of the kidneys, resulting in water reabsorption and urine concentration. Other VP effects include vasoconstriction, stimulation of glycogenolysis, and augmentation of corticotropin release from the anterior pituitary.

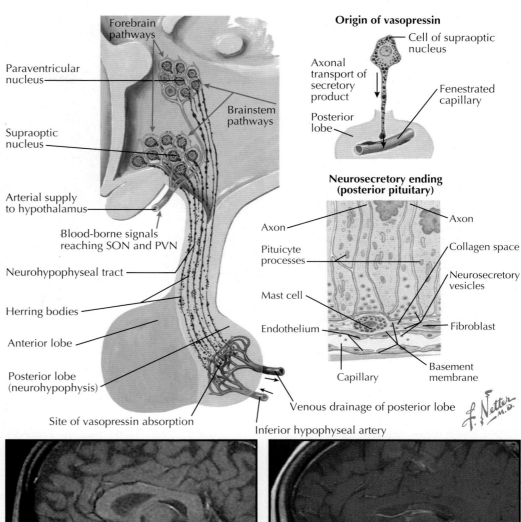

Forebrain pathways

Paraventricular nucleus

Brainstem pathways

Supraoptic nucleus

Arterial supply to hypothalamus

Blood-borne signals reaching SON and PVN

Neurohypophyseal tract

Herring bodies

Anterior lobe

Posterior lobe (neurohypophysis)

Site of vasopressin absorption

Inferior hypophyseal artery

Venous drainage of posterior lobe

Origin of vasopressin

Cell of supraoptic nucleus

Axonal transport of secretory product

Fenestrated capillary

Posterior lobe

Neurosecretory ending (posterior pituitary)

Axon

Pituicyte processes

Mast cell

Endothelium

Axon

Collagen space

Neurosecretory vesicles

Fibroblast

Capillary

Basement membrane

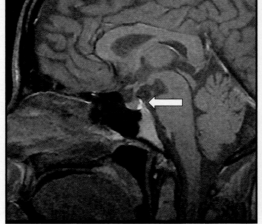

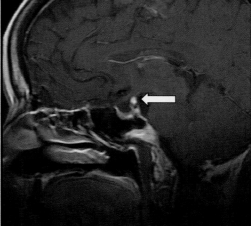

Posterior pituitary bright spot. Sagittal T1-weighted MRI showing hyperintensity (*arrow*) in the posterior aspect of the sella turcica.

Ectopic posterior pituitary. Sagittal T1-weighted MRI showing hyperintensity (*arrow*) along the posterior aspect of the pituitary infundibulum.

MR images from Young WF. The Netter Collection of Medical Illustrations, Vol. 2: Endocrine System. Elsevier; 2011.

Failure of VP synthesis and secretion is the cause of *central diabetes insipidus,* (arginine vasopressin deficiency) which is characterized by passage of large volumes of dilute urine, driving increased thirst. Dehydration and hypernatremia may generally occur if access to water is limited in untreated patients. Although diverse space-occupying lesions in the hypothalamus or within the sella may lead to central diabetes insipidus, it may also be noted that pituitary adenomas only rarely cause this condition preoperatively. The "posterior bright spot" is generally absent on MRI in patients with central diabetes insipidus.

The release of OXY occurs in response to neural inputs during parturition, suckling, and intercourse. Animal data have suggested a role for OXY in propagation of labor and milk let-down during breastfeeding. However, females who are deficient in OXY may experience normal labor and successful lactation, suggesting that the physiologic role of OXY in humans remains incompletely understood. A possible role of OXY in behavior, including social bonding, empathy, and appetite, is under study. There is also evidence in animals that OXY as a central neurotransmitter may promote maternal behavior and social interaction.

Plate 5.27

Brain: PART I

ANATOMIC RELATIONSHIPS OF THE PITUITARY GLAND

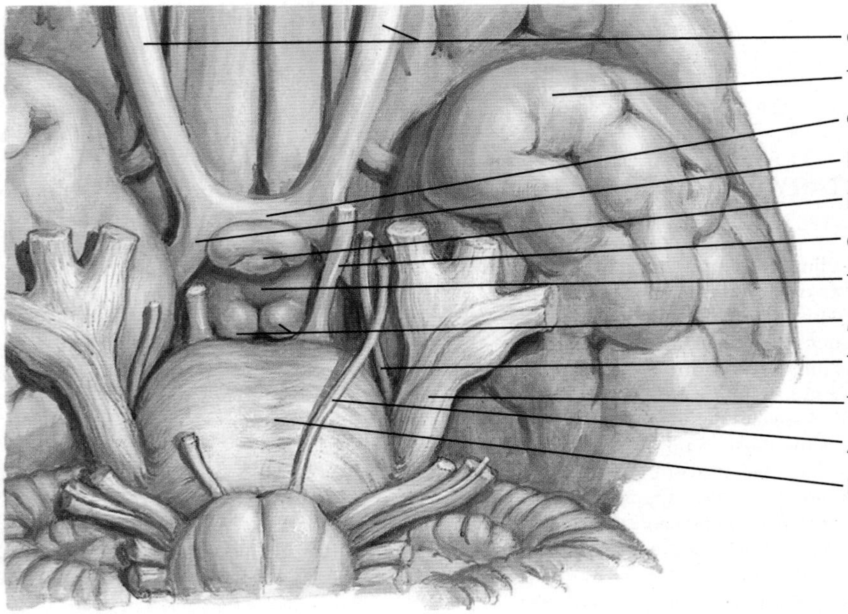

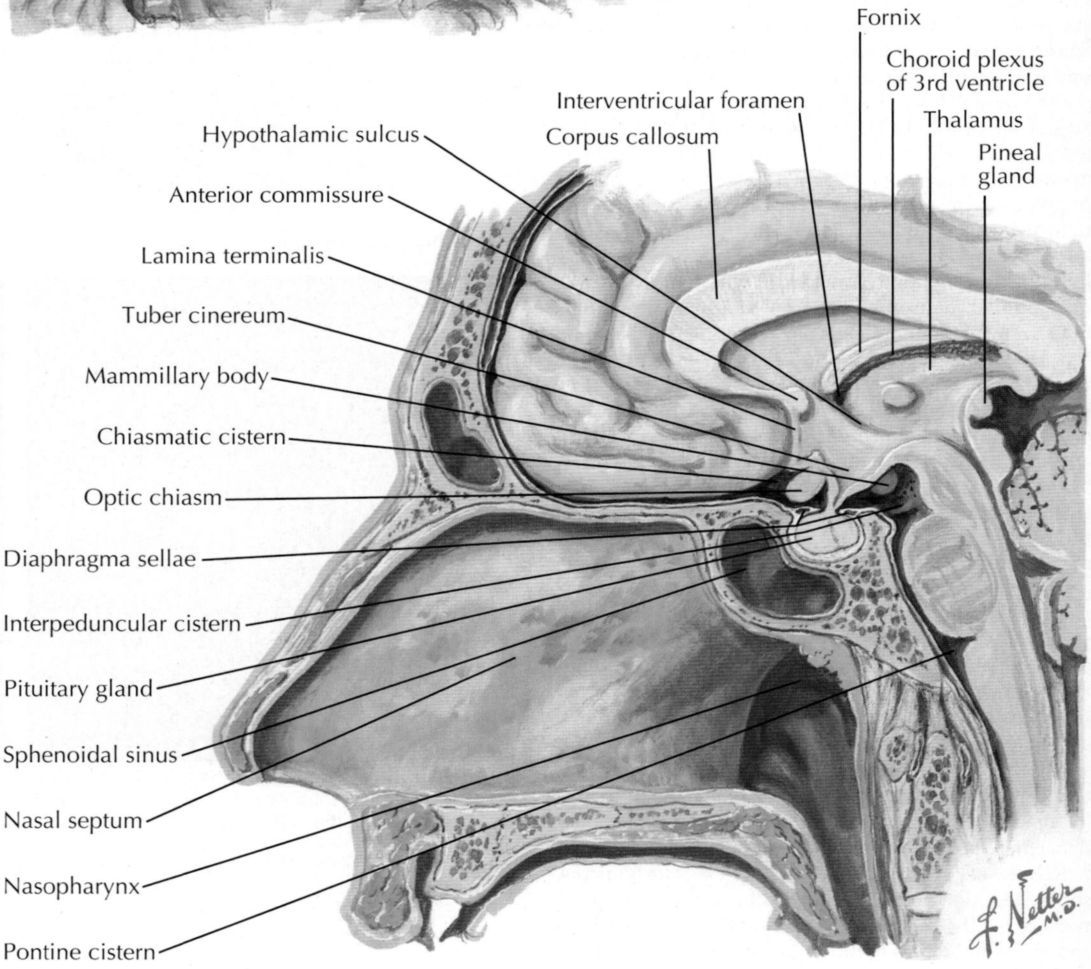

The pituitary gland resides in a depression (fossa) in the body of the sphenoid bone, termed the *sella turcica*. The tuberculum sellae forms the anterior wall of the sella, and the dorsum sellae forms its posterior wall. The pituitary is covered superiorly by a circular fold of dura mater, the diaphragma sellae. This sellar diaphragm is pierced by the pituitary stalk and the hypophyseal vessels. A fold of the arachnoid may herniate through the sellar diaphragm in some patients, thus extending the subarachnoid space within the sella (see MRI in Plate 5.26 for an example). Chronic pulsatile pressure exerted by the cerebrospinal fluid may expand the sella, leading to the appearance of an enlarged "empty sella," which may be associated with hypopituitarism in a minority of these patients.

The *optic chiasm* rests superiorly to the diaphragma sellae. Nerve fibers originating in the nasal portion of each retina cross at the chiasm to the contralateral side and join ipsilateral nerve fibers originating in the temporal portion of each retina, which do not cross at the chiasm, to form each optic tract. The anatomic relationship between the pituitary gland and the optic chiasm is clinically important, because mass lesions within the pituitary may compress either the chiasm or other portions of the optic apparatus, giving rise to a variety of visual field defects. Specific places where the arachnoid separates from the pia mater form cisterns filled with cerebrospinal fluid, including the *chiasmatic cistern* and the *interpeduncular cistern*. These spaces can be distorted by space-occupying sellar lesions growing superiorly from the pituitary.

The *hypothalamus* is located superiorly to the pituitary gland and is bounded between the *optic chiasm* anteriorly, the caudal border of the *mammillary bodies* posteriorly, and the hypothalamic sulcus superiorly. Distinct *hypothalamic nuclei* regulate anterior pituitary function through the synthesis of several stimulating hormones (GH–releasing hormone, CRH, thyrotropin-releasing hormone, and gonadotropin-releasing hormone) and inhibiting hormones (somatostatin and dopamine), released at neuronal axon terminals present in the *median eminence* and the *infundibulum*. These hormones are carried via the hypophyseal portal system to the adenohypophysis, where they regulate hormone secretion in a specific manner. The interrelationships between the hypothalamus and the posterior pituitary are detailed in Plate 5.26. Large lesions arising above the sella may impinge on the hypothalamus, interfering with its functions.

The *cavernous sinuses* are located laterally to the pituitary gland and receive blood from the pituitary via the hypophyseal veins. Each cavernous sinus contains several important structures, including the cavernous portion of the ipsilateral *internal carotid artery,* the *oculomotor, trochlear,* and *abducens nerves,* as well as the first two divisions (ophthalmic and maxillary) of the *trigeminal nerve.* Each of these nerves may be impinged upon by space-occupying lesions arising in the sella that extend into the cavernous sinus. Examples of such

lesions include *meningiomas, chondrosarcomas,* and *sellar metastases.* Characteristically, *pituitary adenomas* only rarely cause dysfunction of cranial nerves within the cavernous sinuses, with the notable exception of adenomas undergoing hemorrhagic necrosis (pituitary apoplexy).

The *circular sinus* lies between the pituitary gland and the underlying sphenoid bone in the sella, forming interconnections between the two cavernous sinuses.

The thin *sellar floor* separates the pituitary gland from the underlying *sphenoid sinus.* The sellar floor can be expanded by slowly growing sellar masses, leading to remodeling of the sella, or eroded by sellar masses growing inferiorly. The close relationship between the sella, the sphenoid sinus, and the nasopharynx provides an important access route to pituitary surgeons. Using a *transsphenoidal* approach, many sellar masses can be resected with low morbidity.

Optic nerves
Temporal pole of brain
Optic chiasm
Right optic tract
Pituitary gland
Oculomotor nerve (III)
Tuber cinereum
Mammillary bodies
Trochlear nerve (IV)
Trigeminal nerve (V)
Abducens nerve (VI)
Pons

Fornix
Choroid plexus of 3rd ventricle
Interventricular foramen
Thalamus
Hypothalamic sulcus
Corpus callosum
Pineal gland
Anterior commissure
Lamina terminalis
Tuber cinereum
Mammillary body
Chiasmatic cistern
Optic chiasm
Diaphragma sellae
Interpeduncular cistern
Pituitary gland
Sphenoidal sinus
Nasal septum
Nasopharynx
Pontine cistern

Plate 5.28

Hypothalamus, Pituitary, Sleep, and Thalamus

EFFECTS OF PITUITARY MASS LESIONS ON THE VISUAL APPARATUS

The close anatomic relationship between the pituitary and the optic apparatus, notably the optic chiasm, but also the *prechiasmatic optic nerves* and the *postchiasmatic optic tracts,* accounts for the frequent occurrence of visual deficits in patients with large pituitary mass lesions extending superiorly. At the optic chiasm, axons of the retinal ganglion cells that originate in the nasal portion of each retina cross to the contralateral side. In contrast, nerve fibers from the temporal portion of each retina remain on the ipsilateral side past the chiasm to form each optic tract, accompanied by nerve fibers crossing from the nasal portion of the contralateral retina.

A variety of mass lesions may arise within the sella. In addition to benign pituitary adenomas, which account for approximately 90% of mass lesions in surgical series, there are many pathologic sellar mass lesions. These include benign (craniopharyngioma, meningioma) and malignant (chondrosarcoma, lymphoma, metastases, or the exceedingly rare primary pituitary carcinoma) neoplasms, cystic lesions (Rathke's cleft cyst; arachnoid, dermoid, and epidermoid cysts), vascular pathologies (aneurysms, arteriovenous malformations), inflammatory lesions (primary hypophysitis or secondary hypophysitis arising secondary to systemic disease or certain medications), infection, or pituitary hyperplasia.

Mass lesions extending superiorly from the sella often impinge on the optic chiasm, which is generally located directly above the diaphragma sellae (in approximately 90% of individuals). Early abnormalities that occur because of chiasmatic compression include loss of color perception as a result of optic neuropathy, which can be documented using standard Ishihara chart testing, as well as variable loss of peripheral (temporal) field vision. Among patients with mass lesions growing from the sella, vision is generally lost first in either or both superior temporal quadrants. In contrast, mass lesions arising at the base of the hypothalamus, which compress the optic chiasm from above, may lead to early loss of vision in the inferior temporal quadrants.

Compression of the prechiasmatic optic nerves may lead to ipsilateral optic neuropathy, giving rise to a central scotoma. Lesions that compress the anterior portion of the chiasm on one side may give rise to ipsilateral optic neuropathy (central scotoma) and loss of peripheral vision in the contralateral superior temporal quadrant, a constellation termed *junctional scotoma.* More posteriorly located lesions may impinge upon one of the optic tracts, leading to contralateral homonymous hemianopsia.

Preliminary visual field testing may be conducted using bedside confrontation testing, but definitive evaluation of peripheral vision requires formal perimetry, using either an automated (Humphrey) or manual (Goldmann) method. Primary optic atrophy is present in cases of long-standing nerve fiber compression. Papilledema may rarely occur in patients with very large tumors extending toward the third ventricle, causing obstructive hydrocephalus. Consultation with an experienced neuro-ophthalmologist is advised for patients with mass lesions abutting or compressing the optic apparatus. Obtained preoperatively, optical coherence tomography of the retinal nerve fiber layer provides helpful prognostic information in patients with compressive optic neuropathy. Recovery of visual function occurs with relief of compression of the optic apparatus in most patients (approximately 70%–75% of cases). However, the likelihood and extent of visual recovery are generally higher with shorter duration of nerve fiber compression. Thus early diagnosis and prompt decompression (generally via surgery, but also medical therapy in patients with prolactin-secreting adenomas) are very important to optimize visual outcomes in these patients.

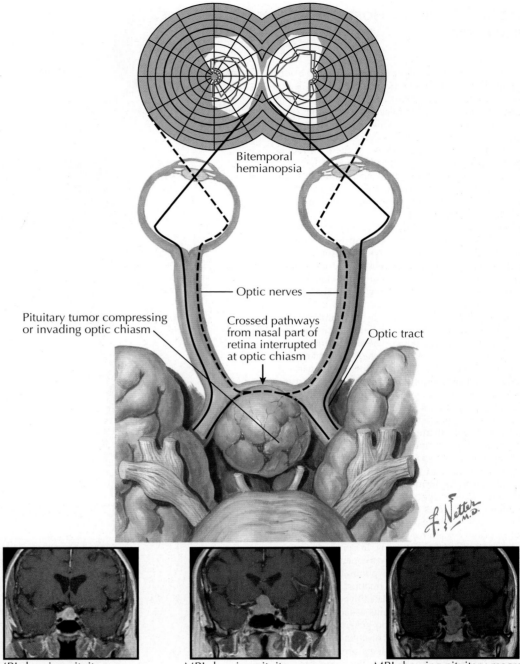

Bitemporal hemianopsia

Optic nerves

Pituitary tumor compressing or invading optic chiasm

Crossed pathways from nasal part of retina interrupted at optic chiasm

Optic tract

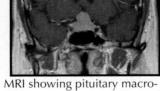

MRI showing pituitary macroadenoma with suprasellar and right cavernous sinus extension. Optic chiasm is raised slightly, but visual fields are normal.

MRI showing pituitary macroadenoma with suprasellar and bilateral cavernous sinus extension. The optic chiasm is compressed, causing bitemporal superior quadrant vision loss.

MRI showing pituitary macroadenoma with suprasellar, bilateral cavernous, and sphenoid extensions. The optic chiasm is markedly compressed, causing complete bitemporal hemianopsia.

MR images from Young WF. The Netter Collection of Medical Illustrations, Vol. 2: Endocrine System. Elsevier; 2011.

Plate 5.29

Brain: PART I

Anterior Pituitary Hormone Deficiencies

There are six types of secretory cells present in the adenohypophysis: somatotrophs (synthesizing GH), lactotrophs (producing prolactin), mammosomatotrophs (synthesizing both GH and prolactin), thyrotrophs (producing thyrotropin), corticotrophs (synthesizing corticotropin), and gonadotrophs (synthesizing both FSH and LH). The synthesis and release of these hormones are well orchestrated under the influence of hypothalamic hormones (most of which are stimulatory and some of which are inhibitory) as well as systemic (endocrine) negative feedback mechanisms, aimed at maintaining homeostatic control.

A wide variety of conditions may cause dysfunction of the hypothalamus or pituitary, leading to selective or universal, partial or complete, acute or chronic loss of adenohypophyseal hormone secretion (anterior hypopituitarism). Any space-occupying lesion impinging on the anterior pituitary, pituitary stalk, or hypothalamus may lead to hypopituitarism. In adults, the most common mass lesion around the sella is a benign pituitary adenoma. However, many other neoplasms (including craniopharyngioma, meningioma, chordoma, metastases, or lymphoma); cystic lesions (including Rathke's cleft cyst or arachnoid cyst); infiltrative (hemochromatosis), inflammatory (hypophysitis, sarcoidosis), or infectious disorders; aneurysm; infarction; primary empty sella; radiation therapy; trauma; surgery; or genetic conditions may cause hypopituitarism. Immune checkpoint inhibitors, which have led to improvements in the outcomes of many patients with advanced malignancies, represent an emerging etiology of hypophysitis and hypopituitarism.

The underlying cause of hypopituitarism may influence the pattern of hormone loss. Gonadotropin deficiency and GH deficiency tend to occur first in patients with pituitary adenomas or those who have received radiation therapy to the hypothalamus and sella, whereas thyrotropin and corticotropin function tend to be spared until later during these conditions. In contrast, corticotropin and thyrotropin deficiency frequently occur first in patients with lymphocytic hypophysitis. Persistent corticotropin deficiency occurs in most patients with immune checkpoint inhibitor–related hypophysitis.

Gonadotropin deficiency presents as lack of pubertal development in adolescents, who generally develop a eunuchoid habitus. If the onset of gonadotropin deficiency occurs in adulthood, patients present with loss of gonadal function, including oligomenorrhea or amenorrhea in women and erectile dysfunction in men. In addition, patients may have low libido and infertility, loss of body hair (particularly in the presence of concurrent thyrotropin deficiency), fine facial wrinkling, loss of bone calcium leading to increased fracture risk, and hot flashes. Females may also experience breast atrophy, vaginal dryness, and dyspareunia. Males may note loss of stamina, increased body fat, decreased lean body mass, and decreased testicular size. *Prolactin deficiency* may result in failure of lactation postpartum.

GH deficiency leads to decreased linear growth if it occurs in childhood or adolescence. In adulthood, loss of GH secretion is more subtle but may be associated with fatigue, decreased exercise capacity and muscle strength, abnormal body composition (decreased lean body mass, loss of bone calcium, and gain in body fat), dyslipidemia, insulin resistance, increased cardiovascular risk, and poor quality of life.

Thyrotropin deficiency leads to central hypothyroidism, including fatigue, lethargy, weight gain, bradycardia,

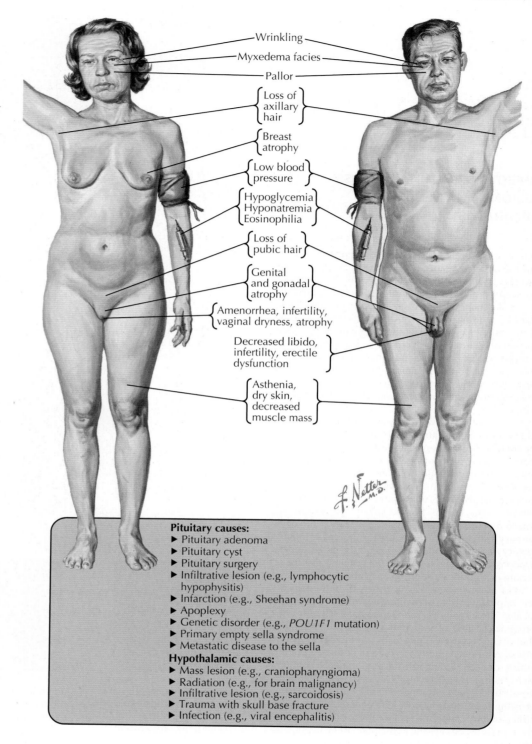

Wrinkling
Myxedema facies
Pallor
Loss of axillary hair
Breast atrophy
Low blood pressure
Hypoglycemia Hyponatremia Eosinophilia
Loss of pubic hair
Genital and gonadal atrophy
Amenorrhea, infertility, vaginal dryness, atrophy
Decreased libido, infertility, erectile dysfunction
Asthenia, dry skin, decreased muscle mass

Pituitary causes:
► Pituitary adenoma
► Pituitary cyst
► Pituitary surgery
► Infiltrative lesion (e.g., lymphocytic hypophysitis)
► Infarction (e.g., Sheehan syndrome)
► Apoplexy
► Genetic disorder (e.g., *POU1F1* mutation)
► Primary empty sella syndrome
► Metastatic disease to the sella

Hypothalamic causes:
► Mass lesion (e.g., craniopharyngioma)
► Radiation (e.g., for brain malignancy)
► Infiltrative lesion (e.g., sarcoidosis)
► Trauma with skull base fracture
► Infection (e.g., viral encephalitis)

dry skin, myxedema, anemia, constipation, muscle aches, slow relaxation phase of Achilles reflexes, and cold intolerance.

Corticotropin deficiency leads to central hypoadrenalism, which is potentially the most life-threatening of all pituitary hormone deficiencies. These patients often exhibit fatigue, weight loss, nausea and vomiting, orthostatic hypotension and dizziness, and diffuse arthralgias. Notable is the lack of cutaneous and mucosal hyperpigmentation, in contrast to patients with primary adrenal insufficiency (Addison disease). These patients may also present acutely with shock unresponsive to volume expansion and pressors. Eosinophilia and hyponatremia may be present. However, hyperkalemia is absent because aldosterone deficiency does not occur.

Once diagnosed, target organ hormone replacement therapies are instituted. In particular, glucocorticoid replacement may prove lifesaving in patients presenting in adrenal crisis and should be administered without awaiting diagnostic confirmation if hypoadrenalism is suspected. Levothyroxine is used to treat central hypothyroidism, and sex steroid replacement is used to treat patients with central hypogonadism. However, if fertility is of interest, gonadotropin therapy is used, including human chorionic gonadotropin and FSH. GH replacement may also be considered. Despite seemingly adequate replacement therapies, patients with hypopituitarism are at increased risk of cardiovascular mortality, the underlying reasons still being a matter of considerable debate.

Plate 5.30   Hypothalamus, Pituitary, Sleep, and Thalamus

SEVERE ANTERIOR AND POSTERIOR PITUITARY HORMONE DEFICIENCIES (PANHYPOPITUITARISM)

Extensive space-occupying lesions within the sella or hypothalamus may lead to complete loss of anterior pituitary function. Of note, the term *panhypopituitarism* is indicative of complete loss of both anterior and posterior lobe function.

Pituitary macroadenomas, which, by definition, exceed 10 mm in greatest diameter, may cause multiple anterior pituitary hormone deficiencies but only rarely cause diabetes insipidus preoperatively. In contrast, large suprasellar tumors that impinge on the hypothalamus, pituitary, pituitary stalk including craniopharyngiomas, may disrupt both anterior and posterior lobe function. Similarly, pituitary surgery or trauma may lead to panhypopituitarism.

Gonadotropin deficiency leads to lack of pubertal development if it occurs before adolescence. Of note, a eunuchoid habitus is unlikely to develop in young patients with concurrent GH deficiency. In adults, severe gonadotropin deficiency leads to central hypogonadism. Severe long-standing gonadotropin deficiency leads to gonadal atrophy, including decreased size of the ovaries in women and testes in men. In addition, there is a decrease in size of the uterus, vagina, and breasts in females, including thinning of the endometrium and vaginal epithelial atrophy. In males, there is a decrease in size of the penis and prostate.

Thyrotropin deficiency leads to central hypothyroidism. The thyroid gland becomes atrophic, including thinning of the follicular epithelium. Corticotropin deficiency leads to *central hypoadrenalism,* involving loss of cortisol and adrenal androgen secretion. Portions of the adrenal cortex, including the zona fasciculata and the zona reticularis, become atrophic in these patients. In contrast, the zona glomerulosa remains structurally intact, and aldosterone secretion is unaffected. These patients may often exhibit pallor as a result of anemia and decreased skin pigmentation resulting from lack of corticotropin action on skin melanocytes.

GH deficiency leads to a decrease in growth velocity in children or adolescents, resulting in short stature if untreated. Hypoglycemia may occur in early childhood and appears to be a consequence of GH and glucocorticoid deficiency. Adults with GH deficiency may exhibit low exercise capacity, abnormal body composition (decrease in lean body mass and bone mass and increase in fat mass), dyslipidemia, insulin resistance, increased cardiovascular risk, and impaired quality of life. Prolactin deficiency leads to failure of lactation in females and has no discernible effects in males.

Lack of VP (antidiuretic hormone) secretion leads to central diabetes insipidus. The presence of diabetes insipidus signifies extensive damage to the hypothalamus or pituitary stalk. Of note, disruption of the pituitary stalk below the diaphragma sellae is less likely to cause diabetes insipidus than injury to the stalk at the level of the median eminence. In cases where the stalk is damaged distally, some VP–secreting axon terminals are spared and may secrete sufficient VP to prevent the development of central diabetes insipidus. It may also be noted that central diabetes insipidus may be

clinically latent in patients with corticotropin deficiency because glucocorticoids have an important role in increasing free water clearance in the kidneys. In these patients, glucocorticoid replacement may precipitate the clinical onset of central diabetes insipidus. Lack of OXY secretion may lead to low empathy. Its role in humans is under study.

Once clinically suspected, the presence of pituitary hormone deficiencies can be established through hormone testing. Assays for systemic levels of target gland hormones (morning cortisol, free thyroxine, and testosterone) are most helpful in the diagnosis of hypopituitarism. In the case of some hormones, including GH and cortisol, stimulation testing is used to evaluate secretory reserve. Either water deprivation testing or measurements of serum copeptin during infusion of hypertonic saline can be used to diagnose central diabetes insipidus.

Replacement therapies are available for all pituitary hormone deficiencies except prolactin and OXY. The respective target gland hormone is administered in patients with central hypoadrenalism (hydrocortisone or prednisone) and central hypothyroidism (levothyroxine). Sex steroid replacement (testosterone in men and estrogen-progestin in women) is generally advised, if not contraindicated. If fertility is of immediate interest, gonadotropin therapy is recommended. GH replacement is advised in children, if not contraindicated. Although not essential for life, GH replacement in adults is available in the United States and several other countries and may improve exercise capacity, body composition, several cardiovascular risk factors, and overall quality of life. Desmopressin, an analog of antidiuretic hormone that is devoid of vasopressor activity, is recommended in patients with central diabetes insipidus.

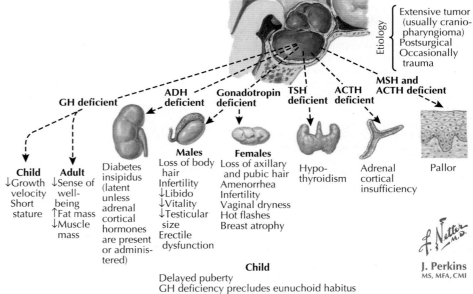

Severe anterior pituitary deficiency

Etiology: Extensive destructive macroadenoma or craniopharyngioma / Postpartum necrosis / Occasionally trauma / Postsurgical

GH deficient — Gonadotropin deficient — TSH deficient — ACTH deficient — MSH deficient

Child
↓Growth velocity
Short stature

Adult
↓Sense of well-being
↑Fat mass
↓Muscle mass

Males
Loss of body hair
Infertility
↓Libido
↓Vitality
↓Testicular size
Erectile dysfunction

Females
Loss of axillary and pubic hair
Amenorrhea
Infertility
Vaginal dryness
Hot flashes
Breast atrophy

Hypothyroidism

Adrenal cortical insufficiency

Pallor

Child
Delayed puberty
GH deficiency precludes eunuchoid habitus

Panhypopituitarism

Etiology: Extensive tumor (usually craniopharyngioma) / Postsurgical / Occasionally trauma

GH deficient — ADH deficient — Gonadotropin deficient — TSH deficient — ACTH deficient — MSH and ACTH deficient

Child
↓Growth velocity
Short stature

Adult
↓Sense of well-being
↑Fat mass
↓Muscle mass

Diabetes insipidus (latent unless adrenal cortical hormones are present or administered)

Males
Loss of body hair
Infertility
↓Libido
↓Vitality
↓Testicular size
Erectile dysfunction

Females
Loss of axillary and pubic hair
Amenorrhea
Infertility
Vaginal dryness
Hot flashes
Breast atrophy

Hypothyroidism

Adrenal cortical insufficiency

Pallor

Child
Delayed puberty
GH deficiency precludes eunuchoid habitus

J. Perkins
MS, MFA, CMI

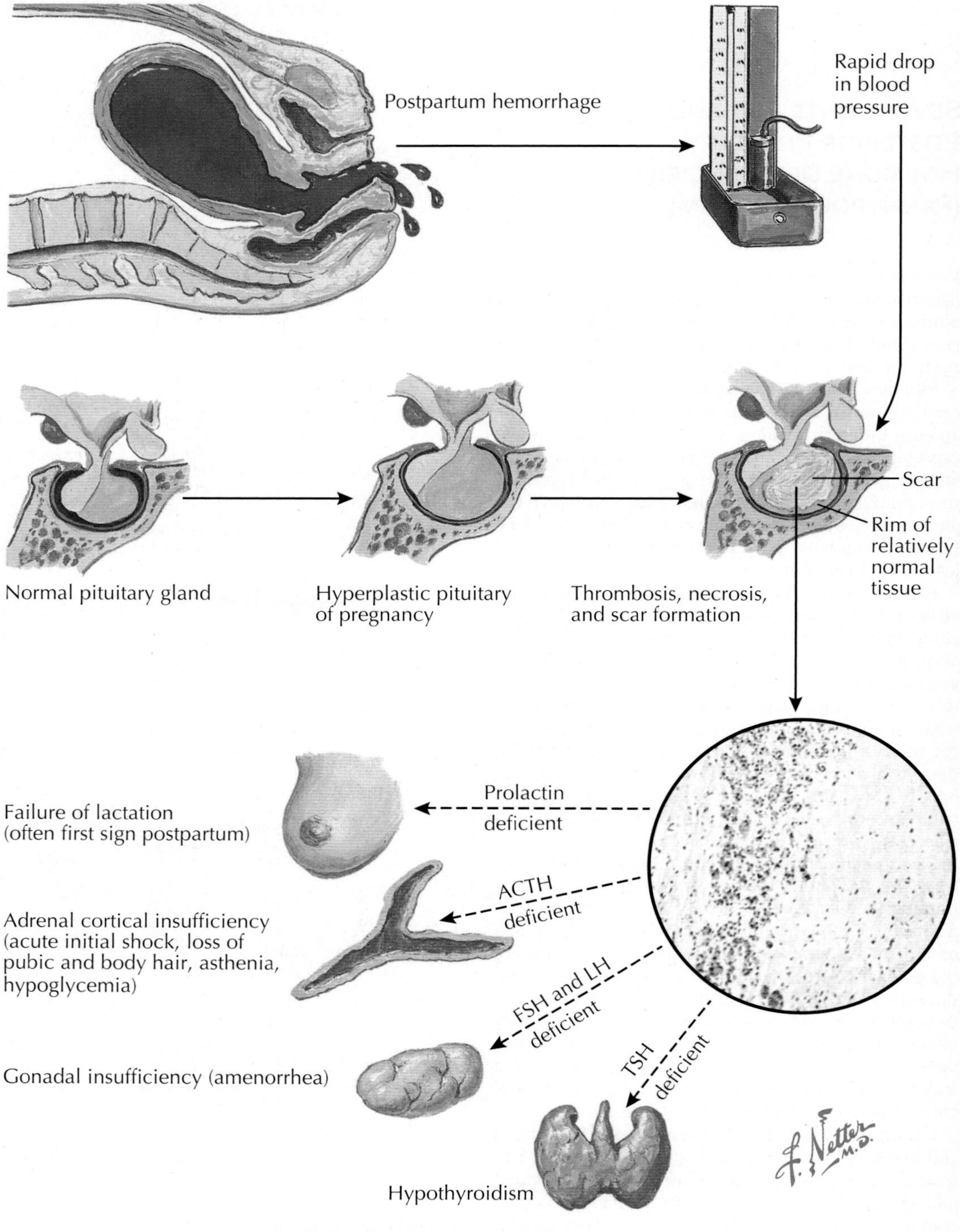

Plate 5.31

Brain: PART I

Postpartum hemorrhage

Rapid drop in blood pressure

Normal pituitary gland

Hyperplastic pituitary of pregnancy

Thrombosis, necrosis, and scar formation

Scar

Rim of relatively normal tissue

POSTPARTUM PITUITARY INFARCTION (SHEEHAN SYNDROME)

In 1937, Sheehan first described the development of pituitary infarction in the setting of hemorrhagic shock occurring after delivery. This entity is much less commonly seen in developed countries today, likely because of modern advances in obstetric care.

The development of postpartum pituitary infarction is based on the fact that the pituitary gland becomes hyperplastic (approximately doubling in mass) during pregnancy as a result of progressive lactotroph hyperplasia occurring until term. Because there is no concurrent increase in blood supply to the pituitary, lactotroph hyperplasia makes the gland more vulnerable to vascular insults during pregnancy and the peripartum period. To highlight the important role of pituitary hyperplasia in the pathogenesis of infarction, it may be noted that pituitary infarction is very rare in nongravid patients in shock. The precise role of vascular spasm, thrombosis, and vascular compression as causative factors in the pathogenesis of Sheehan syndrome is still debated, but the condition ultimately involves infarction of the anterior pituitary lobe as a result of severe decrease in blood flow through the gland.

In addition, the anterior lobe of the pituitary is more vulnerable to ischemia than the posterior lobe because the former receives blood supply through a low-pressure portal system. In contrast, the posterior pituitary receives direct arterial blood supply through the inferior hypophyseal arteries. Consequently, the pars tuberalis and the posterior pituitary lobe are usually spared in these patients, who generally do not develop central diabetes insipidus.

Infarction of the anterior pituitary lobe leads to a gradual decrease in the size of the pituitary gland, which is partly replaced by fibrous scar tissue. On MRI, there is a gradual decrease in the size of the pituitary gland, often culminating in the development of an "empty sella."

Anterior hypopituitarism of varying severity occurs in patients with Sheehan syndrome, depending on the extent of anterior lobe infarction. Loss of 90% of adenohypophyseal cells frequently leads to life-threatening pituitary failure, whereas loss of 50% to 70% of anterior pituitary cells generally leads to partial hypopituitarism. Central hypoadrenalism may result in shock that is refractory to volume expansion and vasopressor administration. If loss of pituitary function is partial and/or less severe, initial symptoms may be

Failure of lactation (often first sign postpartum)

Prolactin deficient

Adrenal cortical insufficiency (acute initial shock, loss of pubic and body hair, asthenia, hypoglycemia)

ACTH deficient

Gonadal insufficiency (amenorrhea)

FSH and LH deficient

TSH deficient

Hypothyroidism

Pituitary insufficiency of variable degree usually *without* diabetes insipidus

more subtle, including failure to lactate and involution of breasts, followed by postpartum amenorrhea. Other symptoms may include fatigue, weight loss, lack of appetite, nausea, dizziness, and loss of axillary and pubic hair.

Sheehan syndrome should be considered in women with severe postpartum blood loss requiring blood transfusion or vasopressor support in an intensive care unit. Additional risk factors include type 1 diabetes and sickle cell disease. In developed countries, lymphocytic hypophysitis, occurring in the third trimester of pregnancy or the postpartum period, has become more common

than Sheehan syndrome as a cause of new-onset hypopituitarism in pregnancy and the puerperium.

Once suspected, the diagnosis involves assays of systemic levels of target gland hormones, including morning serum cortisol, free thyroxine, estradiol, and gonadotropins. Serum prolactin levels may be very low in these patients. Stimulation testing may be needed to examine adrenocortical reserve and is essential to evaluate GH secretion. Standard replacement therapies for pituitary hormone deficiencies are advised. In particular, prompt glucocorticoid replacement can be lifesaving. However, recovery of pituitary function is very uncommon.

Plate 5.32

Hypothalamus, Pituitary, Sleep, and Thalamus

PITUITARY APOPLEXY

Pituitary apoplexy denotes the presence of hemorrhagic necrosis of the pituitary, which generally occurs within a pituitary macroadenoma. In some cases, hemorrhage may occur within a cystic lesion (including Rathke's cleft cyst). Rarely, pituitary apoplexy may occur as a result of hemorrhage within the pituitary gland in the absence of an adenoma or cyst. Pituitary apoplexy is a rare condition. In contrast, asymptomatic hemorrhage within a pituitary adenoma is not uncommon (occurring in approximately 15% of patients with pituitary adenomas).

Patients with pituitary apoplexy present with severe headache of acute onset, which is typically considered as the "worst headache ever" experienced. Nausea and vomiting are very common. The rapid expansion of intrasellar contents frequently leads to compression of the optic chiasm, causing visual field defects. Lateral expansion resulting in compression of the nerves coursing through the cavernous sinuses (including cranial nerves III, IV, V, and VI), frequently leads to diplopia, ptosis, facial pain, or numbness. Increased intracranial pressure may occur, leading to impairment in the level of consciousness. Interference with hypothalamic function may lead to manifestations of sympathetic nervous system dysfunction, including arrhythmias or disordered breathing.

In addition, some of the blood may enter the subarachnoid space, leading to meningeal irritation. Fever and neck stiffness may thus occur. Analysis of the cerebrospinal fluid may reveal the presence of red cells and increased protein content. It is therefore apparent that pituitary apoplexy should be considered in the differential diagnosis of patients with suspected subarachnoid hemorrhage or meningitis.

Life-threatening pituitary failure may occur as a result of central hypoadrenalism (adrenal crisis). Anterior hypopituitarism has been reported in up to 90% of patients with pituitary apoplexy. In contrast, central diabetes insipidus is uncommon.

Pituitary apoplexy is often spontaneous and may occur at presentation of a pituitary adenoma. Identified risk factors for the development of pituitary apoplexy include trauma, anticoagulant use (including heparin or warfarin), coagulation disorders, and administration of dopamine agonists (including bromocriptine or cabergoline) or hypothalamic-releasing hormones. Infection with COVID-19 may be also associated with pituitary apoplexy.

MRI typically reveals a focus of hyperintensity (on noncontrast T1-weighted images) within a sellar mass. A fluid-fluid level may also be evident. Impingement on the optic chiasm or the cavernous sinuses is frequently present. Laboratory testing usually reveals evidence of hypopituitarism.

Pituitary apoplexy is a medical and neurosurgical emergency. These patients should be hospitalized and receive, at minimum, a stress dose glucocorticoid coverage to prevent the development of adrenal crisis. Of note, pharmacologic doses of glucocorticoids are often administered to minimize acute pressure effects from the hemorrhagic sellar mass on neighboring structures.

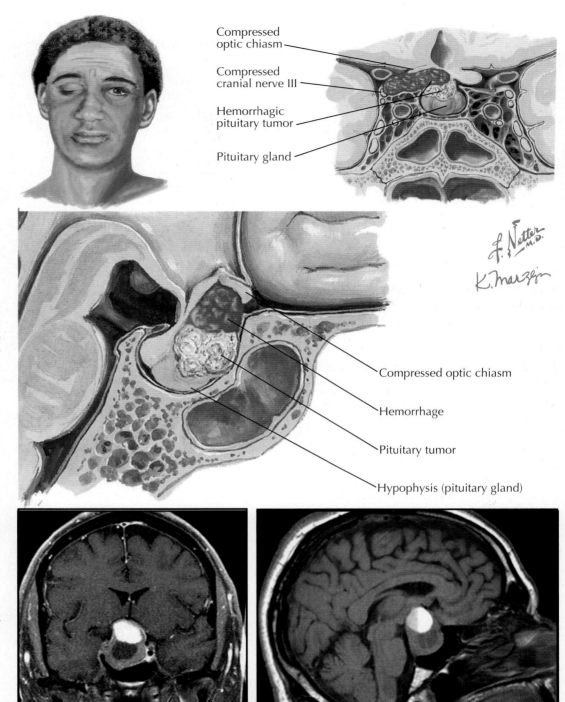

Compressed optic chiasm

Compressed cranial nerve III

Hemorrhagic pituitary tumor

Pituitary gland

Compressed optic chiasm

Hemorrhage

Pituitary tumor

Hypophysis (pituitary gland)

MRI showing pituitary tumor apoplexy. Coronal image *(left)* shows the partially cystic pituitary tumor in the sella with the hemorrhagic component extending above the sella. Sagittal image *(right)* shows fluid-fluid level within the area of recent hemorrhage.

MR images from Young WF. The Netter Collection of Medical Illustrations, vol. 2: Endocrine System. Elsevier; 2011.

Careful attention to electrolyte abnormalities is also advisable.

Patients with impaired level of consciousness or other evidence of increased intracranial pressure, visual field defects, diplopia, or ptosis should be considered for early (within 1 week) neurosurgical decompression, generally performed via the transsphenoidal route. Early pituitary surgery is associated with more complete recovery of visual field deficits than observation. In contrast, patients who maintain a normal level of consciousness and show no evidence of increased intracranial pressure, visual field defects, or ophthalmoplegia may be observed. These patients may be considered for pituitary surgery if the sellar mass fails to regress considerably after the hemorrhage is reabsorbed. Pituitary function needs to be monitored and hormone replacement therapies advised as required. Hypopituitarism is often permanent, regardless of whether surgery is performed.

Plate 5.33

Brain: PART I

THALAMIC NUCLEI AND THALAMOCORTICAL RADIATIONS

Thalamocortical radiations

Central sulcus

Thalamic nuclei

CM	Centromedian
LP	Lateral posterior
MD	Medial dorsal
PO	Posterior
VA	Ventral anterior
VI	Ventral intermedial
VL	Ventral lateral
VPL	Ventral posterolateral
VPM	Ventral posteromedial

Laterodorsal nucleus

Anterior nuclei

Internal medullary lamina

Intralaminar nuclei

Other medial nuclei

Midline (median) nuclei

Interthalamic adhesion

Pulvinar

Medial geniculate body

Acoustic pathway

Lateral geniculate body

Optic tract

Somesthetic from head (trigeminal nerve)

From globus pallidus and substantia nigra

Reticular nucleus (pulled away)

From cerebellum

Somesthetic from body (spinothalamic tract and medial lemniscus)

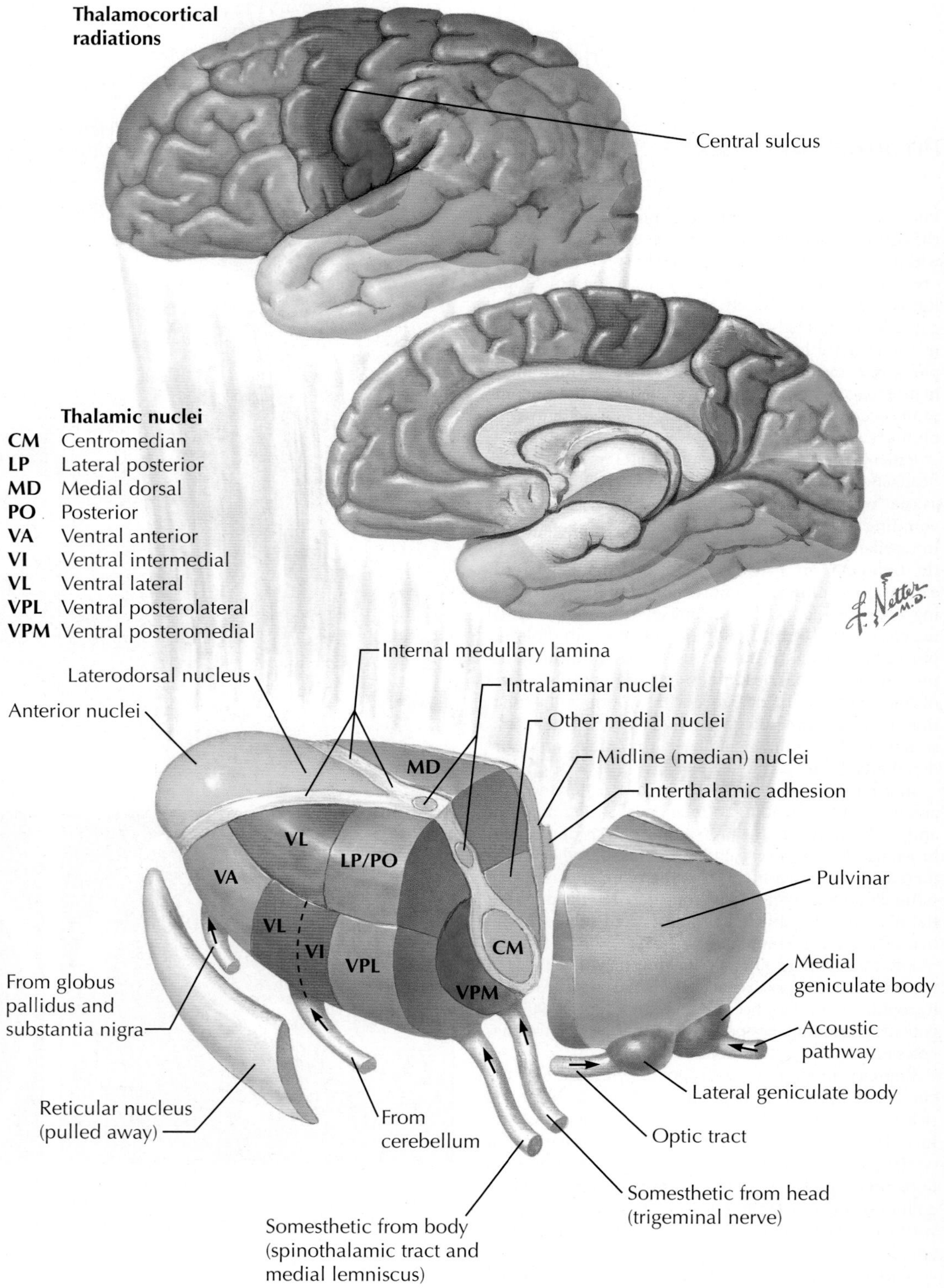

THALAMIC ANATOMY AND PATHOLOGY

THALAMIC ANATOMY

The thalamus, along with the hypothalamus and subthalamus, form the diencephalon. Anatomically, the thalamus sits above the hypothalamic sulcus in the third ventricle and consists of an egg-shaped structure, one on each side of the brain, connected by a bridge in the middle, the massa intermedia. The thalamus is divided by a white matter sheet, known as the internal medullary lamina, into the anterior, medial, and lateral groups of relay nuclei. The lateral group in turn is divided into a ventral tier of nuclei and the lateral nuclei proper. The relay nuclei project to a specific territory in the cerebral cortex, and in turn neurons in layer VI of each neocortical area project back to the same specific thalamic relay nucleus. The relay nuclei typically innervate layer IV of the cerebral cortex and provide most of the sensory information to the cerebral cortex.

In addition, several cell groups are either embedded along the midline (midline nuclei) or in the internal medullary lamina (the intralaminar nuclei). These nuclei send projections more diffusely in the cerebral cortex, with projections favoring layer V, and some project to the striatum as well. They are sometimes viewed as having a more generalized arousal function.

By contrast, the reticular nucleus sits like a thin sheet along the surface of the thalamus. Although nearly all the other thalamic neurons use the excitatory neurotransmitter glutamate, reticular neurons all use GABA and are inhibitory. They sample input both from the cerebral cortex and from the relay nuclei and send inhibitory axons to the relay nuclei, which put the relay neurons into a state where they burst rhythmically but do not transmit sensory information. This bursting behavior underlies the appearance of waxing and waning runs of rhythmic waves in the 12- to 14-Hz range in the EEG, called *sleep spindles,* as an individual enters slow-wave sleep. It is also thought to be involved in causing the characteristic 3-Hz spike-and-wave pattern of EEG seen during absence seizures, in which subjects, usually children, lose contact with the external world for brief intervals, during which they may stare and smack their lips. The reticular nucleus is thought to be important in directing attention to discrete sensory stimuli and inhibiting competing stimuli.

Among the relay nuclei, the largest component of the anterior group is the *anterior nucleus.* The most caudal part of the anterior group is called the *laterodorsal nucleus.* These nuclei send axons mainly to the cingulate gyrus.

The medial group includes the *mediodorsal nucleus* (MD) as well as several other smaller medial nuclei. The MD provides input to most of the frontal lobe and much of the temporal lobe, whereas the other medial nuclei innervate the orbitofrontal and medial temporal lobes.

The lateral group is much more complicated. The ventral tier consists of a series of nuclei related to regions of the motor and sensory cortices. The *ventral anterior nucleus* (VA) receives input from the globus pallidus internal segment and the substantia nigra pars reticulata, concerned with initiation of movement, and projects to the premotor cortex. The *ventrolateral nucleus* (VL) is the terminus of the cerebellar output (the dentatorubrothalamic tract), which carries information about body movement and innervates the primary motor cortex. The *ventroposterior lateral nucleus* (VPL) receives sensory input from the spinal cord for the

Plate 5.34

Hypothalamus, Pituitary, Sleep, and Thalamus

THALAMIC ANATOMY AND PATHOLOGY (Continued)

arms, legs, and trunk, and the *ventroposterior medial nucleus* (VPM) serves the same function for the face. They project topographically to the primary somatosensory cortex. Just medial to VPM is the *ventroposteromedial parvicellular nucleus*, a small area (not pictured) that receives taste information from the tongue and projects to a gustatory region in the anterior insular cortex. Most caudally in the ventral tier are the *medial geniculate nucleus,* which conveys auditory information from the inferior colliculus to the primary auditory cortex, and the *lateral geniculate nucleus,* which relays visual information from the optic tract to the primary visual cortex.

The dorsal tier of the lateral group includes a series of nuclei that project to progressively more posterior parts of the parietal lobe temporal lobe. The *lateroposterior nucleus* (LP) and *posterior nucleus* (PO) send axons to the region just caudal to the primary somatosensory cortex. The *pulvinar nucleus* sends axons to the posterior parietal lobe and the lateral surface of the temporal lobe. The neurons in these cell groups relay integrative information that relates the visual and auditory map of the world to the personal space of the individual.

THALAMIC PATHOLOGY

The most common neurologic disorders involving the thalamus are small infarcts, sometimes called *lacunar infarcts*. These are believed to be due to the occlusion of small thalamic perforating arteries that arise from the posterior cerebral and posterior communicating arteries. The infarctions are often as small as a single nucleus, causing sensory loss on the contralateral body or face if the VPL or VPM nuclei are damaged; memory impairment if the MD and anterior nuclei are involved; or motor weakness if the VL or VA nuclei are injured. The lateral geniculate nucleus may be involved by an occlusion of the anterior choroidal artery, resulting in homonymous hemianopsia. After a pure sensory thalamic infarct involving VPL or VPM, some patients go on to develop pain in the deprived region, known as the Dejerine-Roussy syndrome.

The thalamic perforating arteries may also hemorrhage. This often produces a thalamic syndrome similar to ischemic infarction. However, as the hemorrhage grows it may press downward on the midbrain, causing impairment of consciousness or a cluster of eye movement problems known as Parinaud syndrome. In Parinaud syndrome there is loss of pupillary light reflexes, upgaze, and vergence eye movements due to pressure on the pretectal area and dorsal midbrain.

The thalamus is also characteristically involved in fatal familial insomnia, a prion disorder that causes rapid onset of dementia, ataxia, and brainstem dysfunction, including almost complete inability to sleep in some cases. However, the pathology involves the cerebral cortex and brainstem as well, and it is difficult to determine how much of the symptomatology is due to the thalamic degeneration. Eastern equine encephalitis also preferentially involves the thalamus and basal ganglia.

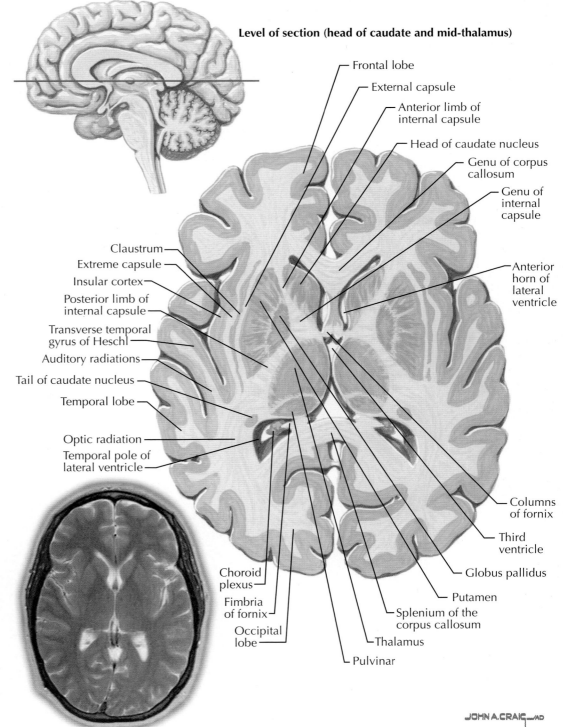

AXIAL (HORIZONTAL) SECTIONS THROUGH THE FOREBRAIN:
LEVEL 6—CAUDATE AND MID-THALAMUS

Level of section (head of caudate and mid-thalamus)

- Frontal lobe
- External capsule
- Anterior limb of internal capsule
- Head of caudate nucleus
- Genu of corpus callosum
- Genu of internal capsule
- Anterior horn of lateral ventricle
- Claustrum
- Extreme capsule
- Insular cortex
- Posterior limb of internal capsule
- Transverse temporal gyrus of Heschl
- Auditory radiations
- Tail of caudate nucleus
- Temporal lobe
- Optic radiation
- Temporal pole of lateral ventricle
- Columns of fornix
- Third ventricle
- Globus pallidus
- Putamen
- Choroid plexus
- Fimbria of fornix
- Occipital lobe
- Splenium of the corpus callosum
- Thalamus
- Pulvinar

JOHN A. CRAIG—AD

DISORDERS OF CONSCIOUSNESS (COMA)

Plate 6.1

Brain: PART I

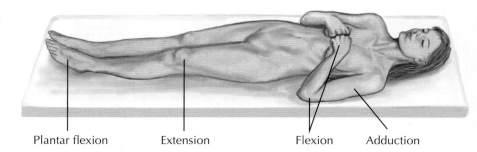

Decorticate rigidity

Plantar flexion · Extension · Flexion · Adduction

Decerebrate rigidity

Plantar flexion · Extension · Flexion · Pronation · Extension · Adduction

COMA

The term *consciousness* refers to a state of awareness of self and one's environment. Assessing consciousness in another person relies on judging that individual's performance or behavior in some mental function and arousal or response of awakening to a stimulus. The word *coma* originates from the Greek *kôma* (genitive, *komatos*), meaning deep sleep. In this section, "coma" is used to describe a potentially reversible state of unarousable unresponsiveness, which is not sleep at all. By this strict definition, there should not be grades of coma, but many physicians recognize the usefulness of describing and summating a patient's behavioral response using a scoring system. The most used score follows three domains of function: motor and verbal response and eye opening (see Plate 14.15 on the Glasgow Coma Scale score). An alternative scoring system extends the components of the Glasgow Coma Scale score and uses four components: eye and motor response, brainstem reflexes, and respiratory pattern (see Plate 6.3 on the Full Outline of UnResponsiveness [FOUR] score). However, equating the degree of abnormal motor response with a depth of coma is confusing because the neural structures regulating motor function and consciousness are independent. That said, it is common practice to use the clinical integrity of the motor cortex and brainstem nuclei, and their respective projections, as an indication of the level of impairment.

Appropriate localizing and flexor responses in a comatose patient imply that sensory pathways are functioning and that the pyramidal tract from the cerebral cortex to effector is functioning at least partially (also see Plate 6.2). When both sides are tested, unilateral absence of responses is consistent with interruption of the corticospinal tract somewhere along its length. Loss of response on both sides may reflect a lesion in the brainstem that interrupts the corticospinal tracts bilaterally or indicates injury to the pontomedullary reticular formation and associated extrapyramidal pathways. *Inappropriate motor responses* depend on the level of brainstem injury, as demonstrated by three main responses to a painful stimulus: decorticate rigidity, decerebrate rigidity, and decerebrate changes in the arms combined with flexor responses in the legs.

Decorticate rigidity consists of flexion of the arms, wrist, and fingers, with adduction in the upper extremity and extension, internal rotation, and plantar flexion in the lower extremity. This motor pattern occurs if brainstem activity is impaired *above the level of the red nucleus* because the red nucleus has a strong influence on upper limb flexion. It occurs with lesions involving the corticospinal pathways at the internal capsule, cerebral hemisphere, or rostral cerebral peduncle.

Decerebrate rigidity consists of opisthotonus with the teeth clenched; the arms extended, adducted, and hyperpronated; and the legs extended with the feet plantar flexed. This motor pattern occurs if brainstem activity

Red nucleus

Oculomotor nerve (III)

Decorticate

Decerebrate

CN V and ganglion (gasserian)

CN IV

CN VII

CN VIII

CN VI

CN IX

CN XII

CN X

CN XI

The motor pattern of decorticate rigidity occurs if brainstem activity is impaired above the level of the red nucleus, indicated by the dashed line. The motor pattern of decerebrate rigidity occurs if brainstem activity is impaired between the levels of the rostral poles of the red nucleus and vestibular nuclei.

Efferent fibers
Afferent fibers
Mixed fibers

is impaired *between the levels of the rostral poles of the red nucleus and vestibular nuclei* (rostral midbrain to midpons), as seen during rostral-caudal deterioration with transtentorial herniation, expanding posterior fossa lesions, or neurotoxicity of the upper brainstem. It occurs because of the reduction in extensor inhibition normally exerted on the reticular formation by the cerebral cortex. As a result, the spinal extensor motor neurons are driven by extensor-facilitating parts of the

reticular formation that are activated by a painful stimulus. The lateral vestibular nuclei are also intimately involved because, experimentally, extensor posturing is greatly reduced when the lateral vestibular nuclei are ablated. Decerebrate rigidity or posturing in the arms combined with either flaccidity or weak flexor responses in the legs is a motor pattern that is found in patients with extensive brainstem damage extending down to or across the pons at the trigeminal level.

Plate 6.2

Disorders of Consciousness (Coma)

RETICULAR FORMATION: NUCLEI AND AREAS IN THE BRAINSTEM AND DIENCEPHALON

DISORDERS OF CONSCIOUSNESS

Consciousness is a state of wakefulness and awareness of self and surroundings. In describing the state between normal consciousness and coma (unarousable unresponsiveness), many clinicians refer to a spectrum or gradation of states of diminished consciousness leading to coma. *Lethargy* has been used to describe a state of reduced wakefulness with deficits in attention; *obtundation,* a reduction in alertness and interaction with the environment; and *stupor,* a state of unresponsiveness with little or no spontaneous movement, from which the patient can be aroused temporarily with vigorous stimulation. These descriptions are imprecise and have, in general, been applied to diffuse metabolic pathologies causing brain dysfunction. Other terminology may be more specific. For example, the *vegetative state,* which may follow coma, describes a state in which the individual is unaware but has sleep-wake cycles without detectable cerebral cortical dysfunction. *Unresponsive wakefulness syndrome* and the *minimally conscious state* describe severely altered consciousness in association with minimal awareness of self or environment. *Akinetic mutism* is a condition of extreme slowing or absence of bodily movement, with loss of speech. Wakefulness and awareness are preserved, but cognition is slowed because of bilateral lesions to the inferior frontal lobes, cerebral hemispheres, paramedian mesencephalic reticular formation, or posterior diencephalon. *Locked-in syndrome* is a state of preserved consciousness and cognition with complete paralysis of the voluntary motor system because of complete destruction of corticospinal and corticobulbar pathways at or below the pons or severe peripheral nervous system disease. Eye movements may be preserved, allowing for some communication, and cortical function is intact.

The anatomic substrate for a disorder in consciousness is dysfunction in the *reticular formation* and the *ascending reticular activating system* (ARAS) because activation of the cerebral cortex during arousal and wakefulness depends on the influence of these structures. In the absence of the ARAS, stimulation of any of the sensory pathways (e.g., somatosensory, auditory, and visual) cannot arouse the cerebral cortex. Three groups of nuclei in the brainstem (locus coeruleus, raphe, and ventral tegmental) contribute to the modulating effect of the ARAS. An additional group of nuclei in the basal forebrain (basal nucleus of Meynert) also contributes to the diffuse modulating system.

The main nuclei of the reticular formation are present in the medulla, pons, and midbrain. The *locus coeruleus* is located beneath the lateral part of the floor of the rostral pontine fourth ventricle. Its axons are distributed to the cerebral cortex, thalamus, hypothalamus, cerebellar cortex, brainstem, and spinal cord. These norepinephrine-containing neurons are involved in the regulation of attention, cortical arousal, and the sleep-wake cycle. The *raphe nuclei* are clustered in the midline of the medulla, pons, and midbrain and constitute the serotonergic projections involved in the sleep-wake cycle. The nuclei near the pontomedullary junction constitute the *nucleus raphe magnus,* which projects to the spinal cord for the modulation of slow pain. The nuclei in the rostral pons and midbrain project to the thalamus, the limbic

A. Thalamus and hypothalamus

Thalamus:
Intralaminar nuclei
Reticular nucleus of thalamus
Midline nuclei
Lateral hypothalamic area through septal nuclei

B. Midbrain

Lateral RF of the midbrain
Substantia nigra
Interpeduncular nucleus
Periaqueductal gray matter
Raphe nuclei (dorsal, central superior)
Ventral tegmental nucleus

C. Pons

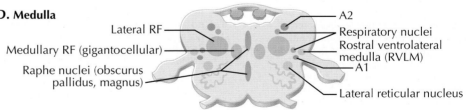

Locus coeruleus
A5
Raphe nuclei (pontis)
Lateral RF
Parabrachial nucleus
Parapontine RF (lateral gaze center)
Pontine RF (pontis, caudalis, ovalis)

D. Medulla

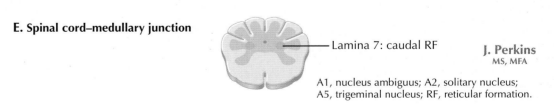

Lateral RF
Medullary RF (gigantocellular)
Raphe nuclei (obscurus pallidus, magnus)
A2
Respiratory nuclei
Rostral ventrolateral medulla (RVLM)
A1
Lateral reticular nucleus

E. Spinal cord–medullary junction

Lamina 7: caudal RF

J. Perkins
MS, MFA

A1, nucleus ambiguus; A2, solitary nucleus; A5, trigeminal nucleus; RF, reticular formation.

system, and cerebral cortex. The *ventral tegmental area* is located posteromedial to the compact nigra, and its dopaminergic neurons project chiefly to the accumbens, amygdala, and prefrontal cortex. Lastly, cholinergic neurons in the pons and midbrain project to the thalamus and regulate the excitability of the thalamic nuclei. Taken together, the outputs from all of these nuclei funnel through the paramedian midbrain reticular formation and divide into posterior and lateral

anterior roots in the diencephalon. The posterior root projects to relay nuclei and to intralaminar and other nuclei that have widespread cortical connections. The anterior root enters the lateral hypothalamic zone and is joined by projections from other neurons in the hypothalamus and basal forebrain. Lesions in the medulla or pons do not affect arousal and wakefulness. However, paramedian tegmental lesions in the rostral midbrain interrupt the ARAS and result in coma.

Plate 6.3

Brain: PART I

FULL OUTLINE OF UNRESPONSIVENESS SCORE (FOUR)

Eye response

4 = eyelids open or opened, tracking, or blinking to command
3 = eyelids open but not tracking
2 = eyelids closed but open to loud voice
1 = eyelids closed but open to pain
0 = eyelids remain closed with pain

Motor response

4 = thumbs-up, fist, or peace sign
3 = localizing to pain
2 = flexion response to pain
1 = extension response to pain
0 = no response to pain or generalized myoclonus status

Brainstem reflexes

4 = pupil and corneal reflexes present
3 = one pupil wide and fixed
2 = pupil or corneal reflexes absent
1 = pupil and corneal reflexes absent
0 = absent pupil, corneal, and cough reflex

Respiration

4 = not intubated, regular breathing pattern
3 = not intubated, Cheyne-Stokes breathing pattern
2 = not intubated, irregular breathing
1 = breathes above ventilator rate
0 = breathes at ventilator rate or apnea

Interpretation: Minimum score = 0, maximum score = 16. The lower the score, the greater the coma.

From Wijdicks EFM, Bamlet WR, Maramattom BV. Validation of a new coma scale: the FOUR score. Ann Neurol 58:585-593, 2005.

EMERGENCY MANAGEMENT AND ASSESSMENT AND NEUROLOGIC EXAMINATION

EMERGENCY MANAGEMENT AND ASSESSMENT

The many causes of coma are described elsewhere in this atlas (see Sections 9, Cerebrovascular Circulation and Stroke; 11, Infections of the Nervous System; 12, Neuro-oncology; and 14, Head Trauma). Immediate care, regardless of the cause of diminished consciousness, must include attention to adequacy of spontaneous ventilation and blood pressure to maintain homeostasis. Thereafter, the *emergency treatment* of comatose patients follows accurate diagnosis that depends on history taking, examination findings (including the evolution of neurologic symptoms and signs), and accompanying nonneurologic problems.

COMA SCALES

The Glasgow Coma Scale score (see Plate 14.14) for *best motor response* in either the upper or lower limbs is rated on a scale of 1 (no response) to 6 (patient obeys commands). If there is no response or an incomplete reaction to verbal stimuli, a noxious stimulus is applied, preferably to the medial side of the arms or legs, to differentiate a localizing response from abnormal flexor or extensor posturing. If the patient moves the limb toward (rather than away from) the noxious stimulus, the response is not consistent with localization. The patient's reaction is classified as fending-off movements with localization of pain (score 5), fending-off movements without localization of pain (4), abnormal flexion (3), abnormal extension (2), and no response (1). A *localizing response* indicates that the stimulus at more than one site causes a limb to move so as to attempt to remove it. A *flexor response* in the upper limb may vary from rapid withdrawal, associated with abduction of the shoulder, to a slower decorticate posture, with adduction of the shoulder. An *extensor response* is abnormal and usually associated with adduction, internal rotation of the shoulder, and pronation of the forearm. *No response* is usually associated with hypotonia. The Glasgow Coma Scale score alone is not an adequate assessment of brainstem function. Further, it does not assess vital signs (blood pressure, heart rate, body temperature, blood sugar) or ability to protect the airway and clear any airway obstruction (cough and gag) or suggest what support or intervention is required to restore homeostasis. A newer FOUR scoring system measures impaired consciousness and specific brainstem responses (Plate 6.3). The four variables

assessed are eye and motor responses, brainstem reflexes, and respiratory pattern. The acronym additionally reflects the number of categories and the maximum number of potential points in each category.

After immediate assessment, the next step is to initiate necessary emergency interventions for life support. For example, an adequate airway must be ensured, and an intravenous line should be placed. If the patient is hypoventilating, endotracheal intubation with assisted mechanical respiration should be considered. Intravenous

fluid bolus and vasopressors may be needed to treat hypotension. Blood samples should be drawn for measurement of electrolytes, glucose, toxicology, and arterial acid-base and blood gases. Serum is saved for further study if necessary. When bedside testing shows the patient to be hypoglycemic, an intravenous bolus of dextrose should be administered. If narcotic abuse is suspected or if the patient does not respond to supportive measures, an opiate receptor antagonist, such as naloxone, can be given intravenously.

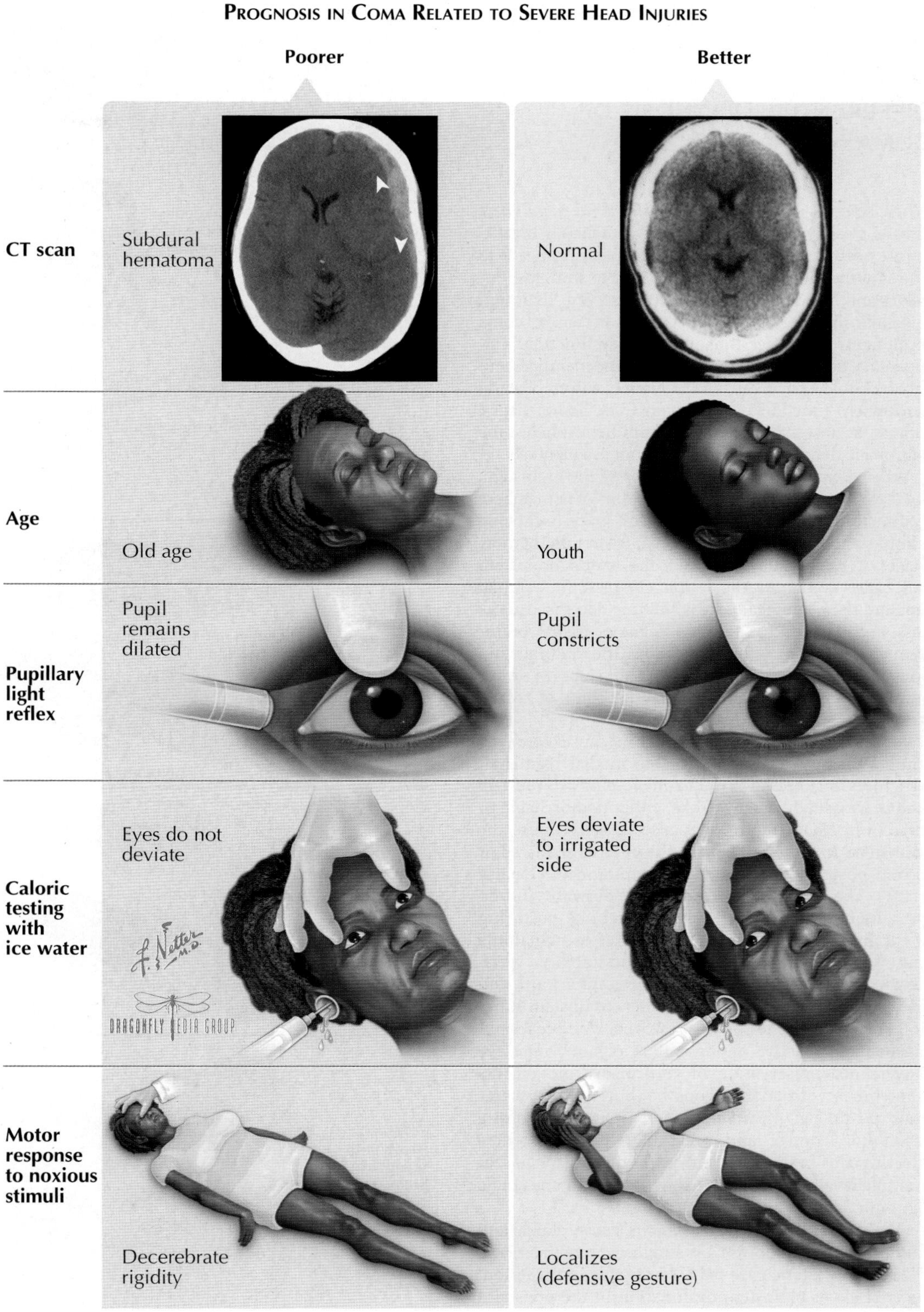

Plate 6.4

Disorders of Consciousness (Coma)

EMERGENCY MANAGEMENT AND ASSESSMENT AND NEUROLOGY EXAMINATION (Continued)

Next, after any necessary immediate treatment is instituted, steps are taken to determine the cause of coma with a robust and thorough history and appropriate investigation. The patient's family, friends, or physician can often supply useful diagnostic information. Inquiries may elicit a history of diabetes; previous renal, hepatic, or cardiac disease; severe depression; or drug use or abuse. It is important to know what prescription medications have been used and whether the patient had experienced any prodromal symptoms, such as headache, unilateral weakness, and ataxia, or previous episodes of stupor.

NEUROLOGIC EXAMINATION

It is important to carry out careful physical and neurologic examinations. Evaluation of the patient's spontaneous limb and bulbar movements, pupillary reactions, eye movements, and response to painful stimuli usually indicates the level of brain lesion causing coma. If the patient is able to blink, yawn, lick, and swallow, which are complex brainstem reflexes, lower brainstem function is preserved.

Pupillary size depends on the balance between sympathetic function (descending sympathetic fibers course in the lateral brainstem tegmentum) and parasympathetic function (parasympathetic fibers exit with the oculomotor [cranial nerve III] in the midbrain).

Pupillary reaction depends on the afferent light stimulus reaching the superior colliculus as well as efferent transmission through the oculomotor nerve. The light reflex arc is located in the diencephalon and midbrain.

Eye movements are observed by retracting the upper eyelids and watching spontaneous activity. When the head is rotated to one side—a maneuver to be performed only when it is clear that the cervical spine is not injured—the eyes should move fully and conjugately in the opposite direction if the appropriate brainstem oculomotor and vestibular centers are preserved (doll's eye phenomenon, or oculocephalogyric reflex). When the head is moved to the right, the eyes move conjugately to the left; when the head is moved downward, the eyes should roll upward. Ice water introduced into one ear canal with the patient's head of bed elevated to 30 degrees should evoke conjugate eye movements toward the side of the stimulation

(vestibulo-ocular reflex). In this position, the horizontal semicircular canal is in a vertical position, and the endolymph falls within the canal, thereby decreasing the rate of vestibular afferent firing. The eyes turn toward the ipsilateral ear, with horizontal nystagmus to the contralateral ear. Horizontal reflex eye movements are controlled by the oculomotor, trochlear (cranial nerve IV), and abducens (cranial nerve VI) nerves and their nuclei; the medial longitudinal

fasciculus and parapontine reticular formation (pontine lateral gaze center); and the vestibular nuclei and nerves (cranial nerve VIII). All these structures are located within the pontine tegmentum. Vertical movements are controlled by centers in the rostral midbrain and caudal diencephalon.

Lastly, spontaneous limb movements should be observed. If absent, testing for a response to a noxious stimulus is appropriate.

PROGNOSIS IN COMA RELATED TO SEVERE HEAD INJURIES

	Poorer	Better
CT scan	Subdural hematoma	Normal
Age	Old age	Youth
Pupillary light reflex	Pupil remains dilated	Pupil constricts
Caloric testing with ice water	Eyes do not deviate	Eyes deviate to irrigated side
Motor response to noxious stimuli	Decerebrate rigidity	Localizes (defensive gesture)

Plate 6.5

Brain: PART I

DIFFERENTIAL DIAGNOSIS OF COMA

When coma is caused by *bilateral cerebral hemisphere disease,* swallowing, yawning, and spontaneous breathing are normal. The eyes rove spontaneously from side to side, and the limbs move symmetrically to stimulus. Pupillary and oculomotor reflexes are preserved. Toxic and metabolic disorders are the most common cause of coma resulting from bilateral hemisphere dysfunction. Encephalitis, hemorrhage, or infection in the meninges and subarachnoid space can also adversely affect bilateral hemisphere function. Although infarcts, hemorrhages, tumors, or abscesses can involve both hemispheres, the neurologic deficit becomes bilateral only sequentially.

When a *hemispheric lesion* compresses the brainstem, the patient usually has signs or symptoms of hemisphere dysfunction, such as hemiparesis. Any space-occupying lesion, such as subdural hematoma, infarction, hemorrhage, or tumor, may compress the rostral brainstem and cause coma. As the lesion enlarges, intracranial pressure rises, and headache, vomiting, decreased alertness, and papilledema develop. Signs of rostral brainstem diencephalic dysfunction follow. The midbrain and pons are disrupted sequentially, and signs of lower brainstem failure are added to dysfunction of rostral structures.

An intrinsic brainstem lesion can cause coma by compromising the function of the medial tegmental structures bilaterally. Primary *diencephalic brainstem lesions* are usually due to stroke, either hemorrhagic or infarction. Head trauma may also directly injure the brainstem. In *midbrain lesions,* the pupils are dilated or in mid-position, and bilateral oculomotor nerve palsy occurs. The eyes rest downward and outward and do not adduct or move vertically. Decerebrate posturing of the limbs is present. Pontine infarct or hematoma cause small, poorly reactive pupils and impaired vertical gaze. The eyes may rest downward and inward, and one eye may be lower than the other. Brainstem function rostral to the lesion is preserved. *Pontine lesions* cause small, reactive pupils; failure of horizontal eye movements; preservation of vertical eye movements (sometimes with spontaneous bobbing); and decerebrate posturing. *Medullary lesions* may compromise vasomotor control and breathing. Toxic disorders affecting the brainstem and cerebral hemispheres at multiple levels cause signs inconsistent with any single anatomic locus.

Cerebellar space-occupying lesions cause ataxia and vomiting, often followed by abducens (cranial nerve VI) nerve or lateral gaze palsy to the side of the lesion. Signs of lower brainstem dysfunction in the pons and medulla then develop.

Treatment. If a cerebral or cerebellar lesion compresses the brainstem, immediate treatment is required to avoid irreversible injury. With a primary brainstem lesion, the situation is equally urgent. Neuroradiologic investigations are critical in determining the nature and extent of pathology. Endotracheal intubation, controlled mechanical ventilation, and osmotic diuresis are undertaken, and emergency cranial computed tomography (CT) is performed to determine whether the patient requires immediate surgical decompression, cerebrospinal ventricular drainage, or hematoma evacuation as lifesaving measures. Brain magnetic resonance imaging (MRI)

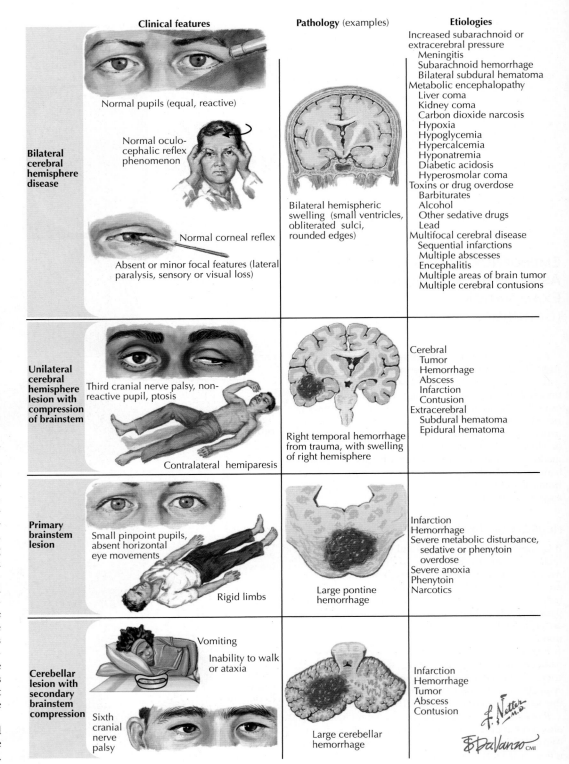

Clinical features	Pathology (examples)	Etiologies
Bilateral cerebral hemisphere disease — Normal pupils (equal, reactive); Normal oculocephalic reflex phenomenon; Normal corneal reflex; Absent or minor focal features (lateral paralysis, sensory or visual loss)	Bilateral hemispheric swelling (small ventricles, obliterated sulci, rounded edges)	Increased subarachnoid or extracerebral pressure — Meningitis, Subarachnoid hemorrhage, Bilateral subdural hematoma; Metabolic encephalopathy — Liver coma, Kidney coma, Carbon dioxide narcosis, Hypoxia, Hypoglycemia, Hypercalcemia, Hyponatremia, Diabetic acidosis, Hyperosmolar coma; Toxins or drug overdose — Barbiturates, Alcohol, Other sedative drugs, Lead; Multifocal cerebral disease — Sequential infarctions, Multiple abscesses, Encephalitis, Multiple areas of brain tumor, Multiple cerebral contusions
Unilateral cerebral hemisphere lesion with compression of brainstem — Third cranial nerve palsy, nonreactive pupil, ptosis; Contralateral hemiparesis	Right temporal hemorrhage from trauma, with swelling of right hemisphere	Cerebral — Tumor, Hemorrhage, Abscess, Infarction, Contusion; Extracerebral — Subdural hematoma, Epidural hematoma
Primary brainstem lesion — Small pinpoint pupils, absent horizontal eye movements; Rigid limbs	Large pontine hemorrhage	Infarction; Hemorrhage; Severe metabolic disturbance, sedative or phenytoin overdose; Severe anoxia; Phenytoin; Narcotics
Cerebellar lesion with secondary brainstem compression — Vomiting; Inability to walk or ataxia; Sixth cranial nerve palsy	Large cerebellar hemorrhage	Infarction; Hemorrhage; Tumor; Abscess; Contusion

provides more detailed anatomy and may even reveal the likely cause for coma, but the imperative is to utilize immediately available imaging that leads to time-saving, and potentially lifesaving, interventions. This approach is certainly relevant in emergency cerebrovascular stroke care when time from onset of symptoms determines use of thrombolytic therapy. Here CT scan can exclude hemorrhagic stroke and point to the appropriate treatment. An MRI would help in determining the ischemic penumbra but would be of no use if it delayed the start of thrombolysis.

Bilateral cerebral hemisphere disease is usually treated medically rather than surgically. It is often the result of metabolic encephalopathy from *exogenous intoxication,* such as drug overdose, alcohol intoxication, or overmedication. *Endogenous intoxication* is caused by organ failure (the lungs and carbon dioxide narcosis, the liver and hyperammonemia, the kidney and uremia), hyperglycemia, hypercalcemia, hypernatremia, or insufficiency of endogenous or exogenous substances such as hypoglycemia, hypothyroidism, hypocalcemia, or hyponatremia.

Plate 6.6

Disorders of Consciousness (Coma)

Border zone ischemia (shock, circulatory insufficiency)

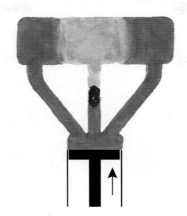

Pump with three outflows,
one outflow blocked.
Deficit occurs in zone
supplied by it.

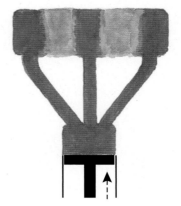

If pump is weak,
deficit is between
zones supplied by
three outflows.

Cerebral artery zones

Anterior   Middle   Posterior

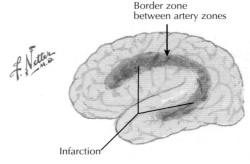

Border zone
between artery zones

Infarction

Infarction

If brain artery is
blocked, infarction
occurs in zone
supplied by that vessel.

If total blood flow is
inadequate, deficit is
mostly at border zone
between supply zones.

HYPOXIC-ISCHEMIC BRAIN DAMAGE

At a national level, out-of-hospital cardiac arrests are an all-too-frequent occurrence. One-quarter of individuals experiencing such an arrest will receive emergency cardiopulmonary resuscitation. However, fewer than 20% of these events will lead to survival at hospital discharge even with the combined efforts of emergency and hospital critical care services. Of those who do survive, many will have profound neurologic injury and disability.

HYPOXIC-ISCHEMIC ENCEPHALOPATHY

Hypoxic-ischemic encephalopathy describes injury after cardiac arrest or severe hypoxia causing global injury, or prolonged hypotension causing arterial border zone injury. Many variables determine the extent and location of injury: the completeness of circulatory collapse (full cardiac arrest or hypotension, with some preserved cardiac output), the duration of circulatory compromise accompanying circulatory failure, and the blood glucose level at the time of the event. *Apnea* or *hypoxia* (as in carbon monoxide poisoning or strangulation) with preserved circulatory function often results in pallidal and thalamic necrosis with preservation of cerebral cortex. *Persistent hypotension* leads to arterial border zone ischemic lesions at the limits of the anterior and middle cerebral artery territories and the middle and posterior cerebral artery territories.

Cardiac arrest can cause hippocampal damage, basal ganglia injury, middle laminar necrosis of the cerebral cortex, and lesions of the cerebellum and brainstem nuclei. The order in these regions of the brain also represents the hierarchy of injury. The most vulnerable region to brief cerebral ischemia is the hippocampus, and the phrase often used to describe this phenomenon is *hippocampal regional vulnerability*. Arterial border zone ischemia results in arm weakness, incoordination during visually directed behavior, and defective visual and spatial perception. In children, severe hypotension can lead to more extensive injury, with severe impairment of motor development and function. *Loss*

Diffuse cortical necrosis; persistent vegetative state

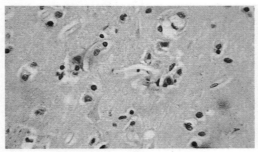

Few anoxic neurons in early anoxia

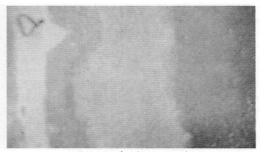

Extensive laminar necrosis

of Purkinje cells in the cerebellum leads to ataxia and action myoclonus.

HYPOTHERMIA TREATMENT

Many drug and anesthetic treatments have been tested in the setting of cardiac arrest. The idea has been to use agents that reduce brain metabolism or limit the cascade of cellular events that lead to neuronal death. Currently, no single drug therapy has been found to provide significant clinical benefit. The only treatment that has been shown to improve the probability of a good outcome in adults after ventricular fibrillation or pulseless ventricular tachycardia cardiac arrest, or in babies with birth asphyxia, is physical

treatment with the control or "targeting" of temperature. In newborn infants with birth asphyxia, at least 35 weeks old and treated within 6 hours of birth, the therapeutic target temperature is 33.5°C to 34.5°C, which is used for the first 72 hours of intensive care and is followed by slow rewarming (0.5°C/hour). In adults and children resuscitated after out-of-hospital or in-hospital cardiac arrest, the randomized controlled trial data are less robust for indicating a specific target in temperature, the duration of hypothermia, and the rate of rewarming. It appears that avoidance of too low a temperature (i.e., <32°C) or too high a temperature (>36°C in adults, >37.5°C in children) in the first 24 hours after resuscitation is important. More research is ongoing.

Plate 6.7

Brain: PART I

The vegetative state. The condition is called *persistent* when it lasts without change for more than 1 month.

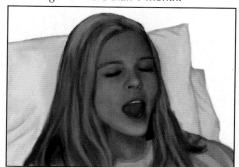

This patient is yawning but not in conscious response. Such patients may startle, look about, or yawn, but none of these actions is in conscious response to a specific stimulus.

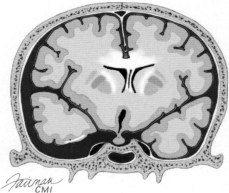

Subarachnoid hemorrhage was the cause of the patient's state.

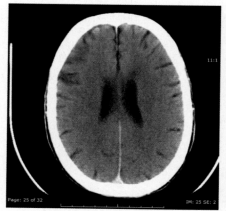

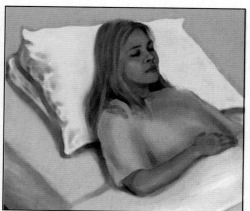

Noncontrast brain CT demonstrating ominous sign of diffuse brain injury and possible prelude to a persistent vegetative state: subtle disappearance of normal differentiation between gray and white matter

VEGETATIVE STATE, MINIMALLY CONSCIOUS STATE, AND UNRESPONSIVE WAKEFULNESS SYNDROME

Survivors of some severe circulatory event who are initially comatose may pass through a spectrum of clinical conditions before partially or fully recovering consciousness. If, after having been in a coma, the patient opens the eyes but remains unable to initiate voluntary motor activity, this behavior marks the transition to what is called the *vegetative state* (VS). The further transition to *unresponsive wakefulness syndrome* (UWS) or *minimally conscious state* (MCS) is characterized by reproducible evidence of simple voluntary behavior. Emergence from MCS is signaled by the return of functional communication or object use. Further developments lead to outcomes ranging from severe disability to a good recovery. If, however, the patient remains in the VS for more than 1 month after the occurrence of brain damage, this condition is called the *persistent vegetative state*. This state is not necessarily irreversible. Reversibility is much less likely in patients in the *permanent vegetative state*; that is, in VS lasting more than 3 months after hypoxic-ischemic damage or 1 year after traumatic brain injury.

To date, VS and the MCS/UWS have both been defined by clinically observed behavioral responses. For example, VS is characterized by wakefulness in the absence of any awareness of self or environment. Typically, such a person retains autonomic functions with variable preservation of cranial and spinal reflexes but exhibits no clinical evidence of sustained, reproducible, purposeful, or voluntary behavioral responses to multisensory stimulation, nor evidence of language comprehension or response to command. MCS describes a spectrum of behavior that, at its most basic description, requires evidence of visual pursuit and, at best, involves intermittent responses to command. However, it has now become apparent using newer technologies, such as functional MRI, that the distinction between VS and MCS cannot be based purely on observation. A notable proportion of patients considered to be in VS retain some awareness that is not consistent with their externally observable behavior.

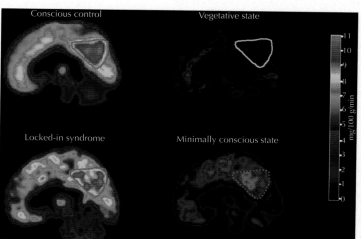

Color-coded cerebral metabolic rate for glucose scans in the sagittal plane showing reduced metabolism in the precuneus in a patient in a vegetative state (*top right*) and in a patient in a minimally conscious state (*bottom right*). The red area in the conscious control (*top left*) and locked-in syndrome (*bottom left*) scans indicate normal metabolism. (*From Laureys S, Owen AM, Schiff ND. Brain function in coma, vegetative state, and related disorders. Lancet Neurol 3:537-546, 2004.*)

The neuropathology of postanoxic VS and MCS/UWS is indistinguishable. There is characteristically little or no damage in the brainstem, but such patients commonly have evidence of diffuse necrosis in the cerebral cortex, variable abnormalities in the basal ganglia and cerebellum, and severe thalamic damage. At a functional level, cerebral metabolic studies and MRIs have identified that the behavior during VS and MCS/UWS represents a functional disconnection syndrome in a large-scale frontoparietal network as a result of damage to long-range connectivity. The structures involved include the lateral and medial frontal regions, parietotemporal and posterior parietal areas, and posterior cingulate and precuneal cortex.

Plate 6.8

Disorders of Consciousness (Coma)

BRAIN DEATH OR DEATH BY NEUROLOGIC CRITERIA

Severe hypoxic-ischemic encephalopathy may result in brain swelling of such severity that all blood flow into the cranium is blocked, thereby worsening the ischemia to a terminal stage. There is only one death that may be determined by cardiac criteria or neurologic criteria. The term *brain death* (BD) refers to the determination of *death by neurologic criteria* (DNC); more recently, the latter terminology has been used to avoid any confusion about there being two forms of death. Worldwide, the determination of BD/DNC is based on a clinical diagnosis using absence of neurologic function in the context of a diagnosis that has resulted in irreversible coma. In the United States and countries that have a similar code of practice, BD/DNC indicates death of the "entire" or "whole" brain. In the United Kingdom and countries that have a similar code of practice, BD/DNC refers to a state in which there is coexistence of unresponsive and irreversible coma with apnea and absence of brainstem reflexes. A complete neurologic examination that includes the elements outlined in Plates 6.4 to 6.8 is mandatory to determine BD/DNC, with all components appropriately documented. The current recommendation in adults is that a single evaluation suffices for the determination of BD/DNC. In children, two assessments should be performed, with the duration of interval between tests varying with age.

Before starting the assessment for determination of BD/DNC, reversible conditions or conditions that can interfere with the neurologic examination must be excluded. For example, hypothermia, hypotension, and metabolic disturbance that could affect the neurologic examination must be corrected. After cardiopulmonary resuscitation or use of therapeutic targeted temperature management (e.g., hypothermia), determination of BD/DNC should be deferred for 24 to 48 hours, or longer if there are concerns or inconsistencies in the examination. Sedatives, analgesics, neuromuscular blockers, and anticonvulsant agents should be discontinued for a reasonable period, based on the elimination half-life of the pharmacologic agent, to ensure that they do not affect the examination; blood or plasma levels can be used to confirm that the drug is in the low to middle therapeutic range.

The components of the clinical neurologic examination consistent with the determination of BD/DNC include presence of unresponsive and irreversible coma, loss of all brainstem reflexes, apnea (Plate 6.8), and absence of spontaneous or induced movements but exclude spinal cord events such as reflex withdrawal or spinal myoclonus.

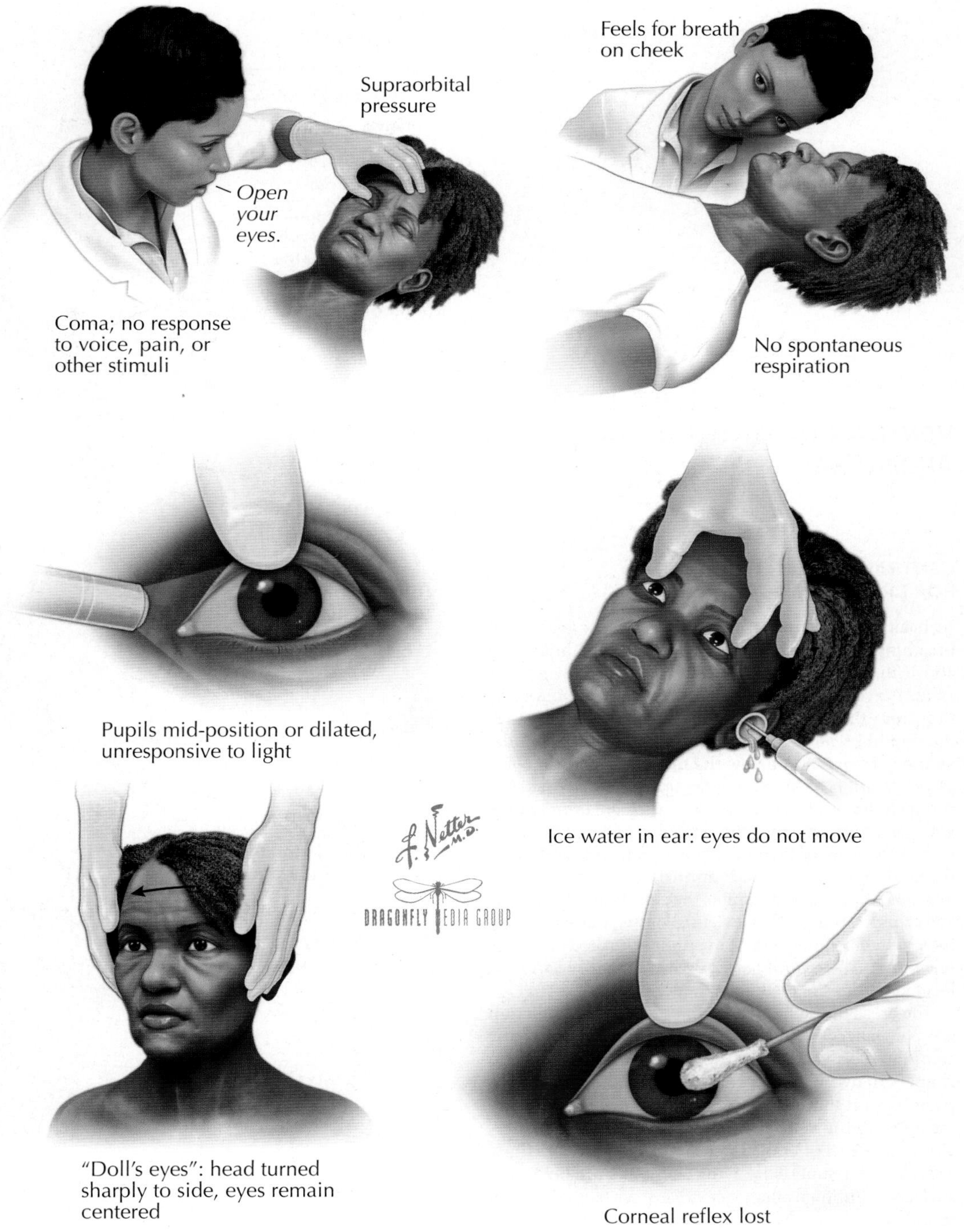

IRREVERSIBLE COMA

The patient must exhibit complete loss of consciousness, vocalization, and volitional activity. Noxious stimuli should produce no eye opening or eye movement and no motor response other than spinal-mediated reflexes.

LOSS OF ALL BRAINSTEM REFLEXES

The patient exhibits the following: mid-position or fully dilated pupils that do not respond to light, either directly or consensually (assessment 1); absence of movement of bulbar musculature, including facial and oropharyngeal muscles, such as in response to deep pressure on the condyles at the level of the temporomandibular

~Open your eyes.

Supraorbital pressure

Coma; no response to voice, pain, or other stimuli

Feels for breath on cheek

No spontaneous respiration

Pupils mid-position or dilated, unresponsive to light

Ice water in ear: eyes do not move

"Doll's eyes": head turned sharply to side, eyes remain centered

Corneal reflex lost

joints and over the supraorbital ridge (assessment 2); absent corneal reflexes so that touching the cornea with a sterile cotton swab does not elicit any eyelid movement (assessment 3); absent oculovestibular reflexes (assessment 4); and absence of gag and cough on stimulation of the posterior pharynx with a tongue blade or suction catheter (assessment 5). Assessment of these brainstem functions should be carried out sequentially and systematically because they relate to different levels of brainstem functioning (see Plate 6.9). The oculovestibular reflex is tested by irrigating each ear with ice water (caloric testing) after first checking that the external auditory canal is not occluded by wax and that the eardrum is intact. The head of the bed is elevated to 30 degrees, and the patient's head is kept in the midline. Each ear is irrigated with 50 to 60 mL of ice water, which

should elicit no movement of the eyes during 1 minute of observation. The aim is to reduce local temperature at the tympanic membrane so that there is a gradient with core body temperature. Both sides are tested with an interval of several minutes. In normal individuals, nystagmus is induced in both eyes. The fast phase is toward the side opposite that which is being irrigated with cold water and is triggered by the cerebral cortex. The slow phase of nystagmus is caused by the oculovestibular reflex. In comatose patients with an intact response, cold water will turn both eyes slowly toward the side being irrigated. These movements are comparable with the slow phase of the nystagmus induced in normal individuals. Caloric-induced movements are absent when the midbrain or rostral pons is impaired and the oculovestibular path is no longer intact.

Plate 6.9

Brain: PART I

VENTILATORY PATTERNS AND THE APNEA TEST

CENTRAL PATTERN GENERATOR FOR BREATHING

In health, the anatomic origin of the cyclic pattern of breathing is the brainstem. Sectioning the brainstem above the pons leaves breathing unaffected when the vagus nerve (cranial nerve X) carrying afferent information from the lungs is intact. Vagotomy results in a reduction in breathing frequency and an increase in tidal volume. Transection below the medulla results in complete cessation of breathing. Sectioning above the central medulla results in rhythmic but irregular breathing, with vagotomy slowing the irregular pattern. Transection at the level of the upper pons leads to a slowing of respiration and an increase in tidal volume. If both vagus nerves are cut, the result is the cessation of breathing at full inspiration (called *apneusis*) or inspiratory spasms interrupted by intermittent expirations (called *apneustic breathing*). The *central pattern generator for breathing* is located within the medullary center.

The areas of the brainstem that modulate ventilation are colocalized to the same structure containing the central pattern generator. The areas that are sensitive to changes in hydrogen ion concentration and blood composition of respiratory gases (chemosensitive areas) are localized to the ventral surface of the medulla, bilaterally, at the level of cranial nerve roots VIII to XI. These areas are very superficial, lying about 200 μm below the surface. Additional chemosensitive areas have also been found caudally in the area of the XII cranial nerve root (hypoglossal nerve). All of these central chemoreceptors are sensitive to local changes in cerebrospinal fluid pH induced by rising partial pressure of carbon dioxide in arterial blood ($Paco_2$). Failure to respond to an adequate $Paco_2$ stimulus indicates a failure in the medullary respiratory centers.

The *apnea test* is performed if the brainstem reflexes are *all* absent, and it is a requirement of testing in the determination of BD/DNC (see Plate 6.8). A number of techniques are used to perform this test in the intensive care unit. However, the essential feature in BD/DNC is that the patient must have complete absence of respiratory effort by formal testing using the endogenous increase in $Paco_2$ as the stimulus to breathing. At baseline, the patient should start with a $Paco_2$ of approximately 40 mm Hg. The stimulus to breathing is considered adequate when there has been a rise in $Paco_2$ by 20 mm Hg to some value greater than 60 mm Hg.

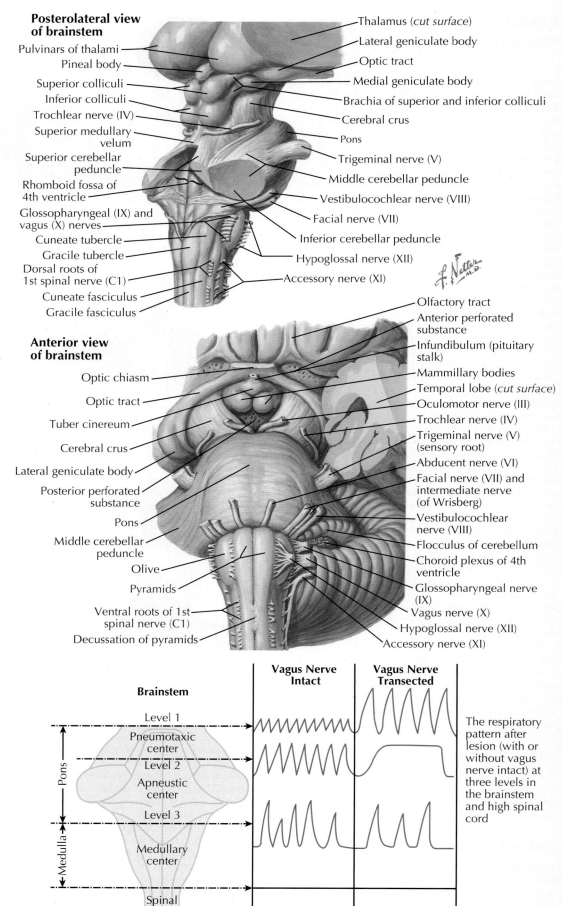

BASAL GANGLIA AND MOVEMENT DISORDERS

Plate 7.1

Brain: PART I

BASAL NUCLEI (GANGLIA)

Horizontal sections through cerebrum

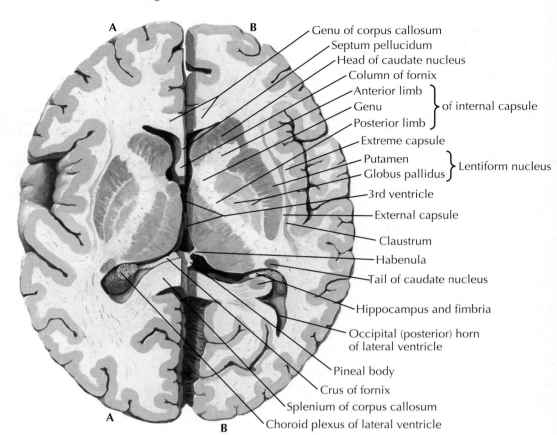

- Genu of corpus callosum
- Septum pellucidum
- Head of caudate nucleus
- Column of fornix
- Anterior limb
- Genu } of internal capsule
- Posterior limb
- Extreme capsule
- Putamen
- Globus pallidus } Lentiform nucleus
- 3rd ventricle
- External capsule
- Claustrum
- Habenula
- Tail of caudate nucleus
- Hippocampus and fimbria
- Occipital (posterior) horn of lateral ventricle
- Pineal body
- Crus of fornix
- Splenium of corpus callosum
- Choroid plexus of lateral ventricle

ANATOMY OF THE BASAL GANGLIA AND RELATED STRUCTURES

OVERVIEW OF MOVEMENT DISORDERS

Movement disorders encompass a group of conditions characterized by poverty of movement, the *akinetic-rigid syndromes,* and those with excessive movements, the *hyperkinetic movement disorders* (tremor, dystonia, myoclonus, chorea/ballism, tics, and others). This traditional view, in which basal ganglia disorders resulted in these syndromes, has now expanded to include the *ataxias and disorders of gait and posture.* Advances in surgical techniques and imaging studies have broadened the clinical horizon and catchments of the movement disorders specialist. With the increasing indications for botulinum toxin therapy, *spasticity* and other disorders are now managed by many movement disorder neurologists.

Abnormal involuntary movements should be viewed as clinical signs with many causes. For example, parkinsonism may be the clinical manifestation of various conditions with different or unclear etiologies. *Defining* the broad category of the movement disorder in an individual patient precedes the classic approach to neurologic diagnosis: *localizing* the lesion and determining the etiology of the condition. A careful history with particular attention to family background, pregnancy, labor and delivery, early developmental milestones, trauma, infections, medical and psychiatric comorbidities, and use of illicit drugs and medications, especially neuroleptics, is particularly important when first evaluating a patient with abnormal involuntary movements and may suggest the underlying cause. A detailed general medical examination with emphasis on eye movements, presence of Kayser-Fleischer rings (suggesting Wilson disease), and funduscopic examination looking for retinopathy and optic nerve abnormalities (papillitis, papilledema, or optic nerve atrophy suggesting demyelinating diseases, metabolic disorders, or mitochondrial cytopathies), organomegaly (betraying metabolic or storage diseases), and skin discolorations or deposits (defining phakomatosis, xeroderma pigmentosum, vitaminosis, gastrointestinal disease, malabsorption, calcinosis, or cholesterol deposits, especially at the

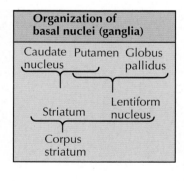

Organization of basal nuclei (ganglia)

Caudate nucleus — Putamen — Globus pallidus
Striatum — Lentiform nucleus
Corpus striatum

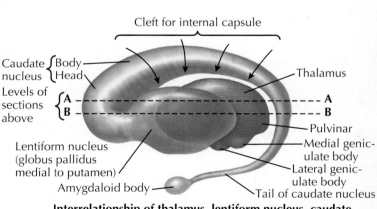

- Cleft for internal capsule
- Caudate nucleus { Body, Head
- Levels of sections above { A, B
- Thalamus
- A
- B
- Pulvinar
- Medial geniculate body
- Lateral geniculate body
- Lentiform nucleus (globus pallidus medial to putamen)
- Amygdaloid body
- Tail of caudate nucleus

Interrelationship of thalamus, lentiform nucleus, caudate nucleus, and amygdaloid body: left lateral view

muscle tendons) may prove rewarding. A carefully performed neurologic examination may reveal additional clues that help in understanding the patient's condition.

Once the abnormal movements have been classified and the neurologic accompaniments documented and placed in context, the cause may become apparent, and proper ancillary testing may be undertaken.

ANATOMY OF THE BASAL GANGLIA AND RELATED STRUCTURES

Anatomically, the basal ganglia constitute a complex circuitry that includes neurons of the caudate nucleus, putamen, subthalamic nucleus (STN), globus pallidus, and substantia nigra (SN). The basal ganglia output is directed at the motor thalamus (and from there to the frontal cortex), superior colliculus, and the pedunculopontine nucleus (PPN).

Plate 7.2

Basal Ganglia and Movement Disorders

ANATOMY OF THE BASAL GANGLIA AND RELATED STRUCTURES (Continued)

GLOBUS PALLIDUS

Divided by the internal medullary lamina into an external (GPe) and internal (GPi) segments, the *globus pallidus* borders laterally with the putamen, dorsomedially with the internal capsule and optic tract, and ventrally with the substantia innominata, which, in turn, contains three major functional anatomic systems: the ventral striatopallidal system, the extended amygdala, and the nucleus basalis of Meynert. With its cholinergic and γ-aminobutyric acid (GABAergic) projections, this latter nucleus plays an essential role in memory disorders and the treatment of dementias. The GPi is a central efferent structure of the basal ganglia, using three major projection systems: the ansa lenticularis, the lenticular fasciculus, and the pallidotegmental tract. The ansa lenticularis sweeps ventromedially around the internal capsule, joining the lenticular fasciculus to form the thalamic fasciculus, which, in turn, projects to different thalamic nuclei, especially the ventral anterior, ventral lateral, centromedian, and parafascicular intralaminar nuclei of the thalamus. The pallidotegmental tract terminates in the pedunculopontine nucleus.

CAUDATE NUCLEUS

The caudate nucleus resembles an elongated and curved exclamation mark. Its main part is an expanded head directly continuous with a smaller and attenuated body that merges into an elongated tail. The *head* bulges into the anterior horn of the lateral ventricle and forms its sloping floor. The caudate nucleus is separated from the lentiform nucleus by the anterior limb of the internal capsule, but the separation is incomplete because the head of the caudate nucleus and the putamen are connected, especially anteroinferiorly, by bands of gray matter traversing the white matter of the anterior limb. This admixture of gray and white matter produces the striated appearance that justifies the term "corpus striatum" applied to these nuclei. The head tapers into the narrower *body* that lies in the floor of the central part of the lateral ventricle, lateral to the superior surface of the thalamus and separated from it by a shallow sulcus lodging the stria terminalis and thalamostriate

vein. The *tail* turns downward along the outer margin of the posterior surface of the thalamus, with the stria terminalis still lying in a slight groove between them. It then curves forward into the roof of the inferior horn of the lateral ventricle, where it separates from the thalamus and lentiform nucleus by the inferior part of the internal capsule and by fibers (including some from the anterior commissure) that spread into the temporal lobe.

AMYGDALOID BODY

The tail of the caudate nucleus ends in a small, almond-shaped expansion, the amygdaloid body, which is a complex of several small nuclei located in the forepart of the roof of the inferior horn of the lateral ventricle. The *stria terminalis* issues from the amygdaloid body and runs along the medial side of the caudate nucleus until it reaches the vicinity of the ipsilateral

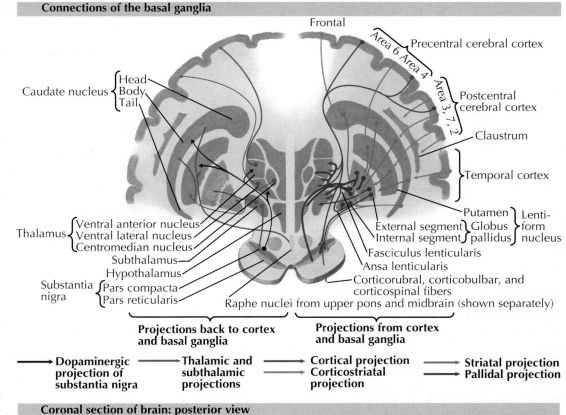

BASAL GANGLIA AND RELATED STRUCTURES

Connections of the basal ganglia

Frontal

Precentral cerebral cortex
Area 6, Area 4, Area 3, 7, 2
Postcentral cerebral cortex
Claustrum
Temporal cortex

Caudate nucleus: Head, Body, Tail

Putamen — Lentiform nucleus
External segment / Internal segment — Globus pallidus

Thalamus: Ventral anterior nucleus, Ventral lateral nucleus, Centromedian nucleus
Subthalamus
Hypothalamus
Substantia nigra: Pars compacta, Pars reticularis

Fasciculus lenticularis
Ansa lenticularis
Corticorubral, corticobulbar, and corticospinal fibers
Raphe nuclei from upper pons and midbrain (shown separately)

Projections back to cortex and basal ganglia | Projections from cortex and basal ganglia

→ Dopaminergic projection of substantia nigra
→ Thalamic and subthalamic projections
→ Cortical projection / Corticostriatal projection
→ Striatal projection / Pallidal projection

Coronal section of brain: posterior view

Corpus callosum
Septum pellucidum
Lateral ventricle
Body of caudate nucleus
Choroid plexus of lateral ventricle
Stria terminalis
Superior thalamostriate vein
Body of fornix
Internal cerebral vein
Tela choroidea of 3rd ventricle
Choroid plexus of 3rd ventricle
Thalamus
Putamen
Globus pallidus } Lentiform nucleus
Internal capsule
3rd ventricle and interthalamic adhesion
Hypothalamus
Tail of caudate nucleus
Optic tract
Choroid plexus of lateral ventricle
Temporal (inferior) horn of lateral ventricle
Fimbria of hippocampus
Hippocampus
Dentate gyrus
Mammillary body
Parahippocampal gyrus

White arrow in left interventricular foramen (of Monro)
— Ependyma
— Pia mater

Plate 7.3

Brain: PART I

SCHEMATIC AND CROSS SECTION OF BASAL GANGLIA
Simplified schematic diagram of basal ganglia circuitry

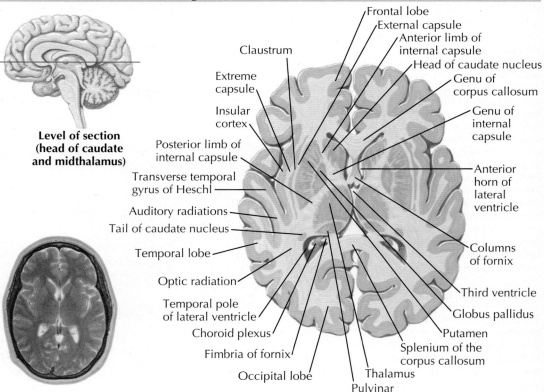

— Glutamatergic
— GABA
— Acetylcholine
— Dopamine

Cerebral cortex

Caudate nucleus

Putamen

Globus pallidus (external segment)

Globus pallidus (internal segment)

Subthalamic nucleus

Substantia nigra (pars compacta)

Substantia nigra (pars reticularis)

Pedunculopontine nucleus

Centromedian parafascicular complex

Pons

Axial (horizontal) sections through the forebrain

Level of section (head of caudate and midthalamus)

Claustrum

Extreme capsule

Insular cortex

Posterior limb of internal capsule

Transverse temporal gyrus of Heschl

Auditory radiations

Tail of caudate nucleus

Temporal lobe

Optic radiation

Temporal pole of lateral ventricle

Choroid plexus

Fimbria of fornix

Occipital lobe

Frontal lobe

External capsule

Anterior limb of internal capsule

Head of caudate nucleus

Genu of corpus callosum

Genu of internal capsule

Anterior horn of lateral ventricle

Columns of fornix

Third ventricle

Globus pallidus

Putamen

Splenium of the corpus callosum

Thalamus

Pulvinar

ANATOMY OF THE BASAL GANGLIA AND RELATED STRUCTURES (Continued)

interventricular foramen. Here, some of its fibers join the anterior commissure. Others pass to the "septal" region adjacent to the lamina terminalis. The remainder descends to the hypothalamus and anterior perforated substance.

A nuclear midbrain complex, the *substantia nigra*, is divided into a pigmented and dopamine-containing pars compacta (SNc) and a cell-poor, pigment-free pars reticularis (SNr). Most dopaminergic projections go to the striatum, and a smaller proportion of SNc axons terminate in the prefrontal cortex. The SNr is a major primary efferent structure of the basal ganglia along with GPi. SNr projects primarily to the thalamus, PPN, and the superior colliculus.

A biconvex structure, the *subthalamic nuclei* receives glutamatergic inputs from the cerebral cortex and GABA inhibition from the GPe and provides glutamatergic innervations to the GPe, GPi, SN, and PPN. The STN has become a structure of interest because of its pivotal role in basal ganglia function.

The postsynaptic dopamine receptors are divided into two major broad categories, D1-like family (D1/D5) and D2-like family (D2, D3, D4), which can be segregated into two main pathways. The *direct pathway*, subserved by D1 dopamine receptors, sends projections to the thalamus via the GPi. The *indirect pathway*, via the D2 family of receptors, influences the STN via the GPe.

New data suggest that dopamine receptors may be modulated via adenosine in the direct and indirect pathways. Adenosine A2A receptors can be found in striatopallidal neurons that express D2 receptors. When activated, these receptors inhibit D2 receptor signaling, resulting in increased GABA activity in these neurons. In addition, the A1 receptor has been demonstrated to interact with the D1 receptor in the direct pathway; however, the potential role of this finding has yet to be fully understood.

Recently the excitatory-inhibitory interplay between the direct and indirect pathways has been conceptualized as focused selection and tonic inhibition (surround inhibition hypothesis). By suppressing excitability in an area surrounding an activated neural network, neuronal

activity selects desired responses. Simultaneously, other pallidal neurons projecting to the thalamus act to permit desired movements. By decreasing their discharge through focused striatal output chiefly via the direct pathway, tonic inhibition to the thalamus is removed, releasing the cortical generators for normal or desired movement to occur. Therefore abnormal involuntary movements result from either failure of inhibition or excessive excitation of the surrounding structures.

Based on these models, it is important to recognize the pallidum as the major outflow structure of the basal ganglia. Most fugal pathways pass through the fields of Forel. Presently, the STN is the preferred target for the surgical treatment of idiopathic Parkinson disease (iPD), the VIM thalamus for the treatment of essential and certain other types of tremor, and the GPi for dystonia, with deep brain stimulation (DBS) being the favored surgical procedure.

Plate 7.4

Basal Ganglia and Movement Disorders

PARKINSONISM: EARLY MANIFESTATIONS

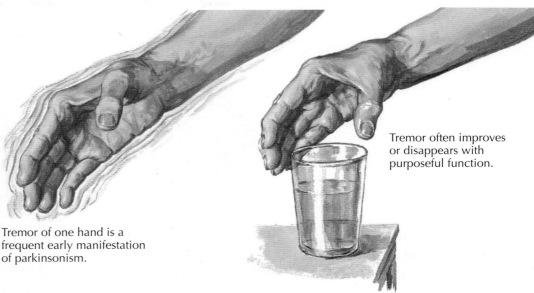

Tremor of one hand is a frequent early manifestation of parkinsonism.

Tremor often improves or disappears with purposeful function.

AKINETIC-RIGID SYNDROME, PARKINSONISM, OR PARKINSONIAN SYNDROME

The parkinsonian syndrome is operationally defined by the presence of *t*remor, *r*igidity, *a*kinesia, and *p*ostural/gait disturbances (mnemonic: TRAP). The diagnosis of parkinsonism is readily made if a given individual has two of the four cardinal features at the time of presentation. Although there are many causes for parkinsonian syndrome, iPD is by far the most common cause, affecting 1% of the population older than 50 years. It has an insidious onset and progresses slowly at a variable rate for 10 to 20 years or more before culminating in severe disability.

IDIOPATHIC PARKINSON DISEASE

The characteristics of iPD are the presence of tremor, rigidity, or bradykinesia early in the course of the illness, with postural and gait disturbances developing late in the course of the disease. The presence of atypical symptoms and the rate of disease progression are important in distinguishing Parkinson disease (PD) from other parkinsonian syndromes. For example, early-onset postural instability, falls, and gait disturbances characterize progressive supranuclear palsy (PSP); marked autonomic disturbances, such as erectile dysfunction in men or urinary bladder incontinence in women, may herald the onset of multiple system atrophy (MSA). Stooping, masked facies, decreased blinking, micrographia, and hypophonia are common features of parkinsonism but are not unique to PD and may be present in other parkinsonian syndromes. Severe anterocollis and camptocormia (bent spine) are more likely to be due to MSA or paraspinal muscle fatty atrophy/myopathy rather than PD (see Plate 7.5). Excessive neck rigidity, primarily when accompanied by marked oculomotor disturbances, such as hypometric slowed saccades in downward gaze or an evident defect of voluntary ocular excursion to command or pursuit but a normal excursion on the doll's eye maneuver, particularly in the vertical plane, suggest PSP. Other oculomotor disturbances, such as saccadic intrusions (principally square wave jerks or ocular flutter), nystagmus, or ocular impersistence, may be present in PSP, MSA, corticobasal degeneration, Huntington disease, and the cerebellar ataxias in variable combinations and degrees of severity.

It is estimated that approximately 80% of the dopaminergic neurons in the substantia nigra have been lost

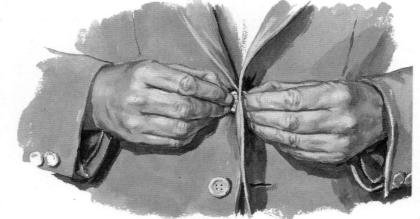

Difficulty in performing simple manual functions may be initial symptom.

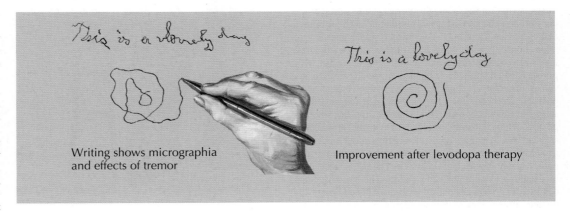

Writing shows micrographia and effects of tremor

Improvement after levodopa therapy

by the time that PD is first diagnosed; hence the initial degenerative process leading to parkinsonism begins several years before the clinical diagnosis is made. Although it is usually difficult to diagnose PD in the preclinical (premotor) stage, anosmia, constipation, and mood and personality changes may precede the onset of motor symptoms by a few years. For most patients, the onset of motor symptoms is subtle and may be evident first to family members or coworkers.

Dopamine deficiency is responsible for the pathophysiology of motor symptoms in PD. Although symptoms improve with dopaminergic replacement therapy, tremor and postural and gait disturbances tend to have only a partial response to treatment, particularly in the later stages of the disease, suggesting that the substrate of such symptoms may lie somewhere else within the central nervous system. Indeed, it has been shown that the PPN, a cholinergic structure closely linked to

Plate 7.5

Brain: PART I

PARKINSONISM: SUCCESSIVE CLINICAL STAGES

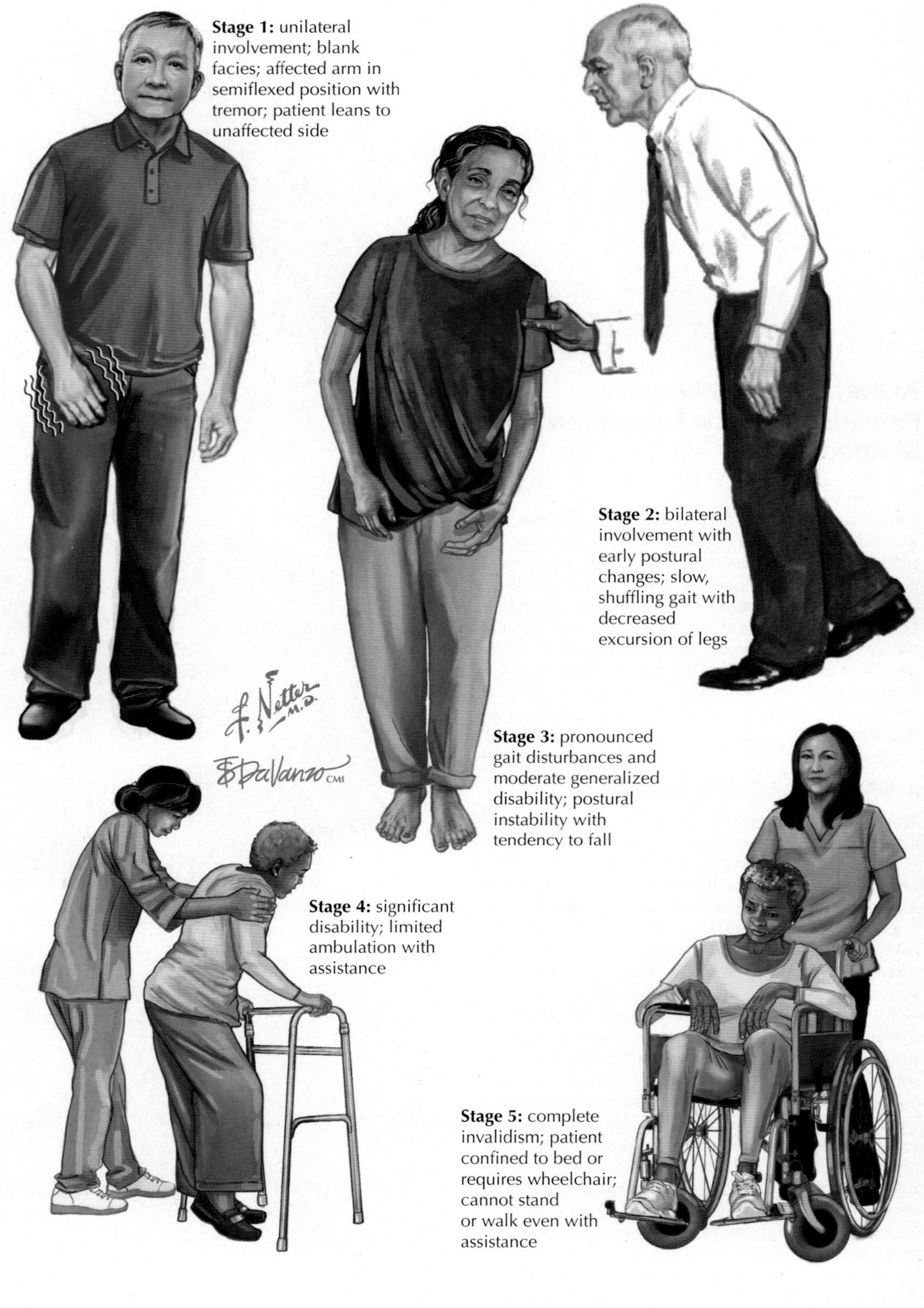

AKINETIC-RIGID SYNDROME, PARKINSONISM, OR PARKINSONIAN SYNDROME (Continued)

the striatonigral system, may play a significant role in gait control. In addition, preliminary studies using PPN-targeted neuromodulation have shown mild improvements in gait difficulties and freezing in some patients, but the outcomes of such studies are currently unclear.

Tremor is a classic feature of parkinsonism. Typically it is a rest tremor, disappearing with movement but resuming when a static posture is achieved with a 3-Hz frequency. Although it is most commonly seen in PD, it may occur in other parkinsonian conditions, such as MSA and states induced by dopamine-blocking or dopamine-depleting medications. Its origin is unclear, but some evidence suggests that the inferior olives or the cerebellum acts as the central oscillator, driving tremors via the cerebellothalamocortical loop as a reverberating system.

Untreated PD may be divided into five stages. *Stage 1* is characterized by mild unilateral disease. Tremor may be the only visible sign, but other subtle findings, including slowness or rigidity, may be noted on examination. Gait is usually normal, but there may be a mild decrease in arm swing on the most symptomatic side, and the upper limb may be carried slightly abducted at the shoulder and flexed at the elbow. Diminished facial expression, hypophonic speech, reduced manual dexterity, impaired rapid alternating movements, and micrographia with poorly formed letters may be present. As the disease advances to *stage 2*, there is bilateral involvement with postural changes. The more classic phenotype is observed in this stage, with reduced facial mobility, stooped posture when standing, reduced arm swing on walking, and en bloc turning; rapid alternating movements are impaired. Movements become slow and deliberate, and patients may report fatigue and weakness. Fatigue may be disabling in up to 75% of patients. The hand assumes the so-called striatal posture with dorsiflexed wrist, adducted fingers, flexed metacarpophalangeal and distal interphalangeal joints, and extended proximal interphalangeal joints. A "striatal foot" may be present in some patients, consisting of a varus position with clawing of toes. In *stage 3* disease, retropulsion and propulsion reflect increasing impairment of postural reflexes and righting responses. Gait is festinating and shuffling.

In this stage, the symptoms become increasingly pronounced, and the patient may require assistance in the activities of daily living. A more advanced stage is reached *(stage 4)*, with severe disability, rigidity, bradykinesia, and gait disturbances. Standing

is unsteady; a slight push precipitates severe retropulsion, culminating in a fall if the patient is not caught or is left unattended. Eventually, the patient becomes markedly bradykinetic, rigid, and confined to bed or requires a wheelchair *(stage 5)*. Drs. Melvin Yahr and Margaret Hoehn studied the natural progression of patients with PD, developing a staging scale that bears their names. This classification, known as the Hoehn and Yahr staging scale, emphasizes

the disease by the progression of symptoms; it is arbitrarily divided into five stages of disease progression, and although widely used, it provides only a crude estimate of disease severity.

PATHOLOGY

The pathologic hallmark of PD is the loss of pigmentation of the substantia nigra, decreased neuromelanin-containing

Stage 1: unilateral involvement; blank facies; affected arm in semiflexed position with tremor; patient leans to unaffected side

Stage 2: bilateral involvement with early postural changes; slow, shuffling gait with decreased excursion of legs

Stage 3: pronounced gait disturbances and moderate generalized disability; postural instability with tendency to fall

Stage 4: significant disability; limited ambulation with assistance

Stage 5: complete invalidism; patient confined to bed or requires wheelchair; cannot stand or walk even with assistance

Plate 7.6

Basal Ganglia and Movement Disorders

NEUROPATHOLOGY OF PARKINSON DISEASE

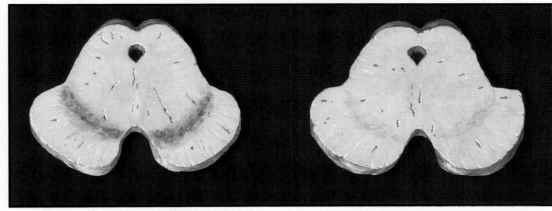

Normal: section through cerebral peduncles and substantia nigra

Parkinson disease: substantia nigra depigmented

AKINETIC-RIGID SYNDROME, PARKINSONISM, OR PARKINSONIAN SYNDROME (Continued)

neurons, and deposition of a Lewy body in the motor nucleus of the vagus, locus coeruleus, and substantia nigra (see Plate 7.6). The Lewy body is an intracytoplasmic, eosinophilic inclusion composed primarily of ubiquitin, neurofilaments, and alpha-synuclein, an important component protein generally found throughout the brain, particularly at the synapse. The role that alpha-synuclein plays in the pathogenesis of PD is not well understood. Point mutations, duplications, or amplifications in the region of chromosome 4q21 containing the gene encoding for alpha-synuclein have been found in some familial, early-onset cases. Excessive alpha-synuclein leads to protein aggregation and clumping. Other mutations affecting the genes encoding for parkin, an important protein of the ubiquitin/proteasome system (*DJ-1* and *PINK1*), may affect mitochondrial function leading to impaired free radical handling and energy production. The high concentration of iron in the substantia nigra and striatum increases cell vulnerability to oxidative stress. Recently the progression of PD and Lewy body deposition with degeneration has been conceptualized as beginning in the olfactory bulb and lower brainstem, progressing over time to the diencephalon, amygdala, and entorhinal and neocortex.

An example of a fully developed clinical syndrome due to generalized diffuse Lewy deposits is diffuse Lewy body disease/dementia complex.

MULTIPLE SYSTEM ATROPHY

In *multiple system atrophy* (MSA), the unifying pathologic feature is the oligodendroglial cytoplasmic inclusion bodies (GCIs), which are present in striatonigral degeneration, sporadic olivopontocerebellar atrophy (OPCA), and Shy-Drager syndrome, nosologic entities once considered unrelated disorders but now grouped under the rubric of MSA. The autonomic abnormalities that characterize Shy-Drager syndrome are found eventually in both disorders. Thus MSA is divided into two major groups, MSA-C (cerebellar) and MSA-P (parkinsonism). Other pathologic features include variable neuronal cell loss with gliosis in the putamen and, to a lesser degree, the pallidum, brainstem (particularly the basis pontis and inferior olive), cerebellum, intermediolateral columns of the spinal cord, and peripheral nerves. When OPCA/MSA-C is present, atrophy is

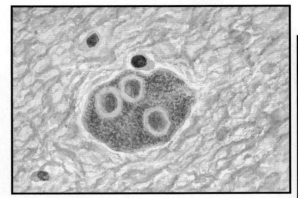

Lewy inclusion bodies in cell of substantia nigra in Parkinson disease; may also appear in locus coeruleus and tegmentum, cranial motor nerve nuclei, and peripheral autonomic ganglia

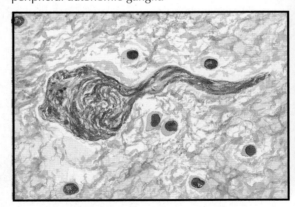

Neurofibrillary tangle in nerve cell of substantia nigra as seen in postencephalitic parkinsonism, progressive supranuclear palsy, and parkinsonism-dementia complex

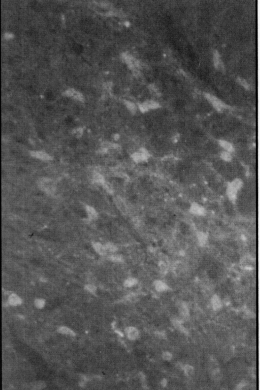

Section of substantia nigra of normal animal: treatment of section with formaldehyde vapor causes formation of polymers with monoamines (dopa and norepinephrine) that fluoresce to bright green under ultraviolet light

predominant in the pons, cerebellum, and medullary olives. Tau and alpha-synuclein are the predominant components of GCIs. The appearance on magnetic resonance imaging (MRI) is sometimes characteristic (see Plate 7.8).

PROGRESSIVE SUPRANUCLEAR PALSY

Progressive supranuclear palsy is characterized by oculomotor disturbances, parkinsonism, and gait disturbances

with postural instability, the latter a common early manifestation of the disease, preceding in most cases the typical downward gaze and horizontal paresis characteristic of the disease (see Plate 7.7). Pathologically, there is neuronal cell loss and gliosis in the periaqueductal gray, with deposition of tau-containing globose neurofibrillary tangles with ubiquitin immunoreactivity, and atrophy of the diencephalon, globus pallidus, subthalamic nucleus, and mesencephalon. This atrophy leads to the "Mickey

Plate 7.7

Brain: PART I

PROGRESSIVE SUPRANUCLEAR PALSY

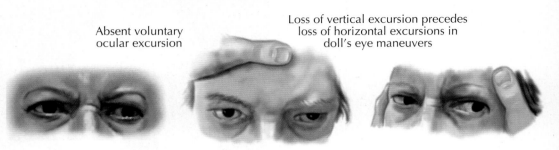

Absent voluntary ocular excursion

Loss of vertical excursion precedes loss of horizontal excursions in doll's eye maneuvers

AKINETIC-RIGID SYNDROME, PARKINSONISM, OR PARKINSONIAN SYNDROME (Continued)

Mouse" midbrain sign on axial views or the penguin or hummingbird sign on sagittal views in brain MRI.

CORTICOBASAL DEGENERATION

Corticobasal degeneration (CBD) is characterized by asymmetric cortical atrophy, neuronal cell loss, gliosis, and ballooned neurons in the central sulcus region (primary motor/primary sensory cortex), with achromatic intracytoplasmic neuronal inclusions similar to the Pick bodies seen in Pick disease/frontotemporal dementia and primary progressive aphasia. These inclusions with corresponding neuronal cell loss are found predominantly in the diencephalon, thalamus, substantia nigra, locus coeruleus, and cerebral cortex. Tau protein, ubiquitin, phosphorylated neurofilaments, and, to a lesser degree, alpha-synuclein are components of such inclusions, sharing immunoreactive properties similar to that found in Pick bodies. CBD (see Plate 7.8) is characterized clinically by asymmetric dystonic posturing with superimposed stimulus-sensitive and action-induced myoclonus, giving the affected hand or limb a tremulous appearance, and by the alien limb phenomena, limb apraxia, parkinsonism, and gait and postural instability, with dementia and oculomotor disturbances manifesting later in the course of the disease.

LEWY BODY DISEASE

Lewy body disease, also known as *dementia with Lewy bodies,* operationally may be viewed as typical dopa-responsive parkinsonism with early-onset dementia, fluctuating alertness and attention, confusion, sleep disturbances, marked sensitivity to neuroleptic or dopamine-blocking agents, and vivid and well-formed visual hallucinations. In most autopsy series, Lewy body dementia is second after Alzheimer disease as the cause of dementia, with vascular dementia a close third. The Lewy body, which is structurally and morphologically similar to that found in iPD, is found throughout the cerebral cortex to a variable degree and in the substantia nigra. Ubiquitin, neurofilament protein, and alpha-synuclein are components of Lewy bodies. In the nucleus basalis and hippocampal formation, scattered senile plaques and neurofibrillary tangles are found

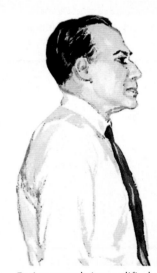

Patient stands in modified hyperextension in contrast to flexed position in Parkinson disease.

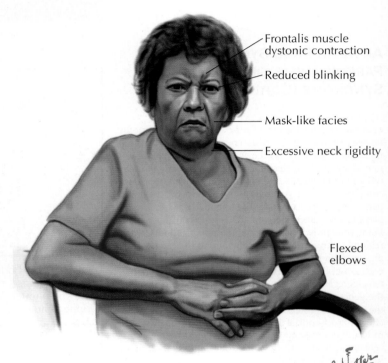

Frontalis muscle dystonic contraction

Reduced blinking

Mask-like facies

Excessive neck rigidity

Flexed elbows

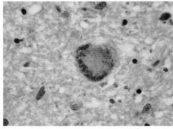

Neurofibrillary tangles (NFTs) in substantia nigra (stained with hematoxylin and eosin)

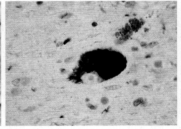

NFTs in substantia nigra (stains with tau)

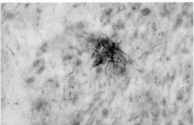

Astrocytic tuft in pallidum (Gallyas stain)

with granulovacuolar degeneration simulating that observed in Alzheimer disease.

DRUG-INDUCED PARKINSONISM

Although not a degenerative disorder of the basal ganglia, drug-induced parkinsonism (DIP) can mimic iPD and may be difficult to differentiate in a given individual. Therefore the clinician should have a high index of

suspicion and must obtain a thorough drug history. DIP is discussed here because of the importance in making the diagnosis. Treatment is readily available, and in most instances identifying the offending medication(s) is all that is needed to explain the symptoms and proceed with treatment. At the most basic level, DIP results from either dopamine receptor blockade, such as that observed with neuroleptic medications, metoclopramide, or certain calcium channel

Plate 7.8

Basal Ganglia and Movement Disorders

CORTICOBASAL DEGENERATION

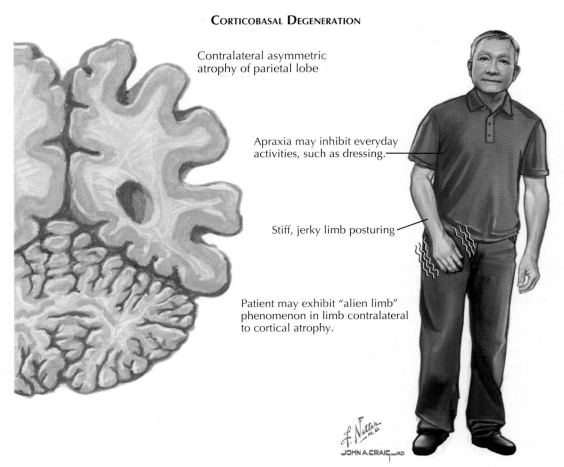

Contralateral asymmetric atrophy of parietal lobe

Apraxia may inhibit everyday activities, such as dressing.

Stiff, jerky limb posturing

Patient may exhibit "alien limb" phenomenon in limb contralateral to cortical atrophy.

AKINETIC-RIGID SYNDROME, PARKINSONISM, OR PARKINSONIAN SYNDROME (Continued)

blockers (flunarizine, cinnarizine), or when using dopamine-depleting agents (reserpine, tetrabenazine). Atypical neuroleptics (clozapine, olanzapine, risperidone, quetiapine, ziprasidone), once believed to be free of extrapyramidal side effects, are now clearly implicated in some cases of DIP. Interactions with dopaminergic (D1, D2), histaminergic, muscarinic, alpha-adrenergic, and serotonergic receptor binding may account for the phenomenology observed. The most commonly prescribed antidepressants, selective serotonin reuptake inhibitors, may result in DIP by serotonergic downregulation of dopamine synthesis. Other medications, such as valproic acid and lithium, may result in DIP by poorly understood mechanisms. Elimination of the offending agent, dose adjustments, or identification of drug interactions (effect potentiation) may result in symptom improvement. Patients should be educated on the side effects of medications, particularly when parkinsonism may result as a consequence of their use.

TREATMENT

Despite recent advances in our understanding of the chemical and pathologic changes and the development of novel therapies for PD, levodopa continues to be the gold standard (see Plate 7.9). Orally administered levodopa is absorbed into the circulation principally from the proximal small intestine. It may be detected in blood for several hours after administration, reaching maximum peak levels in 2 to 3 hours after ingestion. Levodopa is available in different formulations (oral, enteral suspension, inhalation powder) with no superiority among them. The inhalation powder provides an attractive alternative because it bypasses the gastrointestinal tract, being useful in patients with sudden offs or freezing episodes.

Once levodopa reaches the bloodstream, it is rapidly converted to dopamine by the enzyme dopa decarboxylase (DDC; L-amino-acid decarboxylase). Approximately 1% of the oral dose penetrates the cerebral capillaries to diffuse through the brain parenchyma, where it is picked up and converted to dopamine in the remaining dopamine-producing cells. Once secreted into the synaptic cleft, dopamine is rapidly deactivated, principally to homovanillic acid by catechol-O-methyltransferase (COMT) and monoamine oxidase (MAO). To increase available levodopa and to diminish

MULTIPLE SYSTEM ATROPHY

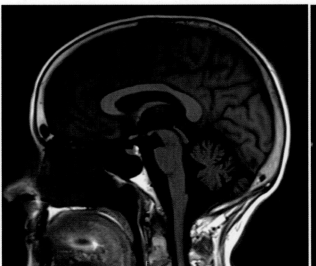

MRI brain in T1 sequence in sagittal plane shows severe brainstem and anterior and posterior cerebellar vermis atrophy.

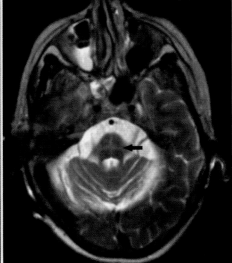

"Hot cross bun" sign typical for MSA

unwanted peripheral dopamine side effects (nausea, vomiting, arterial hypotension), DDC is inhibited peripherally with carbidopa. The inhibition markedly reduces the conversion of levodopa to dopamine in the medullary vomiting center or trigger zone, preventing its activation. With long-term levodopa use, coupled with the intrinsic pathologic changes occurring in parkinsonism, late motor complications develop in approximately 75% of patients, particularly after 10 years

of illness. Wearing off, freezing of gait, unpredictable responses, and levodopa-induced abnormal involuntary movements or dyskinesias may complicate medical management.

Certain agents, namely dopamine agonists (ropinirole, pramipexole, rotigotine, pergolide, cabergoline, and bromocriptine), have been developed to eliminate or delay the need for levodopa. These agents stimulate dopamine receptors and thus act like dopamine.

Plate 7.9

Brain: PART I

PARKINSONISM: HYPOTHESIZED ROLE OF DOPAMINE

AKINETIC-RIGID SYNDROME, PARKINSONISM, OR PARKINSONIAN SYNDROME (Continued)

A dopamine agonist may provide symptomatic improvement and may delay the development of motor complications, chiefly by postponing the need to introduce levodopa. Dopamine agonists are often used as the initial monotherapy in early stages in selected, usually young (<60 years) patients. Nonetheless, most patients will require levodopa at some point in the course of their disease. The dopamine agonists can be divided into ergoline and non–ergoline-derived agonists. The most commonly used are the non-ergoline agonists because they have fewer side effects. Their presentation includes an oral formulation, a skin patch, and a subcutaneous infusion (apomorphine), which can be useful as a rescue medication.

Another strategy has been the use of COMT enzyme inhibitors to block COMT. Consequently, dopamine remains at the synaptic cleft, leading to increased duration of on-time (time during which clinical benefit is obtained from levodopa) by 1 to 2 hours and stable plasma levodopa levels. With the progressive loss of neurons and its attendant decline in buffering capacity, plasma levodopa levels become the primary driver of the clinical response and motor complications. Of the two currently available COMT inhibitors, entacapone, a peripheral COMT inhibitor, is the most commonly used. Tolcapone, a peripheral and central COMT inhibitor, is not widely used in the United States because of concerns of severe and potentially fatal liver failure occurring as an idiosyncratic reaction to it.

Although antiparkinsonian medication is centered on dopaminergic therapy, an adenosine receptor A2A antagonist (istradefylline) has also been developed as an adjunctive treatment to help with the off-periods. Pimavanserin may be useful in patients with PD taking dopaminergic agents who have hallucinations. This medication was approved for PD–associated hallucinations and blocks the 5-HT2A receptors.

The hope of "neuroprotective treatments"—that is, treatments to slow disease progression—has been marred by controversies and methodologic flaws in most studies performed to date. Interpretation of the data has been conflicting; instruments used for data collection have proven insensitive, and results of studies in animal models have correlated poorly with findings in humans. Therefore, at present, no clear indication and consensus exist for the use of MAO inhibitors (e.g., rasagiline, selegiline, or safinamide), vitamins (e.g., vitamin E),

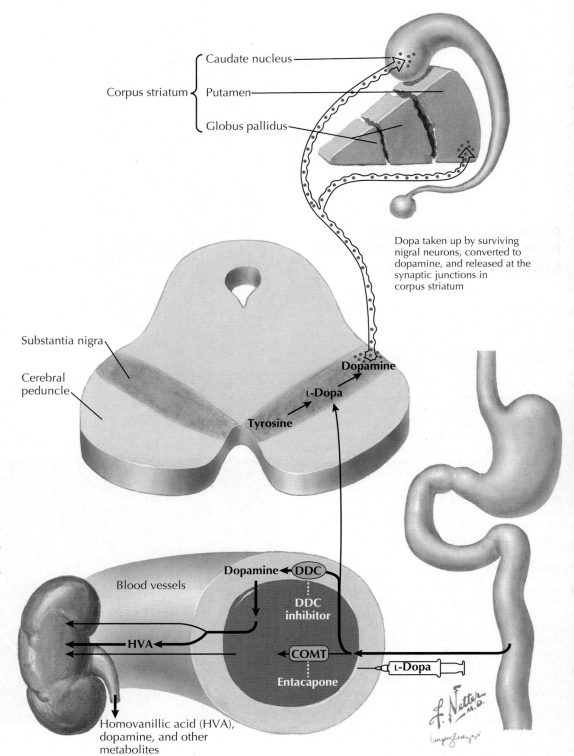

or other elements (coenzyme Q10). Rasagiline, selegiline, safinamide, and amantadine produce mild symptomatic improvement in some patients, thus allowing a delay in levodopa use.

Surgery

By the middle of the 20th century, a handful of surgical procedures had been developed to treat PD and other movement disorders (see Plate 7.10). Cortical excisions,

capsulotomies, caudotomies, ansotomies, pedunculotomies, and pyramidotomies were performed with variable results; unfortunately, most procedures were fraught with severe side effects and poor outcomes. In 1952, while performing a planned pedunculotomy on a 39-year-old patient with postencephalitic parkinsonism, Irving Cooper, a New York neurosurgeon, accidentally ligated the anterior choroidal artery (this type of insult results in a medial globus pallidus infarction).

Plate 7.10

Basal Ganglia and Movement Disorders

SURGICAL MANAGEMENT OF MOVEMENT DISORDERS

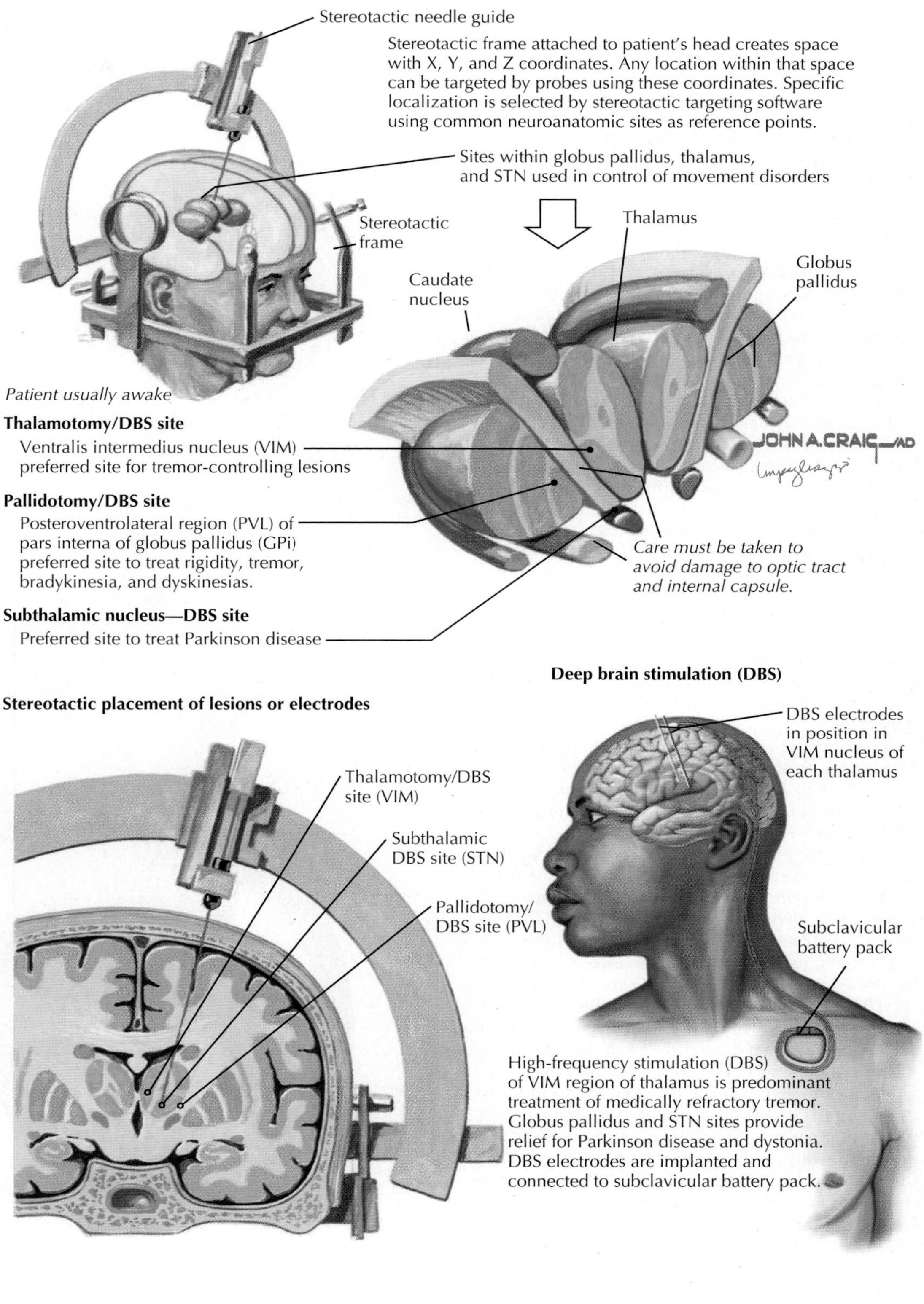

Stereotactic needle guide

Stereotactic frame attached to patient's head creates space with X, Y, and Z coordinates. Any location within that space can be targeted by probes using these coordinates. Specific localization is selected by stereotactic targeting software using common neuroanatomic sites as reference points.

Sites within globus pallidus, thalamus, and STN used in control of movement disorders

Stereotactic frame

Patient usually awake

Thalamus

Caudate nucleus

Globus pallidus

JOHN A. CRAIG—AD

Thalamotomy/DBS site
Ventralis intermedius nucleus (VIM) preferred site for tremor-controlling lesions

Pallidotomy/DBS site
Posteroventrolateral region (PVL) of pars interna of globus pallidus (GPi) preferred site to treat rigidity, tremor, bradykinesia, and dyskinesias.

Subthalamic nucleus—DBS site
Preferred site to treat Parkinson disease

Care must be taken to avoid damage to optic tract and internal capsule.

Stereotactic placement of lesions or electrodes

Deep brain stimulation (DBS)

DBS electrodes in position in VIM nucleus of each thalamus

Thalamotomy/DBS site (VIM)

Subthalamic DBS site (STN)

Pallidotomy/DBS site (PVL)

Subclavicular battery pack

High-frequency stimulation (DBS) of VIM region of thalamus is predominant treatment of medically refractory tremor. Globus pallidus and STN sites provide relief for Parkinson disease and dystonia. DBS electrodes are implanted and connected to subclavicular battery pack.

AKINETIC-RIGID SYNDROME, PARKINSONISM, OR PARKINSONIAN SYNDROME (Continued)

To Cooper's amazement, the patient survived with resolution of the incapacitating tremor and rigidity that had hampered his quality of life up to that point. This event led to an interest in the pallidum as a surgical target. It was not until advances had occurred in understanding the physiology of the basal ganglia, in surgical and imaging techniques, and in intraoperative recording devices that the current era of lesioning and later neuromodulation techniques developed.

DEEP BRAIN STIMULATION AND LESIONING PROCEDURES

With few exceptions, lesioning procedures such as pallidotomies or thalamotomies are rarely performed. These have been replaced by deep brain stimulation (DBS) using implantable quadripolar brain electrodes in three main targets, namely the medial globus pallidus (GPi), STN, and ventral intermediate nucleus of the thalamus (VIM nucleus). Although STN is the preferred DBS target for the surgical treatment of PD, there is no conclusive evidence that STN-DBS is superior to GPi-DBS.

DBS does not improve symptoms that are resistant to levodopa, and, consequently, careful documentation of an adequate response to levodopa is important in surgical candidates. A positive symptomatic benefit from levodopa exposure predicts a better surgical outcome than otherwise. There is no clear age cutoff for the procedure. Octogenarians undergoing the procedure have done well. Surgery is reserved for those with a confirmed clinical diagnosis of iPD who have developed motor fluctuations and drug-induced dyskinesias despite optimal medical therapy. Patients should have no general medical contraindications to surgery and should be without dementia or psychiatric comorbidities. In patients with atypical symptoms or a Parkinson-plus syndrome, a poor response to levodopa, dementia, severe autonomic dysfunction, or marked psychiatric disease, DBS is associated with an increased risk for poor outcome and is generally contraindicated. All parkinsonian symptoms improve with surgery, particularly tremors and medication-related abnormal involuntary movements on the side contralateral to the procedure. Rigidity and bradykinesia respond well but to a lesser degree. Postural instability and gait disturbances are less likely to respond. However, the development

of DBS targeting neurons in the PPN might be useful for patients with gait issues.

It is not clear how DBS works in PD. What is evident is that DBS provides a nondestructive and reversible means by which to disrupt neuronal function via electrical stimulation and thereby modulate neuronal firing. DBS continues to evolve as an important and established treatment for neurologic diseases, with new indications being added continuously. A

multidisciplinary approach to management provides the best chances for a good outcome in those who are candidates for surgery.

Today, the use of MRI–guided focused ultrasound for the treatment of essential or parkinsonian tremors is gaining popularity due to its ability to provide a reasonable outcome without requiring a craniotomy. Its final role in the armamentarium for treating PD will become clearer as experiences accrue.

Plate 7.11

Brain: PART I

HYPERKINETIC MOVEMENT DISORDER–IDIOPATHIC TORSION DYSTONIA

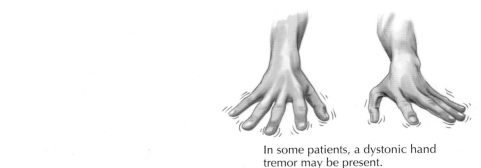

In some patients, a dystonic hand tremor may be present.

Dystonic trunk and head tremor

Hypertrophic neck muscles may be observed.

Tremor may abate with the finger-to-nose maneuver.

Truncal dystonia may lead to lordosis.

Bilateral foot dystonia

HYPERKINETIC MOVEMENT DISORDERS

DYSTONIA

Dystonia is characterized by sustained muscle contractions causing twisting and repetitive movements or abnormal postures. Dystonia may be a symptom, a syndrome, or a disease and may be classified by distribution, age at onset, and etiology. By definition, no cause for dystonia is apparent in primary dystonia. Genetic and chromosomal abnormalities have been identified in a small proportion of patients with dystonia.

Childhood-onset primary generalized dystonia, also known as Oppenheim dystonia or idiopathic torsion dystonia, is characterized by involuntary, repetitive, sustained muscle contractions or postures, beginning in the foot and leg during childhood and progressing to a more generalized distribution by the second decade of life (see Plate 7.11). It was first described in Ashkenazi Jews expressing the *DYT1* mutation on chromosome 9. A GAG deletion mutation in the *DYT1* gene, which encodes for the protein torsin A, has been associated more frequently with the disease. The estimated prevalence is 3.4 per 100,000 individuals. This mutation is also found in non-Ashkenazi individuals throughout the world.

Other genetic mutations causing childhood-onset generalized dystonia have been described more recently. Next to *DYT1*, perhaps the most important is *DYT6*, which is associated with a mutation in the *THAP1* gene.

Adult-onset primary dystonia is usually focal or segmental in distribution and may be a forme fruste of idiopathic generalized dystonia. It may develop in susceptible individuals who perform repetitive tasks, such as instrumentalists, typists, dental hygienists, and writers, or appear without known precipitating factors. Examples of *focal dystonia* are writer's cramp, cervical dystonia (spasmodic torticollis), blepharospasm (bilateral, involuntary, synchronous, forceful eye closure), oromandibular dystonia (forceful involuntary jaw opening or closure), spasmodic dysphonia (adductor or abductor dysphonia), and musician's dystonia. In *segmental dystonia,* characteristically, two or more adjacent body parts are involved. *Hemidystonia* involves an arm and leg on the same side of the body. *Axial dystonia* affects midline structures (trunk and neck muscles) and may cause speech and swallowing difficulty or arching of the back or neck. *Multifocal dystonia* refers to abnormal posturing affecting two or more nonadjacent body parts. Involvement of both legs and at least one arm or axial involvement in combination with at least one affected limb is usually observed in *generalized dystonia.* Deep tendon reflexes may be normal or exaggerated, particularly in patients with a secondary cause or cervical dystonia who have developed compressive myelopathy due to severe and often early degenerative spine disease. A *dystonic tremor* or myorhythmia may be noted in some patients.

In *secondary dystonias,* a cause is identified, such as cerebral infarction, tumors, brain trauma, infections, and medication exposure, particularly to dopamine-blocking agents (neuroleptics, metoclopramide). Secondary dystonia can be focal, likely contralateral to the lesion, or may be due to minor peripheral trauma resulting from the severe causalgia-dystonia syndrome. It may be hemidystonic or segmental when two or more contiguous body parts are affected or generalized when the trunk and two other contiguous body parts are involved. Secondary generalized dystonia may result from trivial trauma or, in the appropriate setting, psychogenic factors may be the sole cause. Dopamine receptor–blocking medications, such as neuroleptics and phenothiazine-based antiemetics, can produce *acute dystonia* after a single dose or *tardive dystonia* after chronic usage.

Cervical dystonia, probably the most common focal dystonia, results in involuntary contraction of the neck muscles, causing chin deviation, anterocollis or retrocollis, lateral flexion, and, in many patients, shoulder elevation (see Plate 7.12). The continuous activity may result in muscle hypertrophy, particularly

Plate 7.12

Basal Ganglia and Movement Disorders

CERVICAL DYSTONIA

HYPERKINETIC MOVEMENT DISORDERS (Continued)

the sternocleidomastoid and neck flexors. Many patients may notice that specific sensory stimuli or sensory tricks, the *geste antagoniste*, transiently suppress or attenuate spasms. Examples of sensory tricks include touching the face, chin, or elsewhere on the head with a hand, finger, or object. For many years, this phenomenon and the higher prevalence of cervical dystonia in women were mistakenly taken to support the belief that the disorder is psychogenic. In approximately 75% of patients, pain is the most prominent feature. Degenerative cervical spine disease is a common complication and is occasionally associated with compressive myelopathy.

Dystonia-plus syndromes include dystonia accompanied by other neurologic findings on examination. *Dopa-responsive dystonia* (DRD), an autosomal dominant condition with incomplete penetrance, is due to a defect in chromosome 14 encoding for the guanosine triphosphate–cyclohydrolase enzyme responsible for the biosynthesis of tetrabiopterin, which, in turn, is an essential cofactor in the production of dopamine by tyrosine hydroxylase. Tyrosine hydroxylase is the rate-limiting step in the synthesis of dopamine and other catecholamines. DRD, also known as Segawa disease, typically manifests in the first decade of life as a gait disorder mimicking cerebral palsy. In adolescents, dystonia is characterized by diurnal symptom fluctuations and can be accompanied by mild parkinsonism, tremor, spastic or scissoring gait, and scoliosis. One key feature in the clinical examination of adolescents or young adults with DRD is the marked loss of postural stability noted when performing the pull-push test. The disorder has an excellent response to levodopa, which is the treatment of choice.

CHOREA/BALLISM

Chorea is characterized by random jerky movements jumping from one body part to another. They are irregularly timed, nonrepetitive, and abrupt, varying in severity. In mild cases, they may lead to restlessness, intermittent exaggeration of facial expression, or fidgetiness of the hands or toes. In more severe cases, the gait has a dancing quality, and limbs exhibit violent and ballistic movements. It can involve proximal and distal muscles. Patients often attempt to mask such movements by incorporating them into voluntary activities. *Ballism* can be conceptualized as a severe form of chorea affecting the proximal limb muscles. The most common form of ballism is seen in patients with parkinsonism and severe levodopa-induced abnormal involuntary movements (dyskinesias) or patients with contralateral subthalamic lesions (e.g., infarct, demyelination). Patients may have difficulties maintaining a sustained posture. When asked to grip the examiner's hand, pressure cannot be sustained, resulting in the "milkmaid's grip"; when asked to protrude the tongue, the tongue will pop out, resulting in the "catch fly

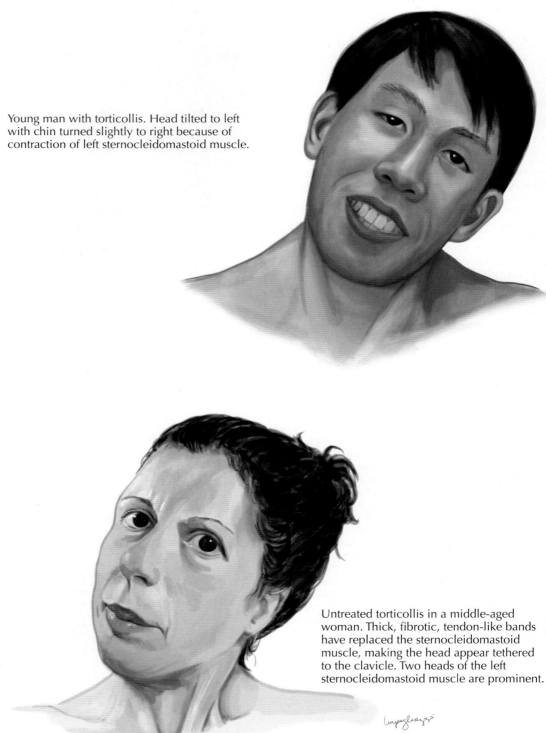

Young man with torticollis. Head tilted to left with chin turned slightly to right because of contraction of left sternocleidomastoid muscle.

Untreated torticollis in a middle-aged woman. Thick, fibrotic, tendon-like bands have replaced the sternocleidomastoid muscle, making the head appear tethered to the clavicle. Two heads of the left sternocleidomastoid muscle are prominent.

sign" or "harlequin's tongue." The "bon-bon sign" may be present (the tongue moves involuntarily inside the mouth, hitting the inside wall of the cheeks). This latter sign is particularly prominent in patients with drug-induced orolingual chorea (neuroleptic-induced tardive dyskinesia).

There are many causes of chorea, such as pregnancy (chorea gravidarum), Huntington disease, benign hereditary chorea, neuroacanthocytosis, Sydenham chorea,

systemic lupus erythematosus, focal vascular lesions, medications (particularly the chronic use of neuroleptics and oral contraceptives), various metabolic and endocrine disorders (hyperthyroidism, hypoparathyroidism, or hyperparathyroidism and hypoglycemia or hyperglycemia), and others.

In adults, the most common cause of chorea is medication, especially the use of levodopa in patients with PD or the long-term use of neuroleptic drugs or

Plate 7.13

Brain: PART I

HYPERKINETIC MOVEMENT DISORDERS (Continued)

metoclopramide, which causes tardive dyskinesia. In children, Sydenham chorea remains the most common cause.

The second most common cause of chorea in adults is *Huntington disease.* First described by George Huntington in 1872, this autosomal dominant neurodegenerative disorder, with a 100% penetrance, has an abnormal trinucleotide (CAG) gene expansion, with the defective gene located in the short arm of chromosome 4. The disorder is characterized by choreiform movements and dementia or behavioral changes. In the United States the estimated prevalence is 5 to 10 cases per 100,000 people. Age at onset is in the fifth to sixth decades of life, with a duration of illness of 15 years in the adult and 8 to 10 years with the Westphal variant. Because of its insidious onset, the onset of symptoms is often not recognized, and abnormal movements are erroneously attributed to anxiety. Patients often have personality and behavioral changes early in the disease, which may be the initial manifestation in more than 50% of cases. Eventually, symptoms become prominent and disabling. Speech becomes dysarthric. Oculomotor alterations are common, such as impaired saccade initiation, particularly an inability to initiate saccadic eye movement without blinking or head thrusts. Loss of optokinetic nystagmus can occur after some years. The only laboratory study available to confirm the diagnosis is genetic testing. In the early stages of the disease, brain MRI may show nonspecific changes in the neostriatum, caudate, and putamen; striatal atrophy, most notably the caudate head, occurs later in the disease.

Benign hereditary (familial) chorea, an autosomal dominant disorder, begins in childhood. Mild generalized chorea, affecting the distal extremities more than the proximal muscle groups, is the characteristic movement disorder. When present, minor neuropsychiatric features, such as mildly lower scores on cognitive tests, complete the clinical picture. Benign hereditary chorea has been associated with mutations in the *TITF1* gene.

Sydenham chorea is a manifestation of acute rheumatic fever. It is also called St. Vitus's dance, acute chorea, chorea minor, or rheumatic chorea. Although more common in adolescent girls, it is also seen in adults. The clinical features of chorea are similar to those described for Huntington disease. Obsessive-compulsive and impulsive disorders and emotional lability may also occur. Prophylaxis with antibiotics is recommended until adulthood for children with Sydenham chorea because rheumatic fever recurs in up to one-third of patients.

Athetosis is a slow, writhing movement of the fingers and toes, seen most often in patients with cerebral palsy, particularly when excited or when trying to communicate. Dystonic posturing, tremor, ataxia, or scissoring gait usually accompanies athetotic movements.

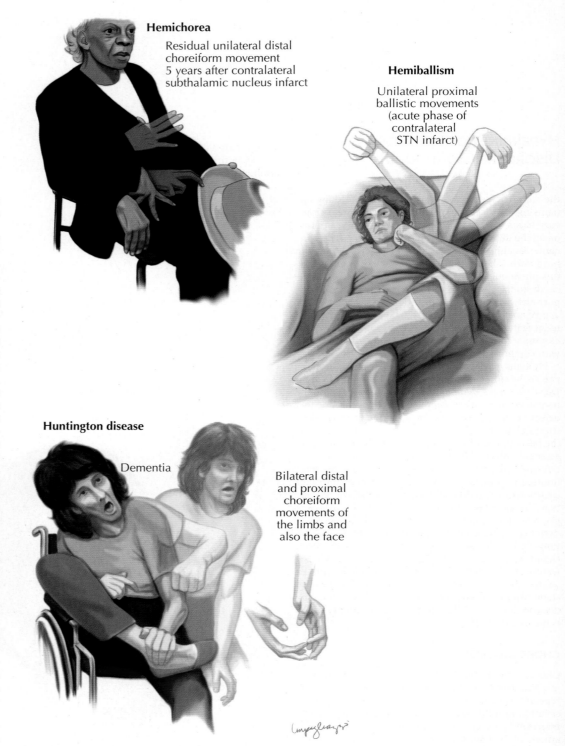

Hemichorea
Residual unilateral distal choreiform movement 5 years after contralateral subthalamic nucleus infarct

Hemiballism
Unilateral proximal ballistic movements (acute phase of contralateral STN infarct)

Huntington disease
Dementia

Bilateral distal and proximal choreiform movements of the limbs and also the face

TREMOR

Tremor is a rhythmic, oscillatory, involuntary movement caused by the alternating activation of agonist and antagonist muscles. The etiology of tremor is diverse and includes *hereditary* (familial tremor), *degenerative* (PD), *metabolic* (thyroid, parathyroid, or hepatic disorders and hypoglycemia), *toxins* (nicotine, mercury, lead, carbon monoxide, manganese, arsenic, toluene), *illicit drug use or medication-induced* (neuroleptics, tricyclics, lithium, cocaine, alcohol, adrenaline, bronchodilators, theophylline, caffeine, steroids, valproate, amiodarone, thyroid hormones, vincristine), *peripheral neuropathies* (Charcot-Marie-Tooth disease, Roussy-Levy syndrome, complex regional pain syndrome), and *psychogenic disorders.*

Based on its relation to activity, tremor may be classified as *rest, postural,* or *intentional.* Rest tremor is best seen when the upper limbs are relaxed, resting in the patient's lap; when necessary, mental exercises may help "bring out" the tremor. A 3- to 5-Hz rest tremor is a characteristic feature of PD ("pill-rolling" tremor) and often starts asymmetrically. A critical feature of this type of tremor is its disappearance or improvement with limb movement. Although the tremor may become bilateral

Plate 7.14

Basal Ganglia and Movement Disorders

HYPERKINETIC MOVEMENT DISORDERS (Continued)

with disease progression, it commonly remains more severe on the initially affected side.

Postural tremor is seen when the limbs are actively maintained in a particular posture against gravity and disappears when the limbs are at rest. Examples of postural tremors are *essential tremor*, drug- or toxin-induced tremor, metabolic conditions, and alcohol withdrawal states. *Physiologic tremors* are also postural in nature and are seen in all individuals at a frequency of 8 to 12 Hz. They are enhanced by caffeine, fear, or anxiety.

Essential tremor is sporadic, but a family history may be elicited in approximately 50% of those affected (*familial tremor*). Typically, a 5- to 8-Hz tremor is present bilaterally in the hands or arms. A tremor of the head or vocal cords is also common. Patients often notice an improvement in tremor after drinking a small quantity of alcohol. Most cases are mild and do not require treatment, but propranolol, primidone, or certain antiepileptic drugs (gabapentin, topiramate) may be effective. Surgical treatment is indicated in refractory cases. DBS is the most common option targeting the thalamic VIM nucleus either unilaterally or bilaterally. Thalamotomy procedures can be done by radiofrequency ablation, stereotactic radiosurgery, or MRI-guided focused ultrasound (vide supra).

Intention tremor is the tremor most commonly associated with disease of the cerebellum and its associated pathways, but it may be seen in patients with advanced essential or familial tremor. The tremor, which occurs during movement, can be unilateral or bilateral, depending on the cerebellar lesion, and may affect upper and lower limbs. It has a frequency of 2 to 4 Hz and characteristically worsens as the limb approaches its target (endpoint accentuation). Another term used for cerebellar outflow tremor is rubral tremor. This term is discouraged, however, because it is not specific for lesions found only at the red nucleus. The term *cerebellar outflow tremor* is preferred to describe intention, rubral, or cerebellar tremor.

A "wing beating" tremor has been described in patients with Wilson disease, multiple sclerosis, or stroke involving the superior cerebellar peduncular region. In these patients, the tremor is most prominent when flexing the forearms at the elbows and elevating the shoulders laterally to reach a 90-degree angle in the fully abducted position. This phenomenology is similar to that in cerebellar outflow tremor, particularly when severe, and probably represents the involvement of cerebellothalamofugal pathways.

TICS AND TOURETTE SYNDROME

Tics are sudden, rapid, stereotyped, repetitive, nonrhythmic movements or vocalizations affecting discrete muscle groups. Most experts agree and clinical experience dictates that tics are preceded by a sensory component, described by patients as an "urge." When patients

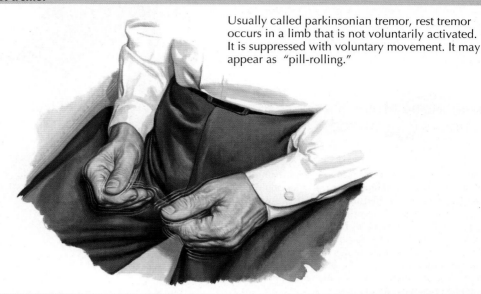

Rest tremor

Usually called parkinsonian tremor, rest tremor occurs in a limb that is not voluntarily activated. It is suppressed with voluntary movement. It may appear as "pill-rolling."

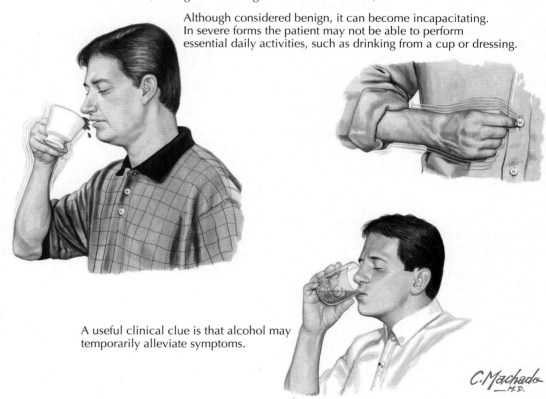

Action tremor (example: essential tremor)

Typically bilateral, essential tremor is the most common movement disorder. It may be accentuated with goal-directed movement of the limbs. Essential tremor affects the hands and cranial musculature (in this order of prevalence). Most common presentation is the association of hand tremor and a tremor in the cranial musculature (leading to a nodding or no-no head tremor).

Although considered benign, it can become incapacitating. In severe forms the patient may not be able to perform essential daily activities, such as drinking from a cup or dressing.

A useful clinical clue is that alcohol may temporarily alleviate symptoms.

are asked to prevent movements from occurring, an uncomfortable inner sensation builds, and an urge to "release" develops, resulting in the expression of the tics.

The spectrum of tics includes *transient tics of childhood* when present for less than 1 year, *chronic motor or vocal tics* when tics are present for more than 12 months, and *Tourette syndrome*, defined by the presence of both motor and vocal tics for more than 12 months.

Tics may be classified according to the complexity of symptoms as *simple motor or vocal tics* when involving only a few muscles or simple sounds, such as eye blinking, shoulder shrugging, facial grimacing, whistling, grunting, throat clearing, snorting, chirping, or sniffing. Many such youngsters are initially mistakenly diagnosed as having chronic rhinitis or "allergies" or punished unnecessarily for loud behaviors. Once considered rare, schoolteachers now easily identify tics

Plate 7.15

Brain: PART I

HYPERKINETIC MOVEMENT DISORDERS (Continued)

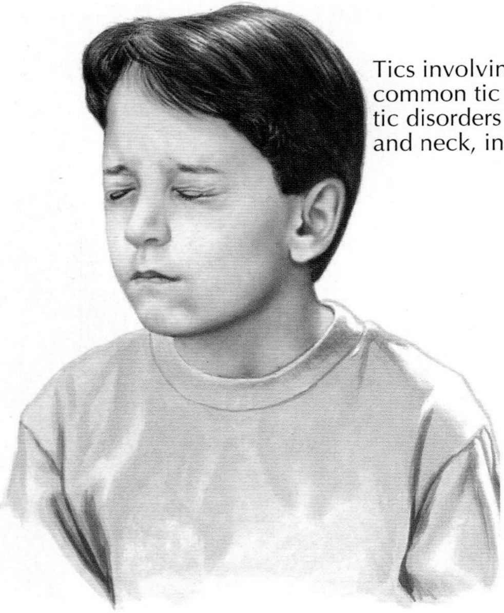

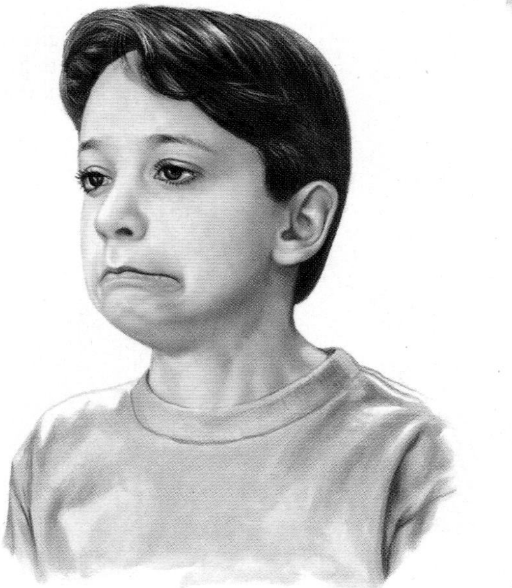

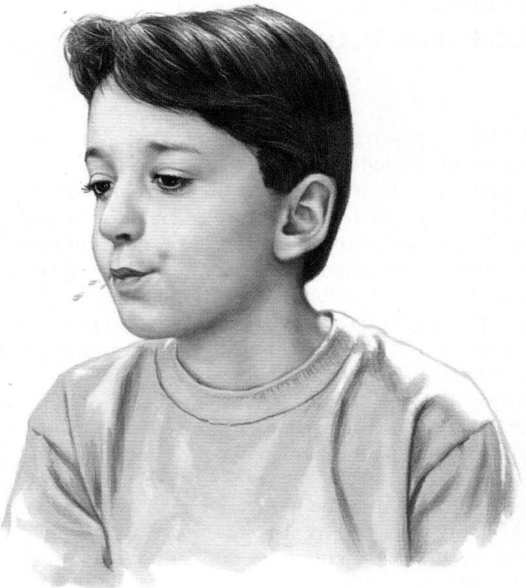

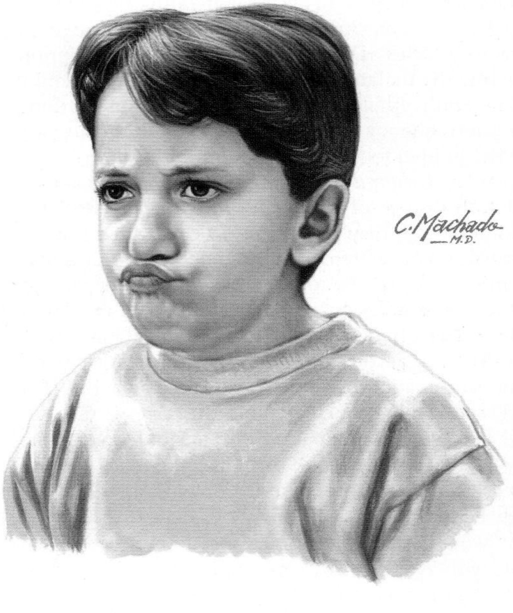

and may be the first to call attention to a child's unique behavior. In *complex motor or vocal tics,* multiple muscle groups are recruited in orchestrated bouts of involuntary movements or utterances of words and sentences or phrases. Examples include hand gestures, jumping, touching, pressing, shouting words, or speech blocking. Some individuals may exhibit *copropraxia,* the sudden performance of obscene gestures or *echopraxia,* the involuntary spontaneous imitation of someone else's movements.

Multiple motor *and* vocal tics characterize *Tourette syndrome* (TS). In many patients with TS, obsessive-compulsive behaviors and attention deficit disorder, or both, may be present. Anxiety, depression, and self-injury behaviors may complicate the clinical picture.

Tics may be primary or "idiopathic," or *secondary,* in which a definable cause is found. Primary tics are by far more common in children and adolescents, with secondary disorders in that age group being rare. In adults, trauma, encephalitis, stroke, carbon monoxide poisoning, neurosyphilis, Creutzfeldt-Jakob disease, and central nervous system injury from hypoglycemia may result in tics or tourettism. Some genetic disorders in which tics have been described include Huntington disease, neuroacanthocytosis, neuroferritinopathy (Hallervorden-Spatz disease), dystonia with tics, tuberous sclerosis complex, and some cases of Duchenne muscular dystrophy. Patients with Down syndrome, autism spectrum disorder, and fragile X tremor syndrome have also been reported to have tics. The use of illicit drugs or medications may result in tics, tourettism, or punding, particularly the use of cocaine, amphetamines, and antiepileptic medications (phenobarbital, phenytoin, and carbamazepine). Less commonly, opioids, lithium, levodopa, and antidepressants may induce or worsen tics.

The substrate for tics and Tourette syndrome seems to reside in the basal ganglia and related structures. Supporting evidence for this concept includes the clinical observation of tic improvement when patients are treated with dopamine-blocking or dopamine-depleting agents. Other evidence comes from functional imaging studies demonstrating volumetric striatal changes and increased dopamine synaptic content. DBS has led to improvement of tics when focused on different targets of the corticostriatothalamic and limbic pathways/structures. The preferred target for DBS in these patients includes the ventromedial thalamus and globus pallidus internus.

The aim of treatment of tics and Tourette syndrome is to relieve some of the more pressing symptoms. Tics may be the most bothersome aspect of their illness. Obsessive-compulsive behaviors and attention deficit with hyperactivity, anxiety, or depression may be more distressing. There is no general agreement as to the best treatment for tics. Most authors recommend α_2-agonists as first-line therapy, such as guanfacine or clonidine. Dopamine-blocking agents are the most potent anti-tic medications but are also associated with

Tics involving the eyes, such as eye-blinking, are the most common tic in childhood-onset tic disorders. Patients with tic disorders frequently develop other motor tics of the head and neck, including grimacing and frowning.

a high incidence of side effects. Tetrabenazine, a dopamine-depleting drug, may be useful in some cases. A stimulant such as methylphenidate does not worsen tics as previously thought. Therefore it can be safely used in tics and attention deficit disorder. The serotonin reuptake inhibitors are helpful in treating anxiety, depression, or obsessive-compulsive disorder in patients with tics or Tourette syndrome. Botulinum toxin therapy has proven to be of some value when used in patients with dystonic tics. A behavioral therapeutic approach using habit reversal therapy has been shown to be effective in a recent large multicenter study.

MYOCLONUS

Myoclonus is a brief, shock-like muscle jerk, classified according to *origin* (cortical, subcortical, brainstem, and spinal myoclonus) and *distribution* (focal, segmental, multifocal, or generalized). Cortical myoclonus may be epileptic (as in Baltic myoclonus or progressive myoclonic epilepsy, photosensitive myoclonus, epilepsia partialis continua) or part of a neurodegenerative disorder (corticobasal degeneration, Alzheimer dementia, diffuse Lewy body disease, and others). Myoclonus can be classified according to *etiology* as idiopathic/genetic

Plate 7.16

Basal Ganglia and Movement Disorders

HYPERKINETIC MOVEMENT DISORDERS (Continued)

(familial myoclonus, myoclonus-dystonia), physiologic (hypnic jerks or diaphragmatic myoclonus/hiccups), or secondary/symptomatic when a cause for the myoclonus is identified. Examples of the latter group may include encephalitis, hypoxia, toxins, storage diseases, and basal ganglia degenerations, as in Huntington disease, Wilson disease, and certain other disorders. Myoclonus may be *positive* due to a brief muscle contraction or *negative* when muscle tone is briefly lost, as in asterixis.

Anoxic brain injuries may result in myoclonus, which, in turn, may be *cortical, diencephalic,* or *reticular in* origin; *stimulus sensitive* or *action induced;* and *segmental, generalized,* or *multifocal* in distribution. This type of myoclonus may be focal, preferentially affecting the distal limb muscles, or multifocal with spontaneous, reflexive, or stimulus-sensitive jerks accentuated by movement. Frequently, anoxic-induced myoclonus is accompanied by secondary seizures, particularly after cardiopulmonary arrest. Status epilepticus is found in 32% of patients who are postanoxic, and in many, *multifocal myoclonus* alone or in combination with generalized tonic-clonic seizures is frequently observed. The incidence of myoclonic seizures is bimodal, with most occurring within 12 hours after cardiopulmonary resuscitation and the remaining occurring several days later. Electroencephalogram (EEG) is helpful when evaluating these patients, particularly when status epilepticus is suspected. The most frequent EEG findings include diffuse slowing with or without spike or polyspike complexes that are sometimes time locked to the myoclonic jerks. A burst-suppression EEG pattern, when recorded, has a poor prognostic significance. Brain MRI may show diffusion restriction in the cortical and subcortical gray matter between 24 hours and 13 days. Isolated myoclonus generally does not require treatment unless it interferes with mechanical ventilation or nursing care. Myoclonus status is refractory to treatment, may require multiple antiepileptic drugs, and, when accompanied by convulsive status epilepticus, is best controlled with deep anesthesia.

Electrophysiologically, myoclonus is characterized by muscle bursts that are less than 75 msec in duration. When the cerebral cortex is affected, a "giant" somatosensory-evoked cortical response time locked to the onset of the jerk in back-averaged EEG may be obtained.

Levetiracetam, valproic acid, and clonazepam are usually the drugs of choice for treating these patients. Botulinum toxin can be considered an alternative treatment for segmental and peripheral myoclonus that is refractory to medications.

POSTANOXIC MYOCLONUS

In 1963, James Lance and Raymond D. Adams reported a series of patients with the syndrome of intention or action myoclonus as a sequel a to hypoxic encephalopathy. In *postanoxic myoclonus,* axial and proximal muscle

Essential myoclonus

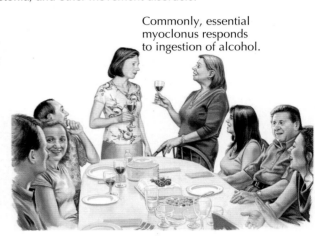

Usually multifocal in distribution, often familial, typically induced by voluntary movements causing a single jerk of the extremity (action myoclonus). Symptoms begin before age 20 and frequently are associated with tremor, dystonia, and other movement disorders.

Commonly, essential myoclonus responds to ingestion of alcohol.

Lance-Adams syndrome (posthypoxic myoclonus)

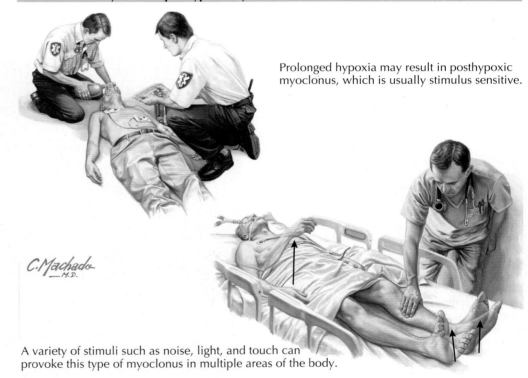

Prolonged hypoxia may result in posthypoxic myoclonus, which is usually stimulus sensitive.

A variety of stimuli such as noise, light, and touch can provoke this type of myoclonus in multiple areas of the body.

groups are particularly affected; the myoclonus often occurs when patients perform an action, such as reaching for an object (action myoclonus). Limb and truncal ataxia, cerebellar outflow tremor, and dysarthria are other common accompaniments. The exact substrate of postanoxic myoclonus generation is not clear. Postanoxic myoclonus may result from cortical or subcortical injury or be due to alterations in brainstem serotonergic pathways. The serotonergic raphe nuclei have frequently been implicated.

Some forms of myoclonus, particularly those of subcortical origin, are believed to arise from the reticular system, primarily from the *nucleus reticularis gigantocellularis.* This *reticular reflex myoclonus* is characterized

by a brief electromyographic burst lasting 10 to 30 msec, with generalized bilateral synchronous activation of muscles following a distribution suggesting spread up the brainstem and down to the cord.

Essential myoclonus may be idiopathic or familial, beginning in the first to second decades of life. The neurologic examination fails to demonstrate other deficits in patients with essential myoclonus. In a few families, lower verbal scores have been reported and occasionally intellectual disability. Similar to essential tremor, alcohol may help ameliorate symptoms. In patients with *myoclonus-dystonia,* there is an autosomal pattern of inheritance, males are more affected than females, and there is a higher incidence of alcoholism and behavioral disturbances.

Plate 7.17

Brain: PART I

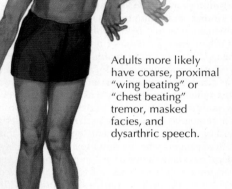

Degenerative changes in lenticular nuclei

Kayser-Fleischer ring

Adolescents more likely have generalized dystonia, with involvement of neck (torticollis) and face (grimacing), occasionally focal; hypertonicity and choreoathetosis may coexist.

Adults more likely have coarse, proximal "wing beating" or "chest beating" tremor, masked facies, and dysarthric speech.

WILSON DISEASE

Also known as hepatolenticular degeneration, Wilson disease is an autosomal recessive disorder that occurs in 1 per 30,000 individuals. The abnormal gene, *ATP7B* (adenosine triphosphate), is located on chromosome 13. The defective protein, adenosine triphosphatase, is involved in the transport and incorporation of copper into ceruloplasmin and the vesicular compartment near the canalicular membrane for further bile excretion.

Although a neurologic disorder, it affects multiple organs, with the liver being the most common and earliest affected. Approximately 40% of newly diagnosed cases have hepatic involvement. Neurologic manifestations include dysarthria, dystonia, rigidity, wing beating tremor, and choreoathetosis. Children younger than 10 years rarely present with neurologic involvement. Progressive dementia, antisocial behavior, impulsivity, and decreased intellectual performance further complicate the disease and are important manifestations. The *Kayser-Fleischer ring*, the classic ophthalmologic sign of the disease, is a yellow-brown discoloration of the Descemet membrane, best demonstrated by slit-lamp examination. In addition, sunflower cataracts may be noted. Careful bedside ophthalmologic evaluation may reveal Kayser-Fleischer rings in suspected cases. Other features include hemolytic anemia, renal failure with tubular dysfunction, nephrolithiasis, cardiomyopathy, hypoparathyroidism, amenorrhea, and testicular atrophy.

Diagnosis requires a strong index of suspicion and should be considered in all patients, particularly those younger than 40 years, those presenting with abnormal involuntary movements, and those presenting with

Brain MRI in FLAIR sequence showing bilateral symmetric abnormally increased FLAIR signal involving the bilateral basal ganglia and anterior lateral thalami

abnormal liver function. Although not specific, 24-hour urinary copper excretion and serum copper and ceruloplasmin levels are useful screening tests. The single best confirmatory test for the diagnosis is elevated hepatic copper levels, but this requires a liver biopsy, which is performed only in cases where the diagnosis is unclear but the index of suspicion is high. On neuroimaging, a brain MRI shows atrophy of the cerebrum, brainstem, and, less commonly, cerebellum. The "face of the giant panda" sign (globus pallidus hypointensity) is a characteristic finding on T2-weighted MRI seen in 34% of cases.

The copper-chelating agent D-penicillamine has been considered the gold standard of therapy. Trientine,

another copper-chelating agent, has been used in patients who cannot tolerate penicillamine. Liver transplantation is the only option in patients with cirrhosis or fulminant hepatic failure. The benefits of liver transplantation for severe neurologic symptoms remain uncertain. New data from a cohort study have shown promising results that liver transplant might reverse symptomatology to some extent or at least does not appear to cause clinical worsening.

In some cases, the MRI brain findings of hyperintensity improve or disappear. The mechanism is unknown because studies are limited.

Plate 7.18

Basal Ganglia and Movement Disorders

PSYCHOGENIC MOVEMENT DISORDERS

Psychogenic (also called functional) movement disorders are disorders without evidence of an organic etiology and for which an underlying psychiatric illness is held responsible. They have been recognized in many cultures and for many centuries. Perhaps one-third of patients diagnosed with *psychogenic disorders* eventually are found to have an organic neurologic illness but one not necessarily related to the movement disorder. A movement disorder must not be attributed to psychogenic causes simply because a definitive organic diagnosis cannot be made. It is important to await developments if a diagnosis is not apparent. With time, new features may suggest the correct diagnosis or additional information from the patient or family may suggest the relevance of psychogenic factors.

Certain features suggest a nonorganic basis for the movement disorder. These include the abrupt onset of symptoms, their variability over a short time, and their suggestibility and distractibility. Furthermore, there is often a marked disparity between symptom severity and the functional limitation to which they reportedly lead. Patients may claim that they are unable to work because of their abnormal movements, and yet they can perform activities of daily living, such as using a personal computer, shopping, cooking, and the like. In other words, any disability is selective. It is also important to enquire about a past history of psychiatric or psychogenic illness and to seek any possible secondary gain, as from pending litigation or workers' compensation, that may result from the current symptoms.

The examination findings may also be helpful, especially the general appearance and affect of the patient. There may be a combination of different dyskinesias that vary markedly in nature and distribution over time and worsen when formally examined. Other signs of nonorganic neurologic deficits may be present, such as a nonanatomic sensory loss or a lurching unsteady gait that never results in falls.

Psychogenic tremor is typically of variable frequency and can be entrained by such maneuvers as foot tapping. With mental distraction, tremors or other *hyperkinetic movement disorders* may become more intermittent, variable, or irregular. During skilled movements with the affected limb, they may cease. Loading the limb with weights may increase rather than diminish tremor amplitude. Patients with *psychogenic dystonia* sometimes report that their symptoms are especially troublesome at rest, whereas organic dystonia is often more conspicuous with volitional activity. In a *psychogenic gait disorder*, the gait is often very slow, with excessive gesturing and sometimes wild or bizarre motor activity. It typically is quite variable in severity, lessening with distraction and worsening when the patient is observed overtly.

No anatomic correlation can be made, and the neurochemical basis of the movement disorder is unknown. Patients with psychogenic movement disorders typically are unresponsive to appropriate medications, but remission may occur with treatment of the underlying psychiatric disorder. The psychiatric diagnosis may include various somatoform and factitious disorders, depression, anxiety, and histrionic personality disorders. A specific psychiatric diagnosis cannot always be made, and the neurologist and psychiatrist may differ in their assessments of the underlying problem.

Investigations should exclude possible organic causes for the patient's symptoms. These may have developed

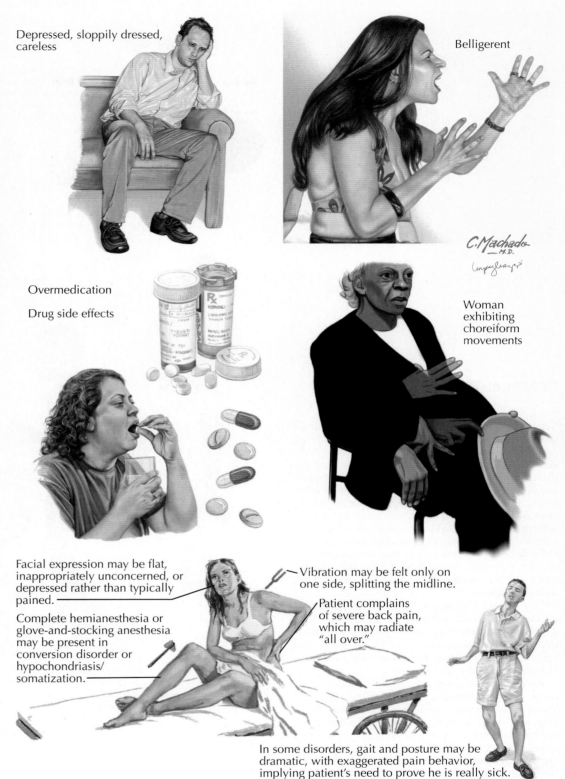

Depressed, sloppily dressed, careless

Belligerent

Overmedication

Drug side effects

Woman exhibiting choreiform movements

C. Machado — M.D.

Facial expression may be flat, inappropriately unconcerned, or depressed rather than typically pained.

Complete hemianesthesia or glove-and-stocking anesthesia may be present in conversion disorder or hypochondriasis/somatization.

Vibration may be felt only on one side, splitting the midline.

Patient complains of severe back pain, which may radiate "all over."

In some disorders, gait and posture may be dramatic, with exaggerated pain behavior, implying patient's need to prove he is really sick.

on an organic basis and then been perpetuated and elaborated psychogenically. Studies may include brain MRI, serum copper and ceruloplasmin levels, 24-hour urine copper excretion, thyroid function studies, and other tests based on clinical suspicion. The diagnostic evaluation may also include a trial of medications used for organic movement disorders. Psychiatric referral is then required, with careful follow-up of the patient.

Prognosis is variable. Features suggesting a good prognosis are acute onset, short duration of symptoms, healthy premorbid functioning, absence of other organic or psychogenic disorders, and presence of an identifiable precipitant. Treatment is difficult and individualized. It involves provision of a clear diagnosis, explanation of the nature of the disorder and of how symptoms arise, and their reversal with physical and psychologic treatments.

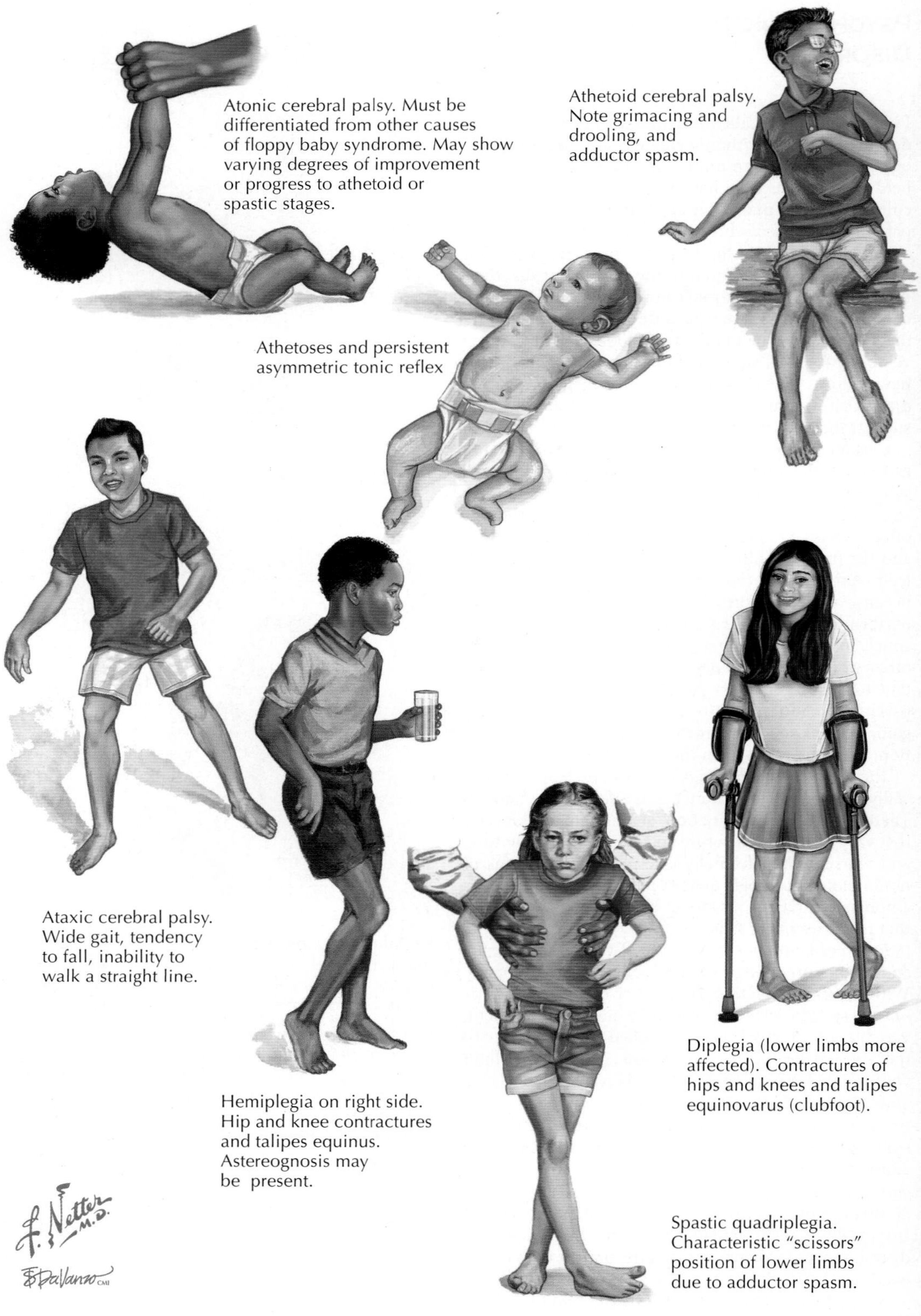

Plate 7.19

Brain: PART I

Atonic cerebral palsy. Must be differentiated from other causes of floppy baby syndrome. May show varying degrees of improvement or progress to athetoid or spastic stages.

Athetoid cerebral palsy. Note grimacing and drooling, and adductor spasm.

Athetoses and persistent asymmetric tonic reflex

Ataxic cerebral palsy. Wide gait, tendency to fall, inability to walk a straight line.

Hemiplegia on right side. Hip and knee contractures and talipes equinus. Astereognosis may be present.

Diplegia (lower limbs more affected). Contractures of hips and knees and talipes equinovarus (clubfoot).

Spastic quadriplegia. Characteristic "scissors" position of lower limbs due to adductor spasm.

CEREBRAL PALSY

Cerebral palsy (CP) is the term applied to a group of slow or nonprogressive motor impairment syndromes resulting from a variety of lesions or congenital brain anomalies. Although the initial lesion may be fixed, the clinical pattern of presentation might vary with growth and development. Its incidence is 2 to 2.5 per 1000 live births. The causes are diverse. Approximately 75% of cases are due to prenatal injury, with less than 10% due to birth trauma or asphyxia. Low birth weight and prematurity are important risk factors for the occurrence of CP. Other risk factors include chorioamnionitis, teratogenic exposures, hyperbilirubinemia, and hypoglycemia. CP has a higher incidence in twins and triplets than in singletons.

CP is a clinical diagnosis. Delays in developmental milestones are usually the earliest clue. Milestones acquired do not show regression. Other early signs include hand preference, prominent fisting, the persistence of neonatal reflexes, and delay in the emergence of protective and postural reflexes.

The topographic classification of CP includes *monoplegic, diplegic, hemiplegic,* and *quadriplegic.* Cases can also be classified into *spastic, dyskinetic, ataxic, hypotonic,* and *mixed.* Of these, spastic CP with diplegia of the lower extremities and scissoring gait is the most common, accounting for 70% to 75% of cases. Imaging demonstrates *periventricular leukomalacia* around the lateral ventricles, with ischemia as the most common pathologic finding. Mild cases manifest with toe walking, whereas severe cases have flexion of the hips, knees, and elbows.

In hemiplegic CP, the upper limb is predominantly affected. Palmar grasp reflexes may be present and can persist for years. Quadriplegic CP, the most severe form, is characterized by polyporencephaly, polymicrogyria, and schizencephaly on neuroimaging studies. Pseudobulbar signs and optic atrophy are usually present in up to 50% of affected children.

Intellectual disability (60%), visual impairment, and oculomotor impairments are common. In children who develop CP as a consequence of kernicterus, deafness, dystonia, choreoathetosis, and, to a lesser extent, ataxia are the most common clinical findings, in addition to corticospinal tract involvement in a smaller proportion of patients. These are key points to remember when assessing adults who come for an evaluation of a new movement disorder and have a history of neonatal hyperbilirubinemia. Among children with CP, 35% to 60% will have some form of epilepsy. Feeding difficulties, swallowing dysfunction, and drooling may complicate the clinical picture.

Botulinum toxin can improve the functionality and gait of these children. Injections in the upper extremities may help maintain posture or relieve contractures. There are different preparations of botulinum toxin (BoNT); however, two types of BoNT-type A are frequently used in CP, namely onabotulinum toxin A (Botox) and abobotulinum toxin A (Dysport).

CEREBELLUM AND ATAXIA

Plate 8.1

Brain: PART I

CEREBELLUM AND THE FOURTH VENTRICLE

The *fourth ventricle* lies posterior to the pons and upper half of the medulla oblongata and anterior to the cerebellum (see Plate 8.1). Its upper and lower ends become continuous, respectively, with the cerebral (sylvian, or mesencephalic) aqueduct and the central canal of the spinal cord in the lower half of the medulla. On each side, a narrow prolongation, the lateral recess, projects outward from its widest part and curves around the brainstem above the corresponding inferior (caudal) cerebellar peduncle; its lateral aperture (foramen of Luschka) lies below the cerebellar flocculus and behind the emerging rootlets of the glossopharyngeal (IX) and vagus (X) nerves. The fourth ventricle has lateral boundaries, a roof, and a floor.

The lateral boundaries are formed on each side from above down by the superior cerebellar peduncle, the inferior cerebellar peduncle, and the cuneate and gracile tubercles.

ROOF OF FOURTH VENTRICLE

The upper and lower parts of the V-shaped roof are formed by the superior and inferior medullary vela, which are thin laminae of white matter between the superior and inferior cerebellar peduncles. The lower part of the inferior velum has a median aperture (foramen of Magendie); cerebrospinal fluid escapes through this opening and the lateral aperture (foramina of Luschka) into the subarachnoid space. Because these are the only communications between the ventricular and subarachnoid spaces, their blockage can produce hydrocephalus.

The lower part of the roof and the posterior walls of the lateral recesses are invaginated by vascular tufts of pia mater, which form the T-shaped choroid plexus of the fourth ventricle.

The floor of the fourth ventricle is rhomboid shaped and is divided into symmetric halves by a vertical median sulcus. Its upper (pontine) and lower (medullary) parts are demarcated by delicate transverse strands of fibers, the striae medullares of the fourth ventricle.

On each side of the median sulcus is a longitudinal elevation, the medial eminence, lateral to which runs the sulcus limitans. Its superior part is the locus coeruleus, colored bluish-gray from a patch of deeply pigmented nerve cells. Also lateral to the upper part of the medial eminence is a slight depression, the superior fovea, and just below and medial to this fovea is a rounded swelling, the facial colliculus, which overlies the nucleus of the abducens (VI) nerve and the facial (VII) nerve fibers encircling it; the motor nucleus of the facial nerve lies more deeply in the pons. Inferolateral to the superior fovea is the upper part of the vestibular area, which overlies parts of the nuclei of the vestibulocochlear (VIII) nerve.

The lower (medullary) part of the medial eminence overlies the 12th cranial nerve nucleus and is called the hypoglossal trigone. Lateral to it is a slight depression, the inferior fovea, which, together with the neighboring vagal trigone, overlies parts of the dorsal nuclei of the glossopharyngeal and vagus nerves. Lateral to the inferior fovea is the lower part of the vestibular area, overlying parts of the vestibular nuclei of the vestibulocochlear nerve. On a deeper plane, parts of the trigeminal, solitary tract, and ambiguus nuclei also underlie the floor of the fourth ventricle. Some of the nuclei mentioned, such as the dorsal vagal and nucleus ambiguus, as well as others located in the nearby reticular formation, are concerned with cardiovascular, respiratory, metabolic, and other important functions and are regarded as vital centers. Any lesion in this relatively small area of the brain may produce disastrous results.

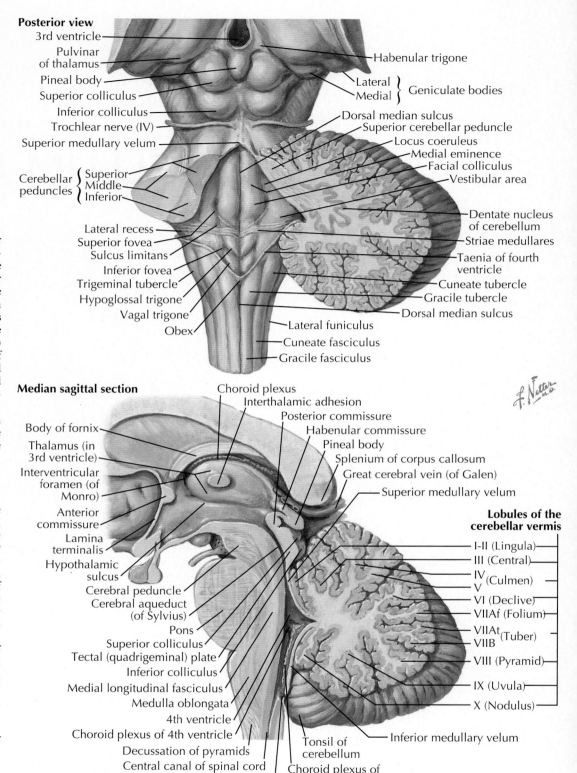

Posterior view

- 3rd ventricle
- Pulvinar of thalamus
- Pineal body
- Superior colliculus
- Inferior colliculus
- Trochlear nerve (IV)
- Superior medullary velum
- Cerebellar peduncles { Superior, Middle, Inferior }
- Lateral recess
- Superior fovea
- Sulcus limitans
- Inferior fovea
- Trigeminal tubercle
- Hypoglossal trigone
- Vagal trigone
- Obex
- Habenular trigone
- Lateral } Medial } Geniculate bodies
- Dorsal median sulcus
- Superior cerebellar peduncle
- Locus coeruleus
- Medial eminence
- Facial colliculus
- Vestibular area
- Dentate nucleus of cerebellum
- Striae medullares
- Taenia of fourth ventricle
- Cuneate tubercle
- Gracile tubercle
- Dorsal median sulcus
- Lateral funiculus
- Cuneate fasciculus
- Gracile fasciculus

Median sagittal section

- Body of fornix
- Thalamus (in 3rd ventricle)
- Interventricular foramen (of Monro)
- Anterior commissure
- Lamina terminalis
- Hypothalamic sulcus
- Cerebral peduncle
- Cerebral aqueduct (of Sylvius)
- Pons
- Superior colliculus
- Tectal (quadrigeminal) plate
- Inferior colliculus
- Medial longitudinal fasciculus
- Medulla oblongata
- 4th ventricle
- Choroid plexus of 4th ventricle
- Decussation of pyramids
- Central canal of spinal cord
- Median aperture (foramen of Magendie)
- Choroid plexus
- Interthalamic adhesion
- Posterior commissure
- Habenular commissure
- Pineal body
- Splenium of corpus callosum
- Great cerebral vein (of Galen)
- Superior medullary velum
- Tonsil of cerebellum
- Choroid plexus of 4th ventricle
- Inferior medullary velum

Lobules of the cerebellar vermis
- I-II (Lingula)
- III (Central)
- IV (Culmen)
- V
- VI (Declive)
- VIIAf (Folium)
- VIIAt (Tuber)
- VIIB
- VIII (Pyramid)
- IX (Uvula)
- X (Nodulus)

Plate 8.2

Cerebellum and Ataxia

CEREBELLUM GROSS ANATOMY

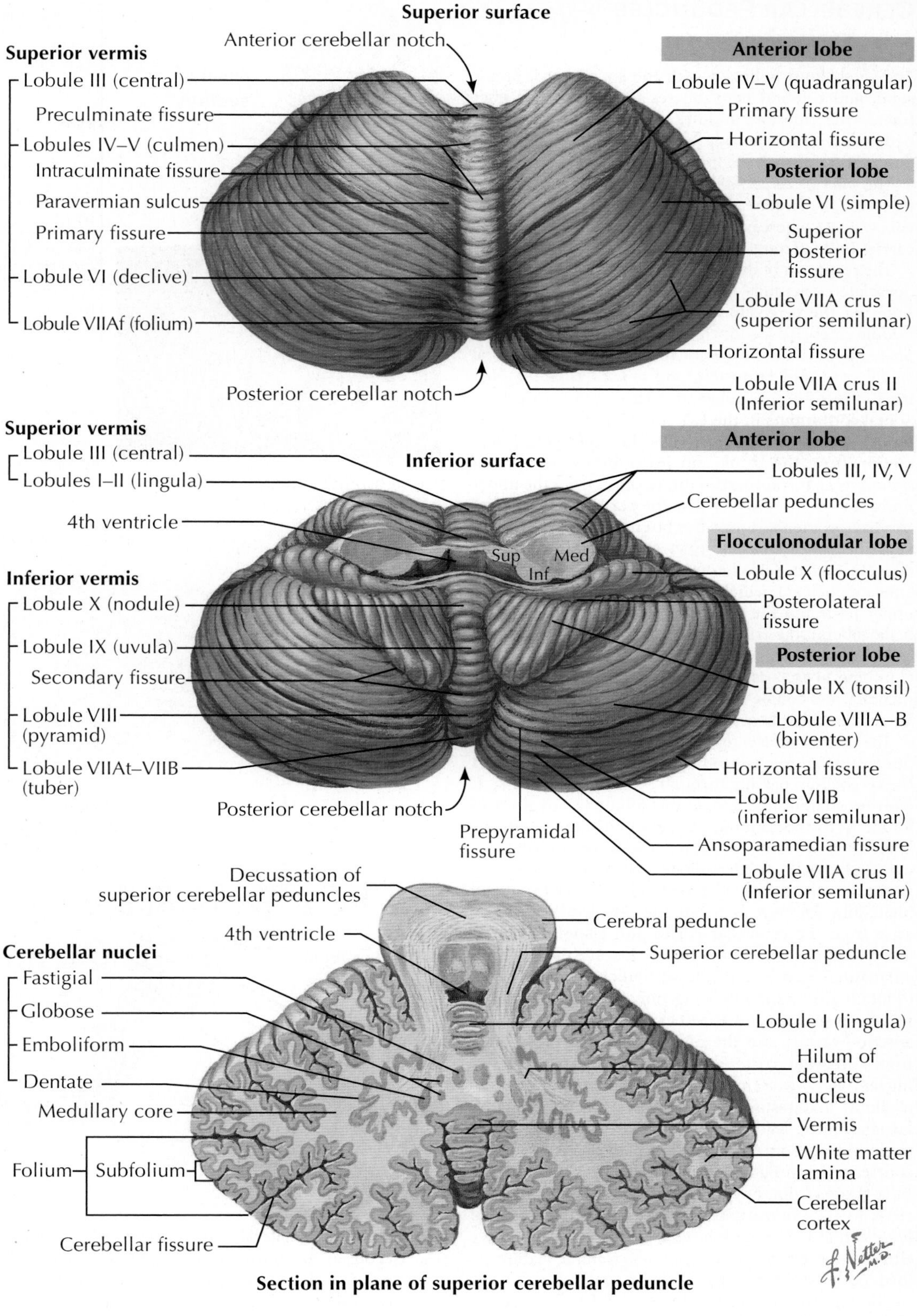

The cerebellum, from the Latin meaning *little brain,* is the largest part of the hindbrain, occupying most of the posterior fossa. In the adult human brain, the cerebellum's volume is about 144 cm³, weighing 150 grams (10% total brain weight). However, its surface area is 40% of the cerebral cortex, containing about 80% the total number of intracerebral neurons. The cerebellum, consisting of two hemispheres situated contiguously with the midline vermis, is separated from the overlying cerebrum by the tentorium cerebelli. The vermis (i.e., from the Latin, meaning *worm*) is visible posteriorly and inferiorly in the vallecula, the deep groove separating the two cerebellar hemispheres. Superiorly, in contrast, the vermis appears as a low ridge straddling the midline, extending up 10 mm bilaterally.

A wide hollow within the anterior cerebellum is occupied by the pons and upper medulla oblongata, which are separated from the cerebellum by the fourth ventricle. Posteriorly, there is a narrow median notch, lodging the falx cerebelli. The cerebellum is connected to the brainstem by three white matter tracts: the superior, middle, and inferior cerebellar peduncles (described more fully in Plate 8.3). The cerebellum's *superior* and *inferior surfaces* meet within the caudal aspect of lobule *crus I.* The cerebellum forms a sphere, and therefore the vermal lobule I/II is separated anteriorly from lobule X by the fourth ventricle.

The cerebellar surfaces include numerous narrow folia separated by parallel, curved, deeply penetrating fissures. Each folium further consists of multiple, small subfolia. The folia are grouped into 10 lobules divided by named fissures. These 10 lobules form three lobes: the *anterior, posterior,* and *flocculonodular* lobes. Lobules I to V are the *anterior lobe,* lobules VI to IX are the *posterior lobe,* and lobule X is the *flocculonodular lobe,* including the *flocculus,* which is a small, semidetached portion lying close to the middle cerebellar peduncle. Earlier cerebellum nomenclatures were not uniform (one version is in the diagrams for comparison). These are replaced by a simplified, coherent numeric system existing across different species' brains. All lobules are identifiable at the vermis; lobules III to X are continuous across the hemispheres.

The *primary fissure* separating the anterior from the posterior lobe is deepest and most evident in the midsagittal plane but not as readily identifiable externally. The *superior posterior fissure* separating lobule VI from lobule VII is well seen on the posterior superior surface. The *horizontal fissure,* prominent on the posterior, inferior, and lateral hemisphere aspects, divides lobule VIIA into two major components: lobule VIIAf at the vermis/crus I in the hemisphere and lobule VIIAt at the vermis/crus II in the hemisphere. The *paravermian sulcus* on each side of the superior cerebellar surface is an indentation formed by the superior cerebellar artery medial branch. The *retrotonsillar groove* at the inferior and medial aspect of the cerebellum is caused by the rim of the foramen magnum and delineates the *tonsil,* a gross morphologic feature comprising lobule IX and part of lobule VIIIB that becomes clinically relevant with herniation syndromes.

The interior of the cerebellum contains a central mass of white matter, the medullary core, surrounded by the deeply folded cerebellar folia. The relationship of the folia to the white matter has a tree branch appearance, hence *arbor vitae.* The *white matter* core extends into the folia as narrow laminae, surrounded by the three-layered cerebellar cortex. The white

matter consists largely of mossy and climbing fibers entering the cerebellum and axons of *Purkinje cells* (PCs) leaving the cerebellar cortex to the nuclei. There are no association fibers in the cerebellum linking cerebellar cortical areas with each other. The *cerebellar nuclei* within the medullary core include, medial to lateral, the *fastigial, globose, emboliform,* and *dentate.* These nuclei, together with other minor nuclei in the medullary core and vestibular nuclei in the posterior pons and medulla, are linked with the cerebellar

cortex and serve as the cerebellum's functional unit, namely, the *corticonuclear microcomplex.* Except for the vestibulocerebellum, these nuclei are the primary source of cerebellar efferents. These have highly organized connections with extracerebellar structures. The large, folded *dentate nucleus* is U-shaped. Its open end, or hilus, points medially, conveying fibers that, together with those from the *fastigial, globose,* and *emboliform* nuclei, form the superior cerebellar peduncle.

Superior surface

Superior vermis
- Lobule III (central)
- Preculminate fissure
- Lobules IV–V (culmen)
- Intraculminate fissure
- Paravermian sulcus
- Primary fissure
- Lobule VI (declive)
- Lobule VIIAf (folium)

Anterior cerebellar notch

Posterior cerebellar notch

Anterior lobe
- Lobule IV–V (quadrangular)
- Primary fissure
- Horizontal fissure

Posterior lobe
- Lobule VI (simple)
- Superior posterior fissure
- Lobule VIIA crus I (superior semilunar)
- Horizontal fissure
- Lobule VIIA crus II (Inferior semilunar)

Inferior surface

Superior vermis
- Lobule III (central)
- Lobules I–II (lingula)

4th ventricle

Inferior vermis
- Lobule X (nodule)
- Lobule IX (uvula)
- Secondary fissure
- Lobule VIII (pyramid)
- Lobule VIIAt–VIIB (tuber)

Sup   Med   Inf

Posterior cerebellar notch

Prepyramidal fissure

Anterior lobe
- Lobules III, IV, V
- Cerebellar peduncles

Flocculonodular lobe
- Lobule X (flocculus)
- Posterolateral fissure

Posterior lobe
- Lobule IX (tonsil)
- Lobule VIIIA–B (biventer)
- Horizontal fissure
- Lobule VIIB (inferior semilunar)
- Ansoparamedian fissure
- Lobule VIIA crus II (Inferior semilunar)

Decussation of superior cerebellar peduncles

4th ventricle

Cerebellar nuclei
- Fastigial
- Globose
- Emboliform
- Dentate
- Medullary core

Folium — Subfolium

Cerebellar fissure

Cerebral peduncle

Superior cerebellar peduncle

Lobule I (lingula)

Hilum of dentate nucleus

Vermis

White matter lamina

Cerebellar cortex

Section in plane of superior cerebellar peduncle

Plate 8.3

Brain: PART I

CEREBELLAR PEDUNCLES

The cerebellum is linked with the spinal cord, brainstem, and cerebral hemispheres by three major fiber tracts—the inferior, middle, and superior cerebellar peduncles. These convey axons into the cerebellum (afferent) or away from it (efferent).

The *inferior cerebellar peduncle* (ICP) has two components. The larger is the *restiform body,* a purely afferent system, whereas the smaller *juxtarestiform body* carries both afferent and efferent fibers.

The restiform body (or ICP proper) is located in the dorsolateral medulla, lateral to the vestibular nuclei. Entering the cerebellum, it is situated medial to the middle cerebellar peduncle, conveying *uncrossed mossy fiber* afferents to the cerebellum from the ipsilateral spinal cord and brainstem and *crossed climbing fiber* inputs from the contralateral inferior olivary nucleus. Spinal cord inputs in the ICP are from the *dorsal (posterior) spinocerebellar tract* (DSCT), conveying information from the trunk and lower limbs. The *rostral spinocerebellar tract* carries information from the upper limbs and the *central cervical tract* arising from upper cervical segments. From the brainstem, the ICP conveys the *cuneocerebellar tract* arising in the external cuneate nucleus (also known as the lateral or accessory cuneate nucleus), which conveys information from the upper limb and the reticular formation (reticulocerebellar fibers), the trigeminal principal sensory nucleus (trigeminocerebellar fibers), and the midline raphe. Climbing fibers arise in the inferior olive, cross in the medulla, and course within the ICP to reach the contralateral cerebellar hemisphere.

The *juxtarestiform body* is a small aggregation of fibers situated medial to the restiform body that enters the cerebellum passing through the vestibular nuclei. It conveys afferent fibers to vermal lobule IX (uvula) and lobule X (the flocculonodular lobe). Primary vestibular afferents arise from the vestibular sense organs (the saccule and utricle) and terminate ipsilaterally; secondary vestibular fibers from the vestibular nuclei terminate bilaterally. Efferent fibers in the juxtarestiform body arise from the cerebellar cortex and fastigial nucleus. Cerebellar cortical axons in the juxtarestiform body emanating from PCs in the vestibulocerebellum (part of lobule IX, and lobule X) terminate in Deiters lateral vestibular nucleus and, together with efferents from the anterior vermis, are the only instance of projections from cerebellar cortex bypassing the deep cerebellar nuclei (DCN) to terminate on a target outside the cerebellum. Juxtarestiform body fibers arising from the fastigial nuclei lead to the vestibular and the reticular nuclei. Axons from the rostral half of the fastigial nucleus course to the ipsilateral brainstem in the *fastigiobulbar tract.* Axons from the caudal half of the fastigial nucleus cross to the contralateral cerebellum in the *uncinate bundle,* that is, the hook bundle of Russell, before traveling to the brainstem in the contralateral juxtarestiform body (see Plate 8.10).

The *middle cerebellar peduncle* (MCP) is a massive tract situated at the lateral aspect of the basis pontis. Axons leave the pontine nuclei, cross to the opposite side of the pons, and course in the contralateral MCP to the cerebellum. The pontine nuclei are an obligatory intermediate link between the ipsilateral corticopontine input via the cerebral peduncle and the contralateral pontocerebellar projections by way of the MCP. A minor projection from cerebellar nuclei back to the pons is also present.

The *superior cerebellar peduncle* (SCP) transmits efferents from and afferents to the cerebellum. It lies

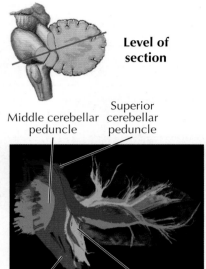

Level of section

Superior cerebellar peduncle

Middle cerebellar peduncle

Corticospinal tract   Inferior cerebellar peduncle

Peduncle	Input (afferents)	Output (efferents)	

Inferior (restiform body)	Spinocerebellar
	  Dorsal
	  Rostral
	  Cuneocerebellar
	Olive-cerebellar
	Reticulocerebellar
	Trigeminocerebellar
	Raphe-cerebellar
		Fastigiobulbar, Uncinate fasciculus	To vestibular and reticular nuclei

Juxtarestiform body	Vestibulospinal (primary, secondary)	Direct cerebellovestibular (to lateral vestibular nucleus)	
Middle (brachium pontis)	Pontocerebellar		

Superior (brachium conjunctivum)	Ventral
	  spinocerebellar
	Trigeminocerebellar
	Tectocerebellar
	  Superior colliculus
	  Inferior colliculus
	Coeruleocerebellar
		Dentatothalamic
		Dentatorubral
		Dentatoreticular
		Interpositus-rubral
		  connections
		  (globose, emboliform)
		Cerebello-olivary	

Image from Takahashi E, Song JW, et al. Detection of postmortem human cerebellar cortex and white matter pathways using high angular resolution diffusion tractography: a feasibility study. Neuroimage. 2013;68:105-11.

Globose nucleus

Fastigial nucleus   **Cerebellum**   Superior cerebellar peduncle   Inferior cerebellar peduncle

Emboliform nucleus   Middle cerebellar peduncle

Dentate nucleus

Fourth ventricle

Medial longitudinal fasciculus

Lateral vestibular nucleus

Tectospinal tract

Genu of CN VII

Medial lemniscus

Nucleus CN VI

Corticospinal tract

Nucleus CN VII

Pontine nuclei

JOHN A. CRAIG—AD   **Pons**

within the posterolateral wall of the fourth ventricle and ascends as the *brachium conjunctivum* to the midbrain, where it decussates and continues rostrally, carrying ascending projections from the cerebellum to the reticular nuclei in the pons and midbrain, red nucleus, hypothalamic area, and thalamus. The hilus of the dentate nucleus is continuous with the SCP, but there are also axons in the SCP arising from the fastigial, globose, and emboliform nuclei. A descending branch of the SCP leaves the larger ascending component in the rostral pons, descends in the pontomedullary tegmentum, and crosses obliquely to the opposite side of the ventral medulla to terminate in the inferior olive (the cerebello-olivary projection). Afferents to the cerebellum coursing in the SCP arise in the spinal cord and

brainstem. These include crossed ventral (anterior) spinocerebellar tract fibers conveying information concerning the contralateral trunk and lower limbs and both crossed and uncrossed fibers in the central cervical tract. Ipsilateral afferents include tectocerebellar projections from the superior and inferior colliculi in the midbrain, trigeminocerebellar fibers from the trigeminal mesencephalic nucleus, and coeruleocerebellar projections from the locus coeruleus in the pons.

The three peduncles are differentially affected by ischemic, compressive, demyelinating, neurodegenerative, and other disorders. Clinically, peduncle lesion manifestations are heterogeneous, reflecting the wide range of functions subserved by the information they convey between the cerebellum and the remainder of the neuraxis.

Plate 8.4

Cerebellum and Ataxia

CEREBELLAR CORTEX AND NUCLEI: NEURONAL ELEMENTS

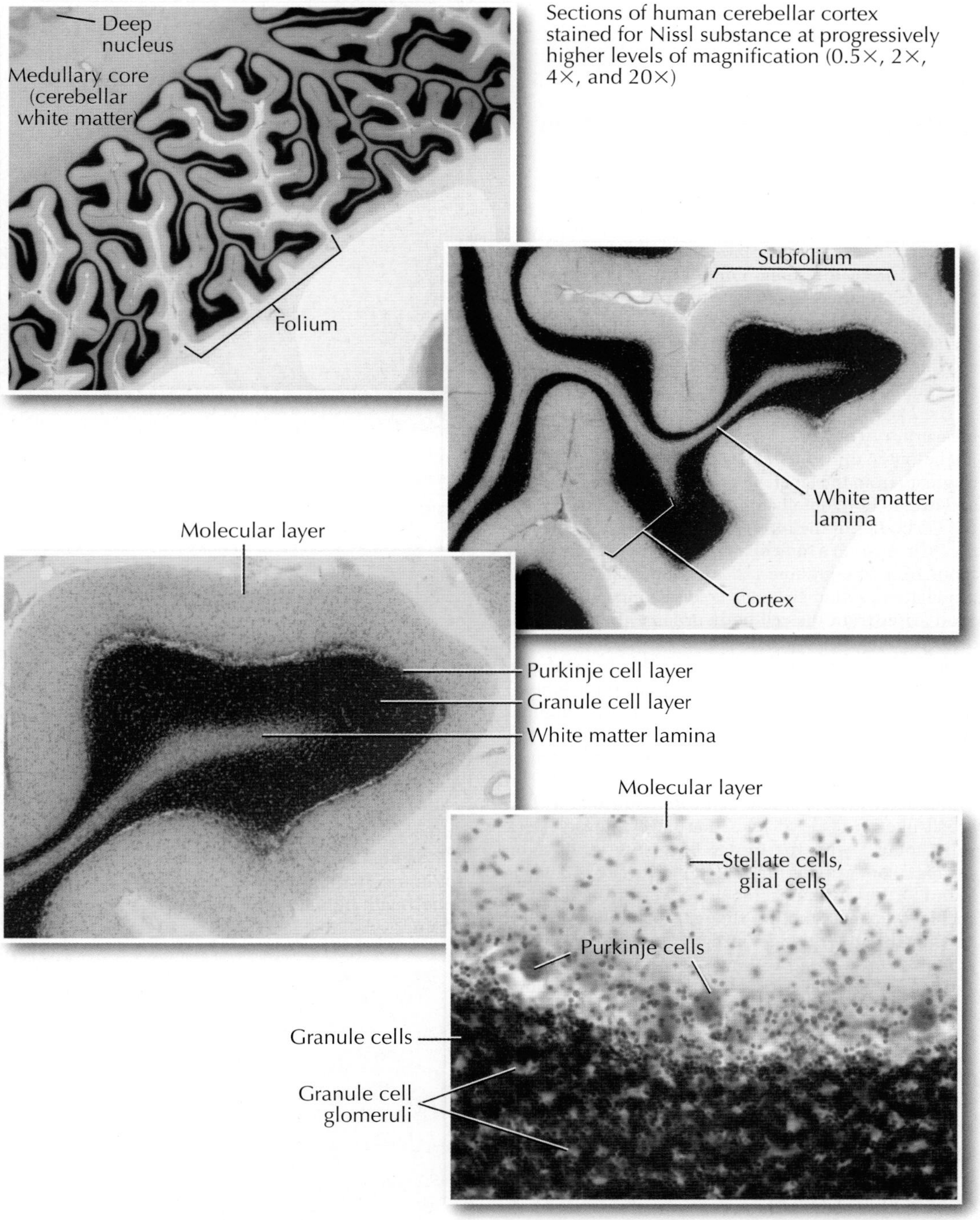

Deep nucleus

Medullary core (cerebellar white matter)

Folium

Sections of human cerebellar cortex stained for Nissl substance at progressively higher levels of magnification (0.5×, 2×, 4×, and 20×)

Subfolium

White matter lamina

Cortex

Molecular layer

Purkinje cell layer

Granule cell layer

White matter lamina

Molecular layer

Stellate cells, glial cells

Purkinje cells

Granule cells

Granule cell glomeruli

CEREBELLAR CORTEX AND NUCLEI

The histology of the cerebellar cortex differs fundamentally from that of the cerebral cortex in that it has essentially the same paracrystalline structure throughout. The trilaminate cortex, the *PC layer* lying between the innermost *granular layer* and the outermost *molecular layer,* is apposed on each side of a white matter lamella conveying fibers to and from the cortex (see Plates 8.4 and 8.5).

The *PC layer* is a monolayer composed entirely of PCs, a 100-μm-thick sheet of 15 million neurons situated between the molecular and granular layers. The PC is the defining neuron of the cerebellum. It is among the largest cells in the nervous system, with a pear-shaped soma (35 × 70 μm) and a fan-like appearance of its dendritic tree. The proximal dendrite divides into two major dendrites that branch multiple times to form a flattened plate (400 × 20 μm) in the parasagittal plane oriented perpendicular to the long axis of the folium. Each PC has over 150,000 spines, with a density 25 times higher on distal dendrites, where parallel fibers (PFs) synapse, than on proximal dendrites, where climbing fibers synapse. The PC is the only neuron with axons leaving the cerebellar cortex. The axon descends through a constricted region surrounded by the pinceau of basket cell axon terminals, acquires a myelin sheath, and descends to the DCN or vestibular nuclei. Recurrent collaterals course back toward the molecular layer, inhibiting interneurons as well as the soma and proximal dendrites of neighboring PCs.

The *molecular layer* is 300 μm thick. It contains *granule cell* axons and PFs, dendritic arborizations of PCs and *Golgi interneurons,* and cell bodies of *basket, stellate,* and *supporting glial cells.*

Parallel fibers are formed when the granule cell axon ascends through the PC layer into the molecular layer and branches in the shape of a T to form the PF, one of the thinnest vertebrate axons. It travels parallel to the long axis of the folium for 1 to 3 mm in the rat and cat and possibly 6 to 8 mm in primates.

The *basket cell* lies in the lower third of the molecular layer just above the PCs. Its dendrites extend up into the molecular layer in a fan-shaped field 30 μm wide in the parasagittal plane (the same plane as the PC dendritic tree), giving off relatively few branches, interdigitating with the dendritic fields of the PCs, and contacting the PFs. Its axon courses in the parasagittal plane among the lower dendrites of 9 or 10 PCs. It emits a succession of descending branches that envelop the PC somata in an axonal sheath with numerous synaptic contacts, giving the basket cell its name. Terminal axonal branches surround the initial segment of the PC axon in a dense fiber plexus with the appearance of an old paintbrush (French, *pinceau*). This axo-axonic complex is unique in the mammalian nervous system. Sparse ascending collaterals from the basket cell axon synapse on secondary and tertiary PC dendrites.

Stellate cells are small, 5 to 10 μm in diameter, with short, profusely branching dendrites contacted by parallel fibers and axons that terminate on PC dendrites. *Superficial stellate cells* in the upper molecular layer have short axons oriented in the parasagittal plane.

Deep stellate cells in the middle part of the molecular layer have long axons up to 450 μm in the parasagittal plane, providing ascending and descending collaterals early in their course, but they rarely enter the pericellular PC plexus and do not participate in the pinceau.

The *granular layer* is 200 to 300 μm deep and contains granule, Golgi, Lugaro, and unipolar brush cells. *Granule cells* number about 50 billion, 3000 per single PC. They have minimal cytoplasm, are among the smallest neurons in the brain (6–8 μm diameter), and are the most numerous. Their density renders the granule cell layer a deep blue on stains such as Nissl, which label nuclear material. The granule cell has three to five claw-like branched dendrites that participate in the

granule cell glomerulus, pale islands between the granule cells containing a complex articulation between terminal rosettes of mossy fiber afferents, arborizations of granule cell dendrites, and Golgi cell axons. The granule cell axon ascends into the molecular layer where its PFs provide excitatory input to the PCs.

Golgi cells are irregularly rounded or polygonal inhibitory interneurons numbering approximately 1 per 1.5 PCs. In contrast to the PC, basket, and stellate cells, the Golgi cell dendritic tree has a three-dimensional configuration. Large Golgi cells, 10 to 24 μm in diameter, lie in the upper half of the granular layer, their dendrites arising as one or two main trunks with subsidiary branches that ascend to the outer zone of the

Plate 8.5

Brain: PART I

CEREBELLAR CORTEX: NEURONAL ELEMENTS

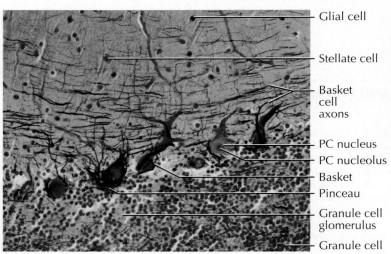

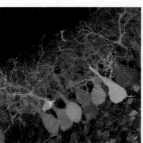

Brainbow image of Purkinje cells and granule cells in mouse, derived by mapping the differential expression of multiple fluorescent proteins in individual neurons. Courtesy Tamily Weissman, PhD. The Brainbow mouse was produced by Livet J, Weissman TA, Kang H, Draft RW, Lu J, Bennis RA, Sanes JR, Lichtman JW. *Nature* 2007;450:56-62.

Cerebellar cortex studied with Bielschowsky silver stain (20×)
Courtesy Dr. Matthew P. Frosch.

CEREBELLAR CORTEX AND NUCLEI (Continued)

molecular layer. Smaller Golgi cells (9 to 18 μm) are in the depths of the granular layer, with dendrites that radiate out from the soma. One to three axons emerge from the Golgi cell body or from proximal dendrites and divide repeatedly, resulting in a multitude of fine branches that form an elaborate, dense plexus extending throughout the granular layer and participating in the granule cell glomerulus.

The *Lugaro cell* is a fusiform inhibitory interneuron measuring 10 by 30 μm, lying horizontally or obliquely in the outer third of the granular layer. Its dendrites originate from the tapering extremities at the two poles and extend horizontally for up to 600 μm at the level of the PC bodies in the infraganglionic plexus formed by the PC recurrent axon collaterals. It receives excitatory input from the granule cell axon and serotoninergic modulation acting through volume transmission. Its axon arises from the cell body or large proximal dendrite, forming two types of axonal plexuses. One parasagittal axon contacts the soma and dendrites of stellate and basket cells in the molecular layer; the other is transverse and contacts Golgi cells in the granular layer.

The *unipolar brush cell* (UBC) is the only excitatory interneuron in the cerebellum. The soma is 9 to 12 μm in diameter, with a single dendrite ending in a tight brush-like tip of dendrioles that have extensive synaptic contact with the mossy fiber rosette. Its axon synapses on granule and Golgi cells. The UBC is found in the vestibulocerebellum, vermis, and dorsal cochlear nucleus, and it is thought to amplify vestibular signals and provide feed-forward excitation to granule cells.

Glial cells in the cerebellum include protoplasmic astrocytes that envelop the PC perikaryon in a neuroglial sheath, Bergmann glial cells in the PC layer that are involved in neural migration and development of the cerebellar cortex and that play a role in regulating glutamatergic neural transmission in the mature cerebellum, and oligodendroglia in cerebellar white matter and in the granular layer.

CEREBELLAR NUCLEI

The fastigial, globose, emboliform, and dentate nuclei are together termed the DCN to differentiate them from the precerebellar nuclei. The fastigial nucleus is the homologue of the medial nucleus in lower primates, whereas the posterior and anterior interpositus nuclei are homologous with the globose and emboliform nuclei, respectively. Among the cerebellar nuclei, the dentate, or lateral nucleus in lower vertebrates, has evolved most. The posterior (dorsal) part with small narrow folds (microgyric) contains large cells and is phylogenetically older. The macrogyric anterior (ventral) and lateral part contains smaller neurons and has expanded greatly in concert with the association cortex of the cerebral hemispheres. This is important from the perspective of anthropology as well as cognitive neuroscience and behavioral neurology. The Deiters lateral vestibular nucleus is located in the dorsal medulla. It

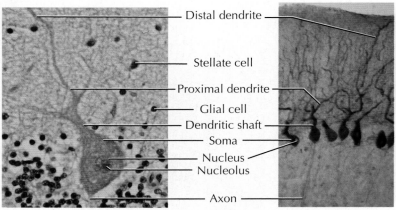

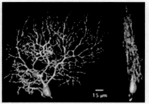

3D reconstruction of Lucifer yellow-filled PC viewed perpendicular to *(left)* and parallel to *(right)* the long axis of the folium. *From Rossi DJ, Alford S, Mugnaini E, Slater NT. Properties of transmission at a giant glutamatergic synapse in cerebellum: the mossy fiber-unipolar brush cell synapse. J Neurophysiol. 1995;74:24-42.*

Purkinje cell and adjacent cortex (20×) stained with hematoxylin and eosin
Courtesy Dr. Matthew P. Frosch.

Cerebellar cortex immunostained with calbindin (10×)

CEREBELLAR NUCLEI

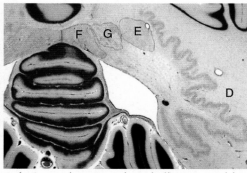

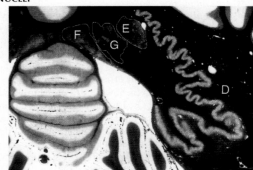

Left: Coronal section of cerebellum stained for Nissl substance shows the fastigial (F), globose (G), emboliform (E), and dentate (D) nuclei. *Right:* Similar section stained for myelin. *From Schmahmann J, Doyon J, Toga A, Petrides M, Evans A. MRI atlas of the human cerebellum. Elsevier; 2000.*

receives PC axons directly from the vestibulocerebellum and part of the anterior vermis and is equivalent to a DCN.

The neurons of the DCN are outnumbered by the PCs of the cerebellar cortex by about 26 to 1. Each PC contacts approximately 35 nuclear neurons, and each DCN neuron receives inputs from more than 800 PCs. The cytologic features of the DCN suggest anatomic subdivisions that may have connectional and functional relevance, but these are not sufficiently definitive to formally subdivide the nuclei further. Neurons in the

DCN are of three types. *Large glutamatergic neurons* convey excitatory output to the thalamus and brainstem and nucleocortical projections back to the cerebellar cortex; small γ-aminobutyric acid (GABA)-ergic neurons are inhibitory to the inferior olivary nucleus; and small glycinergic neurons in the DCN are thought to be inhibitory intranuclear interneurons. It is now possible to identify the DCN on magnetic resonance imaging (MRI) by taking advantage of its iron content, although detailed organization is not apparent with available technology.

Plate 8.6

Cerebellum and Ataxia

CEREBELLAR NEURONAL CIRCUITRY

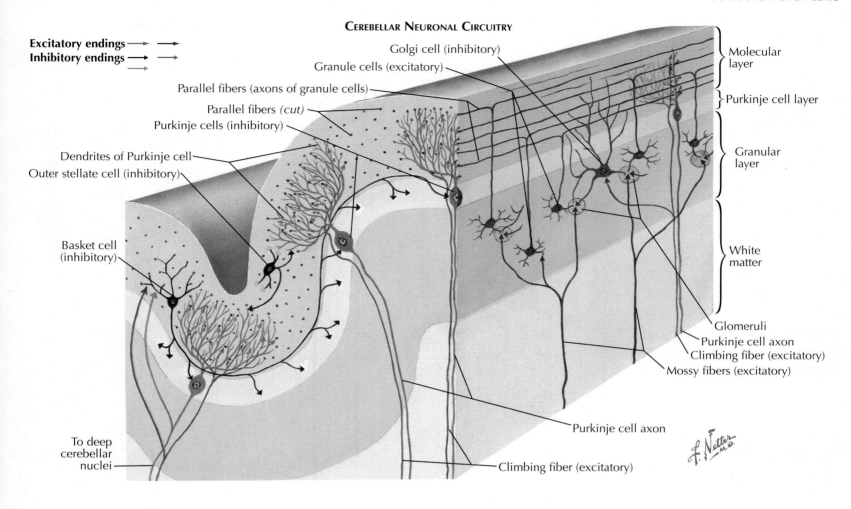

Excitatory endings ⟶
Inhibitory endings ⟶

Golgi cell (inhibitory)
Granule cells (excitatory)
Parallel fibers (axons of granule cells)
Parallel fibers (cut)
Purkinje cells (inhibitory)
Dendrites of Purkinje cell
Outer stellate cell (inhibitory)
Basket cell (inhibitory)
To deep cerebellar nuclei

Molecular layer
Purkinje cell layer
Granular layer
White matter
Glomeruli
Purkinje cell axon
Climbing fiber (excitatory)
Mossy fibers (excitatory)
Purkinje cell axon
Climbing fiber (excitatory)

CEREBELLAR CORTICAL AND CORTICONUCLEAR CIRCUITRY

The neurons of the cerebellar cortex and nuclei are linked together in multiple repeating anatomic microcircuits—corticonuclear microcomplexes—that serve as the essential functional unit of the cerebellum. The key to their elucidation is the dual nature of the cerebellar inputs: the climbing fiber and mossy fiber systems. Monoaminergic fibers from the brainstem are an additional minor source of cerebellar afferents.

Climbing fibers (CFs) arise exclusively from the *inferior olive*. Axons of olivary neurons branch to form 7 to 10 CFs. Each CF provides extensive *excitatory* synaptic contact with the dendritic tree of a single PC (between 1000 and 1500 synaptic contacts between a CF and its PC). CFs enter the cerebellum through the ICP; branch in the white matter, where they emit collaterals to the DCN; and ascend to the molecular layer. In the lower two-thirds of the molecular layer, the CF is tightly wound around the trunk and major proximal branches of the PC dendritic tree. Each varicosity of a CF synapses with several dendritic spines arising from the same dendritic branch. Fine tendrils that branch off the CF in the molecular layer synapse with ascending branches of the basket cell axon and with the dendritic trees of stellate and Golgi cells. The olivocerebellar projection is organized according to a strict mediolateral parasagittal zonal pattern (see Plate 8.12).

Mossy fibers (MFs) are named for their thickened terminals that have thick, short, divergent, varicose branches resembling moss. Their synaptic arborizations are termed *rosettes,* have a variety of shapes, and are located along the course of the MF in the granular layer at the branch points and at their sites of terminations. MFs are heavily myelinated and convey *excitatory afferents* to the cerebellar cortex from the spinal cord, brainstem (except the olive), and the cerebral hemispheres. They enter through all three cerebellar peduncles, giving off 20 to 30 collateral branches in the white matter of the folium as they course toward the granular layer. They also provide collaterals to the DCN. Many MFs terminate bilaterally in the cerebellum after crossing in the cerebellar white matter. Unlike the CF, the MF provides excitatory input to the PC indirectly. The MF rosette is the central component of the granule cell glomerulus, the complex articulation between MF rosettes and the terminal arborizations of granule cell dendrites. Each MF rosette makes excitatory synaptic contact with 50 to 100 dendritic terminals from up to 20 granule cells and receives inhibitory feedback from the descending axons of Golgi cells. The granule cell axon ascends toward the molecular layer, making synaptic contact with dendrites of Golgi cells in the granular layer and spines of the proximal dendrites of PCs in the molecular layer. Upon reaching the molecular layer, the granule cell axon divides to form PFs, the two branches traveling in opposite directions along the folium. The PFs make synaptic contact with one or two spiny branchlets on intermediate and distal

regions of the dendritic trees of up to 300 PCs along the folium.

Each PC receives synaptic inputs from approximately 200,000 PFs. In addition to excitatory inputs to the PCs from MFs and CFs, the PCs participate in a bidirectional corticonuclear projection, receiving excitatory feedback back from those regions of the DCN and vestibular nuclei to which the PC inhibitory projection is directed. The PCs receive inhibitory inputs from interneurons in the molecular layer—stellate cells, basket cells, and Lugaro cells, all of which receive excitatory afferents from the ascending granule cell axon and the PFs. Recurrent axon collaterals of the PCs are also inhibitory. The dendrites of the UBC in the vestibulocerebellum, the only excitatory cerebellar interneuron, receive MF inputs within the granule cell glomerulus. The net effect of these finely balanced interactions is that inputs to cerebellum are excitatory, output from the cortex via the PC is inhibitory, and output from the cerebellum via the DCN is excitatory to the thalamus and brainstem but inhibitory to the inferior olive.

The output from the cerebellar cortex is derived exclusively from PCs, precisely organized, and directed toward the DCN and precerebellar nuclei. PCs in each lobule project to those parts of the DCN closest to them. Thus the vermis projects to the fastigial nucleus, the intermediate cortex to the globose and emboliform nuclei, and much of the lateral hemispheres project to the dentate nucleus. More detail on cerebellar corticonuclear circuits, modules, and microzones is presented in Plate 8.12.

Plate 8.7

Brain: PART I

CIRCUIT DIAGRAM OF AFFERENT CONNECTIONS IN THE CEREBELLUM

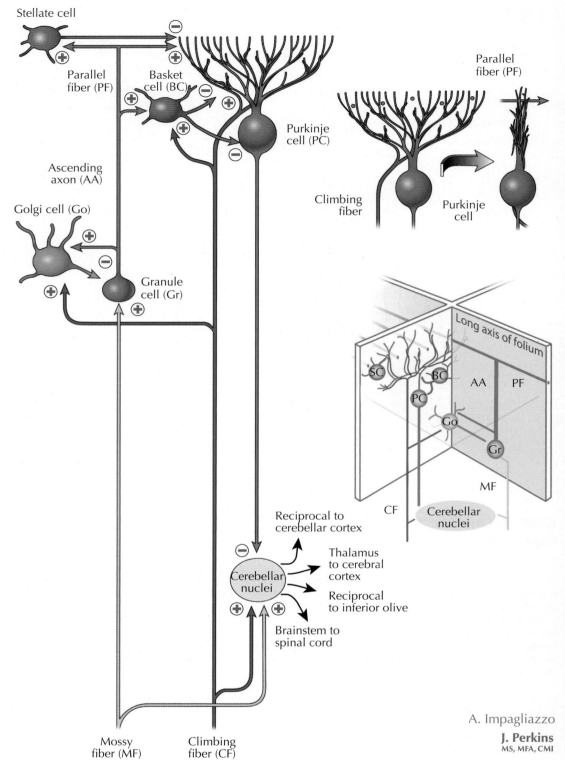

A. Impagliazzo

J. Perkins
MS, MFA, CMI

CEREBELLAR CORTICAL AND CORTICONUCLEAR CIRCUITRY (Continued)

The two major neurotransmitters in the cerebellum are glutamate and GABA. Glutamate is excitatory and is found in the MFs, PFs, CFs, UBCs, and DCN neurons that project to thalamus, brainstem, and cerebellar cortex. GABA is inhibitory and is utilized by the PCs, all remaining cerebellar interneurons (stellate, basket, Golgi, Lugaro), and the DCN neurons that project to the inferior olive. Glycine is present in inhibitory interneurons in the DCN. A number of other peptide neurotransmitters are present also in the afferent fibers and neurons of the cerebellar cortex.

The PC generates two different classes of action potentials in response to its principal afferents. The input of hundreds of MFs produces a brief burst of repetitive simple spikes, 50 to 150 per second. The inhibitory basket and stellate cell interneurons produce inhibition of PCs locally and for some distance lateral to the longitudinal strip of active parallel fibers. Therefore MF-induced PC activity consists of a brief burst of action potentials along the course of active parallel fibers, surrounded by a band of inhibited cells. PC excitation is further restricted by *Golgi cells,* which receive excitatory PF synapses on their apical dendrites and provide a mostly tonic inhibitory input to the glomerulus, decreasing the excitability of granule cells to MF afferents. PF input is thought to provide information about incoming signals, such as direction and speed of limb movement. In the cognitive domain, the PF may provide the PC with the context in which behaviors occur.

CF input to the PC induces a complex spike with the very low frequency of 0.5 to 2 spikes per second, the same rate of firing as the olivary neurons from which the CF originates. The CF input to the PC is thought to signal the occurrence of errors. The MF-CF inputs to the PC are relevant to synaptic plasticity involved in learning and memory. Long-term depression (LTD) is characterized by the persistent depression of synaptic transmission from PFs to the PC that occurs when parallel and CF activation is concurrent. Long-term potentiation (LTP) has also been described. The balance of LTD and LTP enables the cerebellar cortex to adapt to errors by regulating cortical output either down or up.

These corticonuclear circuits and physiology are the basis of theories that the cerebellum functions as an adaptive filter, utilizing internal models to maintain behaviors around a homeostatic baseline, and optimizes cerebellar influence upon motor, cognitive, or limbic behaviors appropriate to the prevailing context. The paracrystalline structure of cerebellar cortical architecture and organization has led to the idea that it has a general signal-transforming ability, a universal cerebellar transform, which is applied to multiple domains of neurologic function. The role of the cerebellum in the nervous system is a result, then, of the combination of the uniform cerebellar structure and function and the complex and varied connections of the cerebellar microcircuits, with extracerebellar areas conveyed by the MF and CF inputs and the corticonuclear outputs.

Plate 8.8

Cerebellum and Ataxia

CEREBELLUM SUBDIVISIONS AND AFFERENT PATHWAYS

The cerebellum is divided into three lobes: anterior, posterior, and flocculonodular (see Plate 8.2). It is also divided into three mediolateral subregions on the basis of phylogeny and function. The *archicerebellum*, or vestibulocerebellum, includes vermal and hemispheric parts of lobule X (flocculonodular lobe), parts of vermal lobule IX (uvula), and lobule I/II (lingula); it is linked with the vestibular nuclei and is concerned with eye movements and equilibrium. The *paleocerebellum*, or spinocerebellum, in vermal and paravermal lobules III through VI and lobule VIII, receives cutaneous and kinesthetic afferents from spinal cord, brainstem, and cerebral hemispheres. The *anterior vermis* is linked with the *rostral fastigial nucleus,* influences the medial motor system through brainstem vestibulospinal and reticulospinal projections, and controls trunk and girdle muscles enabling balance and gait. *Paravermal areas* are linked with the interpositus nuclei, the posterior part of the dentate nucleus, red nucleus, and primary motor cortex, influencing descending lateral motor systems and controlling distal limb movements. The *neocerebellum* (pontocerebellum) includes lobules VI and VII at the vermis and hemispheres. It receives afferents from cerebral cortex through the pons. Lateral *cerebellar hemispheres* project via the ventral dentate nucleus to thalamus and cerebral association areas; the *posterior vermis* is linked through the caudal fastigial nucleus with limbic areas. It appears that the neocerebellum is involved in cognition and emotion.

Knowledge of cerebellar connections with extracerebellar structures is critical to understanding the diverse roles of the cerebellum and the consequences of cerebellar injury. Afferents to cerebellum are conveyed predominantly by MFs and CFs that are organized in a fundamentally different manner (see Plates 8.6 and 8.7).

MOSSY FIBER PATHWAYS

Spinocerebellar Pathways

Sensory afferents from the spinal cord terminate in a somatotopic fashion in the primary sensorimotor representation in lobules III through V and the secondary sensorimotor representation in lobule VIII, with collateral inputs to the DCN. The trunk and lower limbs are subserved by the dorsal and ventral spinocerebellar tracts, and the head, neck, and upper extremities by the cuneocerebellar, rostral spinocerebellar, and central cervical tracts. These are all uncrossed, ascending in the ipsilateral spinal cord, except for the ventral (anterior) spinocerebellar tract (VSCT), which decussates and ascends on the contralateral side.

The dorsal (posterior) spinocerebellar tract (DSCT) and the cuneocerebellar tract (CCT) convey analogous proprioceptive and exteroceptive information from the hindlimb and forelimb, respectively. Both enter cerebellum via the ICP. *Proprioceptive* information comes from (1) muscle spindle afferents that signal *muscle length* (groups Ia and II fibers) and (2) Golgi tendon organs that signal *muscle tension* (group Ib fibers). DSCT or CCT neurons convey information regarding closely related muscles; some relay information from joint receptors. *Exteroceptive* signals provide the cerebellum with cutaneous afferents originating from touch and hair-movement receptors in small areas of skin. The DSCT in the posterolateral funiculus conveys proprioceptive and exteroceptive afferents from the trunk and legs, arising in *Clarke's column* in lamina VII of the

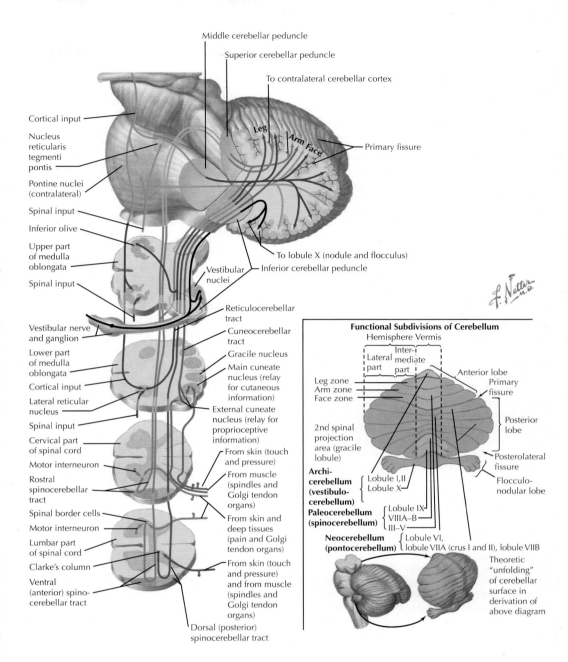

dorsal horn at spinal segments C8 to L3. It terminates in hindlimb projection areas in the intermediate part of the ipsilateral anterior lobe and lobule VIII. The CCT ascends from the medulla, conveying *proprioceptive* afferents from the arms, originating in the external cuneate nucleus, and *exteroceptive* fibers from the main cuneate nucleus.

The *ventral (anterior) spinocerebellar tract* and *rostral spinocerebellar tract* (RSCT) convey information to cerebellum regarding complex motor repertoires. Afferents arise from (1) interneurons within spinal motor centers controlling the hindlimbs (VSCT) and forelimbs (RSCT), (2) group I muscle afferents from Golgi tendon organs in groups of muscles involved in synchronized movements, and (3) multisynaptic spinal pathways activated by cutaneous and high-threshold muscle afferents. The VSCT originates from spinal border cells, mostly in Rexed lamina VII at the posterolateral aspect of the anterior horn of the lumbosacral spinal cord. It decussates

close to the cell bodies, ascends in the contralateral anterolateral funiculus, and enters the cerebellum through the SCP. Most of its fibers cross to the other side; hence the double crossing. It terminates in longitudinal zones in the hindlimb representations in the anterior lobe and, to a lesser extent, in lobule VIII. The RSCT originates from neurons at the base of the posterior spinal horn in Rexed lamina VII at spinal cord levels C4 to C8, ascends in the ipsilateral posterolateral funiculus, and enters the cerebellum via both the ICP and SCP, terminating bilaterally in primary and secondary forelimb sensorimotor representations. The corticospinal system facilitates excitatory or inhibitory effects of cutaneous and muscle afferent fibers in the VSCT and RSCT, whereas the reticulospinal system inhibits them. The rubrospinal and propriospinal pathways produce excitation independent of spinal afferents.

Sensory afferents from C1 through C4 are conveyed in the *central cervical tract.* This arises in the *central*

Plate 8.9

Brain: PART I

CEREBELLUM SUBDIVISIONS AND AFFERENT PATHWAYS (Continued)

cervical nucleus in Rexed layer VII, which integrates information related to head rotation, such as group I afferent input from neck muscles and vestibular input from semicircular canals. The central cervical tract carries information via the ICP and SCP to the anterior lobe and lobule VIII.

Trigeminocerebellar projections from the principal trigeminal sensory nucleus travel in the ICP to the face representation in caudal lobule V and lobule VI; in contrast, cerebellar projections from the *mesencephalic trigeminal nucleus* travel in the SCP. The *tectocerebellar tract* from the superior and inferior colliculi bilaterally projects to lobules VIII and IX (the posterior, or dorsal, paraflocculus and uvula), and the vermal visual area in lobule VII.

Reticulocerebellar projections act over wide areas of the cerebellum and DCN. They originate from the *lateral reticular nucleus* (LRN) and *paramedian reticular nucleus* in the medulla, the *nucleus reticularis tegmenti pontis* (NRTP) in the pons, and the *medial (magnocellular) reticular formation*. Feedback projections arise from the DCN, particularly the fastigial nucleus.

The NRTP receives cerebral cortical afferents from sensorimotor, frontal lobe, and superior parietal regions and subcortical afferents from vestibular and visual- or eye-movement–related nuclei, including the superior colliculus. Inputs from limbic-related structures include the cingulate gyrus and mammillary bodies. NRTP fibers enter cerebellum through the middle cerebellar peduncle and project widely, with a focus in vermal lobules VI and VII and lobule X. The NRTP is involved in ocular vergence and accommodation and the visual guidance of eye movements. The limbic relay provides cerebellum with emotionally salient information (see Plate 8.15).

The *lateral reticular nucleus* receives inputs from the spinal cord, lateral vestibular nucleus, red nucleus, superior colliculus, and cerebral cortex. Its fibers enter the cerebellum through the ipsilateral ICP; many cross to the contralateral side, providing collaterals to the DCN and terminating in multiple parasagittal zones. LRN connections are somatotopically arranged: the ventrolateral parvicellular region conveys afferents from the lumbar cord to primary and secondary hindlimb representations bilaterally; the dorsomedial, magnocellular part conveys inputs from the cervical cord to cerebellar forelimb regions. LRN neurons resemble VSCT or RSCT neurons but lack group I muscle input, are excited by descending vestibulospinal fibers, and respond to stimulation of larger body surface areas.

The *paramedian reticular nucleus* in the medulla receives afferents from the vestibular nuclei and somatosensory regions of the cerebral cortex and projects through the ICP to the vermis.

PERIHYPOGLOSSAL NUCLEI

These medullary nuclei related to the control of extraocular muscles receive vertical and horizontal gaze information from midbrain and pontine nuclei and face regions of the sensorimotor cortex. They are reciprocally interconnected with vermal and hemispheric components of cerebellar lobule X (nodulus and flocculus) and the fastigial and interposed nuclei.

ARCUATE CEREBELLAR TRACT

Fibers from the arcuate nucleus in the ventral medulla form the *striae medullares* visible on the posterior surface of the medulla. They enter cerebellum via the ICP and terminate in ipsilateral hemispheric lobule X. The arcuate nucleus is involved in central reflex chemosensitivity and cardiorespiratory activity.

VESTIBULOCEREBELLAR PATHWAYS

Vestibular input to cerebellum arises from primary vestibular afferent fibers and projections of neurons in the vestibular nuclei. These fibers carry information from receptors of the vestibular labyrinth, which signal the position and motion of the head in space (see Plate 8.11).

PONTOCEREBELLAR PATHWAYS

Basis pontis neurons receive input from multiple areas of the cerebral cortex and project as pontocerebellar fibers via the contralateral MCP to the cerebellar cortex. The organization, somatotopy, and functional relevance of the corticopontocerebellar system are considered in Plate 8.13.

CLIMBING FIBER PATHWAYS

CFs from the inferior olives project via the contralateral ICP to the cerebellar cortex. CF anatomy, connections, and physiology are shown in Plates 8.6 and 8.7.

MONOAMINERGIC FIBERS

Minor dopaminergic inputs to cerebellum arise in the substantia nigra—noradrenergic inputs from the locus coeruleus project diffusely to the vermis and lateral hemispheres, and serotonergic fibers from raphe nuclei project diffusely to most regions of cerebellar cortex.

SOMATOSENSORY SYSTEM: SPINOCEREBELLAR PATHWAYS

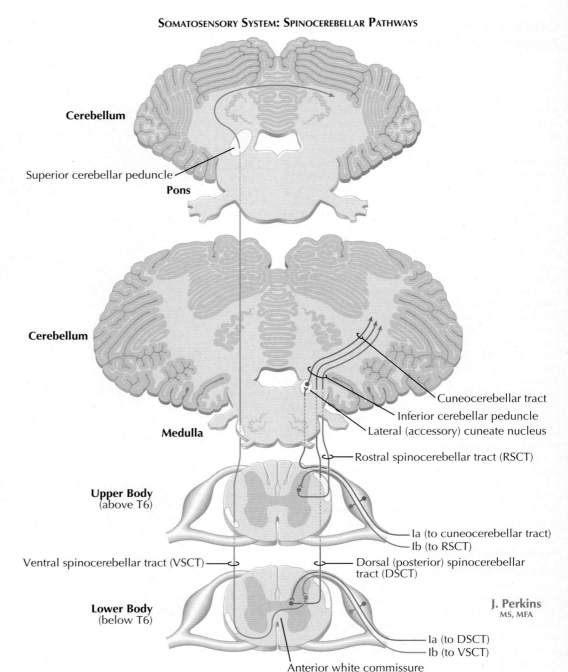

Cerebellum

Superior cerebellar peduncle

Pons

Cerebellum

Cuneocerebellar tract

Inferior cerebellar peduncle

Lateral (accessory) cuneate nucleus

Medulla

Rostral spinocerebellar tract (RSCT)

Upper Body (above T6)

Ia (to cuneocerebellar tract)

Ib (to RSCT)

Ventral spinocerebellar tract (VSCT)

Dorsal (posterior) spinocerebellar tract (DSCT)

J. Perkins MS, MFA

Lower Body (below T6)

Ia (to DSCT)

Ib (to VSCT)

Anterior white commissure

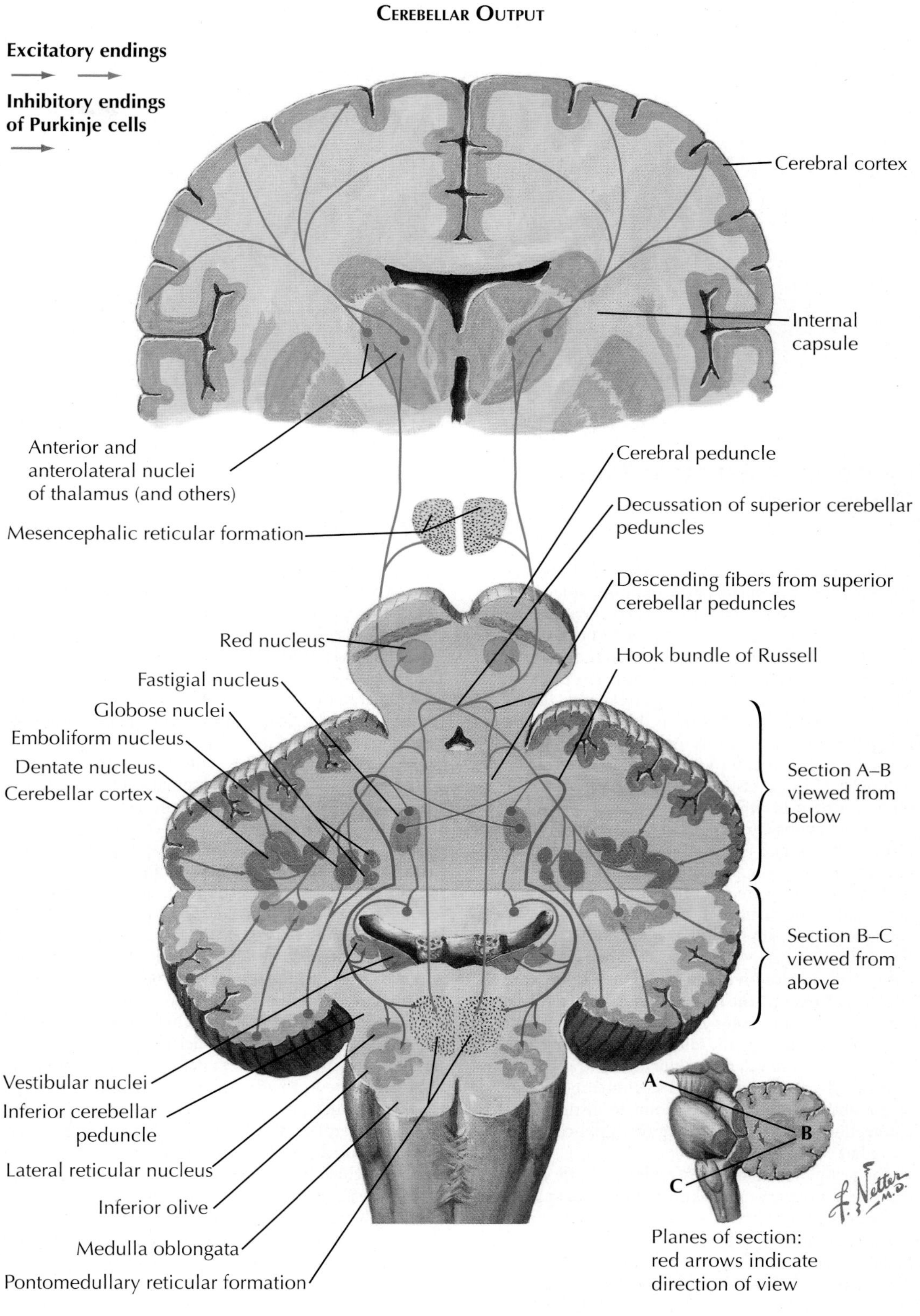

Plate 8.10

Cerebellum and Ataxia

CEREBELLAR OUTPUT

Excitatory endings
⟶   ⟶

Inhibitory endings
of Purkinje cells
⟶

Cerebral cortex

Internal
capsule

Anterior and
anterolateral nuclei
of thalamus (and others)

Cerebral peduncle

Decussation of superior cerebellar
peduncles

Mesencephalic reticular formation

Descending fibers from superior
cerebellar peduncles

Red nucleus

Hook bundle of Russell

Fastigial nucleus

Globose nuclei

Emboliform nucleus

Dentate nucleus

Cerebellar cortex

Section A–B
viewed from
below

Section B–C
viewed from
above

Vestibular nuclei

Inferior cerebellar
peduncle

Lateral reticular nucleus

Inferior olive

Medulla oblongata

Pontomedullary reticular formation

A

B

C

Planes of section:
red arrows indicate
direction of view

CEREBELLAR EFFERENT PATHWAYS

Efferent pathways from cerebellum originate in PCs that project to the DCN. DCN neurons then convey efferents from cerebellum to extracerebral areas in the spinal cord, brainstem, and cerebral hemispheres. DCN neurons receive inhibitory inputs from the PCs and from DCN interneurons and excitatory input from collaterals of MFs and CFs on their way to the cerebellar cortex. The nature of DCN efferents is determined by the interaction of excitation and inhibition governed by the arrival of information in cerebellar afferent pathways and by the processing of that information by the cerebellar cortex. Glutamatergic projection neurons of the DCN are excitatory to all extracerebral areas, whereas GABA-mediated DCN projection neurons to the inferior olive are inhibitory. The PC-DCN interaction is the basis of the corticonuclear microcomplex, the essential component of the parasagittal zones that form cerebellar cortical modules (see Plate 8.12). The reciprocal nucleo-olivary connections are organized with exquisite precision in a closed-loop circuit. The PC-DCN corticonuclear microcomplex receives input from and sends DCN output to essentially the identical cluster of neurons within the inferior olivary complex. The exact pattern of thalamic terminations varies according to the cerebellar module of origin, but the cerebellothalamic projections conform to a general arrangement, whereby focal areas within the DCN project to rod-shaped aggregates of thalamic neurons situated within curved, longitudinally oriented, onion-like lamellae stacked in a mediolateral direction.

The exception to the PC-DCN projection pattern throughout the cerebellum is the vestibulocerebellar cortex (vermal part of lobule IX [uvula], vermal [nodulus], and hemispheric parts [flocculus] of lobule X), which has direct reciprocal connections with vestibular nuclei. In addition, PCs in zone B of the anterior vermis commit their axons directly to the *lateral vestibular nucleus,* the source of the *lateral vestibulospinal tract,* by which the cerebellum regulates the activation

of descending spinal motor systems (see Plates 8.11 and 8.12).

FASTIGIAL NUCLEUS

Corticonuclear projections from the cerebellar vermis are directed to the fastigial nucleus. It has rostral and caudal parts with different connections and functional

significance. The rostral part of the fastigial nucleus sends efferents in the ipsilateral juxtarestiform body to the same side of the brainstem. Axons from its caudal part cross to the contralateral cerebellum in the hook bundle of Russell (the uncinate fasciculus) and project either to the contralateral brainstem in the juxtarestiform body or to the contralateral cerebral hemisphere in the SCP.

Plate 8.10 continued on next page

CEREBELLAR EFFERENT PATHWAYS
(Continued)

Both the rostral and caudal divisions of the fastigial nucleus project to nuclei of the pontomedullary reticular formation from which they receive inputs (see Reticular Afferents, Plate 8.9). They also both project to the vestibular nuclei. Projections from the rostral fastigial nucleus are largely bilateral; those from the caudal fastigial nucleus are mostly contralateral. There are small, crossed projections from the caudal part of the fastigial nucleus to neurons in the posterolateral region of the basis pontis and to the medullary perihypoglossal nuclei. Crossed fastigiospinal projections terminate on motor neurons in the upper cervical spinal cord.

Crossed axons from the caudal division of the fastigial nucleus ascend in the superior cerebellar peduncle and terminate in the pretectal, superior colliculus, and posterior commissure midbrain nuclei concerned with oculomotor and visual control. Connections with periaqueductal gray, anterior tegmental, solitary tract, and interpeduncular as well as parabrachial nuclei impact autonomic, nociceptive, and limbic functions. Fastigial efferents also target the hypothalamus. Thalamic terminations occur in motor-related anterolateral/anterior posterolateral nuclei, the diffusely projecting midline nuclei, and the intralaminar nuclei (central lateral and centromedian). Earlier as well as contemporary physiologic and anatomic studies point to fastigial nucleus connections with the septal region, hippocampus, and amygdala.

The fastigial nucleus connections with the contralateral inferior olivary nucleus are in the caudal part of the medial accessory olive.

Fastigial nucleus efferents influence multiple functional domains: axial and limb girdle musculature (medial motor system) via the vestibular and reticular nuclei; oculomotor systems, including vertical and horizontal gaze centers in the midbrain and pons; autonomic centers through connections with brainstem and hypothalamus; and emotional modulation through links with limbic-related circuits.

GLOBOSE AND EMBOLIFORM NUCLEI

These nuclei are referred to in lower mammals as the nucleus interpositus posterior (NIP) and nucleus interpositus anterior (NIA), respectively. They provide cerebellar efferents in the superior cerebellar peduncle from the predominantly motor-related spinocerebellum that receives proprioceptive and exteroceptive inputs from the spinal cord and brainstem, and sensorimotor information from the cerebral cortex. Fibers leave the interpositus nuclei and travel in the SCP, also known as the brachium conjunctivum, crossing to the contralateral side in the SCP decussation to course through the red nucleus, providing somatotopically arranged terminations in its caudal, magnocellular part. This red nucleus sector provides the origin for rubrospinal fibers that act on the spinal motor apparatus, particularly arm and hand flexor muscles.

Multiple other brainstem connections of the interpositus nuclei include (1) the lateral reticular nucleus and medullary reticular formation giving rise to *reticulospinal tracts,* (2) the vestibular nuclei as source for *vestibulospinal tracts,* (3) the superior colliculus giving rise to the *tectospinal tract,* (4) the oculomotor nuclei (prepositus hypoglossi, Darkschewitsch, and posterior commissures), (5) the sensory (lateral/external cuneate nucleus), and (6) the nociceptive systems (periaqueductal gray, medullary raphe). These rostrally directed fibers from the interpositus nuclei continue to the hypothalamus and zona incerta before reaching the thalamus. Here they provide heavy terminations to nuclei linked with the precentral motor cortex, notably the ventral posterolateral pars oralis (VPLo) and ventrolateral pars caudalis nuclei (VLc), and to the central lateral nucleus, which has widespread connections beyond motor areas. Efferents from the interpositus nuclei coursing within the descending limb of the SCP project back to the contralateral nucleus reticularis tegmenti pontis and to the dorsal and peduncular nuclei of the basis pontis.

The globose nucleus (NIP) is reciprocally linked with the rostral half of the contralateral medial accessory olive, and the emboliform nucleus (NIA) with the rostromedial part of the dorsal accessory olive.

DENTATE NUCLEUS

The large and multiply folded dentate nucleus is the most lateral of the four major DCN. It is divided into a dorsal part with closely packed folds (polymicrogyric) and a ventral part that is less folded (macrogyric). The dorsal part (paleodentate, because of its relationship to the paleocerebellum, or spinocerebellum) is linked with motor regions of the cerebral cortex. The ventral part (neodentate, interconnected with the more recently evolved neocerebellum) is linked with cerebral association areas. Axons from dentate neurons course in the white matter hilum, enter the SCP, cross to the other side in the decussation of the brachium conjunctivum, and terminate in the thalamus. Dorsal dentate nucleus fibers terminate in motor-related thalamic nuclei, including the ventral posterolateral and ventral lateral nuclei, that then project to the primary motor and premotor cerebral cortex. Middle and caudal thirds of the dentate nucleus are linked via the ventral anterior nucleus of thalamus with the premotor cortex and with the frontal eye fields engaged in saccadic eye movements. Ventral and lateral parts of the dentate nucleus project via the dorsal sector of the ventral lateral nucleus and the medial dorsal nucleus to dorsolateral prefrontal, posterior parietal, and other cerebral association areas. Dentate nucleus projections to thalamic intralaminar nuclei provide widespread influence on cerebral cortical areas. These intralaminar nuclei also project to the striatum, providing an indirect link between cerebellum and basal ganglia. The dentate nucleus also projects to the small-celled (parvicellular) part of the red nucleus that feeds back through the central tegmental tract to the inferior olive, which, in turn, is linked with the cerebellum. Lesions in this triangle of Guillain and Mollaret result in palatal tremor. Dentate fibers in the descending limb of the SCP terminate in reticular nuclei in the pons.

The rostral and dorsomedial parts of the dentate nucleus (the paleodentate) project to the dorsal lamina and bend of the principal olive. The ventral and caudal parts of the dentate nucleus (the neodentate) project to the ventral lamina of the principal olive.

The complex and varied destinations of the projections from the DCN and vestibular nuclei underscore the role of the cerebellum in multiple domains of neurologic function. Lesions of these different pathways produce a wide array of impairments, motor and otherwise. Damage to the DCN superimposed upon cerebellar cortical dysfunction appears to have adverse consequences on long-term recovery, as exemplified in patients with cerebellar stroke or tumor.

Plate 8.11   Cerebellum and Ataxia

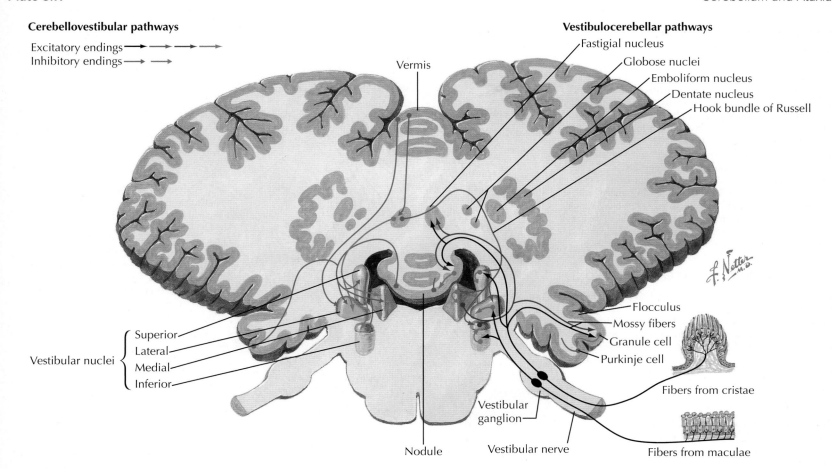

Cerebellovestibular pathways

Excitatory endings ➝ ➝ ➝ ➝
Inhibitory endings ➝ ➝ ➝

Vermis

Vestibulocerebellar pathways

Fastigial nucleus
Globose nuclei
Emboliform nucleus
Dentate nucleus
Hook bundle of Russell

Superior
Lateral
Medial
Inferior

Vestibular nuclei

Flocculus
Mossy fibers
Granule cell
Purkinje cell

Fibers from cristae

Vestibular ganglion

Vestibular nerve

Fibers from maculae

Nodule

Cerebellovestibular Pathways

The vestibular system is closely related to vermal lobule IX (uvula), vermal and hemispheric parts of lobule X (nodulus and flocculus, respectively), and vermal lobule I/II (lingula)—phylogenetically ancient regions that are therefore referred to both as archicerebellum and vestibulocerebellum. The vestibular system is also related to the paleocerebellum (spinocerebellum) through its connections with anterior lobe vermis and the fastigial nucleus.

VESTIBULOCEREBELLAR PROJECTIONS

There are five peripheral vestibular end organs: the cristae in the three orthogonally oriented semicircular canals detect movement in the sense of angular rotation in the horizontal, pitch, and roll planes, and the maculae in the two otoliths sense the effect of the linear acceleration of gravity during roll-tilt (utricle) and pitch (saccule).

Vestibular afferents from these end organs combine in the vestibular nerve. One branch terminates in the ipsilateral cerebellar cortex, providing profuse primary vestibular afferents from otoliths to vermal lobule IX and from semicircular canals to vermal lobule X. The other branch terminates with varying degrees of intensity in different subregions of all four vestibular nuclei: medial, lateral, superior, and inferior. These nuclei, with the exception of the posterior part of the lateral vestibular nucleus (Deiters nucleus), provide cholinergic secondary vestibular afferents bilaterally to the vermal and hemispheric regions of lobules IX and X and to the anterior vermis. Together with the perihypoglossal nucleus, they

also project to the fastigial nucleus as collaterals of vestibulocortical fibers. Axons of both pathways terminate as diffusely projecting MFs in granule cell glomeruli within the cerebellar cortex. Tertiary vestibular afferents reach vermal lobules IX and X as CFs derived from subregions of the medial accessory olive (beta subnucleus and dorsomedial cell column). These olivary nuclei receive inhibitory input from the parasolitary nucleus that, in turn, receives projections from the labyrinth. The olivocerebellar terminations are arranged in discrete parasagittal zones, relaying information from the vertical and anterior semicircular canals.

CEREBELLOVESTIBULAR PROJECTIONS

Projections from vermal and hemispheric parts of lobules IX and X are directed to all the vestibular nuclei. The anterior lobe vermis projects to the fastigial nucleus, and, in addition, PCs in zone B of the anterior vermis project directly to the part of the lateral vestibular nucleus that is devoid of vestibular afferents and gives rise to the lateral vestibulospinal tract. Strong topographically arranged projections to the vestibular nuclei are also derived from the fastigial nucleus. The rostral fastigial nucleus, linked with the spinal recipient anterior vermis, projects to the medial, superior, and perihypoglossal nuclei. The caudoventral region of the fastigial nucleus, devoted to oculomotor control, projects to the inferior vestibular nucleus and to the part of the lateral vestibular nucleus that receives zone B cortical inputs. The projections of the rostral portion of the fastigial nucleus are ipsilateral, whereas fibers from the caudal fastigial nucleus cross in the hook bundle of Russell to excite contralateral vestibular neurons. Thus PCs of the

cerebellar vermis can depress the activity of neurons in the vestibular nuclei either by direct inhibition or by inhibiting the discharge of neurons in the fastigial nucleus, thereby decreasing the excitatory activity reaching vestibular neurons via fastigiovestibular pathways, an example of disfacilitation.

FUNCTIONAL CONSIDERATIONS

The vestibular system is critical for the control of eye movements for orientation in intrapersonal and extrapersonal space and for control of the axial musculature, essential for balance. Vestibulocerebellar connections provide the cerebellum with a topographic map of space, serving as an anatomic substrate for modulation of postural reflexes evoked by vestibular and optokinetic stimulation. The vestibulocerebellum predicts spatial environments and, by modulating the amplitude of movements produced by reflexes such as the vestibulo-ocular reflex, compensates for head movements to optimally guide behavior. The clinical relevance of these vestibulocerebellar circuits is exemplified by the loss of plastic changes in the horizontal vestibulo-ocular reflex in individuals with damage to lobule X (flocculus) and by the inability to remember postural adjustments to a previously maintained head position in space after damage to the vermal lobules IX and X. Acute injury to the vestibular system produces violent nausea, vomiting, and vertigo. The paleocerebellum receives a modest amount of vestibular afferent input but extensive input from spinocerebellar tracts. The principal action of the paleocerebellum on the vestibular system is to regulate vestibular activity in relation to proprioceptive and exteroceptive information about the head, trunk, and extremities. This is critical for posture, balance, and equilibrium.

Plate 8.12

Brain: PART I

CEREBELLUM MODULAR ORGANIZATION

The cerebellar cortex and DCN are linked anatomically in multiple repeating, parasagittally arranged, and histochemically identifiable *corticonuclear microcomplexes*. These channel PC axons from longitudinal PC zones to focal regions within the DCN. The zonal organization is reflected also in the connections of the inferior olive with the cerebellar cortex and DCN. *Cerebellar zones* are further divided into microzones about 0.5 mm wide (four to five PCs), extending many millimeters rostrocaudally. Monoclonal antibody stains show alternating zebrin-positive and -negative stripes in the cortex that correlate with corticonuclear and olivocerebellar connections.

CEREBELLAR CORTICONUCLEAR PROJECTION

Output from the cerebellar cortex to the DCN is derived exclusively from PCs and is inhibitory. The vermis projects to the fastigial nucleus, the intermediate cortex project to globose and emboliform nuclei, and lateral hemispheres project to the dentate nucleus. There is a reciprocal excitatory projection of the DCN neurons back onto the PCs (Plate 8.5).

INFERIOR OLIVARY NUCLEUS

This nuclear complex is a folded sheet of 1.5 million neurons in the medulla, situated between the pyramidal tract and the lateral reticular nucleus. The medial accessory olive (MAO) and the dorsal accessory olive (DAO) each have rostral and caudal components. The principal olive (PO) has dorsal, lateral, ventral, and medial lamellae. Other subnuclei include the beta cell group, dorsomedial cell column (DMCC), and dorsal cap of Kooy. Proximal dendrites of olivary neurons have appendages that form the central core of a complex synaptic structure, the olivary glomerulus. These have gap junctions enabling electrotonic coupling between groups of olivary neurons. Each olivary axon provides 7 to 10 CFs to the cerebellar cortex and DCN, one CF per PC (see Plate 8.6).

OLIVARY AFFERENTS AND PROJECTIONS TO CEREBELLUM

The olive receives multiple excitatory afferents, sends excitatory CFs to discrete longitudinally oriented parasagittal microzones in the cerebellar cortex, and sends collaterals to focal areas within the DCN that are linked to PCs in that cortical microzone. Olivary neurons receive inhibitory feedback projections from those DCN neurons to which they project, forming a closed-loop system.

Spinal cord projections are conveyed directly to the MAO and DAO in the crossed ventral spino-olivary tracts (SOTs) and indirectly in the dorsal SOT that ascends in the ipsilateral dorsal column, synapses in the gracile and cuneate nuclei, decussates to the contralateral olive, and decussates again in the olivocerebellar projection, terminating in the cerebellum ipsilateral to its spinal cord origin. Spino-olivary fibers terminate in primary and secondary arm and leg representations in the spinocerebellum (zones A through C3).

The *trigeminal sensory nucleus* projects to the caudal MAO and rostromedial DAO; these project to lobule VI in zones C1 and C3, with collaterals to the emboliform nucleus.

Cerebral cortex projections are conveyed to the olive and cerebellum via the parvocellular component

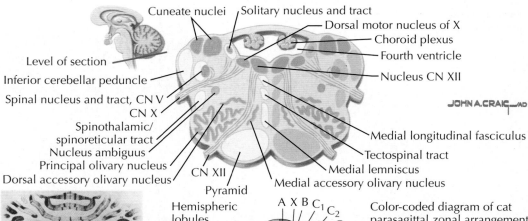

CEREBELLUM MODULAR ORGANIZATION

Cuneate nuclei — Solitary nucleus and tract — Dorsal motor nucleus of X — Choroid plexus — Fourth ventricle — Nucleus CN XII — Medial longitudinal fasciculus — Tectospinal tract — Medial lemniscus — Medial accessory olivary nucleus

Level of section — Inferior cerebellar peduncle — Spinal nucleus and tract, CN V — CN X — Spinothalamic/spinoreticular tract — Nucleus ambiguus — Principal olivary nucleus — Dorsal accessory olivary nucleus — CN XII — Pyramid — Medial accessory olivary nucleus

JOHN A. CRAIG _AD

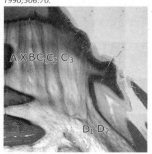

Coronal section through adult rat cerebellum immunostained for zebrin I shows Purkinje cells aligned in parasagittal bands in vermis and hemispheres. *From Leclerc N, Doré L, Parent A, Hawkes R. The compartmentalization of the monkey and rat cerebellar cortex. Brain Res 1990;506:70.*

Transverse section through anterior lobe of monkey cerebellum stained for acetylcholinesterase shows parasagittal compartments within the white matter, from zone A medially to zone D2 most laterally. *From Voogd J, Paxinos G, Mai JK. The human nervous system. Academic Press; 1990.*

Hemispheric lobules: I–V, VI, Crus I, Crus II, VIIIA, VIIIB, IX, X

A X B C_1 C_2 C_3 D_1 Y D_2 A_2

Color-coded diagram of cat parasagittal zonal arrangement of cerebellar cortical connections (zones A through D2) with the deep cerebellar nuclei and with the inferior olivary nuclear complex. *Adapted from Voogd J. Cerebellar zones—a personal history. Cerebellum. 2001;10:334-350.*

Deep cerebellar nuclei:
F (fastigial)
AI (anterior interposed)
PI (posterior interposed)
Dr (rostromedial dentate)
Dc (caudoventral dentate)

Minor nuclei:
ICG (interstitial cell group)
DLP (dorsolateral protuberance)

Vest (vestibular nuclei)
LV (lateral vestibular nucleus)

Inferior olivary nuclear complex:
PO (principal olive)
MAO (medial accessory olive)
DMCC (dorsomedial cell column)
DC (dorsal cap)
DAO (dorsal accessory olive)

r: rostral
int: intermediate
c: caudal

DLP — AI — Dr — F — Dc — PI — ICG

LV — vest — Ventral lamina — Dorsal lamina — DMCC — r — int — c — DC — Beta — c — r

MAO — PO — DAO

of the red nucleus (RNpc). Primary motor and premotor cerebral cortex are linked somatotopically with the caudolateral RNpc; this projects to the PO dorsal lamina and bend, which sends efferents to the lateral cerebellar D2 zone and dorsomedial dentate nucleus (paleodentate) and to the rostral MAO that targets cerebellar zone C2 and the globose nucleus. Frontal eye fields, premotor areas, and prefrontal areas project via the dorsomedial RNpc and the PO ventral lamina to the medial cerebellar D1 zone and the caudoventral dentate nucleus (neodentate). The inferior olive also conveys information to cerebellum from the cerebral cortex via the zona incerta in the mesodiencephalic junction.

Optokinetic information from pretectal nuclei, including the nucleus of the optic tract and accessory optic nuclei, is conveyed to the dorsal cap and the ventrolateral outgrowth and relayed to lobule X (flocculonodular lobe).

Vestibular information is conveyed to vestibular nuclei, including the parasolitary nucleus, which project via DMCC and nucleus B to vermal and hemispheric

regions of lobules IX (uvula, paraflocculus) and X (nodulus and flocculus).

Visual information from the superior colliculus is relayed through the caudal MAO to the vermal visual area in lobule VII and fastigial nucleus. Other afferents originate in midbrain regions concerned with oculomotor control (nuclei of Darkschewitsch, Cajal, Edinger-Westphal, perihypoglossal) and are conveyed to vermal lobules IX and X. The lateral reticular nucleus, periaqueductal gray, and zona incerta convey motor, nociceptive/autonomic, and associative information to the olive.

Together with their connections with the inferior olive, the corticonuclear microcomplexes comprise cerebellar modules that are also linked with pontine and other afferents and efferents. The paracrystalline architectural uniformity of the modules likely supports a neural computation, the universal cerebellar transform, common to all cerebellar areas, which can be applied to multiple domains of neurologic function by virtue of the precise connections of each module with extracerebellar structures.

Plate 8.13

Cerebellum and Ataxia

Cerebrocerebellar Connections

There are massive, reciprocal, topographically arranged connections between the cerebral cortex and the cerebellum. Each cerebral hemisphere communicates predominantly with the contralateral cerebellar hemisphere. The cerebrocerebellar circuit has a two-stage feed-forward limb and a two-stage feedback limb. Ipsilateral corticopontine projections originate in cortical layer Vb in sensorimotor areas as well as association and limbic-related cortices concerned with cognition and emotion (posterior parietal, superior and middle temporal, dorsolateral and medial prefrontal and cingulate areas, and posterior parahippocampal gyrus). Corticopontine projections terminate around neurons in the basis pontis. Pontocerebellar pathways decussate in the middle cerebellar peduncle, conveying corticopontine afferents to the contralateral cerebellum. Feedback to cerebral cortex is via crossed cerebellothalamic projections in the superior cerebellar peduncle, and ipsilateral thalamocortical projections to cortical areas from which the feed-forward projections arose, thereby completing the closed-loop systems.

In the *cerebral peduncle,* prefrontal fibers are most medial, sensorimotor fibers intermediate, and fibers from the parietal, temporal, and occipital lobes are lateral. In the monkey, terminations in the pons from motor and association areas are topographically arranged. The *caudal pons* preferentially receives sensorimotor inputs and projects mostly to the cerebellar anterior lobe and lobule VIII, containing primary and secondary sensorimotor representations, respectively. The *dorsolateral pons* projects to visual areas in the vermal and hemispheric lobule IX. *Medial parts of the rostral pons* project to crus I. *The medial, anterior,* and *lateral pons* project to crus II. By way of these projections, lobules III through V of the anterior lobe and lobule VIII receive sensorimotor afferents. In contrast, much of lobule VI, crus I and crus II of lobule VIIA, and lobule VIIB receive inputs from association areas and limbic-related regions of the cerebral cortex.

Clinicopathologic studies in patients show that *speech* is represented medially in the rostral pons, *hand coordination* medially and anteriorly in the rostral and mid-pons, the *arm* anteriorly and laterally to the hand, *leg coordination* mostly laterally in the caudal pons, and *gait* is distributed in medial and lateral locations throughout.

In the feedback system, the primary motor cortex receives projections via the thalamus from dorsal parts of the dentate nucleus and caudal portions of the anterior interpositus nucleus, where neurons activate with arm movement. The *premotor cortex* receives input from the midrostrocaudal dentate nucleus. Frontal eye field–projecting neurons are in the caudal third of the dentate nucleus activated by saccadic eye movements. The *dorsolateral prefrontal cortex* (areas 46 and 9 lateral) receives projections from the ventral dentate. Projections to parietal, temporal, and cingulate association areas also appear to arise in ventral and lateral parts of the dentate nucleus. Fastigial nucleus projections to intralaminar thalamic nuclei have widespread influence on the cerebral hemisphere.

These connectional patterns are matched by MRI studies in humans using resting state functional connectivity and experiments performed while subjects are actively engaged in tasks. The cerebellum, like the cerebral cortex, is topographically arranged into functional domains. The *primary sensorimotor cerebellum* is in lobules III, IV, and V of the anterior lobe and adjacent

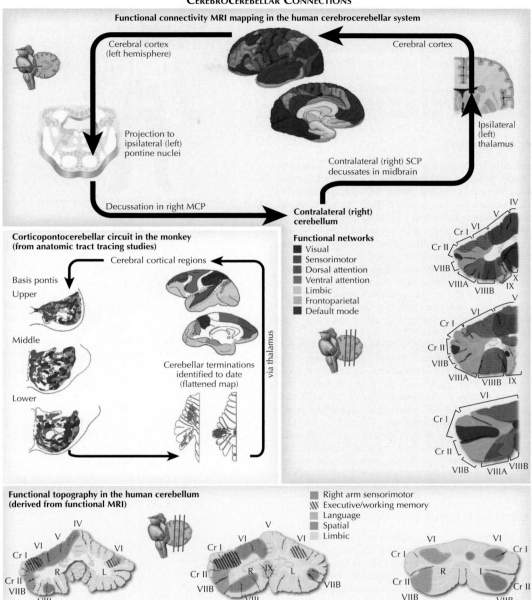

Modified from Schmahmann JD, Pandya DN. The cerebrocerebellar system. Int Rev Neurobiol. 1997;41:31-60; Kelly RM, Strick PL. Cerebellar loops with motor cortex and prefrontal cortex of a nonhuman primate. J Neurosci. 2003;23:8432-8444; Middleton FA, Strick PL. Cerebellar output channels. Int Rev Neurobiol. 1997;41:61-82; Buckner RL, Krienen FM, Castellanos A, Diaz JC, Yeo BT. The organization of the human cerebellum estimated by intrinsic functional connectivity. J Neurophysiol. 2011;106:2322-2345; Stoodley CJ, Schmahmann JD. Functional topography in the human cerebellum: a meta-analysis of neuroimaging studies. NeuroImage. 2009;44:489-501; and Stoodley CJ, Valera EM, Schmahmann JD. Functional topography of the cerebellum for motor and cognitive tasks: an fMRI study. NeuroImage. 2012;59:1560-1570.

parts of lobule VI; the secondary sensorimotor representation is in lobule VIII. The *motor cerebellum* is functionally coupled with sensorimotor cerebral areas and engaged in motor tasks: leg and foot are in lobules II, III, and VIII; hand representation in lobules IV, V, and VIII; and orofacial movements in paravermal anterior lobe and medial lobule VI. The *supramodal, or cognitive, cerebellum* is linked with cerebral association cortices but not with sensorimotor areas. These posterior lobe regions are lobule VI, lobule VIIA at the vermis and in crus I and crus II in the hemispheres, and lobule VIIB. The *cognitive cerebellum* is differentially linked with the various subdivisions of the prefrontal cortex and other cerebral association areas. *Lobules VI, crus I and crus II, and lobule IX* also correlate with an executive control network in the cerebral hemispheres;

lobule VI with a salience network; and lobule IX with the default network. Working memory and executive functions engage lobules VI and VII, language recruits posterolateral cerebellum on the right, and spatial tasks recruit it on the left. Affective/emotional processing and pain and autonomic functions involve lobules VI and VII in the vermis more than the hemispheres. The anterior lobe is not engaged in cognitive tasks; the posterior lobe is not involved in motor tasks, with the exception of parts of lobule VI and the second sensorimotor representation in lobule VIII.

These anatomic and imaging findings demonstrate a high degree of functional topography in cerebrocerebellar loops, and they provide the anatomic and functional foundations for the cerebellar modulation of sensorimotor, cognitive, and limbic domains.

Plate 8.14

Brain: PART I

CEREBELLAR MOTOR EXAMINATION

Cerebellar incoordination is characterized by disturbed rate, rhythm, and force of movements. This manifests as impaired oculomotor control; articulation (dysarthria); stance, equilibrium, and gait (ataxia); and motion of the limbs (dysmetria). Severity of involvement can be graded using ataxia rating scales.

EYE MOVEMENTS

Cerebellar lesions produce unsteady ocular fixation in primary position, microsaccadic oscillations, square wave jerks, ocular flutter, ocular bobbing, and opsoclonus. Pursuit eye movements show saccadic intrusions—jerkiness following a moving target. Volitional gaze (saccade) is hypermetric (overshoot) or hypometric (undershoot/catch-up). Gaze-evoked, direction-beating nystagmus has a fast phase in the direction of eccentric gaze and a slow phase in the opposite direction. Downbeat nystagmus in primary gaze points to mass lesions of the cervicomedullary junction or neurodegenerative disorders affecting the flocculonodular lobe, and upbeat nystagmus to midline lesions or drug toxicity.

The *vestibulo-ocular reflex* (VOR) maintains visualized image stabilization on the retina during head movement. With passive trunk and head rotation while focusing on their own hand, the patient's eyes should not move relative to the head. Failure of this VOR cancellation from lesions of the vestibulocerebellum manifests as saccadic eye movements.

Slowing of eye movements leading to ophthalmoplegia occurs in spinocerebellar ataxias and mitochondrial disorders. Patients with oculomotor apraxia cannot direct gaze voluntarily and perform head thrusts to initiate these movements.

SPEECH/SWALLOWING

Cerebellar dysarthria is described as "scanning speech." Syllables are poorly articulated, cadence is slowed and irregular, and rapid or alternating buccal, palatal, and lingual consonants are degraded. Dysarthria is compounded by deficient volume control. Ataxic respiration affects quality of speech. Impaired control of muscles of deglutition leads to dysphagia and aspiration risk.

MOTOR CONTROL

Resting tone in pure cerebellar disease is generally decreased, or *hypotonic*. There may be a spastic catch or frank spasticity when spinal cord pathology is also present in some inherited ataxic disorders. Cerebellar lesions do not produce weakness, but there may be slowed initiation and generation of force. Truncal ataxia occurs with midline lesions, including titubation; that is, oscillations of the head and trunk. The patient has a widened stance and is unable to stand in tandem position or on one foot. Cerebellar ataxic gait is staggering, uneven, irregular, and veers from side to side. Unilateral lesions cause stumbling toward the affected side.

COORDINATION OF ARMS AND LEGS

Dysmetria (from the Greek *dus* [bad] and *métron* [measure]) is the disordered ability to regulate, judge, and control behavior, both with motor and cognitive

Brainstem and/or cerebellar manifestations

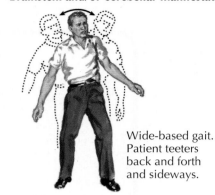

Wide-based gait. Patient teeters back and forth and sideways.

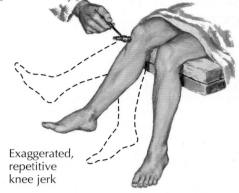

Exaggerated, repetitive knee jerk

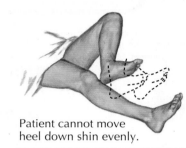

Patient cannot move heel down shin evenly.

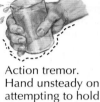

Action tremor. Hand unsteady on attempting to hold glass, write, etc.

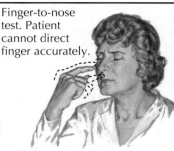

Finger-to-nose test. Patient cannot direct finger accurately.

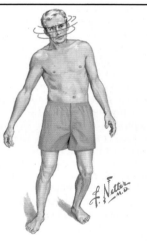

Acute cerebellar lesions produce headache, nausea, vomiting, and vertigo, along with gait ataxia, dysarthria, and sometimes diplopia. Hiccups and tinnitus may also occur.

domains (see Plate 8.15). The cerebellar motor syndrome causes difficulty judging distances, trajectory of intended movements, and force required for movements. Compound movements (across more than one joint) are particularly affected. Visual guidance improves outcome minimally.

Postural tremor is assessed with arms extended in pronated position. Rebound is tested by the examiner displacing the arm downward, observing for overshoot above the starting point. Dysmetria characteristics include end-point tremor, overshooting targets (hypermetria) or undershooting (hypometria), and oscillation at the elbow. These are assessed with finger-to-nose testing; the patient brings the index finger to their nose and then to the examiner's finger held steady at arm's length. Tremor increases with proximity to the target; tremor direction is generally perpendicular to direction of movement. The finger chase/mirror test measures overshoot/undershoot. The patient points to the examiner's finger held at arm's length, following their sequential moves horizontally and vertically. Dysdiadochokinesia is degradation of rapid alternating movements, tested by forearm pronation/supination. Tapping the index finger on the crease of the thumb assesses fine

motor control. Dysrhythmia is an inability to generate normal rhythms, assessed by rapidly tapping the hand on a surface or the heel on the ground.

The heel-to-shin test, performed with the patient supine, assesses leg coordination. The heel is placed on the opposite knee and moved down the shin. In patients who use a wheelchair, the heel is brought to the knee of the opposite leg held parallel to the ground. Proximal overshoot occurs as the heel is placed on the knee, and tremor occurs as the heel is maintained in that position. Slowing, jerking, or side-to-side movements are noted as the heel moves down the shin. In the draw-a-circle test, the supine patient traces a circle in the air; decomposition manifests as irregular or chaotic motions.

Cerebellar tremor is large amplitude, 2 to 3 Hz, and may involve many body parts. *Rubral tremor* from red nucleus lesions and its connections involves multiple joints and direction changes and is frequently rotatory. *Palatal tremor* is slow and semirhythmic, resulting from Guillain-Mollaret myoclonic triangle lesions of this neuronal brainstem/cerebellum network (dentate nucleus to red nucleus and inferior olivary nucleus).

Plate 8.15

Cerebellum and Ataxia

CEREBELLAR COGNITIVE AFFECTIVE SYNDROME

The cerebellum is organized into a primary sensorimotor region in the anterior lobe and adjacent part of lobule VI and a second sensorimotor region in lobule VIII. The cognitive and limbic regions are in the posterior lobe (lobule VI, lobule VIIA [which includes crus I and crus II], and lobule VIIB); and lobule IX is also part of this network. Cognitively relevant areas are situated more laterally in these lobules, whereas the limbic cerebellum is represented in the vermis. Lesions of the sensorimotor cerebellum result in cerebellar motor incoordination (see Plate 8.14). Lesions of the cognitive and limbic cerebellum lead to the cerebellar cognitive affective syndrome (CCAS, or Schmahmann syndrome). This constellation of deficits is characterized by impairments in (1) executive function, (2) visual-spatial processing, (3) linguistic deficits, and (4) affective dysregulation. CCAS occurs in adults and children after many types of injury. It can be prominent after acute lesions, including stroke, hemorrhage, and infectious or postinfectious cerebellitis, but relatively subtle in late-onset hereditary ataxias.

Executive function deficits include problems with working memory, as tested with reverse digit span; mental flexibility is tested using tasks of set shifting; and perseveration is demonstrated using bedside tests of mental control. Patients may have concrete thinking, poor problem-solving strategies, and impaired ability to multitask, with trouble planning, sequencing, and organizing their activities.

Mental representation of visual-spatial relationships can be impaired. Visuospatial disintegration is apparent when attempting to copy or recall visual images. Identification of multiple features within a complex diagram (simultanagnosia) is difficult.

Expressive language can be abnormal, characterized by long response latency, brief responses, reluctance to engage in conversation, and word-finding difficulties. Verbal fluency is decreased, affecting phonemic (letter) more than semantic (category) naming. Mutism occurs postoperatively for vermis tumors, particularly in children but also in adults subsequent to cerebellitis, infarction, and hemorrhage. Speech may have abnormal syntax, resulting in agrammatism. Degraded control of volume, pitch, and tone can produce high-pitched, hypophonic speech.

Short-term memory impairments include difficulty learning and spontaneously recalling new information, reflecting deficient strategies for organizing verbal or visual-spatial material, and difficulty locating information in memory stores. Successful recall is aided by a structured approach to the task, using clues and other prompts. Conditional associative learning is degraded, as shown in studies of classic conditioning in patients with cerebellar dysfunction (as well as in animals). Mental arithmetic is impaired. Ideational apraxia and hemi-inattention have been reported.

The affective component of CCAS occurs when lesions involve the limbic cerebellum in the vermis and fastigial nucleus. Patients exhibit difficulty modulating behavior and personality style, have flattened affect or disinhibition manifesting as overfamiliarity, and display flamboyant or impulsive actions. Behavior may be regressive and childlike, sometimes with obsessive-compulsive traits. Patients can be irritable, with labile affect and poor attentional and behavioral modulation. Acquired panic disorder is described in this setting as well.

CEREBELLAR COGNITIVE AFFECTIVE SYNDROME

CCAS following tumor resection in adult

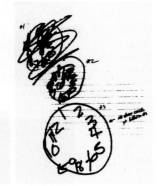

MRI after resection of ganglioglioma

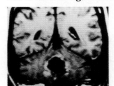

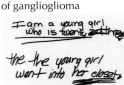

Patient writing sample demonstrates agrammatism ("twenty 3rd"), perseveration ("the the"), and disinhibition (underlining)

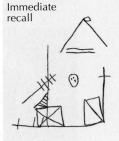

Patient clock drawing reveals impaired visual-spatial strategy and execution

Postinfectious cerebellitis following Epstein-Barr virus infection

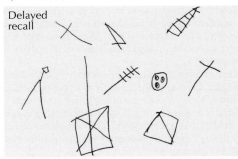

Patient's copy of Rey diagram showing poor visual-spatial planning

CCAS following resection of left cerebellar cystic astrocytoma in child

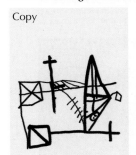

Copy

Immediate recall

Delayed recall

Severely impaired Rey diagrams

CCAS following cerebellar infarction

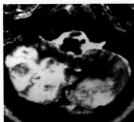 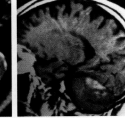

Axial and parasagittal MRI showing bilateral PICA and left SCA infarcts, respectively

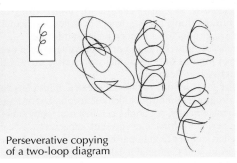

Perseverative copying of a two-loop diagram

From Schmahmann JD, Sherman JC. The cerebellar cognitive affective syndrome. Brain. 1998;121(Pt 4): 561-579; and Levisohn L, Cronin-Golomb A, Schmahmann JD. Neuropsychological consequences of cerebellar tumour resection in children: cerebellar cognitive affective syndrome in a paediatric population. Brain. 2000;123(Pt 5):1041-1050.

Current evidence indicates five domains of behavioral dysregulation caused by cerebellar damage. These are impairments of attentional control or emotional control, autism spectrum disorder, psychosis spectrum disorders, and difficulties with social skills. Within each of these domains, there are hypometric/diminished behaviors and hypermetric/exaggerated behaviors, consistent with the dysmetria of thought theory of the cerebellar role in nervous system function.

The intellectual and emotional impairments from damage to the cognitive and limbic posterior lobe of the cerebellum may be more disabling than motor deficits, and when the anterior lobe is spared, these occur in the absence of the motor syndrome. Recognizing the nonmotor manifestations of cerebellar lesions can lead to earlier diagnosis of cerebellar damage and facilitate treatment of cognitive emotional consequences of disrupted cerebellar modulation of higher function. The nature of these deficits provides new avenues for conceptualizing mental illnesses, including autism, schizophrenia, bipolar disorder, attention deficit disorder, and dyslexia and for exploring the potential cerebellar role in neurodegenerative disorders. Appreciating the role of the cerebellum beyond motor control therefore has implications for understanding and improving neuropsychiatric disorders. This represents a radical departure from our previous understanding of the functions of the "little brain" and is an area of active investigation in neuroscience. The neural substrates that support this nonmotor cerebellar role are discussed in Plate 8.13.

Plate 8.16

Brain: PART I

Cerebellar Disorders: Differential Diagnosis

Diagnosing the cause of a cerebellar disorder can be straightforward or require sleuthing and special tests. The following principles guide the approach: (1) recognize symptoms and signs of cerebellar disease; (2) determine whether peripheral nerves, spinal cord, brainstem, or cerebral hemispheres are also affected; (3) characterize the timing of onset and progression—that is, the temporal profile; (4) search for risk factors—that is, toxins and drugs, recent infections, and systemic features of neoplasms; (5) document family history and country of origin, a critical feature when considering hereditary disorders; (6) perform brain MRI, which is essential; and (7) review laboratory data, which may clinch the diagnosis.

ACUTE: MINUTES TO HOURS

Ischemic stroke and hemorrhage start abruptly. Both worsen clinically over hours if cerebellar edema develops. Note the posterior fossa mantra of acute cerebellar and brainstem injury: headache, nausea, vomiting, and vertigo, with or without ataxia, dysarthria, diplopia, and nystagmus. Neurologic examination lateralizes to side of injury.

Acute cerebellitis occurs more commonly in children than adults, starting more abruptly than postinfectious cerebellitis; both produce a pancerebellar syndrome.

Thiamine deficiency produces *Wernicke encephalopathy*, a triad of ataxia, confusion, and oculomotor disturbances that is a medical emergency requiring immediate repletion of vitamin B$_1$.

SUBACUTE: DAYS TO WEEKS

Paraneoplastic immune-mediated PC attack from remote tumors (lung, breast, ovary) may develop acutely over days, producing a pancerebellar syndrome.

Cerebellar tumors (benign or malignant) worsen over weeks to months but occasionally present acutely with obstructive hydrocephalus.

Other focal lesions include abscesses, multiple sclerosis, progressive multifocal leukoencephalopathy, and rhombencephalitis. Alcoholic cerebellar atrophy (anterior superior vermis) may present subacutely, as can cerebellar leukoencephalopathy from inhaled solvents and heroin, and Creutzfeldt-Jakob disease, with ataxia, dementia, and myoclonus.

INSIDIOUS, CHRONIC PROGRESSION: MONTHS TO YEARS

Neurodegenerative disorders start insidiously, progressing over years or decades. Autosomal dominant (AD) ataxic disorders pass down through generations. AD spinocerebellar ataxias (SCAs) typically manifest during adulthood. SCA1 and SCA3 have extrapyramidal, corticospinal, and peripheral nerve lesions. SCA2 has slowed eye movements and extrapyramidal features in younger patients. SCA3 is prevalent in individuals with Portuguese Azorean ancestry but is also the most common SCA worldwide; younger patients have dystonia. SCA5 and SCA6 are purely cerebellar. SCA7 has visual failure from rod-cone macular dystrophy. SCA8 includes mild chorea. SCA10 occurs in association with epilepsy in families with Native American ancestry. SCA17 resembles Huntington disease, with cognitive failure and choreoathetosis. Dentatorubro-pallidoluysian

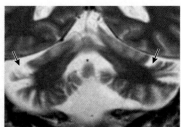

Cerebellar hypoplasia. Underdeveloped cerebellum seen on T2-weighted coronal MRI, with prominent fissures *(arrows)* and fourth ventricle *(asterisk)*.

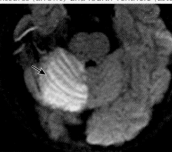

Cerebellar stroke. Acute infarction *(arrow)* in the territory of the superior cerebellar artery seen on axial diffusion-weighted MRI.

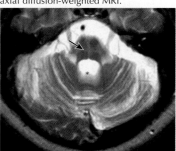

Multiple system atrophy, cerebellar type (MSAc). Axial T2 *(left)* and mid-sagittal T1 MRI *(right)* showing prominent cerebellar volume loss including the white matter, enlarged fourth ventricle *(asterisk)*, and marked pontine volume loss with "hot cross bun" sign *(arrow)*.

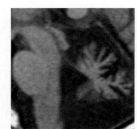

Idiopathic late-onset cerebellar ataxia. Cerebellar volume loss with small vermis and prominent fissures seen on mid-sagittal T1 MRI. The pons is largely spared.

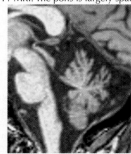

Spinocerebellar ataxia type 2. Cerebellar volume loss and mild pontine volume loss seen on mid-sagittal T1 MRI.

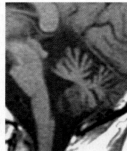

atrophy causes myoclonus, dystonia, and cognitive decline; it is uncommon outside Japan. Currently, there are more than 48 SCAs (see www.ncbi.nlm.nih.gov/books/NBK1138/).

Episodic ataxias (EAs) are AD. EA1, a *potassium channelopathy*, starts in childhood, producing brief duration ataxic episodes and myokymia. EA2 is a *calcium channelopathy*; attacks last for days, sometimes with migraine. The gene causing EA2 is associated with familial hemiplegic migraine and SCA6. Both these EAs improve with acetazolamide. Episodic ataxias 3 through 8 are rare.

Autosomal recessive (AR) disorders manifest in one generation, usually in childhood. Parents are asymptomatic; nonsibling family history is unrevealing. *Friedreich ataxia* is the most common AR cerebellar disorder, with ataxia, peripheral neuropathy, cardiomyopathy, scoliosis, and diabetes. Hearing and visual impairment occur late. Occasionally, it begins in adulthood, resembling SCAs. *Ataxia telangiectasia* often manifests before telangiectasias develop; features include recurrent infections from immunoglobulin A deficiency and radiation sensitivity with risk of neoplasia. *Ataxia with oculomotor apraxia* types 1 and 2 include peripheral neuropathy, choreiform movements, and cognitive difficulties. *AR cerebellar ataxia (ARCA) type 1* commences in early adulthood and progresses over decades, and *AR spastic ataxia of Charlevoix-Saguenay* usually starts in childhood. Both conditions have a founder effect in the French-Canadian population but also occur worldwide.

ARCA2 (ataxia with coenzyme Q10 deficiency) and ataxia with vitamin E deficiency are treatable.

Hereditary spastic paraplegias are AD or AR. Myelopathy may be accompanied by ataxia and dysmetria.

Mitochondrial encephalomyopathies cause ataxia and complex clinical constellations. Most are AR or obey mitochondrial maternal inheritance. *Mitochondrial recessive ataxia syndromes* caused by mutations in polymerase gamma cause ataxia, neuropathy, and hearing loss, particularly in Scandinavian families. *Fragile X–associated tremor ataxia syndrome* is an X-linked polyglutamine disorder usually of older men causing ataxia, tremor, cognitive failure, and erectile dysfunction.

Sporadic ataxias include *multiple system atrophy*, a synucleinopathy with cerebellar ataxia or parkinsonism, autonomic dysfunction (postural hypotension, erectile dysfunction, urinary incontinence), and rapid eye movement sleep behavior disorder. *Idiopathic late-onset cerebellar ataxia* describes adults older than 50 years with isolated cerebellar degeneration in whom a cause cannot be identified even with exome testing.

Isolated downbeat nystagmus points to lesions at the cervicomedullary junction or lobules IX/X. It is also caused by a recently identified intronic repeat disorder in the *FGF14* gene, SCA 27B.

Many disorders of infancy and childhood have cerebellar malformations or disruptions: hypoplasia, agenesis, megacerebellum, and Chiari and Dandy-Walker malformations.

Plate 8.17

Cerebellum and Ataxia

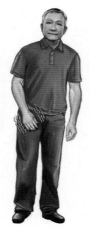
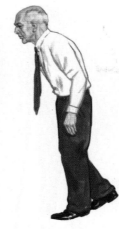
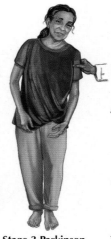
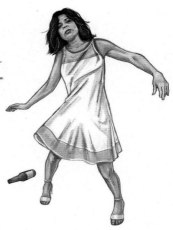

Stage 1 Parkinson disease: unilateral involvement; blank facies; affected arm in semiflexed position with tremor; patient leans to unaffected side

Stage 2 Parkinson disease: bilateral involvement with early postural changes; slow, shuffling gait with decreased excursion of legs

Stage 3 Parkinson disease: pronounced gait disturbances and moderate generalized disability; postural instability with tendency to fall

Typical wide-based gait of alcohol intoxication

Gait Disorders: Differential Diagnosis

Gait is a complex neurologic function that can be degraded by lesions at multiple points in the nervous and musculoskeletal systems. Identifying the location of pathology is essential to establishing the diagnosis. Elicitation of the history is followed by observation of the gait, which facilitates hypothesis-driven examination. Focused imaging and laboratory investigations confirm or refute the clinical impression.

MUSCLE

Myopathy is proximally predominant in inflammatory myopathies, steroid myopathy, and Duchenne and limb girdle dystrophies. Waddling gait results from dropping of the pelvis. Patients have difficulty ascending stairs, arising from chairs, or arising from a seated position on the floor.

NEUROMUSCULAR JUNCTION

Of the various neuromuscular junction (NMJ) disorders, Lambert-Eaton myasthenic syndrome is most likely to present with a gait disorder. Climbing stairs and arising from a chair are impaired. Typically, myasthenia gravis presents with ocular symptoms; gait dysfunction usually does not occur until generalization later in the course. Both NMJ disorders worsen with exertion.

PERIPHERAL NERVE

Peroneal nerve palsy produces foot drop because of tibialis anterior muscle weakness. The leg is lifted high; the foot does not dorsiflex and is slapped down with the ball of the foot hitting the ground first. Femoral neuropathies affect the quadriceps muscles, causing weakness or buckling when navigating stairs, particularly descending as the quadriceps needs to lock to support the after-coming leg.

Generalized peripheral neuropathies are symmetric and length dependent, causing foot slapping because of

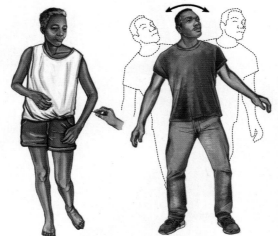
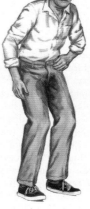
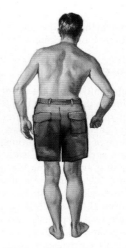

Left hemiparesis with decreased arm swing sometimes associated with limited sensation secondary to a corticospinal tract lesion

Wide-based gait of midline cerebellar tumor or other lesion

Apraxic gait of normal-pressure hydrocephalus

Characteristic posture in left-sided lower lumbar disc herniation

distal weakness and sensory deafferentation, particularly proprioceptive impairment. The proprioceptive loss contributes to increased gait and balance difficulties in darkness; the Romberg test is positive. Muscle stretch reflexes are diminished or absent. Lumbosacral polyradiculopathies or plexopathies produce weakness in multiple myotomes, unilaterally or bilaterally, affecting walking.

SPINAL CORD

With myelopathies, lower extremity hypertonicity causes spastic gait, scissoring (legs tending to cross each other), stiff-legged motions, minimal knee flexion, and circumduction. Strength may be preserved. Reflexes are exaggerated with extensor plantar responses, but the jaw jerk is normal.

CEREBELLUM

Cerebellar gait is wide based and veers from side to side, with a lurching, irregular cadence, and extra steps when turning or making sudden moves. The earliest sign is inability to walk in tandem. Late-stage cerebellar disease destroys truncal stability, making gait impossible without a walker or bilateral support. Unilateral cerebellar lesions produce stumbling and/or ipsilateral falling. Strength is preserved.

BRAINSTEM

Ataxic hemiparesis results from lesions in the basis pontis, midbrain, thalamus, and corona radiata, involving corticospinal and cerebrocerebellar circuits. Mild weakness is accompanied by true cerebellar dysmetria

Plate 8.18

Brain: PART I

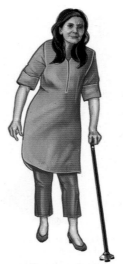

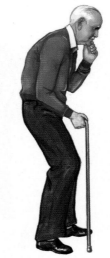

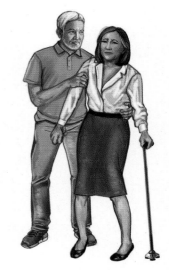

Patient walks gingerly due to loss of position sense and/or painful dysesthesia

Patient with lumbar spinal stenosis with forward-flexed gait

Patient with peripheral neuropathy and loss of proprioception

Gait Disorders: Differential Diagnosis (Continued)

and dysrhythmia. The affected leg circumducts, with inaccurate foot placement.

BASAL GANGLIA

Extrapyramidal movement disorders affect gait, depending on the interplay of inhibition and disinhibition within the basal ganglia circuitry. Parkinsonian syndromes characteristically have small shuffling steps at initiation of stride and through all gait phases, stooped posture, and festination, with the anteriorly displaced center of gravity pulling the patient forward. The patient festinates from one stationery object to another to prevent escalation of speed. Resting tremor occurs in Parkinson disease (see Plate 7.4), anteflexed neck in multiple system atrophy, absent vertical gaze in progressive supranuclear palsy (see Plate 7.7), and limb apraxia in corticobasal degeneration (see Plate 7.7). Chorea, dystonia, and athetosis characterize Huntington disease (see Plate 7.13); dyskinesias occur with dopaminergic excess in treated patients with Parkinson disease; hemiballism is seen after subthalamic lesions and in Tourette syndrome.

CEREBRAL CORTEX AND WHITE MATTER

Frontal lobe gait disorders (gait apraxia) secondary to subcortical small vessel lacunar disease are characterized by a magnetic quality, as if glued to the floor, or slipping clutch. Patients have difficulty initiating stride, taking small repetitive steps before launching a gait that looks almost normal. After stopping, the attempt to restart reproduces the pattern. Confined spaces are particularly troublesome.

NORMAL PRESSURE HYDROCEPHALUS

Normal pressure hydrocephalus (see Plate 8.17) produces a frontal lobe–appearing gait disorder, together with urinary dysfunction, cognitive decline, and ventriculomegaly on imaging.

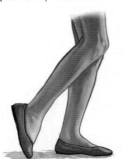

Typical spastic gait, scuffing toe of affected leg

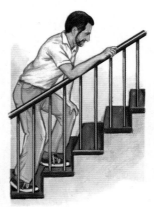

Severe myopathy or NMJ lesion with proximal weakness

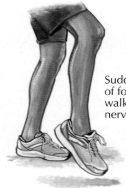

Sudden occurrence of foot drop while walking (peroneal nerve)

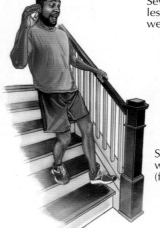

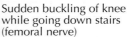

Sudden buckling of knee while going down stairs (femoral nerve)

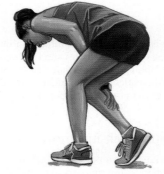

Muscle cramps from defect in energy metabolism (McArdle disease)

Hemiparesis from upper motor neuron lesions produces increased tone in the contralateral limbs, with the leg maintained in extension and the arm in flexion. The leg circumducts because of poor flexion at the hip and knees. The plantar-flexed foot may have clonus, producing a bouncing quality to the gait.

NONNEUROLOGIC DISORDERS

Elderly persons sometimes have a slow cautious gait, reflecting slowing of neural conduction and concern to prevent falls. Nonneurologic disorders producing limp or insecure gait include arthritis, trochanteric bursitis, lumbosacral spine or disc disease, and podiatric conditions (bunions, tenosynovitis, neuromas).

Gait is sometimes irregular in *primary psychiatric disorders,* with stereotypies and mannerisms or extrapyramidal features from chronic psychotropic medications. Functional neurologic gait disorders (*astasia-abasia*) are varying and inconstant, contravening recognized neurologic patterns; this diagnosis is best made by neurologists after careful investigation.

Plate 8.19

Cerebellum and Ataxia

FRIEDREICH ATAXIA

Friedreich ataxia (FRDA) is a unique disorder involving expansion of a trinucleotide repeat (GAA) in the first intron of the disease-related gene, frataxin *(FXN),* leading to loss of function in the unstable frataxin protein. FRDA is AR, unlike other trinucleotide repeat disorders, which are typically AD or X-linked. It differs from CAG repeat disorders (Huntington disease, spinocerebellar ataxias, and Kennedy disease), wherein expansion occurs in the coding region, leading to toxic gain of function by increasing content of glutamine in the relevant protein.

First described in 1863 by Nikolaus Friedreich, FRDA is the most common form of hereditary ataxia. FRDA a progressive spinocerebellar disorder typically having prepubertal onset between ages 5 and 15 years, although exceptions occur with up to 25% having delayed onset into adulthood. Because of spinal cord, peripheral nerve, and, to a lesser extent, cerebellar atrophy, the initial signs are principally ataxia involving gait and limb function (spinocerebellar tracts) and muscle weakness followed by progressive loss of muscle stretch reflexes at the knees and ankles, contrasting with spasticity and extensor plantar responses (pyramidal tracts). Approximately 12% retain their reflexes up to 10 years after onset. In addition, progressive diminution of proprioception and vibratory sensation (posterior columns) occurs as well as slurred speech and swallowing dysfunction. With steady progression of gait and lower limb dysfunction and progressive foot deformities—that is, equinovarus, pes cavus, and clawed toes—wheelchair dependency occurs as early 10 years after onset.

Progressive dysarthria is typical. Abnormal visual and auditory function develops, particularly in later stages. Abnormal oculomotor function is quite common;

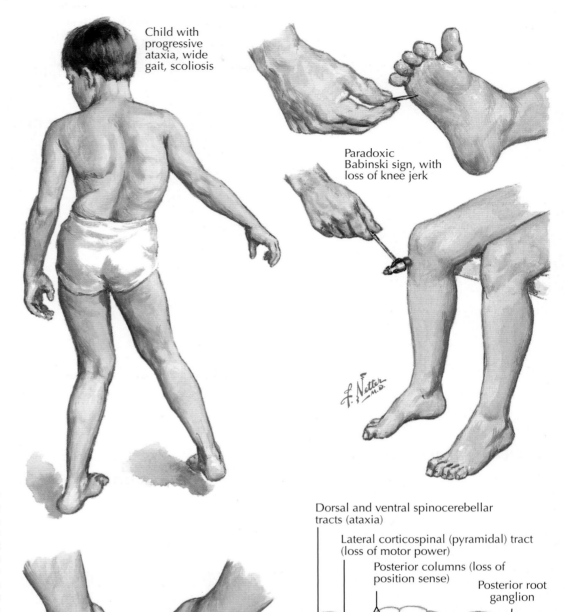

Child with progressive ataxia, wide gait, scoliosis

Paradoxic Babinski sign, with loss of knee jerk

Pes cavus with talipes varus and claw toes

Dorsal and ventral spinocerebellar tracts (ataxia)

Lateral corticospinal (pyramidal) tract (loss of motor power)

Posterior columns (loss of position sense)

Posterior root ganglion

Sites of spinal cord degeneration (and resultant functional deficits)

optic atrophy occurs in 25%. Although cognitive function is not affected overall, the speed of information processing is often slowed, with increasing difficulty in complex reasoning. Scoliosis is present in virtually all individuals, requiring constant surveillance for progression, bracing to slow progress, and surgical intervention in up to 20%.

Systemic involvement is also prominent in the form of cardiomyopathy and progressive cardiac conduction defects (arrhythmia and heart block), representing the most common cause of death. In addition, diabetes

mellitus in 30% and carbohydrate intolerance in 50% require ongoing glucose monitoring.

Assessment of neurologic function should include neuroimaging, clinical electrophysiology (electromyography), radiologic evaluation for scoliosis, and testing for visual and audiometric function. MRI of cerebral hemispheres is normal, but atrophy of the spinal cord, brainstem, and cerebellum is progressive. Motor nerve conduction velocities are generally normal, but sensory nerve studies reveal reduced or absent function. An electrocardiogram is recommended

Plate 8.20   Brain: PART I

Cardiac abnormalities in Friedreich ataxia

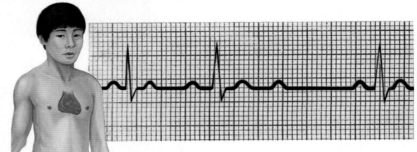

Death often caused by cardiac abnormalities (interstitial myocarditis, fibrosis, enlargement, arrhythmias, murmurs, heart block)

GAA expansion mutation

A

EXPANDED ALLELE

(GAA)   90–1200

Exon 1   Exon 2

PCR PRODUCT

NORMAL ALLELE

(GAA)   <40

Exon 1   Exon 2

PCR PRODUCT

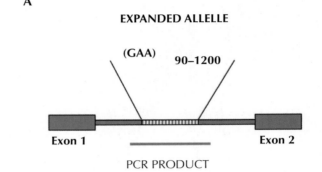
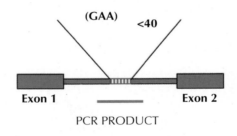

B

N/N 730/1100 N/900

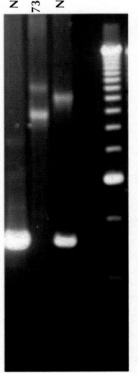

2000bp

Friedreich Ataxia (Continued)

at diagnosis and annually thereafter, and echocardiography is recommended with onset of cardiomyopathy.

FRDA has an incidence in Indo-European populations of approximately 1:50,000, although isolates have been described at 1:25,000. Lower frequencies are reported in Native Americans and residents of sub-Saharan Africa and Southeast Asia.

The normal range of GAA repeats in *FXN* is 5 to 33, with greater than 80% having less than 12. Affected individuals have at least 70 GAA repeats, although expansions up to 1700 are described. Most commonly, repeat length is 600 to 1200. Disease severity is typically related to the size of the expansion. The lower expansion size (40–70 GAA repeats) is regarded as a premutation, the percentage of affected individuals being less than 1%. In the 25% with delayed FDRA onset, the GAA expansion is generally smaller (100–600 repeats), but factors such as genetic background and environmental influences are important variables. FRDA is due to abnormal expansion (equal or different lengths) in both alleles of *FXN* in approximately 98% of affected individuals. The remainder represents individuals with abnormal expansion in one allele and a point mutation or deletion inactivating the gene in the other allele. No individual has been described as lacking an expansion in at least one *FXN* allele.

Diagnosis of FDRA depends on assessment of *FXN* in blood by DNA sequencing methodology capable of detecting GAA expansion and direct assessment of inactivating mutations of nonexpanded regions for the small percentage with a point mutation or deletion. Carrier detection and prenatal diagnosis are recommended for individuals in a family with known disease-producing expansion. Frataxin is a relatively

A, Scheme showing the intronic GAA repeat in the frataxin gene. To determine its length, a polymerase chain reaction (PCR) product containing the repeat is generated between two flanking primers and its size is estimated by gel electrophoresis. **B**, Agarose gel electrophoresis of PCR products containing the GAA repeat in the frataxin gene. The sample in the first lane (N/N) is from a homozygous normal individual; the sample in the second lane is from a patient with FRDA with two expanded GAA repeats (the numbers 730 and 1100 indicate the estimated number of GAA triplets in each allele); the third lane is from a heterozygous individual with one normal (N) and one expanded (estimated at 900 triplets) allele. Such an individual may be a healthy carrier or an FRDA patient, if the chromosome containing the normal size repeat carries a frataxin point mutation. *From Pandolfo M. Friedreich ataxia. In: Darras BT, ed. Neuromuscular Disorders of Infancy, Childhood, and Adolescence. 2nd ed. Elsevier; 2015:984-1002.*

small (210 amino acids) protein that is prevalent in the inner mitochondrial membrane. Frataxin is required in the formation of iron-sulfur clusters that occur in respiratory chain complexes I to III and aconitase; deficiency results in defective mitochondrial function, increased mitochondrial free iron, and abnormal energy production in spinal cord and skeletal and cardiac muscle. Differential diagnosis includes peripheral neuropathy (Charcot-Marie-Tooth disease), SCA, ataxia telangiectasia, abetalipoproteinemia, mitochondrial DNA mutations (myoclonus

epilepsy with ragged-red fibers), and late-onset hexosaminidase deficiency.

In general, survival is significantly shortened in FRDA, with an average longevity of 30 to 40 years after onset. Heart disease is the most common cause of death. Although no cure exists at present, a number of pharmacologic agents are under investigation. Overall quality of life depends on maintaining suitable exercise, a proper diet and healthy body mass index, hearing aids, feeding therapy, and regular counseling. Specific gene therapy is not currently available.

CEREBROVASCULAR CIRCULATION AND STROKE

Plate 9.1

Brain: PART I

ARTERIAL SUPPLY TO THE BRAIN AND MENINGES

OVERVIEW OF THE CRANIOCERVICAL LARGE VESSELS

The brain and meninges are supplied by branches that originate from the aorta. The brachiocephalic trunk (or *innominate artery*) divides behind the right sternoclavicular joint into a right common carotid artery (CCA) and a right subclavian artery that supplies the arm. The next aortic branches are the left CCA and the left subclavian artery (supplying the left arm), arising directly from the aortic arch. The vertebral arteries (VAs) are early branches of the subclavian arteries on each side. The CCAs bifurcate in the neck, usually opposite the upper border of the thyroid cartilage, most often at the level of the body of the fourth cervical vertebra, into the internal carotid artery (ICA) and external carotid artery (ECA). The ICAs are direct extensions of the CCA and supply the brain. The ECAs usually course more anteriorly and laterally and supply branches to the face and its structures.

CERVICAL AND EXTRACRANIAL CIRCULATION

Internal Carotid Artery

The ICAs ascend vertically in the neck, posterior and slightly medial to the ECA. The ICAs are positioned medial to the sternocleidomastoid muscle and travel behind the faucial pillars of the pharynx until they reach the carotid canal at the skull base. They have no branches within the neck. At the skull base, the carotid arteries lie adjacent to the ninth to twelfth cranial nerves, which exit the skull from the jugular and hypoglossal foramina. The ICAs then enter the skull through the carotid canal within the petrous bone. A different classification system for the ICAs distinguishes seven segments, only the first of which is extracranial (C1 cervical).

Vertebral Artery

The first branch of each subclavian artery is the VA. The *thyrocervical and costocervical* trunks originate from the subclavian artery just distal to the VA and could serve as collateral channels should the VA origin become occluded. The first segment (V1) of the VA courses upward and backward until it enters the transverse foramina of the sixth or fifth cervical vertebra. Then the artery ascends as the second segment (V$_2$), which courses within the intravertebral foramina, exiting from the transverse process of the atlas. The third segment (V$_3$) passes posteriorly behind the articular process of the atlas; it lies in a groove on the upper surface of the posterior arch of the atlas, behind the atlas, before piercing the dura mater to enter the foramen magnum and becoming the intracranial and intradural V4 segment. The V$_4$ segment ends at the medullopontine junction, where the two VAs join to form the basilar artery.

Branches. The cervical portion of the VAs gives rise to many muscular and spinal radicular branches. The spinal branches pass through the intervertebral foramina and enter the spinal canal to supply the cervical portion of the spinal cord, and the periosteum and bodies of the cervical vertebra. A small anterior and larger posterior meningeal artery originate from the distal extracranial segments (distal V$_2$ or V$_3$).

External Carotid Artery

The ECAs give off many branches that supply structures within the face and neck. The ECAs extend from the

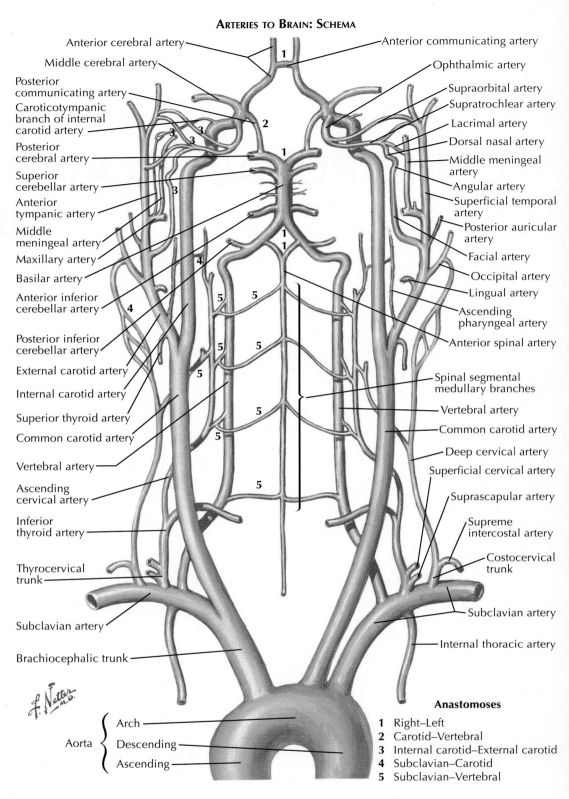

ARTERIES TO BRAIN: SCHEMA

Anterior cerebral artery
Middle cerebral artery
Posterior communicating artery
Caroticotympanic branch of internal carotid artery
Posterior cerebral artery
Superior cerebellar artery
Anterior tympanic artery
Middle meningeal artery
Maxillary artery
Basilar artery
Anterior inferior cerebellar artery
Posterior inferior cerebellar artery
External carotid artery
Internal carotid artery
Superior thyroid artery
Common carotid artery
Vertebral artery
Ascending cervical artery
Inferior thyroid artery
Thyrocervical trunk
Subclavian artery
Brachiocephalic trunk

Anterior communicating artery
Ophthalmic artery
Supraorbital artery
Supratrochlear artery
Lacrimal artery
Dorsal nasal artery
Middle meningeal artery
Angular artery
Superficial temporal artery
Posterior auricular artery
Facial artery
Occipital artery
Lingual artery
Ascending pharyngeal artery
Anterior spinal artery
Spinal segmental medullary branches
Vertebral artery
Common carotid artery
Deep cervical artery
Superficial cervical artery
Suprascapular artery
Supreme intercostal artery
Costocervical trunk
Subclavian artery
Internal thoracic artery

Aorta { Arch, Descending, Ascending

Anastomoses

1 Right–Left
2 Carotid–Vertebral
3 Internal carotid–External carotid
4 Subclavian–Carotid
5 Subclavian–Vertebral

upper border of the thyroid cartilage to the neck of the mandible. There are eight major branches of the ECA. The *superior thyroid, lingual, and facial* arteries arise from the anterior aspect of the ECAs and course medially. The *ascending pharyngeal artery* arises from the medial or deep aspect of the vessel. The *occipital and posterior auricular arteries* arise from the posterior aspect of the artery. Behind the neck of the mandible, the ECA divides into the *superficial temporal and internal maxillary arteries*, usually within the parotid gland. The

internal maxillary artery has mandibular, pterygoid, and pterygopalatine portions supplying the deep structures of the face, including the *middle meningeal artery* branches, which penetrate the skull through the foramen spinosum. The superficial temporal artery has frontal and parietal branches supplying muscles, skin, and pericranium.

The ECAs have several branches that could provide collateral blood flow to the ICA system. The *facial artery* courses along the cheek toward the nasal

Plate 9.2

Cerebrovascular Circulation and Stroke

ARTERIAL SUPPLY TO THE BRAIN AND MENINGES (Continued)

bridge, where it is termed the angular artery. The *internal maxillary, superficial temporal,* and *ascending pharyngeal arteries* can also contribute to the intracranial circulation via small distal collaterals, such as nasoethmoidal to ophthalmic artery branches, and maxillary to cavernous carotid (inferolateral trunk) collaterals.

Anomalous Origin of the Cervical Large Vessels

The right CCA and right subclavian arteries may arise as separate branches directly from the aortic arch. The right VA may arise directly from the brachiocephalic trunk instead of the right subclavian artery. The left VA may also arise from the brachiocephalic trunk or directly from the aortic arch. The right subclavian artery can arise from the aortic arch distal to the left subclavian artery, in which case it then crosses to the right side, which is called an aberrant right subclavian artery. Sometimes the left CCA and the left subclavian artery arise from a common (left brachiocephalic) trunk. Rarely, the VA can arise from the CCA.

INTRACRANIAL CIRCULATION

The internal carotid (anterior) circulation supplies the anterior and most of the lateral portions of the cerebral hemispheres, whereas the vertebrobasilar (posterior) circulation supplies the brainstem, cerebellum, and the posterior portion of the cerebral hemispheres. Approximately 40% of the brain's blood flow comes through each ICA, whereas 20% flows through the vertebrobasilar arterial system.

CIRCLE OF WILLIS

This anastomosis at the base of the brain (more a hexagon than a circle) serves to connect the major arteries of the anterior and posterior circulations, and arteries from both sides. The horizontal portions of the *anterior cerebral artery* (ACA) branches of the ICAs are connected through the *anterior communicating artery,* forming the anterior portion of the circle. The *posterior communicating artery* branches of the ICAs on each side connect to the *posterior cerebral artery* (PCA) branches of the *basilar artery,* forming the lateral sides and posterior portion of the "circle."

ANTERIOR CIRCULATION

Internal Carotid Artery

The ICAs enter the skull through the carotid canal within the petrous bone and form an S-shaped curve on each side. The proximal intracranial portion of the ICAs within this curve is referred to as the *carotid siphon.* There are three divisions of the ICAs within the siphon: an extradural petrous portion, an extradural cavernous portion within the cavernous sinus, and an intradural supraclinoid portion. A more detailed classification system distinguishes seven ICA segments, the first of which is extracranial, and the rest are intracranial: C1 (cervical), C2 (petrous), C3 (lacerum), C4 (cavernous), C5 (clinoid), C6 (ophthalmic), and C7 (communicating).

Branches of the Petrous and Cavernous Segments

Two branches arise from the petrous segment: the caroticotympanic artery supplying the tympanic cavity, and the artery of the pterygoid canal (Vidian artery) supplying the pharynx and the tympanic cavity. The cavernous segment gives off the meningohypophyseal trunk supplying branches to the pituitary gland and meninges, and the inferolateral trunk supplying dura and cranial nerves with extensive internal maxillary and ophthalmic collaterals. Within the cavernous sinus, the ICA lies in close relationship to the nerves that control eye movement (cranial nerves III, IV, and VI) and the ophthalmic and maxillary divisions of cranial nerve V.

Branches of the Supraclinoid Segment

As the ICAs penetrate the dura mater, soon after leaving the cavernous sinus medial to the anterior clinoid process, the supraclinoid segment begins. *The superior hypophyseal artery* arises as the first branch of the supraclinoid portion of the ICAs, giving off branches to the optic chiasm and participating in an anastomosis that supplies the pituitary gland, which is composed of arterial branches from each side and branches of the right and left meningohypophyseal trunk. The ICAs then give off the *ophthalmic artery,* still at the proximal supraclinoid segment. Rarely, this small but important vessel can also arise from the distal cavernous segment. The ophthalmic artery courses from the anterior aspect

ARTERIES TO BRAIN AND MENINGES

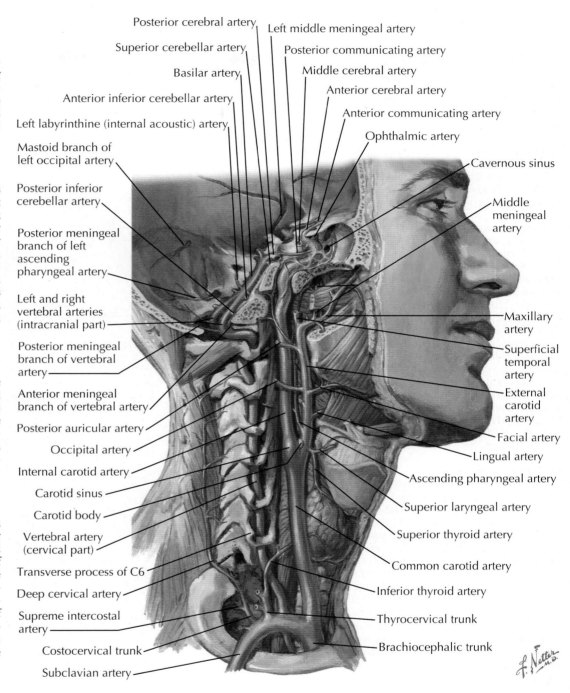

Posterior cerebral artery
Superior cerebellar artery
Basilar artery
Anterior inferior cerebellar artery
Left labyrinthine (internal acoustic) artery
Mastoid branch of left occipital artery
Posterior inferior cerebellar artery
Posterior meningeal branch of left ascending pharyngeal artery
Left and right vertebral arteries (intracranial part)
Posterior meningeal branch of vertebral artery
Anterior meningeal branch of vertebral artery
Posterior auricular artery
Occipital artery
Internal carotid artery
Carotid sinus
Carotid body
Vertebral artery (cervical part)
Transverse process of C6
Deep cervical artery
Supreme intercostal artery
Costocervical trunk
Subclavian artery

Left middle meningeal artery
Posterior communicating artery
Middle cerebral artery
Anterior cerebral artery
Anterior communicating artery
Ophthalmic artery
Cavernous sinus
Middle meningeal artery
Maxillary artery
Superficial temporal artery
External carotid artery
Facial artery
Lingual artery
Ascending pharyngeal artery
Superior laryngeal artery
Superior thyroid artery
Common carotid artery
Inferior thyroid artery
Thyrocervical trunk
Brachiocephalic trunk

Plate 9.3

Brain: PART I

ARTERIAL SUPPLY TO THE BRAIN AND MENINGES (Continued)

of the ICA medial to the anterior clinoid process, projects anteriorly, then passes through the optic canal into the orbit just below and lateral to the optic nerve. The ophthalmic artery is known to have orbital and ocular branches, as well as extensive anastomoses with ECA branches. An important arterial supply of the face also involves the frontal and supratrochlear branches of the ophthalmic artery that supply the medial forehead above the eyebrow and can anastomose with distal ECA branches. Distal to the ophthalmic origin, the supraclinoid segment ascends slightly posteriorly and laterally, passing between the oculomotor and optic nerves.

Distal to the ophthalmic artery, the posterior communicating arteries originate posteriorly and then course medially to join the PCAs on each side about 1 cm from their origins from the basilar artery. Small perforator branches off the posterior communicating artery feed the optic tract and the posterior portion of the optic chiasm, posterior perforated substance, optic tract, pituitary stalk, posterior hypothalamus, and the floor of the third ventricle. The *tuberothalamic (polar) artery* most often arises from the middle third of the posterior communicating artery but may also arise from the proximal segment of the PCA. The polar artery supplies the anteromedial and anterolateral portions of the thalamus. The most notable variant of the posterior communicating artery, present in up to 22% of the population, is the persistent fetal origin PCA (fetal PCA). This variant is defined as a prominent posterior communicating artery that gives rise directly to the P2 segment of the PCA without significant connection to the basilar apex.

The *anterior choroidal arteries* are very small vessels that originate from the posterolateral part of the ICAs, distal to the origins of the ophthalmic and posterior communicating arteries, and then project posteriorly. The anterior choroidal arteries have two main divisions, cisternal and intraventricular. The anterior choroidal artery courses posteriorly and laterally, running along the optic tract, and first gives off penetrating branches to the globus pallidus and posterior limb of the internal capsule. The anterior choroidal artery branches then course laterally to the medial temporal lobe, and medially to supply a portion of the midbrain and the thalamus. The anterior choroidal artery ends in the lateral geniculate body, where they join with lateral posterior choroidal artery branches of the PCAs and in the choroid plexus of the lateral ventricles near the temporal horns.

The termination of the ICA (the T-portion, carotid T, or carotid terminus) is the bifurcation of the vessel into the medially coursing ACA and laterally coursing *middle cerebral artery* (MCA).

Middle Cerebral Artery

The MCA arises from the ICA bifurcation just lateral to the optic chiasm. The mainstem (M1) portion courses horizontally in a lateral direction to enter the sylvian fissure. Three to six medial and lateral lenticulostriate arteries arise from the mainstem MCA and penetrate the anterior perforated substance to supply the basal ganglia and deep portions of the cerebral hemispheres. The *medial lenticulostriate arteries* supply the outer portion of the globus pallidus and the medial parts of the

caudate nucleus and putamen. The *lateral lenticulostriate arteries* supply the lateral portion of the caudate nucleus, the putamen, the anterior portion and genu of the internal capsule, and the adjacent corona radiata. Anterior temporal and frontopolar branches arise from the mainstem MCA after the lenticulostriate origins. Occasionally the mainstem M1 segment of the MCA is short with an early bifurcation, and the lenticulostriate branches may arise from the proximal portion of the superior M2 division.

As the MCA enters the sylvian fissure, it becomes the M2 segment. The MCA typically divides into large superior and inferior M2 divisions. The superior division supplies the lateral portions of the cerebral hemispheres above the sylvian fissure, and the inferior division supplies the temporal and inferior parietal lobes below the sylvian fissure. These main divisions turn upward and around the inferior portion of the insula of Reil to continue upward and backward in the deepest part of the sylvian fissure between the outer

TEMPORAL AND INFRATEMPORAL FOSSAE

Masseteric nerve
Mandibular nerve (CN V₃) (exiting foramen ovale)
Superficial temporal artery
Middle meningeal artery
Condylar process of mandible (cut)
Chorda tympani
Auriculotemporal nerve
Anterior tympanic artery
Deep auricular artery
Maxillary artery
Posterior auricular nerve
Facial nerve (CN VII) (cut)
Internal jugular vein (cut)
Spinal accessory nerve (CN XI) (cut)
Occipital artery
Facial artery
Superior root of ansa cervicalis
Inferior root of ansa cervicalis (cut)
Internal carotid artery
Vagus nerve (CN X)
Ansa cervicalis
Common carotid artery
External carotid artery
Hypoglossal nerve (CN XII) (cut)
Right inferior alveolar nerve
Lingual artery
Right nerve to mylohyoid muscle
Right facial artery
Right submandibular ganglion
Right lingual nerve
Window cut through right medial pterygoid muscle
Submandibular ganglion
Medial pterygoid muscle
Body of mandible (cut)
Nerve to mylohyoid muscle
Mylohyoid branch of inferior alveolar artery
Lingual nerve
Inferior alveolar nerve
Inferior alveolar artery
Posterior superior alveolar arteries
Posterior superior alveolar nerves
Infraorbital artery
Maxillary nerve (CN V₂)
Anterior deep temporal artery
Buccal nerve
Temporalis muscle (cut and reflected superiorly)
Anterior deep temporal nerve
Buccal artery
Superior head of lateral pterygoid muscle (cut)
Posterior deep temporal nerve
Posterior deep temporal artery
Inferior head of lateral pterygoid muscle (cut)

C. Machado M.D.

Plate 9.4

Cerebrovascular Circulation and Stroke

ARTERIAL SUPPLY TO THE BRAIN AND MENINGES (Continued)

surface of the insula and the medial surface of the temporal lobe.

The superior division of the MCA has lateral orbitofrontal, ascending frontal, rolandic, and anterior and posterior parietal branches supplying their corresponding territories. The inferior division provides posterior temporal and angular branches to supply the lateral portions of the cerebral hemispheres below the sylvian fissure.

Anterior Cerebral Artery

The ACA is the smaller of the two terminal branches of the ICAs. The ACA courses medially until it reaches the longitudinal fissures and then run posteriorly over the corpus callosum. The first portion of the ACA is sometimes hypoplastic on one side, in which case the ACA from the other side supplies both medial frontal lobes. The anterior communicating artery connects the right and left ACAs and provides potential collateral circulation from the anterior circulation of the opposite side.

The horizontal segment of the ACA gives rise to multiple branches. Some course inferiorly to supply the upper surface of the optic nerves and the optic chiasm. Dorsally directed branches penetrate the orbital brain surface to supply the anterior hypothalamus, the septum pellucidum, the medial part of the anterior commissure, the columns of the fornix, and the basal frontal lobe structures (called the anterior perforated substance or substantia innominata). The largest horizontal segment branch is called the *recurrent artery of Heubner*. It most often arises from the ACA near its junction with the anterior communicating artery. Most often the "Heubner artery" is a group of parallel small arteries rather than a single vessel. They supply the anteromedial portion of the caudate nucleus and the anterior inferior portion of the anterior limb of the internal capsule.

The proximal interhemispheric portions of the ACAs have medial orbitofrontal branches that travel anteriorly along the gyrus rectus to supply the medial part of the orbital gyri and the olfactory bulbs and tracts, and frontopolar artery branches to the superior frontal gyri. The ACA then passes around the genu of the corpus callosum and, in that general location, divides into callosomarginal and pericallosal branches. The *callosomarginal artery* passes over the cingulate gyrus to course posteriorly within the cingulate sulcus. It supplies anterior, middle, and posterior branches to the medial frontal lobes. The *pericallosal artery* courses posteriorly, below, and parallel to the callosomarginal artery, in a sulcus between the corpus callosum and the cingulate gyrus. It supplies branches to the precuneus and medial superior parietal lobes. The pericallosal artery anastomoses with the pericallosal branch of the PCA variably, usually near the splenium of the corpus callosum.

POSTERIOR CIRCULATION

Vertebral Arteries and Basilar Artery

The intracranial V_4 segment of the VAs gives off posterior and anterior spinal artery branches, penetrating arteries to the medulla, and the large posterior inferior cerebellar arteries (PICAs). The PICAs usually originate

from the V_4 segment of the VA about 16 to 17 mm below the vertebrobasilar junction. They course along the front of the medulla at the level of the inferior olive, then can variably ascend or descend alongside the medulla near or between the origins of the ninth, tenth, and eleventh cranial nerve roots. The next segment of the PICAs courses along the posterolateral surface of the medulla and the inferior cerebellar tonsil, which contains a caudal loop. The next segment courses in the cleft between the tela choroidea and the inferior medullary velum rostrally and the superior pole of the cerebellar tonsil caudally. After that, the vessel supplies

branches to the cerebellar surface. It gives blood supply to the vermis and adjacent hemisphere, the tonsil and hemisphere, and the medullary, choroidal, and cortical arteries.

The intracranial portions (V_4 segment) of the VAs end at the medullopontine junction, where the two VAs join to form the basilar artery. The basilar artery then courses rostrally in a groove closely applied to the anterior surface of the pons, where it is located within the prepontine cistern behind the clivus. The distal segment enters the interpeduncular cistern, where it is often separated from the basal surface of the brainstem. The distal portion of

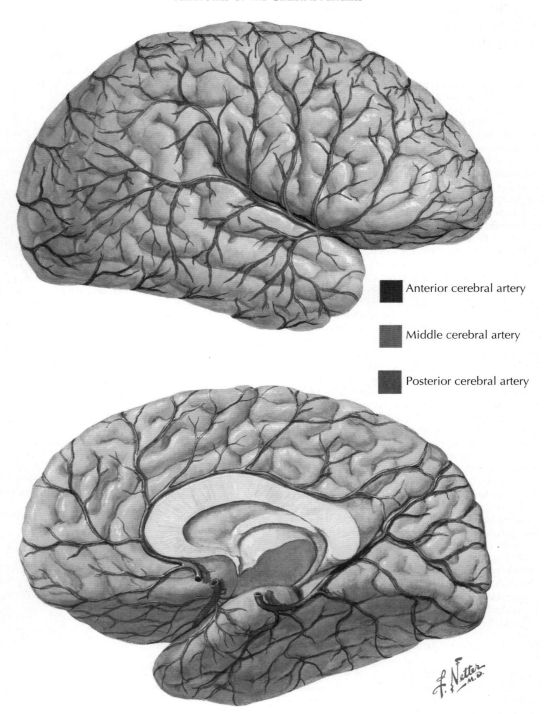

TERRITORIES OF THE CEREBRAL ARTERIES

■ Anterior cerebral artery

■ Middle cerebral artery

■ Posterior cerebral artery

Plate 9.5

Brain: PART I

ARTERIAL SUPPLY TO THE BRAIN AND MENINGES
(Continued)

the artery lies between the cerebral peduncles and ends at the pontomesencephalic junction, just after passing between the two oculomotor nerves, by dividing into the two PCAs. The basilar artery is often curved and tortuous and may deviate from the midline. The basilar artery averages about 33 cm in length, and the average diameter usually is between 4.0 and 4.5 mm and tapers distally. The main branches of the artery are the *anterior inferior cerebellar artery* (AICA) and *superior cerebellar artery* (SCA), paramedian perforator arteries that penetrate directly into the pons, and short circumferential arteries that course around the pons and give off lateral basal and lateral tegmental penetrating arteries.

The AICAs arise from the lower to middle third of the lateral wall of the basilar artery. They usually arise as a single trunk in hemodynamic balance with other cerebellar arteries such as the SCAs and PICAs. However, variations exist, including the rare origin of the artery from the distal VA or duplication of the vessel. The AICAs course posterolaterally, ventral to the pons in the prepontine cistern, then enter the cerebellopontine angle and continue along the anterior cerebellar surface. The main vessel then divides into superior and inferior trunks at the pontomedullary junction adjacent to the exit of cranial nerves VII and VIII from the brainstem. They supply the middle cerebellar peduncle, lower lateral pons, anteroinferior cerebellum, flocculus, and choroid plexus of the lateral ventricle. The labyrinthine artery, supplying the labyrinth and cochlea of the inner ear along with cranial nerves VII and VIII, is mostly a branch of the AICA.

The SCAs can arise as a single or duplicate trunk from the distal basilar artery just before the origin of the PCAs. Initially, the anterior pontomesencephalic segment lies below the oculomotor segment, and the lateral mesencephalic segment courses below the trochlear and above the trigeminal nerves. Then the cerebellomesencephalic segment courses in the groove between the cerebellum and upper brainstem, and eventually the cortical branch is distributed to the cerebellar surface where it supplies the superior part of the cerebellum, vermis, and a small brainstem territory, including the dorsal tegmentum and the tectum of the upper part of the pons.

Posterior Cerebral Artery

The PCAs originate from the terminal bifurcation of the basilar artery rostral to the third cranial nerves and then encircle the midbrain above the level of the tentorium cerebelli. As the PCAs course the dorsal surface of the midbrain, they divide into cortical branches. The arteries are divided into peduncular, ambient, and quadrigeminal segments, named after the cisterns through which they pass. The proximal portion of the arteries, before the posterior communicating artery branch, is referred to as the precommunal, P1 segment, or the mesencephalic artery. A variation in the form of a solitary trunk called the *artery of Percheron* exists in approximately one-third of the population and supplies the rostral midbrain and paramedian thalami bilaterally.

Branches that supply the midbrain and thalamus arise from the proximal peduncular and ambient segments. *Paramedian mesencephalic arteries* arise from the first 3 to 7 mm of the arteries. The thalamic-subthalamic arteries (also called *thalamoperforating*) also arise proximally to supply the paramedian portions of the

posteromedial thalamus. The *medial posterior choroidal arteries* also arise proximally from the peduncular segments and supply the quadrigeminal plate in the midbrain and the choroid plexus of the third ventricle. More distally, the *peduncular perforating* and *thalamogeniculate arteries* originate from the ambient segments. These supply the basolateral midbrain and the anterolateral thalamus, respectively. Each consists of a fan of parallel arteries.

Further in their course, after the PCAs have circled the midbrain, the *lateral posterior choroidal artery* branches arise, which supply the pulvinar, dorsal thalamus, and the lateral geniculate bodies, as well as the

choroid plexus of the temporal horns of the lateral ventricles. There are four main cortical branches of the PCAs: the anterior temporal, posterior temporal, parietooccipital, and calcarine arteries. The *anterior temporal arteries* arise first from the ambient segments, usually as single arterial trunks or as multiple branches to supply the inferior portion of the temporal lobe. The *posterior temporal arteries* course posteriorly on the inferior parietal and occipital lobes. The *parietooccipital and calcarine arteries* are more variable, usually arising independently from the ambient segments and supplying the occipital and medial inferior parietal lobes. The *posterior pericallosal arteries* that circle the posterior

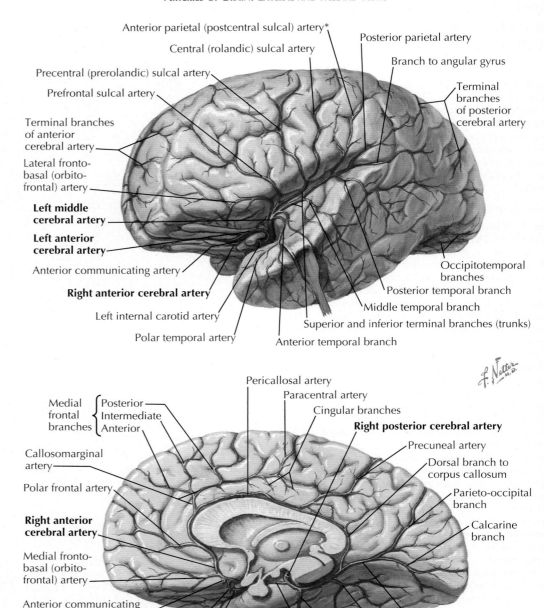

ARTERIES OF BRAIN: LATERAL AND MEDIAL VIEWS

Anterior parietal (postcentral sulcal) artery*
Central (rolandic) sulcal artery
Posterior parietal artery
Branch to angular gyrus
Precentral (prerolandic) sulcal artery
Prefrontal sulcal artery
Terminal branches of posterior cerebral artery
Terminal branches of anterior cerebral artery
Lateral fronto-basal (orbito-frontal) artery
Left middle cerebral artery
Left anterior cerebral artery
Anterior communicating artery
Occipitotemporal branches
Right anterior cerebral artery
Posterior temporal branch
Left internal carotid artery
Middle temporal branch
Polar temporal artery
Superior and inferior terminal branches (trunks)
Anterior temporal branch

Pericallosal artery
Paracentral artery
Medial frontal branches { Posterior, Intermediate, Anterior }
Cingular branches
Right posterior cerebral artery
Callosomarginal artery
Precuneal artery
Polar frontal artery
Dorsal branch to corpus callosum
Right anterior cerebral artery
Parieto-occipital branch
Medial fronto-basal (orbito-frontal) artery
Calcarine branch
Anterior communicating artery (*cut*)
Medial occipital artery
Posterior temporal branch
Distal medial striate artery (recurrent artery of Heubner)
Anterior temporal branch
Right internal carotid artery
Posterior communicating artery

*Note: Anterior parietal (postcentral sulcal) artery also occurs as separate anterior parietal and postcentral sulcal arteries.

Plate 9.6

Cerebrovascular Circulation and Stroke

ARTERIAL SUPPLY TO THE BRAIN AND MENINGES (Continued)

portion of the corpus callosum to anastomose with the anterior pericallosal artery branches of the ACAs usually arise from the parietooccipital arteries within the quadrigeminal cisterns.

MENINGEAL ARTERIES

The meningeal arteries and veins are located along the outer portion of the dura, grooving the inner table of the skull. They supply the dura and the adjacent bony structures, and they form anastomoses across both sides of the skull and with cerebral arteries. Their major clinical importances are that (1) injuries to the skull, especially fractures, can cut across meningeal arteries, leading to epidural hemorrhages that require urgent drainage, and (2) meningiomas, meningeal tumors, and dural arteriovenous fistulas (AVFs) are often fed by meningeal arteries.

The *middle meningeal artery,* originating from the external carotid system via the internal maxillary artery, is the largest of the meningeal arteries. It supplies the major blood supply to the dura mater and ascends just lateral to the external pterygoid muscle to enter the calvarium through the foramen spinosum. The middle meningeal artery then passes forward and laterally across the floor of the middle cranial fossa and divides into two branches below the pterion. The frontal (anterior) branch climbs across the greater wing of the sphenoid and parietal bone, forming a groove on the inner table of the calvaria and then dividing into two branches that supply the outer surface of the dura from the frontoparietal convexity to the vertex and as far posteriorly as the occiput. The smaller parietal (posterior) branch curves backward over the temporal region to supply the posterior part of the dura mater.

The *accessory meningeal artery* may also arise from the internal maxillary artery or from the middle meningeal artery. It ascends through the foramen ovale to supply the trigeminal ganglion and the adjacent dura within the middle cranial fossa.

The bone and dura of the posterior fossa are supplied by (1) the *meningeal branches of the ascending pharyngeal artery,* which pass through the jugular foramen, foramen lacerum, and the hypoglossal canal; (2) the *meningeal branches of the occipital artery,* which pass through the jugular foramen and the condylar canal; and (3) the small *mastoid branch of the occipital artery,* which passes through the mastoid foramen.

Meningeal Branches of the Internal Carotid System

The meningohypophyseal trunk, originating from the cavernous segment of the ICA, has three major branches. The tentorial branch enters the tentorium cerebelli at the apex of the petrous bone, supplying the anterolateral free margin of the tentorial incisura and the base of the tentorium near the attachment to the petrous bone. A dorsal branch supplies the dura mater of the dorsum sella and clivus, sending small twigs to supply the dura around the internal auditory canal. The artery to the inferior portion of the cavernous sinus originates from the lateral aspect of the cavernous segment of the ICA.

As the *ophthalmic artery* passes medially and then above the optic nerve, it gives off a lacrimal branch. The *recurrent meningeal artery* arises from this branch and

passes through the superior orbital fissure to supply the dura of the anterior wall of the middle cranial fossa.

The ophthalmic artery also provides several ethmoidal branches. The *posterior ethmoidal artery* leaves the orbit to supply the posterior ethmoid air cells and the dura of the planum sphenoidale and the posterior half of the cribriform plate. The *anterior ethmoidal artery* passes through the anterior ethmoidal canal to supply the mucosa of the anterior and middle ethmoidal air cells and the frontal sinus. It then enters the cranial cavity, where it gives off an anterior meningeal branch (anterior falx artery) to the dura mater and the anterior portion of the falx cerebri, which runs in the wall of the distal superior sagittal sinus (SSS).

Meningeal Branches of the Vertebral Artery

The meningeal branches enter the skull through the foramen magnum. The anterior meningeal branch originates from the distal part of the second segment of the VA just before its lateral bend at the level of the atlas. It ascends and passes anteromedially to supply the dura of the anterior margin of the foramen magnum. The posterior meningeal branch arises from the third segment of the VA between the atlas and the foramen magnum. It passes between the dura and the calvaria, supplying the posterior rim of the foramen magnum, the falx cerebelli, and the posteromedial portion of the dura of the posterior fossa.

ARTERIES OF BRAIN: FRONTAL VIEW AND SECTION

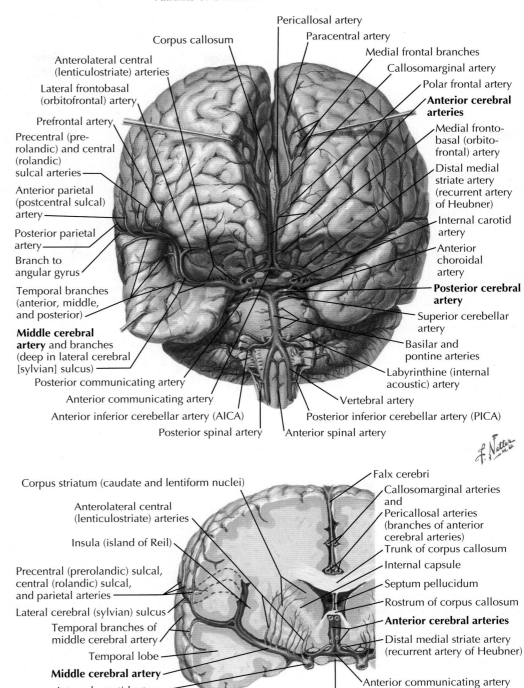

Corpus callosum
Pericallosal artery
Paracentral artery
Medial frontal branches
Callosomarginal artery
Polar frontal artery
Anterior cerebral arteries
Medial frontobasal (orbitofrontal) artery
Distal medial striate artery (recurrent artery of Heubner)
Internal carotid artery
Anterior choroidal artery
Posterior cerebral artery
Superior cerebellar artery
Basilar and pontine arteries
Labyrinthine (internal acoustic) artery
Vertebral artery
Posterior inferior cerebellar artery (PICA)
Anterior spinal artery

Anterolateral central (lenticulostriate) arteries
Lateral frontobasal (orbitofrontal) artery
Prefrontal artery
Precentral (pre-rolandic) and central (rolandic) sulcal arteries
Anterior parietal (postcentral sulcal) artery
Posterior parietal artery
Branch to angular gyrus
Temporal branches (anterior, middle, and posterior)
Middle cerebral artery and branches (deep in lateral cerebral [sylvian] sulcus)
Posterior communicating artery
Anterior communicating artery
Anterior inferior cerebellar artery (AICA)
Posterior spinal artery

Corpus striatum (caudate and lentiform nuclei)
Anterolateral central (lenticulostriate) arteries
Insula (island of Reil)
Precentral (prerolandic) sulcal, central (rolandic) sulcal, and parietal arteries
Lateral cerebral (sylvian) sulcus
Temporal branches of middle cerebral artery
Temporal lobe
Middle cerebral artery
Internal carotid artery
Optic chiasm

Falx cerebri
Callosomarginal arteries and Pericallosal arteries (branches of anterior cerebral arteries)
Trunk of corpus callosum
Internal capsule
Septum pellucidum
Rostrum of corpus callosum
Anterior cerebral arteries
Distal medial striate artery (recurrent artery of Heubner)
Anterior communicating artery

Plate 9.7

Brain: PART I

TYPES OF STROKE

Strokes are divided into two broad categories: *hemorrhagic stroke* and *ischemic stroke*. Hemorrhage is characterized by cerebral bleeding. Hemorrhagic stroke refers to a clinical event from bleeding into the brain, cerebrospinal fluid (CSF), or membranes surrounding the brain. Ischemic stroke refers to a clinical event caused by brain tissue injury or death from insufficient blood flow to the affected brain tissue. Hemorrhagic and ischemic strokes may have different immediate causes, but they may also share common underlying conditions, such as hypertension, angiopathy, and venous sinus thrombosis, among other processes. Ischemia is much more common than hemorrhage in the United States, and about 85% of strokes are ischemic.

HEMORRHAGE

Hemorrhage can be classified according to the site of blood accumulation. Hemorrhage within brain substance (deep to the pia mater) is *intracerebral hemorrhage* (ICH); hemorrhage between the pia mater and arachnoid is *subarachnoid hemorrhage* (SAH). Hemorrhage outside the arachnoid but inside the dura mater is *subdural hemorrhage,* and hemorrhage outside the dura mater but interior to the skull is *epidural hemorrhage.* Subdural and epidural hemorrhages are mainly caused by traumatic brain injury. The term hemorrhagic stroke is typically applied to ICH and SAH.

ICH is usually caused by rupture of small blood vessels, including arterioles and capillaries, or veins. The most common causes are uncontrolled hypertension, coagulopathy, vascular malformations (e.g., arteriovenous malformations, cavernous malformations), vasculopathy, and venous sinus thrombosis causing loss of blood vessel wall integrity. Vasculopathy, in turn, has multiple etiologies, including cerebral amyloid angiopathy, systematic amyloid angiopathy, infection from fungal or bacterial infection, and inflammatory or autoimmune vasculitis. The subsequent extravasation of blood can form a localized hematoma. Hemotomas can exert pressure on brain regions adjacent to the collection of blood and can damage these tissues and interrupt communicating pathways. Hematomas also exert pressure on brain regions adjacent to the collection of blood and can injure these tissues, including vital structure such as the brainstem, leading to death. The extravascular blood can also extend to ventricles, causing intraventricular hemorrhage, which can lead to hydrocephalus from CSF outflow obstruction and increased intracranial pressure (ICP).

Subcortical SAH is usually caused by rupture of an aneurysm with extravasation into the CSF system, most often in proximity to the circle of Willis. The sudden release of blood under arterial pressure increases ICP, causing severe sudden-onset headache, vision

STROKE SUBTYPES

Ischemic ←——— **Stroke** ———→ Hemorrhagic

Thrombosis

Infarct

Clot in carotid artery extends directly to middle cerebral artery

Embolism

Infarct

Clot fragment carried from heart or more proximal artery

Hypoxia

Infarcts

Hypotension and poor cerebral perfusion: border zone infarcts, no vascular occlusion

Subarachnoid hemorrhage
(ruptured aneurysm)

Intracerebral hemorrhage
(hypertensive)

change, ophthalmoparesis, vomiting, confusion, altered alertness, and seizures. Arterial spasm is a complication that narrows and can occlude arterial supply leading to ischemic stroke. Hemorrhage on the cortical surface is more commonly caused by amyloid angiopathy or arterial spasm such as is seen in the reversible cerebral vasoconstriction syndrome (RCVS).

Subdural and epidural hemorrhages are most often caused by head injuries that tear blood vessels.

Subdural hemorrhage usually results from ruptured veins located between the arachnoid and the dura mater. *Epidural hemorrhage* usually results from tearing of meningeal arteries. Arterial bleeding progresses faster than venous bleeding, as do the symptoms after head injury in patients with epidural hemorrhages. In subdural hemorrhage, the bleeding can be slow and may not be symptomatic for weeks after head injury.

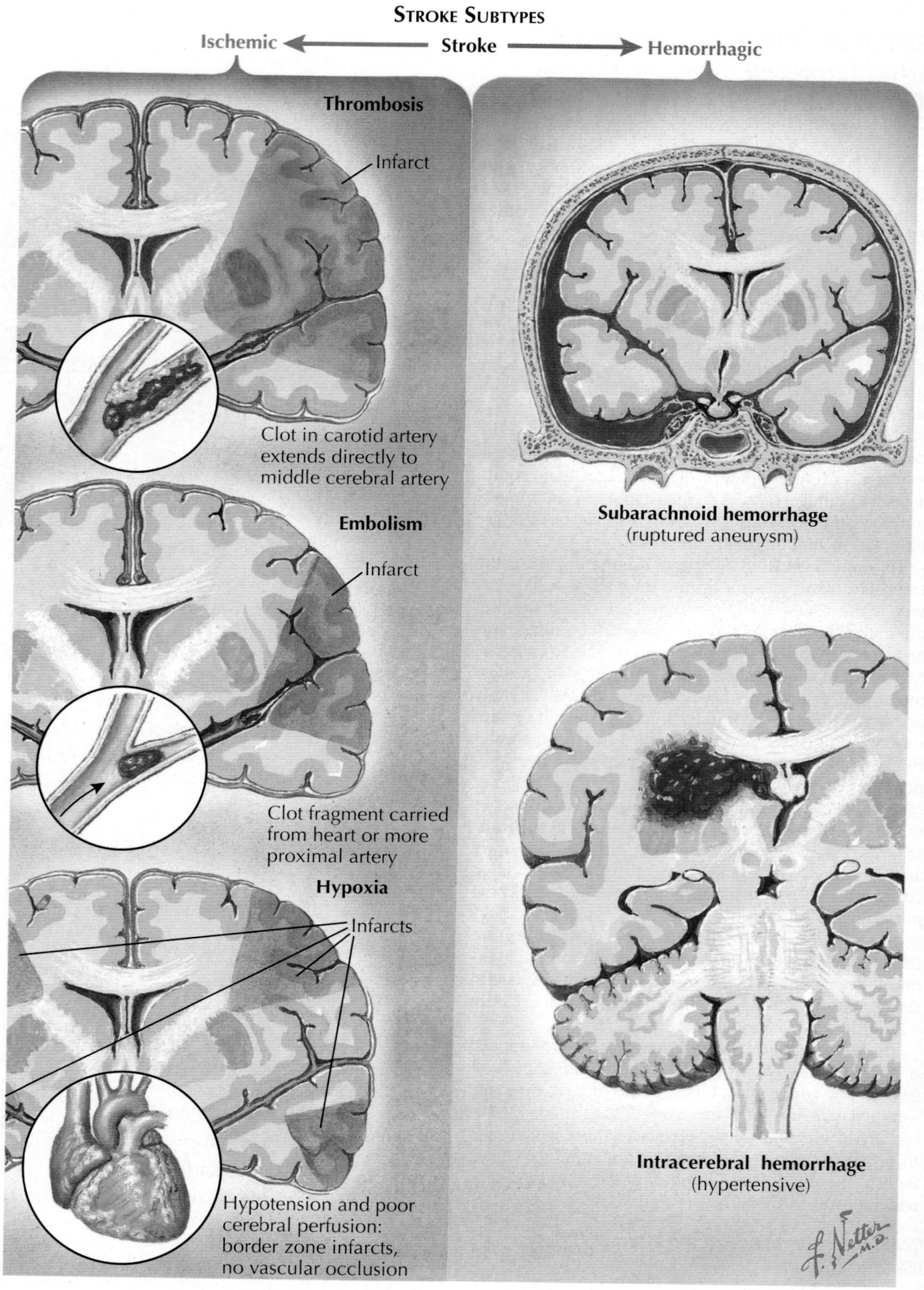

Plate 9.8

Cerebrovascular Circulation and Stroke

TYPES OF STROKE
(Continued)

BRAIN ISCHEMIA

There are multiple etiologies of ischemic stroke. Causes of structural and functional vasculopathy include atherosclerosis, fibromuscular dysplasia, microvasculopathy secondary to hypertension, diabetes, vasculitis, amyloid angiopathy, and RCVS. Causes of central embolic stroke include clot formation in situ (such as thrombus superimposed on unstable plaque from atherosclerosis or hypercoagulation states). Sources of embolism include intracardiac thrombus, septic (bacterial) embolus in the setting of endocarditis, hypercoagulable state, paradoxical clot in the presence of right-to-left shunt with patent foramen ovale, fat embolus from hip fracture, air embolus from penetrating lung injury, and embolus from unstable plaque with or without thrombosis in the aorta. Causes of systemic hypoperfusion include hypotension in the setting of dehydration, blood loss, decreased cardiac output, sepsis, and orthostatic hypotension. Causes of increased outflow resistance include sinus thrombosis or compression venous flow, which includes increased ICP, mass, and compression from bony structures. Similarly, decreased arterial flow can also be caused by compression of an artery due to increased ICP, mass, and compression from bony structures. The compression from bony structures can be static or dynamic (i.e., bow hunter's syndrome). Causes of vascular stenosis/occlusion secondary to compression include increased ICP and compression from bony structures. More than one etiology may coexist to cause ischemic stroke.

Symptoms and signs of ischemic stroke arise from dysfunction of brain secondary to loss of blood flow in specific territories, with resulting specific neurologic deficits. Typical stroke symptoms include altered mentation, speech abnormality (dysarthria or aphasia), weakness, sensory loss, vision abnormality, motor control abnormality, loss of executive or other cortical function (e.g., calculation, perception of bilateral simultaneous stimulation), and gait abnormality. In general, the left side of the brain controls the function of the right side of the body. For example, if a patient has an acute stroke due to left carotid artery occlusion, the result is sudden onset of confusion, right facial weakness, slurred speech, gaze deviation (forced eye deviation toward the left), aphasia (difficulty understanding, repeating, speaking, reading, or writing), right-sided weakness, right-sided sensory loss, and right hemianopia. Seizures due to lack of blood flow can also present at the onset of stroke, which could be focal or focal with secondary generalization.

TRANSIENT ISCHEMIC ATTACK AND ISCHEMIC STROKE WITH COMPLETED INFARCTION

Reversibility of brain ischemia depends on several factors, including severity of the decreased brain perfusion,

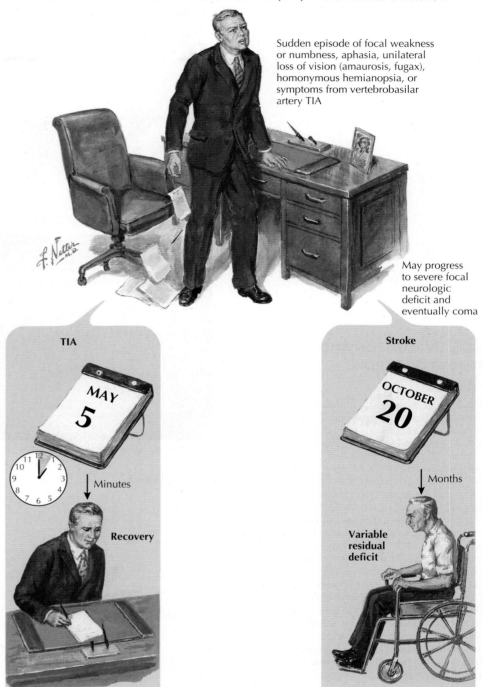

TEMPORAL PROFILE OF TRANSIENT ISCHEMIC ATTACK (TIA) AND COMPLETED INFARCTION

Sudden episode of focal weakness or numbness, aphasia, unilateral loss of vision (amaurosis, fugax), homonymous hemianopsia, or symptoms from vertebrobasilar artery TIA

May progress to severe focal neurologic deficit and eventually coma

TIA

MAY 5

Minutes

Recovery

Stroke

OCTOBER 20

Months

Variable residual deficit

ability of collateral circulation to compensate for blood flow loss, the vulnerability of various brain structures affected, and the length of time of decreased perfusion. Underperfusion can be temporary, resulting in a focal deficit that lasts only a few minutes to hours but less than 24 hours without infarction on brain imaging; these episodes are referred to as *transient ischemic attacks* (TIAs). Studies have shown that patients with TIAs have a high risk of stroke during the succeeding hours and days. The ABCD^2 (Age, Blood Pressure, Clinical Features, Duration, Diabetes) Score can be used to assess the risk for stroke in the setting of TIAs. TIAs demand urgent investigation and management. TIAs provide a window of opportunity for clinicians to intervene before a stroke

occurs. Most TIAs are very brief, lasting minutes to an hour. The distinction between TIA and stroke is whether acute infarction is seen on computed tomography (CT) or magnetic resonance imaging (MRI) studies regardless of whether the symptom is transient or persistent.

TIA and stroke management is a lifelong patient and medical provider commitment. Prevention involves strategies to identify and control potential risk factors before a subsequent stroke occurs. Strategies during acute ischemia involve reperfusion of the ischemic area by IV thrombolysis and/or mechanical thromboectomy. Neuroprotection is currently not available but an important future direction. After a stroke, recovery is facilitated by rehabilitation.

Plate 9.9

Brain: PART I

CLINICAL EVALUATION AND THERAPEUTIC OPTIONS IN STROKE

History (from patient and family, with emphasis on onset and timing)

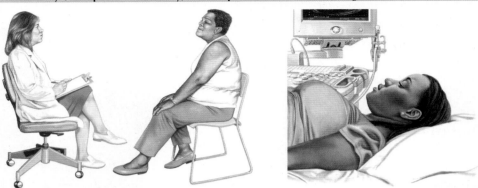

Fundoscopic examination

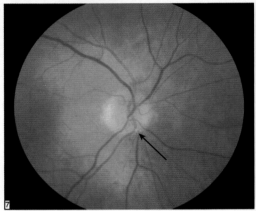

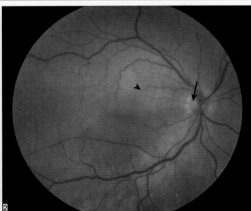

Hollenhorst plaque *(arrow)*

Platelet fibrin emboli *(arrow)* with retinal ischemia *(arrowhead)*

Auscultation

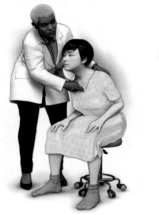

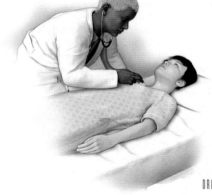

CLINICAL EVALUATION AND TREATMENT OF STROKE

The most important diagnostic information is gained from a thorough history from the patient or someone who witnessed the event, with subsequent thoughtful vascular and neurologic examination that can help localize the lesion. The history is directed to defining the cause and location of the stroke. Information about cause includes (1) the time and activity at and before the onset of symptoms; (2) the course of the symptoms (e.g., transient, gradually progressive, remitting, fluctuating); (3) the past and present known medical and surgical conditions, especially hypertension, diabetes, heart disease, smoking, excess alcohol intake, drug use, peripheral vascular disease, and obesity; (4) past strokes; (5) the presence, nature, and timing of any TIAs; (6) headache before, at, or after stroke onset; (7) the occurrence of a seizure, vomiting, or change in level of consciousness; and (8) the presence of any systemic symptoms or signs.

All patients with suspected stroke require blood tests and brain/vascular imaging. In the acute setting when a decision for intravenous (IV) thrombolytics is being made, brain imaging including CT is done to rule out a hemorrhagic stroke. Although the incidence of hemorrhagic stroke is much lower (15%) compared with ischemic stroke (85%), it is an important exclusion to determine the patient's eligibility for IV thrombolytics like alteplase or tenecteplase. A serum glucose level is required before IV thrombolytic administration. Other laboratory studies, such as coagulation profile and platelet count, may be obtained in patients on therapeutic anticoagulants and those suspected of an underlying blood disorder. Brain and vascular imaging are necessary to (1) verify the presence of a vascular lesion versus other type of brain lesion; (2) assess the location, size, and nature of the lesion(s); and (3) define the relationship between identified vascular perfusion abnormalities and the visualized lesion(s).

Head CT reliably demonstrates the presence or absence of ICH. Immediately after the onset of bleeding, intracerebral hematomas are seen on CT as well-circumscribed areas of high density with smooth borders. Edema develops within the first days and is seen as a dark rim around the high-density signal of the hematoma. Subarachnoid bleeding is demonstrated by a high-density signal within the CSF and brain cisterns. Early signs of brain infarction include obscuring of the basal ganglia density, blurring of the distinction between the gray matter of the cerebral cortex and the underlying white matter, and loss of definition of the insular cortex. In the chronic state, infarction appears as a low-density lesion. High-density signal within arteries may indicate thrombosis, slow flow, or calcific emboli. The signs of infarction on CT are often subtle when images are taken within several hours of the onset of symptoms; modifying the brightness of images during review may uncover early hypodensities.

The Alberta Stroke Program Early CT Score has been established as useful to determine the extent of stroke in the anterior circulation. This tool helps determine candidacy for mechanic thrombectomy in patients with proximal large vessel occlusion by scoring the extent of damage and the amount of surrounding potentially salvageable brain tissue.

Diffusion-weighted MRI images (DWI) and fluid-attenuated inversion recovery MRI images are particularly sensitive for detection of acute brain infarctions. Infarcted areas appear bright on DWI and dark on apparent diffusion coefficient (ADC) images. The location,

Plate 9.10

Cerebrovascular Circulation and Stroke

CLINICAL EVALUATION AND THERAPEUTIC OPTIONS IN STROKE (CONTINUED)

Electrocardiogram

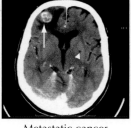
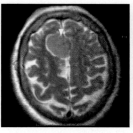

Atrial fibrillation

Myocardial infarction

MRI and CT scans (to rule out other diseases)

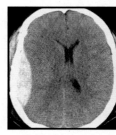
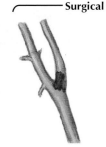

Subdural hematoma   Metastatic cancer   Meningioma   Glioblastoma

Blood analysis followed by angiography

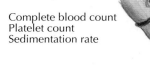

Complete blood count
Platelet count
Sedimentation rate

Glucose level
Calcium level
Serologic test for syphilis

CLINICAL EVALUATION AND TREATMENT OF STROKE (Continued)

pattern, and multiplicity of ischemic lesions seen on DWI help elucidate likely causative stroke mechanisms. DWI positivity wanes during the first 7 to 10 days after stroke onset. Lesions seen on DWI (and confirmed by ADC) usually correspond to areas of infarction. Established infarctions are bright on T2-weighted images. MRI can accurately show ICH, especially when echo-planar gradient-echo susceptibility-weighted (T2*) imaging is performed. T2*-weighted imaging can visualize thrombi within intracranial arteries, dural sinuses, and veins.

Vascular imaging can be performed using CT angiography (CTA), magnetic resonance angiography (MRA), or ultrasound. CTA (using IV iodine dye infusion) and MRA imaging can be performed concurrently with the respective primary brain imaging studies to visualize neck and intracranial arteries and veins. Duplex ultrasound, which includes a B-mode image combined with a pulsed Doppler spectrum analysis, can accurately show occlusive lesions within neck arteries. Transcranial Doppler ultrasound (TCD) involves insonation of intracranial arteries by measuring blood flow velocities using a probe placed on the orbit, temporal bone, and foramen magnum. TCD can detect vascular narrowing or occlusion and monitor in real time embolic materials passing through studied vessels. Digital subtraction angiography (DSA) is currently considered the gold standard for vascular imaging when CTA and MRA do not provide clarity. DSA is used during intravascular interventions such as coiling of aneurysms, stenting, or mechanic thrombectomy.

Management of acute stroke depends on the type and cause. In SAH, aneurysms and vascular malformations can be treated by cranial surgical clipping through craniotomy, direct coiling, stent-assisted coiling, or pipeline embolization using endovascular surgical techniques. In ICH, management can be surgical with clot evacuation or medical with blood pressure control and reversal of underlying bleeding diatheses. Surgical management is determined by the location, timing, and extent of the hemorrhage.

Therapeutic options

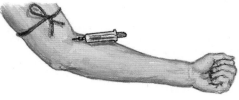

Surgical — | — Medical —

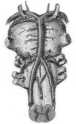
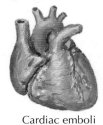

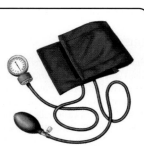

Carotid artery stenosis

Cardiac emboli

Disease of vertebro-basilar artery

Hypertension

In patients with acute brain ischemia, therapy is targeted to achieving early reperfusion either with IV thrombolytics or mechanic thrombectomy. Maximizing collateral blood flow by attention to blood pressure and blood volume can augment perfusion to the ischemic zone. With the advent of advanced imaging modalities, it is possible to determine candidacy of patients for either treatment based on perfusion imaging that can differentiate irreversibly infarcted tissue from at-risk hypoperfused brain tissue known as penumbra. The treatment window for ischemic stroke is evolving to be potentially less time restricted. Currently, CT and magnetic resonance perfusion (MRP) scans are used to select patients with potentially salvageable brain tissue to allow treatment up to 24 hours from the onset of symptoms.

Identification of the etiology of stroke is pivotal to secondary stroke prevention. Work-up should include identifying modifiable risk factors such as hypertension, diabetes mellitus, hyperlipidemia, and atrial fibrillation. CT and MRI can provide insight into the pattern and possible etiology of stroke. Treatment is based on the underlying etiology and can include anticoagulation for cardioembolic- and hypercoagulability-related stroke; antiplatelet therapy for atherosclerosis-related strokes; antiinflammatory agents for inflammatory causes, such as vasculitis; and medications for vascular risk factor control such as antihypertensives, oral hypoglycemics, and lipid-lowering agents.

Plate 9.11

Brain: PART I

UNCOMMON ETIOLOGIC MECHANISMS OF STROKE

Although cardioembolism because of cardiac rhythm disorders and atherosclerotic abnormalities of the arteries of the head and neck supplying blood flow to the brain are the most frequent causes of stroke in the elderly, other etiologies should be considered for young adult patients. When indicated, work-up should be considered for patent foramen ovale that can potentially lead to paradoxical embolism (vein to artery), hypercoagulable state resulting in arterial or venous thrombus formation, infective endocarditis, and inflammatory causes such as vasculitis. Since 2019, an increased incidence of strokes (hemorrhagic and ischemic) has also been seen in patients with active COVID-19 infection in the absence of other typical risk factors. The postulated mechanism of stroke in such patients is thought to be COVID-19–mediated endothelial damage and an inflammatory hypercoagulable state leading to thrombosis.

CARDIAC

Several heart conditions can lead to brain embolism. Valvular conditions can lead to cardioembolic stroke, including rheumatic, calcific, infectious endocarditis, and noninfective fibrotic lesions (Libman-Sacks endocarditis associated with systemic lupus erythematosus [SLE] and similar valvular lesions in patients with cancer and antiphospholipid antibodies [aPL]), mitral annulus calcifications, and artificial surgically implanted mechanic and biologic valves. Myocardial abnormalities such as myocardial infarcts, myocarditis, and myocardiopathies can lead to stroke. Cardiac arrhythmias such as atrial fibrillation and sick sinus syndrome, cardiac neoplasms such as myxomas and fibroelastomas, and septal abnormalities such as atrial septal defects and patent foramen ovale can all lead to cardioembolic stroke. Aside from cardioembolic causes of stroke, cardiac pump failure can lead to ischemic brain damage through systemic hypoperfusion.

ARTERIES

Vascular conditions can predispose to artery-to-artery embolism and can cause localized ischemia due to decreased perfusion. Some vascular lesions promote bleeding. Aortic atheromas, especially those that are mobile and protruding, may occasionally embolize to the brain and lead to ischemic stroke. Arterial dissection of the neck arteries can serve as a nidus for thrombus formation with subsequent embolization and occlusion of intracranial vessels. Vasculitides comprise a heterogenous group of diseases characterized by inflammation of the blood vessel wall. These can either be primary, confined to the central nervous system (CNS) only and not from any secondary causes, or secondary, occurring as a CNS manifestation of systemic vasculitis or because of immune, infectious, neoplastic, or radiation-induced causes. Immune-mediated inflammatory secondary vasculitis can be categorized based on vessel subtype involved, including large vessel (giant cell arteritis, Takayasu arteritis), medium vessel (polyarteritis nodosa), and small vessel (ANCA antibody–mediated vasculitis). Systemic diseases and connective tissue disorders, such as SLE and rheumatoid arthritis, can cause accelerated atherosclerosis leading to atherosclerotic vasculopathy. Infectious etiologies may lead to arterial inflammation including viral agents like HIV, varicella zoster, cytomegalovirus, and parvovirus B19. Bacterial etiologies can include *Treponema pallidum*, *Mycobacterium*

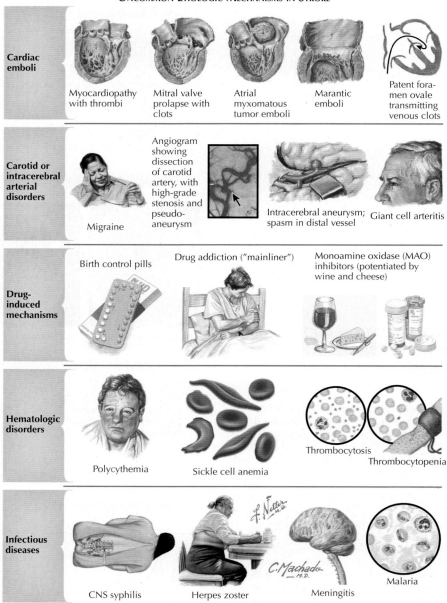

UNCOMMON ETIOLOGIC MECHANISMS IN STROKE

Cardiac emboli
Myocardiopathy with thrombi — Mitral valve prolapse with clots — Atrial myxomatous tumor emboli — Marantic emboli — Patent foramen ovale transmitting venous clots

Carotid or intracerebral arterial disorders
Migraine — Angiogram showing dissection of carotid artery, with high-grade stenosis and pseudo-aneurysm — Intracerebral aneurysm; spasm in distal vessel — Giant cell arteritis

Drug-induced mechanisms
Birth control pills — Drug addiction ("mainliner") — Monoamine oxidase (MAO) inhibitors (potentiated by wine and cheese)

Hematologic disorders
Polycythemia — Sickle cell anemia — Thrombocytosis — Thrombocytopenia

Infectious diseases
CNS syphilis — Herpes zoster — Meningitis — Malaria

tuberculosis, and *Borrelia burgdorferi*. Fungal etiologies can include cryptococcosis, aspergillosis, mucormycosis, and coccidioidomycosis. Rarely, parasitic infection such as Chagas disease, cysticercosis, and schistosomiasis can also lead to stroke. Primary angiitis of the CNS is an inflammatory arterial disease restricted to CNS circulation. It can occur in any vascular distribution but has a predilection for small leptomeningeal vessels. Prompt recognition with appropriate work-up, including CSF analysis and brain and vessel imaging using MRI and MRA with vessel wall imaging, aids in early diagnosis and treatment, which typically involves corticosteroids with transition to steroid-sparing immunosuppressive therapy. Finally, consideration should be made for genetic arteriopathies where appropriate, including cerebral autosomal dominant arteriopathy with subcortical infarcts and leukoencephalopathy (CADASIL), cerebral autosomal recessive arteriopathy with subcortical infarcts and leukoencephalopathy (CARASIL), Ehlers-Danlos syndrome, pseudoxanthoma elasticum, retinal vasculopathy with cerebral leukoencephalopathy with systemic manifestations, or TREX1-mediated vasculopathy.

HEMATOLOGIC

Hypercoagulability can be seen in states of deficiency of protein S, protein C, and antithrombin; activated protein C–resistance; sickle cell disease; other hemoglobinopathies; severe anemia; thrombocythemia; and thrombocytosis. Certain immune-mediated states lead to arterial hypercoagulability associated with lupus anticoagulant (LA), anticardiolipin immunoglobulin (Ig)M/IgG antibodies, and anti–beta II glycoprotein (GP) IgM/IgG antibodies. Bleeding disorders from thrombocytopenia, hemophilia, and prescription of antithrombotic agents can lead to hemorrhagic stroke.

VEINS

Thrombosis of the cerebral dural venous sinuses can lead to brain infarction, brain edema, hemorrhage, and seizures. Occlusion of deep veins is an important cause of stroke in the young owing to venous hypercoagulability disorders such as factor V Leiden (FVL) deficiency. Occlusion of cortical veins on the surface of the brain can also cause cerebral infarction, hemorrhage, and seizures.

Plate 9.12

Cerebrovascular Circulation and Stroke

COMMON SITES OF CEREBROVASCULAR OCCLUSIVE DISEASE

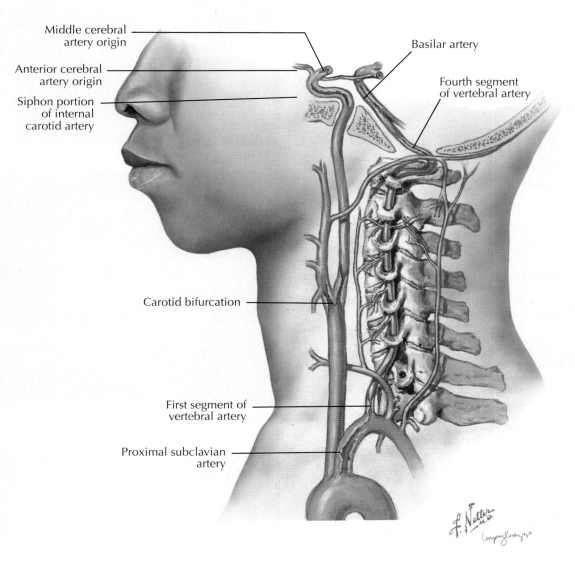

Middle cerebral artery origin

Anterior cerebral artery origin

Siphon portion of internal carotid artery

Basilar artery

Fourth segment of vertebral artery

Carotid bifurcation

First segment of vertebral artery

Proximal subclavian artery

ANTERIOR CIRCULATION ISCHEMIA

Ischemic strokes involving the anterior circulation are common, corresponding to approximately 70% of all ischemic strokes. As the often-used phrase "time is brain" emphasizes, stroke is an emergency, and time is of the essence to decrease its morbidity and mortality. Early recognition of stroke symptoms followed by utilization of appropriate and timely imaging studies and therapeutic interventions are of the utmost importance for optimal outcomes.

PATHOPHYSIOLOGY

The most common etiology of ICA disease is atherosclerosis. Other etiologies include arterial dissection, fibromuscular dysplasia, and giant cell arteritis.

Atherosclerosis causes stenosis or occlusion of extracranial and intracranial arteries and is directly responsible for a significant percentage of cerebral ischemic events. Atheroma formation involves the progressive deposition of circulating lipids and ultimately fibrous tissue in the subintimal layer of the large and medium arteries, occurring most frequently at branching points. Plaque formation is enhanced by blood-associated inflammatory factors, as well as increased shear injury from uncontrolled hypertension. Intraplaque hemorrhage, subintimal necrosis with ulcer formation, and calcium deposition can cause enlargement of the atherosclerotic plaque with consequent worsening of the degree of arterial narrowing.

Disruption of the endothelial surface triggers thrombus formation within the arterial lumen through activation of nearby platelets by the subendothelial matrix. When platelets become activated, they release thromboxane A_2, causing further platelet aggregation. The development of a fibrin network stabilizes the platelet aggregate, forming a "white thrombus." In areas of slowed or turbulent flow within or around the plaque, the thrombus develops further, enmeshing red blood cells (RBCs) in the platelet-fibrin aggregate to form a "red thrombus." This remains poorly organized and friable for up to 2 weeks and presents a significant risk of propagation and embolization. Either the white or red thrombus, however, can dislodge and embolize to distal arterial branches.

The main risk factors for carotid artery atherosclerotic disease are arterial hypertension, diabetes, hypercholesterolemia, and smoking. Frequent sites for anterior circulation atherosclerosis are the origin of the ICA, the carotid siphon, and the mainstems of the MCA and ACA (see Plate 9.12).

Dissection of the extracranial ICA usually occurs in patients between ages 20 and 50 years and commonly involves its pharyngeal and distal segments. Dissection occurring between the intima and media usually causes stenosis or occlusion of the affected artery, whereas dissection between the media and adventitia is associated with aneurysmal dilation (see Plate 9.13, A and B). Congenital abnormalities in the tunica media of the arteries as seen in Marfan syndrome, fibromuscular dysplasia, osteogenesis imperfecta, and cystic medial necrosis can predispose patients to arterial dissection. Although often associated with acute trauma, arterial dissection may result from seemingly innocuous incidents, such as a fall while hiking or skiing, sports activities (particularly wrestling or diving into a wave), and paroxysms of coughing that stretch the artery.

Spontaneous intracranial ICA dissections are uncommon compared with dissections of its cervical portion. Although early reports described a very poor prognosis with extensive strokes and very high mortality, more recent studies have shown a relatively better outcome, with patients surviving with few or moderate deficits. Imaging studies usually show narrowing of the supraclinoid ICA, with extension to the

Plate 9.13

Brain: PART I

OTHER ETIOLOGIES OF CAROTID ARTERY DISEASE

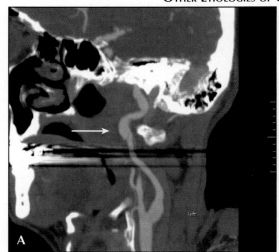
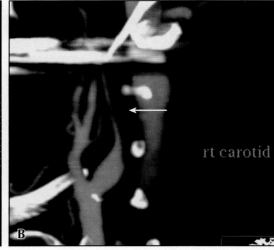

CTA of the neck shows a pseudoaneurysm (**A**) and a string sign of the internal carotid artery (**B**).

ANTERIOR CIRCULATION ISCHEMIA (Continued)

MCA or ACA and, less commonly, aneurysm formation (see Plate 9.13, *C* to *F*).

Fibromuscular dysplasia is a nonatherosclerotic noninflammatory angiopathy characterized by fibrodysplastic changes of unclear etiology. It occurs predominantly in women of childbearing age and often affects the neck arteries, most often the pharyngeal portion of the ICA. Intracranial disease is much rarer. The lesions have a characteristic beaded appearance that can be detected on MRA, CTA, or conventional angiograms (see Plate 9.13, *G*). Fibromuscular dysplasia is a predisposing factor for spontaneous cervical carotid dissections and consequent strokes; however, strokes can also be caused by thromboembolism secondary to the fibromuscular dysplasia.

Giant cell arteritis is a common form of systemic vasculopathy affecting patients older than 50 years. Although it typically involves the temporal, maxillary, and ophthalmic arteries, it can rarely affect the siphon of the ICA, sometimes producing bilateral stenosis.

PRESENTATION AND DIAGNOSIS

Presentation

TIAs in patients with carotid artery disease usually precede stroke onset by a few days or months. TIAs caused by intraarterial embolism from a carotid source are not stereotypical, and symptoms vary depending on which ICA branch is involved. In contrast, hemodynamic "limb-shaking" TIAs are often stereotypical, posturally related, and seen in patients with high-grade ICA stenosis or occlusion. In this classic example of hemodynamic ischemia, patients have recurrent, irregular, and involuntary movements of the contralateral arm, leg, or both, usually triggered by postural changes and lasting a few minutes.

Another important clue to ICA disease is the development of episodes of transient monocular blindness (TMB) (see Plate 9.14). TMB refers to the occurrence of temporary unilateral visual loss or obscuration that is described by careful observers as a horizontal or vertical "shade being drawn over one eye," but most frequently as a "fog" or "blurring" in the eye lasting 1 to 5 minutes. It often occurs spontaneously but at times is triggered by position changes. Positive phenomena, such as sparkles,

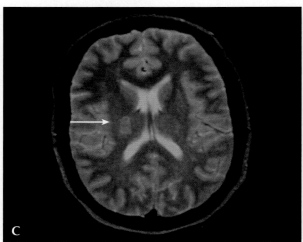

C

T2-weighted MRI shows a right basal ganglia infarct.

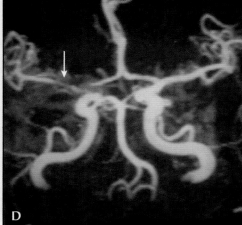

D

MRA of the head demonstrates a filling defect in the distal portion of the right ICA and proximal MCA stem.

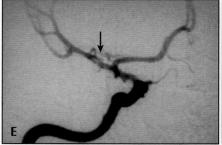
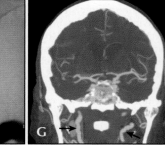

Cerebral angiography shows the presence of a double lumen in the right MCA stem (**E**) and narrowing of the supraclinoid portion of the right ICA, suggestive of intracranial dissection (**F**).

CTA of the head and neck demonstrates areas of fibromuscular dysplasia in both internal carotid arteries.

lights, or colors evolving over minutes, are typical of migraine and help differentiate such benign visual changes from the more serious TMB, a frequent harbinger of cerebral infarction within the carotid artery territory. Rarely, with critical ipsilateral ICA stenosis, gradual dimming or loss of vision when exposed to bright light, such as glare from snow on a sunlit background, can be reported and is due to limited vascular flow in the face of increased retinal metabolic demand.

Strokes from intraarterial embolism from ICA disease are usually cortically based (Plate 9.14). Symptoms depend on whether branches of the MCA, ACA, or both are involved (Plate 9.15). The PCA territory may rarely be affected by intraarterial emboli from ipsilateral ICA stenosis or occlusion in patients with a persistent fetal PCA originating from the ICA.

Neurologic findings vary by the location of the occlusion and the adequacy of collateral circulation. A large MCA territory stroke is usually seen in patients

Plate 9.14

Cerebrovascular Circulation and Stroke

ANTERIOR CIRCULATION ISCHEMIA (Continued)

with MCA mainstem occlusion without good collateral flow, whereas deep or parasylvian strokes are the most common presentation when enough collateral flow is present over the convexities. Contralateral motor weakness involving the foot more than the thigh and shoulder, with relative sparing of the hand and face, is the typical manifestation of distal ACA branch occlusion. Conversely, prominent cognitive and behavioral changes associated with contralateral hemiparesis predominate in patients with proximal ACA occlusions, due to involvement of the recurrent artery of Huebner.

Hemodynamic strokes usually involve the border zone territory between ACA and MCA (anterior border zone), MCA and PCA (posterior border zone), or between deep and superficial perforators (subcortical border zone) and cause the typical clinical symptoms outlined in Plate 9.14.

Although TIAs can occur in intrinsic occlusive disease of the MCA and ACA, they are not as common as in patients with ICA disease and usually occur over a shorter period of hours or days. When strokes occur, initial symptoms are typically noticed on awakening and often fluctuate during the day, supporting a hemodynamic mechanism.

Isolated infarction of the anterior choroidal artery territory is not common. The classic clinical presentation includes hemiplegia, hemianesthesia, and homonymous hemianopsia, but incomplete forms of this syndrome are more frequently seen. Left-sided spatial neglect and mild speech difficulties may accompany right- and left-sided lesions, respectively. Small vessel disease is the most common mechanism of anterior choroidal arteries strokes; however, large strokes in this territory have also been associated with cardioembolism and ipsilateral intracranial carotid artery disease.

Ipsilateral Horner syndrome secondary to involvement of sympathetic fibers along the wall of the ICA and ipsilateral pain involving the eye, temple, or forehead are common in patients with extracranial carotid dissection, and its presence helps with the clinical diagnosis. TIAs and/or strokes usually occur several days after onset of symptoms and are usually caused by intraarterial embolism.

Severe retroorbital or temporal headaches are also frequent in patients with intracranial dissections; however, the neurologic signs, most commonly a contralateral

hemiparesis, tend to follow almost immediately the headache's onset. Neurologic deficits tend to fluctuate within the first 2 weeks of onset of symptoms, probably reflecting cerebral hypoperfusion.

Diagnosis

The diagnosis of anterior circulation ischemia is made in most patients by noninvasive methods, including CT, MRI, and ultrasound techniques (see Plates 9.16 and 9.17). Currently, DSA is rarely used during the stroke work-up, except in selected patients when the diagnosis is still not clear after noninvasive testing.

The most commonly used imaging techniques in the setting of an acute ischemic stroke are CT and MRI. Both can provide information about the brain parenchyma, intra- and extracranial arteries (CTA and MRA), and cerebral perfusion (computed tomography perfusion [CTP] and MRP).

CT modalities are almost universally used in the hyperacute phase of a stroke because of their continuous

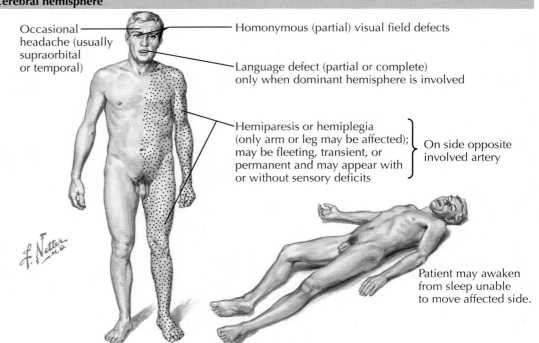

CLINICAL MANIFESTATIONS OF CAROTID ARTERY DISEASE

Stroke location	Clinical symptoms
Anterior border zone	Contralateral weakness (proximal > distal), sparing face, transcortical motor aphasia (left-sided infarcts), mood disturbances (right-sided infarcts)
Posterior border zone	Homonymous hemianopsia, lower-quadrant anopsia, transcortical sensory aphasia (left-sided infarcts), hemineglect, and anosognosia (right-sided infarcts)
Subcortical border zone	Brachiofacial hemiparesis with or without sensory loss, subcortical aphasia (left-sided infarcts)

Plate 9.15

Brain: PART I

OCCLUSION OF MIDDLE AND ANTERIOR CEREBRAL ARTERIES

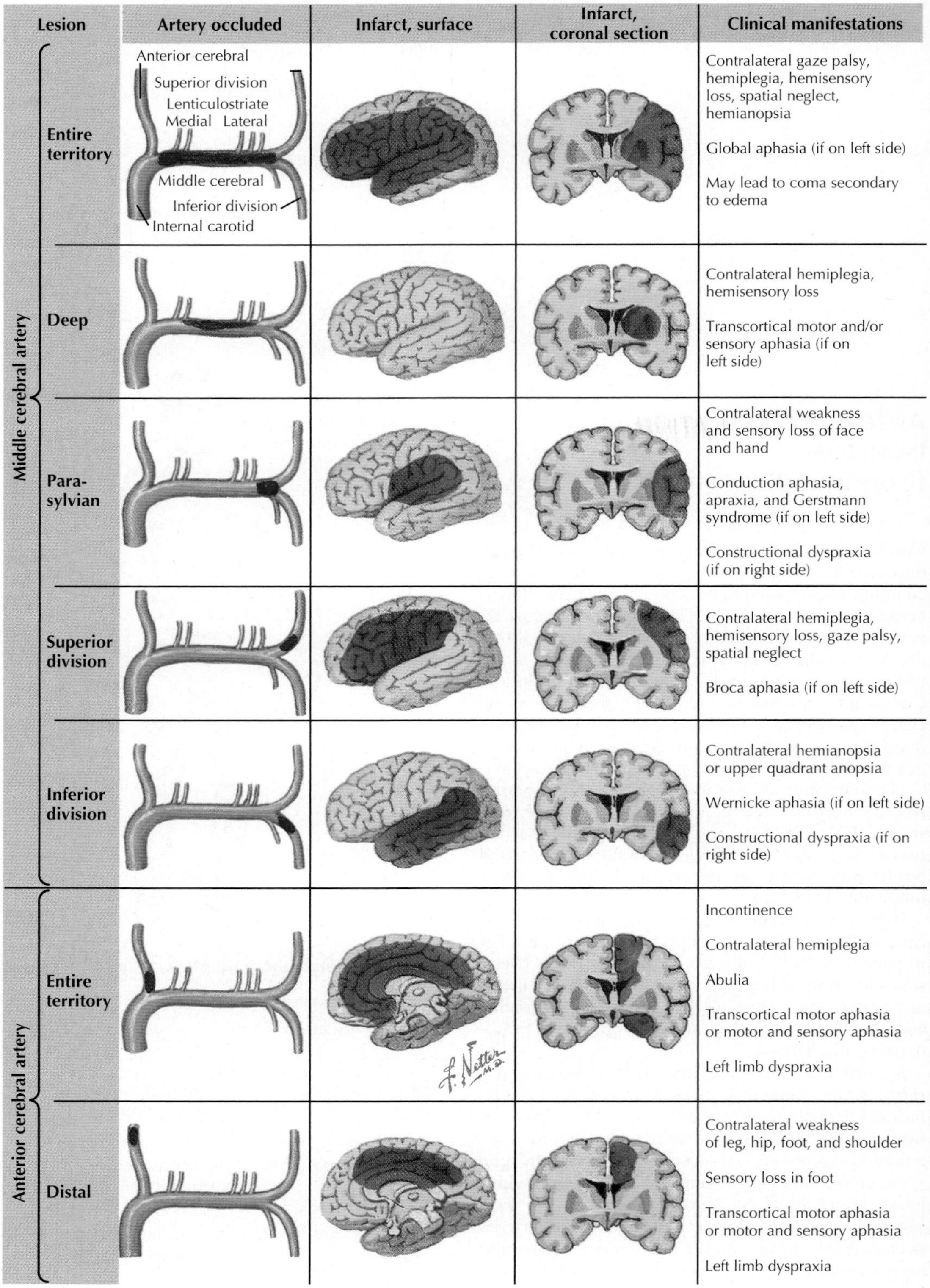

	Lesion	Artery occluded	Infarct, surface	Infarct, coronal section	Clinical manifestations
Middle cerebral artery	Entire territory	Anterior cerebral / Superior division / Lenticulostriate Medial Lateral / Middle cerebral / Inferior division / Internal carotid			Contralateral gaze palsy, hemiplegia, hemisensory loss, spatial neglect, hemianopsia Global aphasia (if on left side) May lead to coma secondary to edema
	Deep				Contralateral hemiplegia, hemisensory loss Transcortical motor and/or sensory aphasia (if on left side)
	Para-sylvian				Contralateral weakness and sensory loss of face and hand Conduction aphasia, apraxia, and Gerstmann syndrome (if on left side) Constructional dyspraxia (if on right side)
	Superior division				Contralateral hemiplegia, hemisensory loss, gaze palsy, spatial neglect Broca aphasia (if on left side)
	Inferior division				Contralateral hemianopsia or upper quadrant anopsia Wernicke aphasia (if on left side) Constructional dyspraxia (if on right side)
Anterior cerebral artery	Entire territory				Incontinence Contralateral hemiplegia Abulia Transcortical motor aphasia or motor and sensory aphasia Left limb dyspraxia
	Distal				Contralateral weakness of leg, hip, foot, and shoulder Sensory loss in foot Transcortical motor aphasia or motor and sensory aphasia Left limb dyspraxia

ANTERIOR CIRCULATION ISCHEMIA (Continued)

availability, quicker acquisition, ease of detecting intracranial hemorrhage (a major contraindication for thrombolysis), and lower cost than MRI. However, DWI is superior to CT for detection of acute ischemic changes in the brain, particularly of small strokes. Therefore a brain MRI is often used as part of the stroke work-up in addition to the initial head CT and CTA of head and neck.

Regarding the imaging of the intra- and extracranial arteries, both CTA and MRA of head and neck (time-of-flight and contrast enhanced) can demonstrate the degree of arterial occlusion and the arterial pathology, such as the presence of atherosclerotic occlusive disease and an arterial dissection.

Compared with conventional angiography, CTA is an accurate method for detection of severe ICA disease with a sensitivity and specificity of 97% and 99%, respectively, whereas MRA sensitivity varies from 91.2% to 94.6% and specificity from 88.3% to 91.9%, depending on the technique used, with higher yield for contrast-enhanced MRA over time-of-flight MRA.

CTA and MRA of the head and neck can also help with plaque characterization in patients with atherosclerotic occlusive disease of the extra- and intracranial vessels; MRI tends to provide more detailed information regarding the plaque features, particularly with the use of vessel wall MRI. This newer technique, often performed on 3T MRI scanners, can detect the presence of intraplaque hemorrhage, lipid-rich necrotic cores, and thin fibrous caps, helping the identification of symptomatic plaques. In addition, this imaging modality can identify the presence of arterial wall enhancement secondary to mural inflammation, a hallmark of cerebral vasculitis. CTA tends to be more helpful in the detection of plaque calcification and ulcerations (see Plate 9.16).

In addition, both CTA and MRA of the head can provide important information about presence or absence of collateral flow in patients with cerebral ischemia with consequent prognostic implications.

In patients with anterior circulation dissection, MRI and MRA of the neck can provide morphologic details and document intraluminal blood flow, respectively. The typical MRI appearance of a dissected artery in cross section is an increased diameter with an eccentric narrowed lumen caused by the presence of an intramural hematoma.

The hematoma can be detected on spin-echo T1- and T2-weighted images and fat-suppressed T1-weighted techniques (see Plate 9.17). The lumen containing a flow void, indicating patency, is usually the true lumen. MRA can show the presence of a double lumen, string sign, wall irregularity, and aneurysmal dilation. The main limitations of this technique are artifacts from swallowing or patient movement, the tendency to overestimate the degree of stenosis, and difficulties distinguishing slow flow and intraluminal thrombus. CTA is another noninvasive

alternative for the diagnosis of arterial dissection, and because it is independent of flow phenomena, small residual lumens and pseudoaneurysms causing slow or turbulent flow can be detected (see Plate 9.13, A and B). However, subtle intimal flaps and intramural thrombi can escape detection with CTA.

CTP is often part of the imaging in acute stroke centers (see Plate 9.16), adding 5 minutes more scan time and an extra 3- to 5-mSv radiation dose. This technique can be helpful in the identification of the infarct core

Plate 9.16

Cerebrovascular Circulation and Stroke

DIAGNOSIS OF INTERNAL CAROTID DISEASE

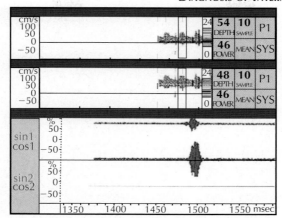

Transcranial Doppler (TCD). Intraarterial embolism in a patient with carotid artery stenosis.

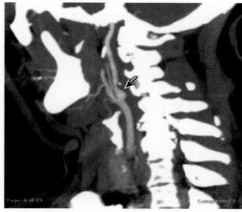

CTA of the head demonstrates an ulcerated plaque.

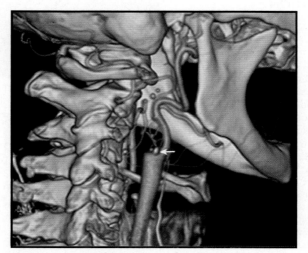

Computer tomographic angiography (CTA). ICA occlusion.

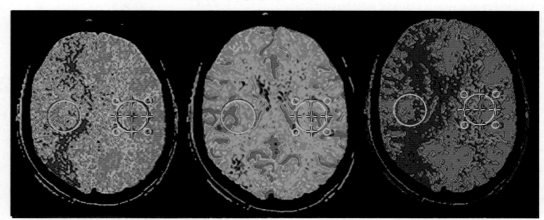

Computer tomography perfusion (CTP). Cerebral hypoperfusion in the right MCA territory in a patient with severe right internal carotid artery (RICA) stenosis.

ANTERIOR CIRCULATION ISCHEMIA (Continued)

and of surrounding salvageable areas (penumbra), guiding the decision of mechanic thrombectomy in patients with large vessel occlusion. MRP can show the same findings as the CTP; however, it is more time-consuming and not as widely available.

The presence of non–MRI-compatible pacemaker devices and renal failure limits the imaging studies performed in patients with ICA disease. MRIs cannot be performed in patients with noncompatible pacemakers, and renal failure is a contraindication for both CTA and MRA with gadolinium.

Ultrasound of the carotid arteries at their bifurcation in the neck can determine the presence of critically stenotic extracranial artery disease, as well as the characterization of carotid plaques as "soft," consisting of cholesterol deposits and clot. "Soft" plaques are more prone to ulcerate and cause artery-to-artery emboli. "Hard" plaques are those that have fibrosed and calcified over time; they are a less common source of emboli. The role of ultrasound in detection of ICA dissection, fibromuscular dysplasia, or giant cell arteritis is more limited because lesions often occur in the pharyngeal portions or distal to it; in these situations only indirect signs of a distal carotid occlusion can be seen with this technique. TCD can assess the patency of the intracranial arteries and patterns of collateral flow through the circle of Willis and can also be used for emboli monitoring (see Plate 9.16). A main limitation of this technique in patients with anterior circulation ischemia is the absence of an adequate temporal acoustic window to allow the insonation of the basal cerebral arteries, common in the elderly population.

TREATMENT AND PROGNOSIS

The treatment of anterior circulation ischemic strokes involves acute reperfusion therapies with IV recombinant tissue plasminogen activator (rTPA) and mechanic thrombectomy when patients are seen within the therapeutic time window. In addition, patients with TIAs and acute ischemic strokes benefit from the identification and treatment of vascular risk factors, antiplatelet therapy or anticoagulants for secondary stroke prevention, carotid vascularization in selected patients, and rehabilitation when residual deficits are present.

Reperfusion Therapies

Reperfusion therapies include IV rTPA and mechanic thrombectomy. IV rTPA was initially approved for the treatment of acute ischemic stroke within 3 hours of symptom onset in 1996, after the publication of the pivotal National Institute of Neurological Disorders and Stroke trial. In 2008 the window for treatment with IV rTPA was extended to 4.5 hours, after the results of the European Cooperative Acute Stroke Study were published. Exclusion criteria have been updated over

time and summarized in the 2018 American Heart Association and American Stroke Association (AHA/ASA) guidelines. Strong contraindications for IV rTPA include, among others, CT evidence of large infarct (more than one-third MCA territory or mass effect); presence of acute cerebral or SAH; previous stroke, serious head trauma, or intracranial/intraspinal surgery within the past 3 months; infective endocarditis; use of direct oral anticoagulants (DOACs) within 48 hours; therapeutic doses of low-molecular-weight heparin

Plate 9.17

Brain: PART I

DIAGNOSIS OF CAROTID ARTERY DISEASE

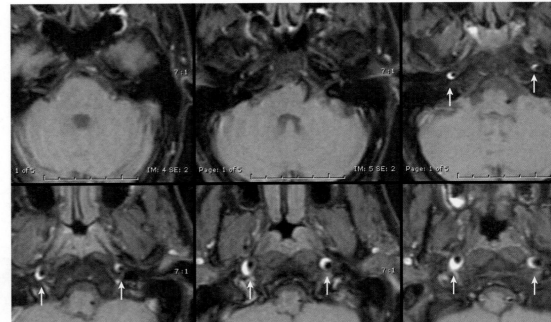

Fat-suppressed T1-weighted imaging showing eccentric narrowed lumen and the presence of an intramural hematoma in both distal ICAs suggestive of bilateral ICA dissection

ANTERIOR CIRCULATION ISCHEMIA (Continued)

(within 24 hours); partial thromboplastin time (PTT) greater than 40 seconds; international normalized ratio (INR) greater than 1.7; and platelet count less than 100,000/mm³. Despite the longer therapeutic window, patients with acute stroke should be treated as soon as possible for better outcome, with current recommended door-to-needle time of 45 minutes.

Despite initial skepticism, mechanic thrombectomy has become standard of care for treatment of large artery occlusions within the first 6 hours of stroke onset after publication of several clinical trials, with meta-analysis showing that the rate of functional independence was better for the interventional group compared with controls (46% vs. 27%, odds ratio 2.35), across different patients' subgroups, including patients with severe strokes and elderly patients, with no significant higher rates of complications. The time window for mechanic thrombectomy has been extended more recently up to 16 to 24 hours in a selected group of patients with acute stroke secondary to proximal MCA or ICA occlusions with evidence of salvageable cerebral penumbra, as defined by the DEFUSE 3 (The Endovascular Therapy Following Imaging Evaluation for Ischemic Stroke) trial and DAWN (DWI or CTP Assessment with Clinical Mismatch in the Triage of Wake-Up and Late Presenting Strokes Undergoing Neurointervention with Trevo) trial, both published in 2018.

Vascular Risk Factors

All patients with TIAs and strokes should be screened for modifiable risk factors, such as hypertension and diabetes, and appropriately treated according to the 2021 AHA/ASA guidelines, which include dietary changes, increased physical activity, and pharmacologic treatment. Smoking cessation is recommended, and avoidance of environmental tobacco smoke for stroke prevention should be considered in all patients. Aggressive reduction in cholesterol levels with a high-intensity statin with a goal low-density lipoprotein (LDL) of 70 mg/dL is also recommended by the 2021 AHA/ASA guidelines for prevention of future ischemic events in all patients with TIA or ischemic stroke and associated atherosclerotic disease (intracranial, carotid, aortic, or coronary). It is also considered reasonable to add ezetimibe and then a proprotein convertase subtilisin/kexin type 9 inhibitor to achieve this LDL goal in high-risk patients. In addition, a

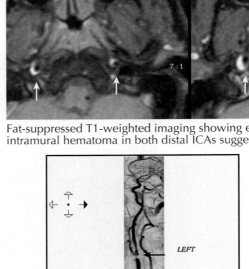

MRA of the neck showing stenosis of the distal left CCA just proximal to ICA and ECA bifurcation

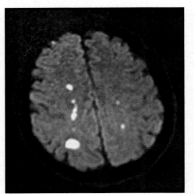

Magnetic resonance imaging (MRI). Anterior border zone strokes, right greater than left, in a patient with bilateral carotid artery disease.

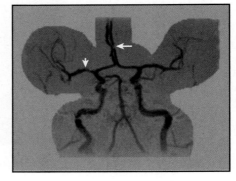

MRA of the head demonstrating stenosis of the right MCA and left ACA

high-dose statin is recommended to reduce stroke recurrence in patients with ischemic strokes and no coronary artery disease or cardiac source for embolism, if LDL is greater than 100 mg/dL. These recommendations do not pertain to patients with cardioembolic stroke and absence of atherosclerotic disease.

Secondary Stroke Prevention

Antiplatelets and anticoagulants are the mainstem therapies for secondary prevention of acute strokes and

TIAs. The benefits of antiplatelet therapy for risk reduction of future cardiovascular events in patients with noncardioembolic strokes or TIA are well established. The most common antiplatelet agents used are aspirin, clopidogrel, and a combination of aspirin and dipyridamole. Inhibition of cyclooxygenase (COX), adenosine diphosphate (ADP)-dependent platelet aggregation, and phosphodiesterase are the mechanisms of action of aspirin, clopidogrel, and dipyridamole, respectively. Ticagrelor, an ADP P2Y12 receptor inhibitor, has also

Plate 9.18

Cerebrovascular Circulation and Stroke

CAROTID ENDARTERECTOMY

Internal carotid artery

External carotid artery

Common carotid artery

Sloping cut through intima

Longitudinal incision to remove atherosclerotic obstruction at carotid bifurcation

Endarterectomy performed

Silastic tube inserted for shunt during endarterectomy. T permits clearance of air from tube.

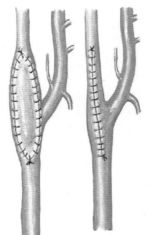

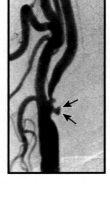

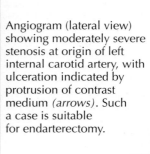

Angiogram (lateral view) showing moderately severe stenosis at origin of left internal carotid artery, with ulceration indicated by protrusion of contrast medium *(arrows)*. Such a case is suitable for endarterectomy.

Vein graft or Dacron velour patch used to widen vessel if necessary. Arteriotomy closed by direct suture.

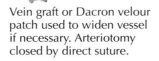

Patient's head turned to side; incision along anterior margin of sternocleidomastoid muscle

ANTERIOR CIRCULATION ISCHEMIA (Continued)

been approved recently for secondary stroke prevention in combination with aspirin.

Both clopidogrel (Clopidogrel versus Aspirin in Patients at Risk of Ischemic Events trial) and the combination of aspirin and dipyridamole (European Stroke Prevention Study 2) have been shown to be superior to aspirin for prevention of cerebral ischemia, whereas no statistical difference was seen between clopidogrel and the combination of aspirin and dipyridamole (Prevention Regimen for Effectively Avoiding Second Strokes trial).

The use of dual antiplatelet treatment with aspirin and clopidogrel is currently recommended to reduce recurrent ischemic strokes in patients with noncardioembolic high risk TIA (ABCD^2 ≥4) or small strokes (NIHSS [National Institutes of Health Stroke Scale] ≤3), after its benefits were shown in the Clopidogrel in High-Risk Patients with Acute Nondisabling Cerebrovascular Events trial and the Platelet-Oriented Inhibition in New TIA and Minor Ischemic Stroke trial. The combined treatment should be initiated early (within 12–24 hours and at least within 7 days of onset of symptoms), continued for the first 21 to 90 days, and followed by antiplatelet monotherapy.

Another dual antiplatelet therapy, using ticagrelor and aspirin, may be used for the initial 30 days in patients with recent noncardioembolic high-risk TIA (ABCD^2 ≥6) or minor to moderate stroke (NIHSS ≤5), as well as in patients with symptomatic intracranial or extracranial stenosis 30% or greater for risk reduction of recurrent strokes. The increase in the risk of serious bleeding, including ICH, should be taken into consideration when using this option.

In extracranial arterial dissections, the best treatment for secondary stroke prevention is unclear. Recent 2021 AHA/ASA guidelines recommend either the use of warfarin or antiplatelet agents for 3 to 6 months and long-term antiplatelet therapy afterward.

The best treatment for stroke prevention is also not established for patients with intracranial dissection. However, in clinical practice, antiplatelet therapy rather than anticoagulation is often preferred because of the potential risk of SAH in intracranial dissection patients.

Carotid Endarterectomy

Carotid endarterectomy (CEA) for prevention of ischemic stroke has been performed since the early 1950s

(see Plate 9.18), but it was only in the 1990s that several large-scale trials were performed comparing this type of surgery against best medical treatment in patients with asymptomatic and symptomatic ICA stenosis.

For patients with asymptomatic ICA stenosis from 60% to 99%, evidence from the ACAS (Asymptomatic Carotid Atherosclerosis Study) and ACST (Asymptomatic Carotid Surgery Trial) showed a modest benefit favoring CEA, with absolute stroke risk reductions at 5 years of 5.9% and 5.4%, respectively. The stroke risk

reduction was more prominent in men and independent of the degree of stenosis or contralateral disease. Therefore it was concluded that CEA should be considered for patients with asymptomatic stenosis of 60% to 99% if the patients have a life expectancy of at least 5 years and the rate of perioperative stroke or death for the institution or surgeon can be reliably kept to less than 3%. Since then, further studies have shown that more intensive medical treatment can decrease the ipsilateral stroke risk to less than 1%. It is possible that the

Plate 9.19   Brain: PART I

ENDOVASCULAR ICA ANGIOPLASTY AND STENTING USING A PROTECTIVE DEVICE

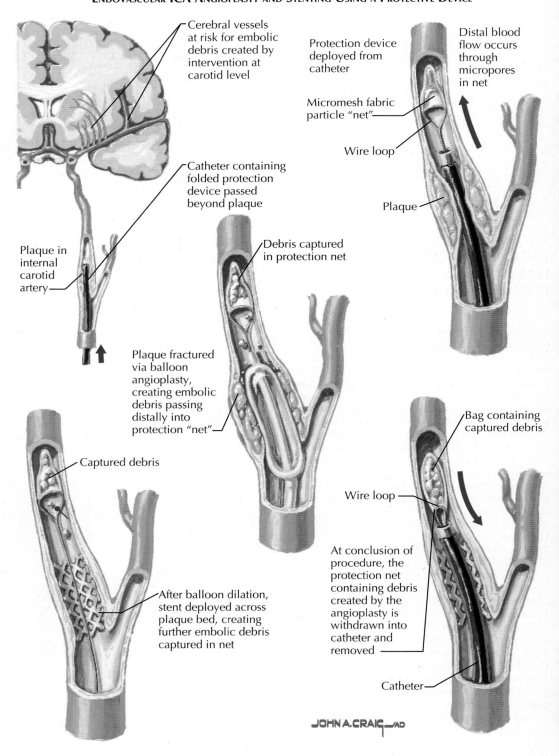

Cerebral vessels at risk for embolic debris created by intervention at carotid level

Protection device deployed from catheter

Distal blood flow occurs through micropores in net

Micromesh fabric particle "net"

Wire loop

Plaque

Catheter containing folded protection device passed beyond plaque

Plaque in internal carotid artery

Debris captured in protection net

Plaque fractured via balloon angioplasty, creating embolic debris passing distally into protection "net"

Bag containing captured debris

Captured debris

Wire loop

At conclusion of procedure, the protection net containing debris created by the angioplasty is withdrawn into catheter and removed

After balloon dilation, stent deployed across plaque bed, creating further embolic debris captured in net

Catheter

JOHN A. CRAIG—AD

ANTERIOR CIRCULATION ISCHEMIA (Continued)

absolute benefit from CEA is even smaller than reported by the ACAS and ACST.

For patients with symptomatic ICA disease, evidence from the NASCET (North American Symptomatic Carotid Endarterectomy Trial) and the ECST (European Carotid Surgery Trial) supports CEA for severe stenosis (70%–99%) over best medical treatment. The NASCET showed an absolute stroke risk reduction at 2 years of 17%, whereas the ECST showed an absolute benefit from surgery of 11.6%. For symptomatic patients with stenosis between 50% and 69%, CEA is moderately useful and can be considered in selected patients. The NASCET showed a 5-year rate of ipsilateral stroke of 15.7% in the surgical group compared with 22.2% among those treated medically in this subgroup of patients. CEA is not indicated for patients with stenosis less than 50%.

Carotid artery stenting (CAS) (see Plate 9.19) has been compared with CEA in several clinical trials of patients with symptomatic ICA disease, including the International Carotid Stenting Study, North American Carotid Revascularization Endarterectomy versus Stenting Trial, Endarterectomy versus Angioplasty in Patients with Symptomatic Severe Carotid Stenosis, and Stent-Supported Angioplasty of the Carotid Artery versus Endarterectomy. CAS is associated with a higher periprocedural stroke rate, but with similar results regarding vascular outcomes compared with CEA beyond the immediate periprocedural period. Therefore CAS is usually considered in patients with symptomatic severe ICA stenosis (≥70%) who have anatomic or medical conditions that increase their surgical risk if submitted to a CEA, granted the anticipated rate of periprocedural stroke or death is less than 6%.

Extracranial-intracranial bypass surgery has shown no therapeutic benefit in patients with recent TIA or stroke ipsilateral to atherosclerotic stenosis or occlusion of the middle cerebral or carotid artery, and it is currently not indicated.

Rehabilitation

Despite the significant advances for treatment of acute ischemic stroke, many patients are left with neurologic deficits. Fortunately, the presence of brain plasticity (brain capacity for recovery after an insult) associated with appropriate rehabilitation can help patients. Newer rehabilitation techniques, such as task-specific,

constraint-induced movement and robotic-assisted therapies, have been shown to promote better and more prolonged motor recovery compared with traditional therapy and have been incorporated into the armamentarium available to patients after a stroke.

Prognosis

The strongest predictors of stroke prognosis are the patient's age and stroke severity. In the evaluation of stroke severity, a combination of the degree of neurologic impairment as identified by the NIHSS and neuroimaging

findings such as stroke location and size are frequently used. Not surprisingly, patients who are older, have a higher NIHSS (NIHSS >22 at 24 hours and >16 at 7–10 days), and have larger strokes involving eloquent areas of the brain tend to have a worse prognosis.

Other factors that may influence prognosis are the presence of patient comorbidities and medical complications during the acute phase of the stroke, in addition to the stroke mechanism, with better prognosis for lacunar and cryptogenic strokes compared with cardioembolic or large artery disease.

Plate 9.20

Cerebrovascular Circulation and Stroke

VERTEBRAL BASILAR SYSTEM DISORDERS

SUBCLAVIAN AND INNOMINATE ARTERIES

The right innominate artery (brachiocephalic trunk) originates from the aortic arch. It branches into the right subclavian artery and right CCA. The left subclavian artery is usually the last major artery that originates from the aortic arch, as it transitions into the descending aorta. The right and left VAs are usually the first branches of their respective subclavian arteries. A hemodynamically significant stenosis, or occlusion of the proximal segment of one subclavian artery, proximal to the VA origin, can result in flow reversal within the ipsilateral VA. This disorder, described as the subclavian steal syndrome, occurs when low pressure in the nonperfused VA results in shunting blood from the contralateral, relatively higher pressure VA at the point where both merge to form the basilar artery at the level of the brainstem. This may result in hypoperfusion of the basilar artery. In a minority of patients, this phenomenon can produce symptoms such as vertigo, diplopia, blurry vision, ataxia, nausea, vomiting, numbness, or syncope. Other symptoms may include exercise-induced ipsilateral arm pain, cooling, paresthesias, and weakness. Atherosclerosis is the most common cause of subclavian artery occlusive disease. Fortunately, most cases are asymptomatic.

Innominate artery occlusive disease is uncommon. When present, it can cause both carotid and VA ischemic attacks and strokes.

VERTEBRAL ARTERIES IN THE NECK

Extracranial VA disease is a common cause of ischemic stroke, accounting for approximately 20% of all posterior circulation ischemic infarcts. Atherosclerosis is the most common etiology of occlusive VA disease. Less common etiologies include dissection, trauma, compressive osteophytes, and rarely vasculitis.

The origin of the VAs is the most common location for atherosclerotic disease in the vertebral system. Atheromas often begin in the subclavian arteries and extend proximally several centimeters up the VAs. Risk factors for proximal VA atherosclerosis are hypertension, smoking, coronary artery disease, and peripheral vascular occlusive disease. Stroke syndromes secondary to extracranial VA disease are usually related to atheroma rupture and artery-to-artery distal thromboembolism to the intracranial vertebrobasilar system. Patients with vertebrobasilar ischemic attacks may present with dizziness, diplopia, oscillopsia, extraocular movement impairment, hemiparesis, or syncope. Hypoperfusion and in situ VA branch occlusion are other potential causes. Symptoms related to vertebrobasilar hypoperfusion are typically transient, stereotypic, and triggered by dehydration or fatigue. The rotational VA occlusion syndrome (bow hunter syndrome) is uncommon and

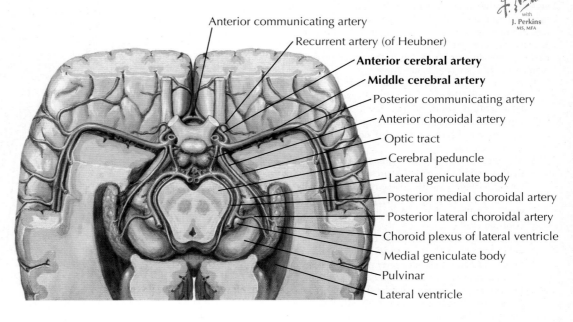

Circle of Willis

Anterior communicating artery
Anterior cerebral artery
Recurrent artery (of Heubner)
Internal carotid artery
Medial and lateral lenticulostriate arteries
Middle cerebral artery
Lateral orbitofrontal artery
Ascending frontal (candelabra) branch
Anterior choroidal artery
Posterior communicating artery
Posterior cerebral artery
Superior cerebellar artery
Basilar artery and pontine branches
Internal auditory (labyrinthine) artery
Anterior inferior cerebellar artery
Vertebral artery
Anterior spinal artery
Posterior inferior cerebellar artery
Posterior spinal artery

Anterior communicating artery
Recurrent artery (of Heubner)
Anterior cerebral artery
Middle cerebral artery
Posterior communicating artery
Anterior choroidal artery
Optic tract
Cerebral peduncle
Lateral geniculate body
Posterior medial choroidal artery
Posterior lateral choroidal artery
Choroid plexus of lateral ventricle
Medial geniculate body
Pulvinar
Lateral ventricle

usually triggered by rotational neck maneuvers in the presence of underlying structural impingement of the VA from spinal osteophyte or fibrous bands.

Intracranial VA occlusive disease can occur, most commonly due to in situ thrombus formation, thromboembolism, or dissection.

Vertebral Artery Dissection

Dissection is the most important cause of stroke in young adults, constituting 10% to 25% of ischemic stroke. VA dissections usually involve portions of the artery that are mobile and rarely occur at the origin. The extracranial VAs are anchored at their origins to the subclavian artery, during their course through bone within the intervertebral foramina (V_2 portion), and by the dura at the point of intracranial penetration. Dissection can involve the proximal most (V_1) segment of the artery above its origin and before it enters the intervertebral foramina at C5 or C6. The distal extracranial segment (V_3) is the most common location for dissection.

Plate 9.21   Brain: PART I

ARTERIES OF POSTERIOR CRANIAL FOSSA

VERTEBRAL BASILAR SYSTEM DISORDERS (Continued)

This segment is relatively mobile and vulnerable to tearing by sudden motion and stretching, as might occur during chiropractic manipulation or trauma. A distal VA dissection may extend into the intracranial VA. Signs and symptoms of VA dissection are most attributable to lateral medullary brainstem or cerebellar ischemia.

INTRACRANIAL VERTEBRAL ARTERY DISEASE

There are three intracranial VA syndromes.

Lateral Medullary Syndrome

Atherosclerosis of the intracranial VAs is most severe in the distal portion of the arteries, often at the vertebrobasilar artery junction, sometimes extending into the proximal basilar artery. Arterial dissection, thromboembolism, or atherothrombotic occlusion of the intracranial VA may result in ischemia affecting the PICA, which arises from the distal VA segment. Patients with ischemia in the distribution of the PICA or adjacent small medullary perforating vessels may present with features of the *lateral medullary syndrome*. The findings are understood best by reviewing the structures in the lateral medullary tegmentum that are specifically involved.

1. *Nucleus and descending spinal tract of CNV.* Paresthesias affecting the ipsilateral eye and face; examination confirms decreased pinprick and temperature sensation on the ipsilateral face as well as an absent or reduced corneal reflex in some patients.
2. *Vestibular nuclei and their connections.* Vertigo or ocular instability may be present; examination shows nystagmus with coarse rotatory eye movements when looking to the ipsilateral side and small-amplitude faster nystagmus when looking contralaterally.
3. *Spinothalamic tract.* There is decreased pinprick and temperature sensation in the *contralateral limbs and body;* a sensory level may be present on the contralateral trunk with pain and temperature loss on the trunk below that level and in the lower extremity. The pinprick and temperature loss can extend to the contralateral face when the crossed *quintothalamic* tract that appends itself medially to the spinothalamic tract is involved. Rarely, the loss of pain and temperature sensation is totally contralateral and involves the face, arm, trunk, and leg.
4. *Inferior cerebellar peduncle.* There is veering or leaning toward the side of the lesion and ataxia of the ipsilateral limbs; examination shows hypotonia and exaggerated rebound of the ipsilateral arm. On standing or sitting, patients often lean or tilt to the side of the lesion.

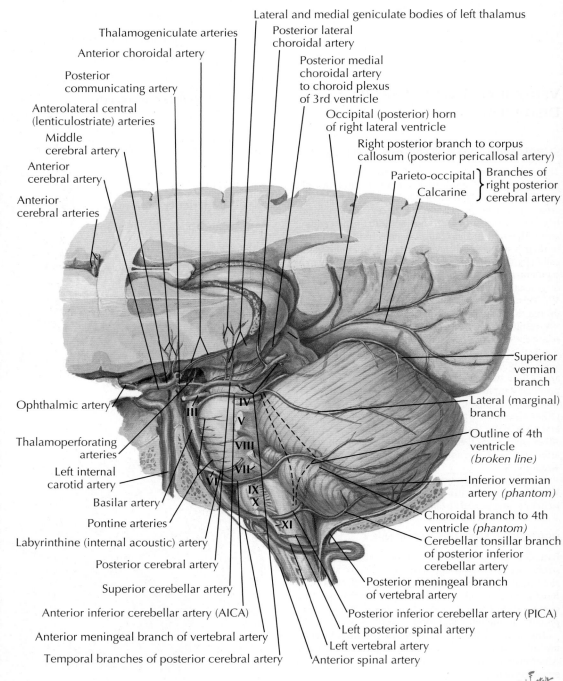

5. *Autonomic nervous system nuclei and tracts.* Descending sympathetic system axons traverse the lateral medulla in the lateral reticular formation; dysfunction causes an ipsilateral Horner syndrome. The dorsal motor nucleus of the vagus nerve is sometimes affected, leading to tachycardia and a labile increased blood pressure.
6. *Nucleus ambiguus.* When the infarction extends medially, it often affects this nucleus, causing hoarseness, dysphagia, and hiccups. The pharynx and palate are weak on the side of the lesion, sometimes causing patients to retain food within the piriform recess of the pharynx. A crow-like cough represents an attempt to extricate food from this area.
7. At times, there is also ipsilateral facial weakness, perhaps related to ischemia of the *caudal part of the seventh nerve nucleus,* just rostral to the nucleus ambiguus, or involvement of corticobulbar fibers going toward the seventh nerve nucleus.

Plate 9.22

Cerebrovascular Circulation and Stroke

CLINICAL MANIFESTATIONS OF VERTEBROBASILAR TERRITORY ISCHEMIA

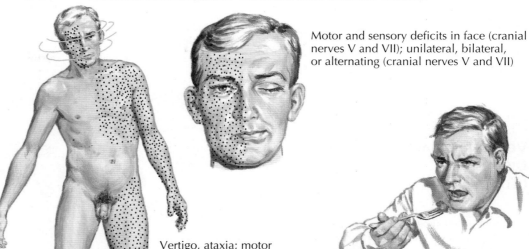

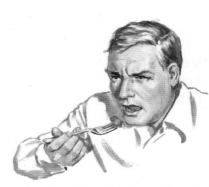

Motor and sensory deficits in face (cranial nerves V and VII); unilateral, bilateral, or alternating (cranial nerves V and VII)

Vertigo, ataxia; motor and sensory deficits, which may be unilateral, or alternating

Dysphagia (cranial nerves IX and X)

VERTEBRAL BASILAR SYSTEM DISORDERS (Continued)

8. Abnormal respiratory control may also be found, especially in *bilateral lateral medullary lesions.* Hypoventilation is probably related to involvement of the nucleus of the solitary tract, nucleus ambiguus, nucleus retroambiguus, and nuclei parvocellularis and gigantocellularis.

Cerebellar Infarction

Another common clinical syndrome resulting from ischemia in the distribution of the PICA is *cerebellar infarction.* Cerebellar infarction may be difficult to diagnose in some patients, as symptoms of central vertigo due to cerebral infarction can resemble peripheral vertigo, requiring specialized bedside testing to detect distinguishing eye movements. Gait ataxia and vomiting are often accompanied by vertigo.

Medial Medullary Infarction

This third syndrome is much less common. The anterior spinal artery supplying the medial medulla arises from the distal intracranial VA. The medial medullary syndrome is characterized by hemiparesis that affects the contralateral arm and leg attributable to ischemia of the medullary pyramid, and ipsilateral weakness of the tongue and contralateral loss of position sense explained by involvement of the hypoglossal nerve and the medial lemniscus. Rarely, in patients with intracranial VA occlusion, ischemia of the medial medulla accompanies lateral medullary infarction, forming a *hemimedullary syndrome.* This occurs more often when an intracranial VA occlusion is extensive, resulting in involvement of the proximal basilar artery, both the lateral medullary penetrators and the anterior spinal artery branches. Rarely, medial medullary infarction is bilateral and can extend caudally into the rostral spinal cord, causing a syndrome of quadriparesis difficult to separate from basilar artery occlusion with bilateral pontine infarction.

PROXIMAL AND MIDBASILAR ARTERY OCCLUSION

The basilar artery forms after merging of the two intracranial VAs at the medullopontine junction and ends at the junction of the pons and midbrain. The major territory of supply of the basilar artery is the pons, especially the basis pontis. The tegmentum of the pons has a rich collateral supply of blood vessels. The SCAs at the distal end of the basilar artery provide much supply to the pontine and midbrain tegmentum. Occlusion of the basilar artery often causes ischemia in the pontine base bilaterally, sometimes extending into the medial tegmentum on one or both sides. The most important

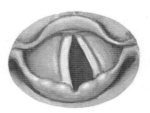

Dysphonia (cranial nerve X)

Headache, vomiting

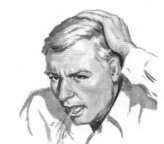

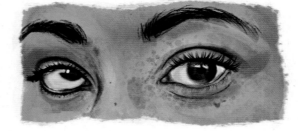

Abnormal eye movements (cranial nerves III, IV, and/or VI). Horner syndrome may be present.

Hemianopsia (bilateral occipital lesions—cortical blindness and Balint syndrome)

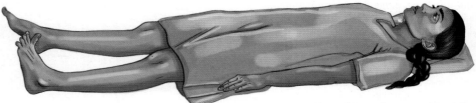

Altered consciousness (partial or complete) may be fleeting, transient, or of long duration

neurologic signs and symptoms that accompany basilar artery occlusion are:

1. *Limb paralysis.* Limb paralysis is usually bilateral but often asymmetric; stiffness, hyperreflexia, and extensor plantar reflexes are found when examining the weak limbs. Some patients present with hemiparesis, but close examination shows weakness and reflex changes in the contralateral limbs.

2. *Bulbar or pseudobulbar paralysis.* Infarction may affect cranial motor nuclei, causing paralysis of the face, palate, pharynx, neck, or tongue on one or both sides. The ninth to twelfth nerve nuclei are located within the medullary tegmentum, which is usually below the level of infarction. Weakness of the cranial musculature innervated by these nuclei causes dysarthria, dysphonia, hoarseness, dysphagia, and tongue weakness. The

Plate 9.23

Brain: PART I

VERTEBRAL BASILAR SYSTEM DISORDERS (Continued)

pontine lesion interrupts corticofugal descending fibers destined for these cranial nerve nuclei. The resulting weakness is referred to as pseudobulbar because it involves the descending pathways controlling the bulbar nuclei rather than the nuclei themselves. Exaggerated jaw and facial reflexes, increased gag reflex, and easily induced emotional lability (pseudobulbar affect) with excessive laughing and/or crying are found. The limb and bulbar paralysis may be so severe that the patient cannot communicate verbally or by gesture. Such patients have been referred to as having the *locked-in syndrome* because of their loss of motor function.

3. *Eye movement abnormalities.* The sixth nerve nuclei, medial longitudinal fasciculi (MLF), and pontine lateral gaze centers are in the paramedian pontine tegmentum and are vulnerable to ischemia in this region. Lesions of the sixth nerve or nucleus cause paralysis of abduction of the eye. An MLF lesion results in loss of adduction of the ipsilateral eye on gaze directed to the opposite side and nystagmus of the contralateral abducting eye. This finding, termed *internuclear ophthalmoplegia,* can be bilateral. Lesions of the paramedian pontine tegmentum may also affect the paramedian pontine reticular formation (PPRF), the so-called pontine lateral gaze center that mediates gaze to the same side. A lesion of this region causes an ipsilateral conjugate-gaze paresis. A unilateral lesion can affect both the PPRF and the MLF on the same side, resulting in the *one-and-a-half syndrome* because only one-half of gaze (scoring 1 for gaze to each side) is preserved. With *nystagmus,* the vestibular nuclei and their connections are also often affected, causing vertical and horizontal nystagmus. Other eye signs, including ptosis, small pupils, and ocular skewing, are also often found.

4. *Reduced level of consciousness.* When the reticular formation is affected bilaterally in the medial pontine tegmentum, lethargy, stupor, or coma may result. Sensory and cerebellar abnormalities are absent or slight because the infarction usually affects the midline and paramedian structures in the basis pontis, sparing the spinothalamic tracts and the cerebellum. Collateral circulation is mainly through the circumferential vessels, which course around the lateral portions of the brainstem to nourish the lateral base, tegmentum, and cerebellum. The cerebellar hemispheres are mostly nourished by the PICA that originates before the basilar artery, and the SCA, which is preserved when a basilar artery thrombosis or

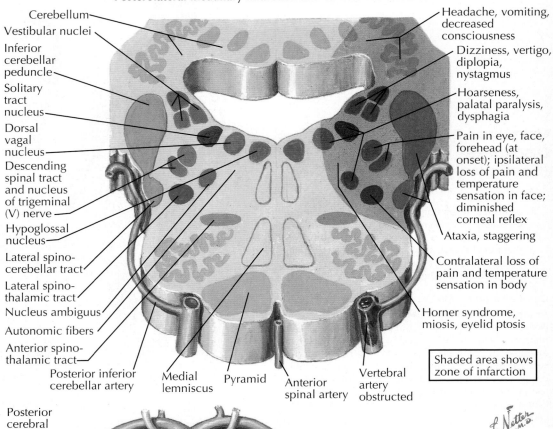

INTRACRANIAL OCCLUSION OF VERTEBRAL ARTERY
Posterolateral medullary infarction and clinical manifestations

Cerebellum
Vestibular nuclei
Inferior cerebellar peduncle
Solitary tract nucleus
Dorsal vagal nucleus
Descending spinal tract and nucleus of trigeminal (V) nerve
Hypoglossal nucleus
Lateral spino-cerebellar tract
Lateral spino-thalamic tract
Nucleus ambiguus
Autonomic fibers
Anterior spino-thalamic tract

Posterior inferior cerebellar artery
Medial lemniscus
Pyramid
Anterior spinal artery
Vertebral artery obstructed

Headache, vomiting, decreased consciousness
Dizziness, vertigo, diplopia, nystagmus
Hoarseness, palatal paralysis, dysphagia
Pain in eye, face, forehead (at onset); ipsilateral loss of pain and temperature sensation in face; diminished corneal reflex
Ataxia, staggering
Contralateral loss of pain and temperature sensation in body
Horner syndrome, miosis, eyelid ptosis

Shaded area shows zone of infarction

Posterior cerebral artery
SCA
Basilar artery
Pons
AICA
Vertebral artery
Medulla
PICA
Dura
Anterior spinal artery

Intracranial obstruction of vertebral artery proximal to origin of posterior inferior cerebellar artery (PICA) may be compensated by preserved flow from contralateral vertebral artery. If PICA origin is blocked, lateral medullary syndrome (shown above) may result. Clot also may extend to block anterior spinal artery branch, causing hemiplegia, or embolization to basilar bifurcation may cause "top of basilar" syndrome.

embolus does not extend to the distal basilar artery.

TOP-OF-THE-BASILAR ARTERY EMBOLISM

Occlusion of the distal basilar artery is most often caused by embolism from the heart or the proximal VA system. Emboli small enough to pass through the VAs seldom lodge in the proximal basilar artery, a vessel larger than each intracranial VA, but reach the distal basilar artery or its terminal branches. The distal basilar artery supplies the midbrain and diencephalon through small vessels that pierce the posterior perforated substance. The findings in patients with top-of-the-basilar embolism include:

1. *Pupillary abnormalities.* The lesion often interrupts the afferent reflex arc by interfering with fibers going toward the Edinger-Westphal nucleus. The third nerve nucleus can also be involved, as well as the rostral descending sympathetic system.

Plate 9.24

Cerebrovascular Circulation and Stroke

OCCLUSION OF BASILAR ARTERY AND BRANCHES

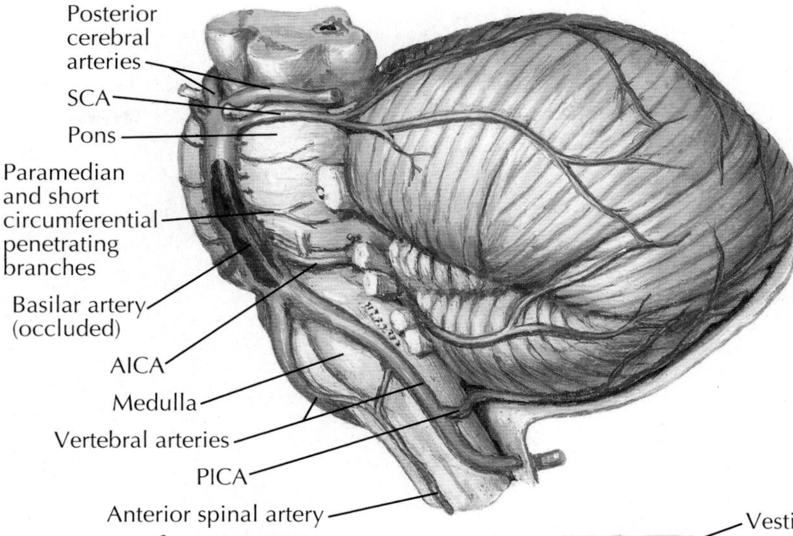

Posterior cerebral arteries

SCA

Pons

Paramedian and short circumferential penetrating branches

Basilar artery (occluded)

AICA

Medulla

Vertebral arteries

PICA

Anterior spinal artery

Collateral circulation via superior cerebellar (SCA), anterior inferior cerebellar (AICA), and posterior inferior cerebellar (PICA) arteries may partially compensate for basilar occlusion. Basilar artery has paramedian, short circumferential and long circumferential (AICA) and (SCA) penetrating branches. Occlusion of any or several of these branches may cause pontine infarction. Occlusion of AICA or PICA may also cause cerebellar infarction.

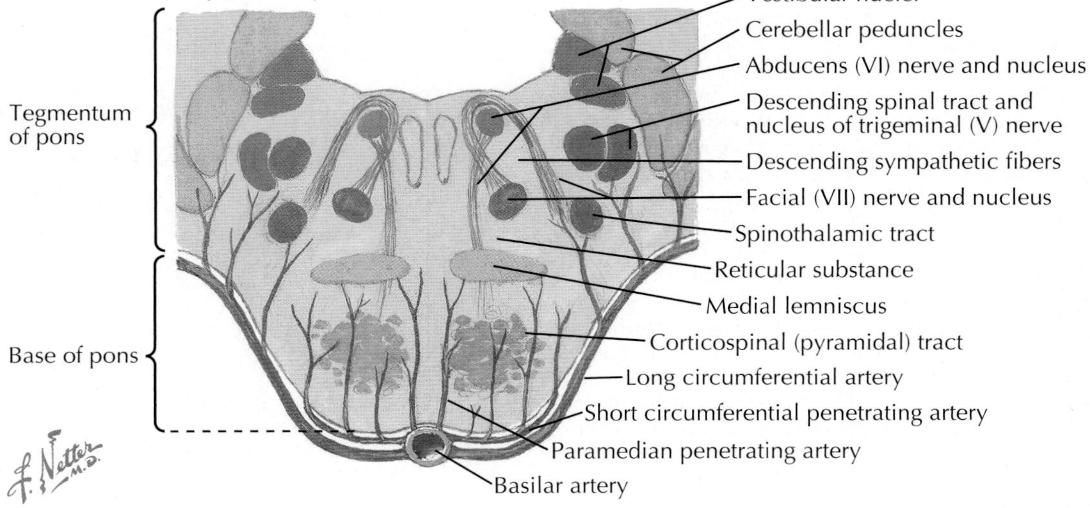

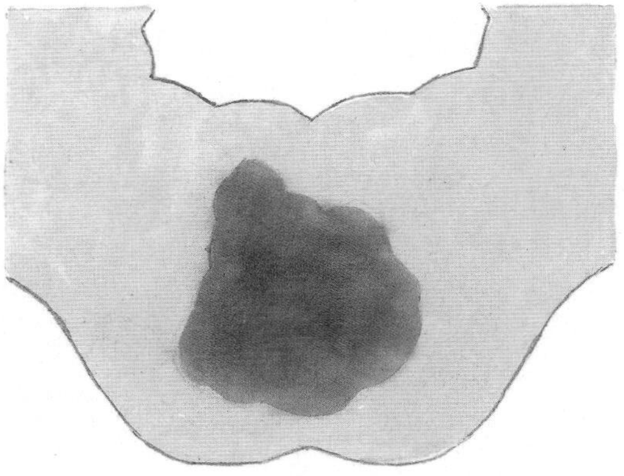

Vestibular nuclei

Cerebellar peduncles

Abducens (VI) nerve and nucleus

Descending spinal tract and nucleus of trigeminal (V) nerve

Descending sympathetic fibers

Facial (VII) nerve and nucleus

Spinothalamic tract

Reticular substance

Medial lemniscus

Corticospinal (pyramidal) tract

Long circumferential artery

Short circumferential penetrating artery

Paramedian penetrating artery

Basilar artery

Tegmentum of pons

Base of pons

Large pontine infarction, resulting in pupillary and other ocular abnormalities, facial weakness, quadriplegia, and coma

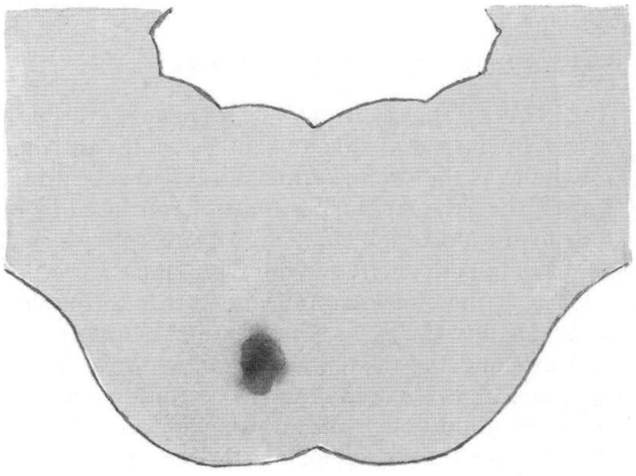

Small infarct in the left base of the pons causing a right hemiparesis

VERTEBRAL BASILAR SYSTEM DISORDERS (Continued)

The pupils are usually abnormal and can be small, midposition, or dilated, depending on the level and extent of the lesion. Decreased pupillary reactivity and eccentricity or an oval shape of the pupil can also be found.

2. *Eye movement abnormalities.* Paralysis of upward or downward gaze is common. The eyes may also be skewed and deviated at rest, most often downward and inward. Hyperconvergence, retraction nystagmus, and pseudo sixth nerve paresis are other oculomotor abnormalities noted. Reduced ocular abduction in patients with pseudo sixth nerve paresis is explained by hyperadduction of the eye. The adduction vector neutralizes the abduction motion, so abduction is incomplete. The lesion is far rostral to the sixth nerve nucleus or fibers.

3. *Decreased alertness.* Lethargy, stupor, or frank coma can result from bilateral paramedian rostral brainstem dysfunction. After the acute phase, the patient may remain relatively inert and apathetic. Some patients may experience hypersomnolence and sleep many hours a day unless stimulated or coaxed into activities.

4. *Memory loss.* Patients are unable to form new memories and may not be able to recall events just preceding their stroke. There are often other behavioral abnormalities, including agitation, hallucinations, and abnormalities that mimic lesions of the frontal lobe.

THALAMIC INFARCTS

The thalamus is supplied by arteries that arise at or near the basilar artery bifurcation and from the proximal PCAs. The *tuberothalamic (polar) artery* arises on each side from the middle third of the posterior communicating artery and supplies the anteromedial and anterolateral thalamic nuclei. Unilateral anterolateral thalamic infarction in the distribution of the polar artery on either side usually causes abulia, facial asymmetry, transient minor contralateral motor abnormalities and, at times, aphasia (left lesions) or visual neglect (right lesions). Abulia, including slowness, decreased amount of activity and speech, and long delays in responding to queries or conversation, is the predominant abnormality. Memory may also be affected.

The *thalamic-subthalamic arteries* (also called thalamoperforating) originate from the proximal PCAs and supply the most posteromedial portion of the thalamus near the posterior commissure. The right- and left-sided arteries usually arise separately but can originate from a single unilateral artery or a common pedicle. Unilateral lesions are usually characterized

by paresis of vertical gaze (upward or both upward and downward) and by amnesia. Motor and sensory signs and symptoms are absent. Memory loss may be severe, with profound difficulty in forming new memories and encoding recent events, particularly with bilateral lesions. Bilateral butterfly-shaped paramedian posterior thalamic infarction can result from a branch occlusion of a single supplying artery or pedicle and cause hypersomnolence and bilateral third nerve palsies.

The *thalamogeniculate group of arteries* arises from the PCAs to supply the ventrolateral thalamus, an area that includes the somatosensory nuclei (ventral posterior lateral and ventral posterior medial) and the ventral lateral and ventral anterior nuclei. The findings in patients with lateral thalamic infarctions are contralateral hemisensory symptoms accompanied by contralateral limb ataxia. At times, hemichoreic movements of the contralateral arm develop, and the hand may assume a fisted position.

Plate 9.25

Brain: PART I

OCCLUSION OF TOP-OF-THE-BASILAR AND POSTERIOR CEREBRAL ARTERIES

Internal carotid artery

Middle cerebral artery

Posterior communicating artery

Thalamoperforating arteries to medial thalamus

Thalamoperforating arteries to lateral thalamus

Posterior cerebral artery

Superior cerebellar artery

Basilar artery and obstruction

Anterior inferior cerebellar artery

Vertebral artery

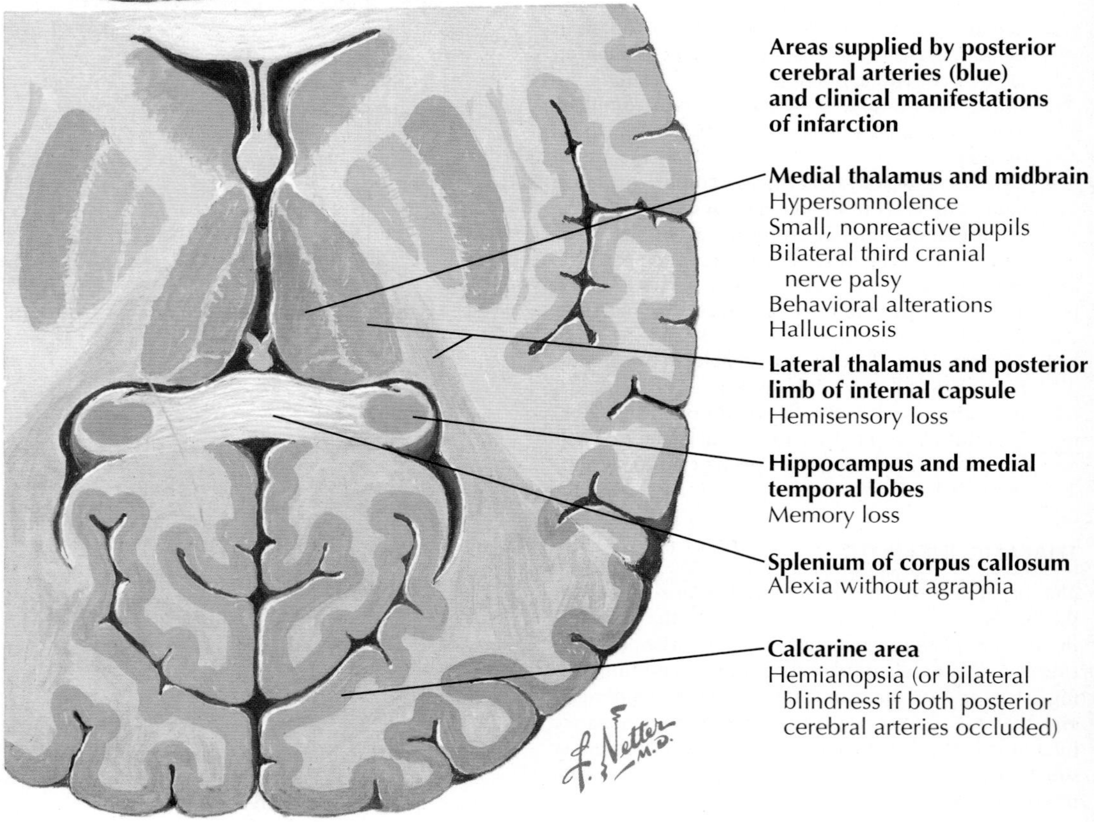

Areas supplied by posterior cerebral arteries (blue) and clinical manifestations of infarction

Medial thalamus and midbrain
Hypersomnolence
Small, nonreactive pupils
Bilateral third cranial
  nerve palsy
Behavioral alterations
Hallucinosis

Lateral thalamus and posterior limb of internal capsule
Hemisensory loss

Hippocampus and medial temporal lobes
Memory loss

Splenium of corpus callosum
Alexia without agraphia

Calcarine area
Hemianopsia (or bilateral blindness if both posterior cerebral arteries occluded)

VERTEBRAL BASILAR SYSTEM DISORDERS (Continued)

Occlusion of branches of the thalamogeniculate arteries supplying the somatosensory nuclei is the leading cause of *pure sensory stroke* (hemisensory symptoms or signs without other abnormalities). The infarctions are usually smaller than those found in patients with lateral thalamic syndrome. Occlusion of thalamogeniculate branches occasionally causes a syndrome referred to as *sensory motor stroke*, characterized by the sensory symptoms and signs of pure sensory stroke accompanied by hemiparesis and pyramidal signs involving the same limbs due to involvement of adjacent fibers of the posterior limb of the internal capsule.

The *posterior choroidal arteries* originate from the PCAs and course forward from caudal to rostral in the thalamus. The lateral posterior choroidal arteries supply mostly the pulvinar, a portion of the lateral geniculate body, and then loop around the superior portion of the thalamus to supply the anterior nucleus. The medial arteries supply the habenula, anterior pulvinar, parts of the center median nucleus, and the paramedial nuclei. Homonymous quadrantanopia, hemisensory symptoms, and behavioral abnormalities most often occur in patients with posterior choroidal artery territory infarcts.

POSTERIOR CEREBRAL ARTERIES

The PCAs are the main terminal branches of the basilar artery. Intrinsic atheromatous disease of the PCA most often affects the origin of the vessel. However, infarction in the PCA territory is most often caused by emboli to the posterior circulation from arteries of the vertebrobasilar system or a more proximal source.

After giving off penetrating branches to the midbrain and thalamus, the PCAs supply branches to the occipital lobes and the medial and inferior portions of the temporal lobes. Infarction in the cerebral territories of the arteries most often affects vision and somatic sensation but seldom causes paralysis. The most common finding is *hemianopia* caused by infarction of the striate visual cortex on the banks of the calcarine fissure or by interruption of the geniculocalcarine tract as it nears the visual cortex. If just the lower bank of the calcarine fissure is involved (the lingual gyrus), a superior quadrant field defect results. An inferior quadrantanopia results if the lesion affects the cuneus on the upper bank of the calcarine fissure. When infarction is restricted to the striate cortex and does not extend into the adjacent parietal cortex, the patient is fully aware of the visual field loss.

Somatosensory abnormalities are also common. The lateral thalamus is the site of the major somatosensory relay nuclei: the ventral posteromedial and lateral nuclei. Ischemia to these nuclei or white matter tracts

carrying fibers from the thalamus to somatosensory cortex produces sensory symptoms and signs, usually without paralysis. Patients report paresthesias or numbness in the face, limbs, and trunk. The combination of hemisensory loss and hemianopia without paralysis is virtually diagnostic of infarction in the PCA territory. Rarely, occlusion of the proximal portion of the artery can cause hemiplegia. Perforating branches from the proximal PCA penetrate the midbrain to supply the cerebral peduncle.

Cognitive and behavioral abnormalities are also common. When the left PCA territory is infarcted, patients may lose the ability to read, although they retain the ability to write and spell. Anomic aphasia and memory loss are also common. When the right PCA territory is involved, disorientation to place may develop.

When the PCA territory is infarcted bilaterally, as may occur with emboli, the most common findings are cortical blindness, amnesia, and agitated delirium.

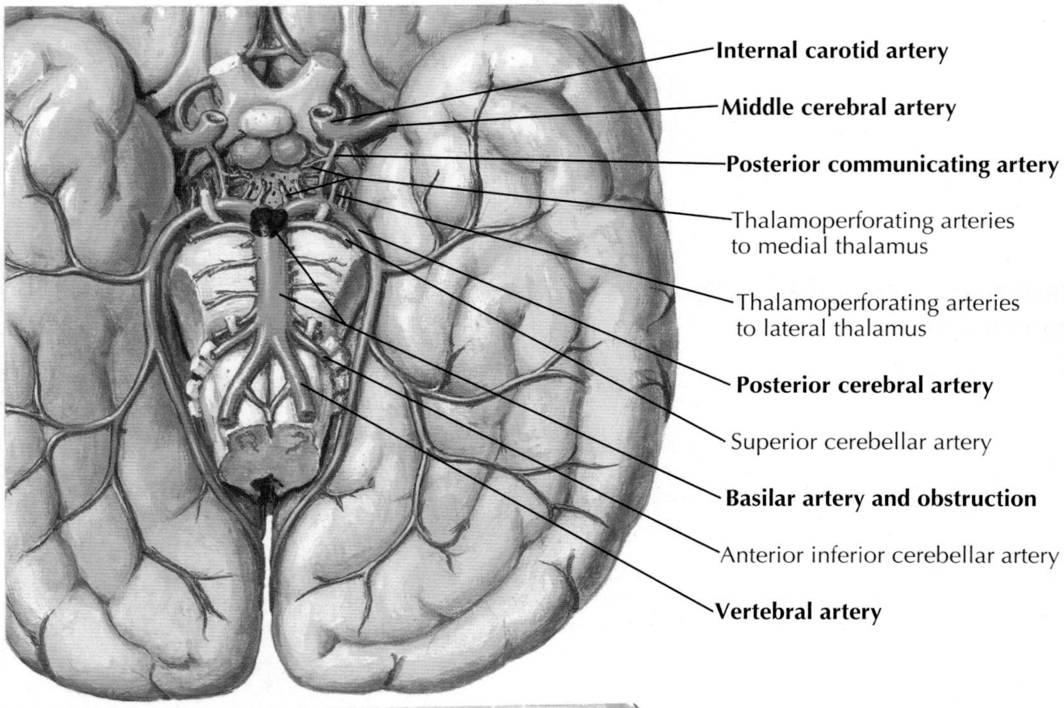

Plate 9.26

Cerebrovascular Circulation and Stroke

BRAIN EMBOLI

There are three main participants in the process of brain embolism: the *recipient artery* that catches and receives the embolic material even temporarily; the *embolic material* itself, the matter that makes up the emboli; and the *donor source* from which embolic material originates.

RECIPIENT ARTERIES

The recipient artery is the main determinant of the clinical symptoms and signs. When a recipient cervical or intracranial artery is blocked, blood flow to the area of brain supplied by the blocked artery suddenly becomes insufficient and normal function stops. The neurologic symptoms that result from the arterial blockage depend on the area of brain that is underperfused. If an embolus blocks a PCA supplying the visual cortex, loss of vision in the opposite visual field might result. If an embolus blocks the left MCA, the right limbs may become weak and numb, and the patient may become aphasic. An embolus to an intracranial VA may cause ataxia. The symptoms do not depend on the nature of the embolic material.

Whether the symptoms are transient or persistent depends on the size and fate of the embolus. Emboli very often move through recipient arteries so quickly that no or very transient obstruction occurs. These passing emboli can be identified as high-intensity transient signals that pass quickly under an ultrasound probe monitoring an intracranial artery. Thus embolic events may lead to no symptoms, transient symptoms (TIAs), or irreversible tissue loss (infarction).

Most emboli traveling through the ICA from the heart or aorta, or from the carotid artery itself, pass into the ipsilateral MCA. From there, emboli may move into superior or inferior divisions of the MCA, or into one of the smaller cortical branches. Less often, emboli move from the carotid artery into other intracranial carotid branches, the ACA, or the anterior choroidal artery.

In the posterior circulation, a common endpoint for an embolus moving through the VA is the PICA. If the embolus travels further, it will reach and possibly obstruct the basilar artery, which can lead to brainstem stroke, including locked-in syndrome in severe cases. From the basilar artery, a small embolus could obstruct the AICAs, the SCAs, or the PCAs that arise from the basilar artery terminus.

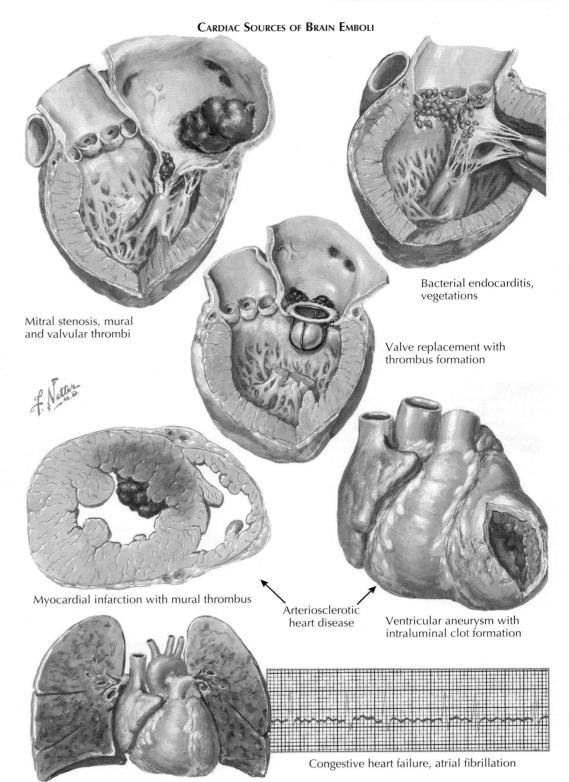

CARDIAC SOURCES OF BRAIN EMBOLI

Mitral stenosis, mural and valvular thrombi

Bacterial endocarditis, vegetations

Valve replacement with thrombus formation

Myocardial infarction with mural thrombus

Arteriosclerotic heart disease

Ventricular aneurysm with intraluminal clot formation

Congestive heart failure, atrial fibrillation

DONOR SOURCES AND THEIR EMBOLIC MATERIALS

The source of the embolic material determines the most likely treatment and prophylaxis.

CARDIAC SOURCES

Emboli that arise from the heart often consist of *red erythrocyte–fibrin thrombi* that form in the atria or on the surface of myocardial infarcts (where the ventricular

wall becomes hypokinetic or akinetic) or within ventricular aneurysms. The most common cause of embolism from the heart are *arrhythmias,* especially atrial fibrillation. Red thrombi form in the inefficiently contracting, dilated left atrium and left atrial appendage. *Valvular disease* is another common cause. *White platelet–fibrin thrombi* form along irregular valvular surfaces and prosthetic valves. Many times white thrombi form the nidus for a superimposed red thrombus so that both are involved in the thromboembolism. In patients with

Plate 9.27

Brain: PART I

UNCOMMON CARDIAC MECHANISMS IN STROKE

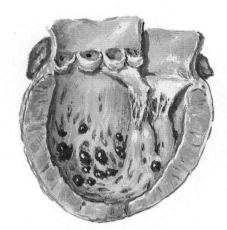

Myocardiopathy with thrombi

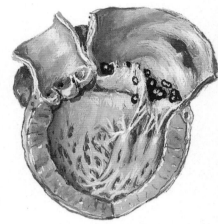

Mitral valve prolapse with clots

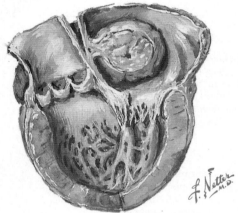

Atrial myxomatous tumor emboli

BRAIN EMBOLI
(Continued)

SLE, antiphospholipid antibody syndrome (APS), cancer, and other hypercoagulable states, nonthrombotic fibrinoid valvulitis develops and serves as a nidus for white clots. Calcium present in *calcific aortic valves* and in *mitral annulus calcifications* can break loose and embolize to the brain. Bacteria and fungi engrafted upon valves in patients with *infective endocarditis* can travel into the bloodstream and into the cranium, causing meningitis, brain abscesses, and infarctions, and can directly infect arteries, causing mycotic aneurysms. Tumor tissue present in *cardiac myxomas* and *fibroelastomas* can form the matter of emboli.

EXTRACARDIAC SOURCES

In some patients red thrombi originate in veins of the limbs and pelvis and embolize to the right heart and then pass through an atrial-septal defect or patent foramen ovale into the left atrium. They then embolize to the brain. This is termed *paradoxical embolism*. A similar process of right-to-left shunting may occur less frequently in patients with arteriovenous malformations in the lungs.

Similarly, emboli arising from the aorta are composed of different substances. White platelet–fibrin thrombi form in crevices and irregular surfaces. These white clots activate the coagulation cascade and promote red thrombi to form on their surface. Red thrombi often form within ulcers or regions of plaque rupture. Red and white thrombi often break off and reach the brain. Large protuberant and mobile plaques often contain red thrombi. Cholesterol crystals within aortic plaques or other complex plaque constituents themselves can travel to the brain. Calcium may also be a component of aortogenic emboli.

Artery-to-artery emboli have the same basic components as those that arise from the aorta: calcium, cholesterol fragments, red and white clots, and so forth. Occasionally, air, fat, and foreign materials enter the bloodstream and embolize to the brain and other viscera.

TREATMENT

Selection of treatment for acute embolic brain ischemia should consider the nature of the embolic material. Thrombolytic drugs, such as rTPA, can lyse red clots but are less effective against white clots. COX, P2Y12 inhibitors, and GP IIb/IIIa inhibitors that are active against platelet-fibrin bridges can potentially lyse white clots. These treatments are likely to be ineffective

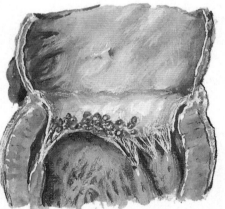

Marantic emboli

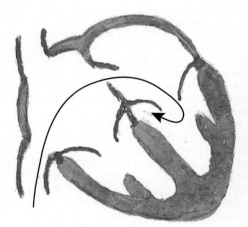

Probe: patent foramen ovale transmitting venous clots

against calcium, cholesterol crystals, tumor fragments, infective agents, and foreign matter. Mechanical methods of retrieving emboli can snare different materials.

Similarly, prophylaxis against reembolization (secondary prevention) must consider the nature of the embolic material. The most effective prophylaxis against embolism in patients with infective endocarditis includes antibacterial and antifungal agents, along with valvular surgery in some circumstances.

Secondary prevention also depends on the donor sources. Atrial fibrillation may respond to antiarrhythmics or cardiac conduction pathway ablation procedures. Prevention of emboli due to atrial fibrillation is

often by use of vitamin K antagonists and newer oral anticoagulants, such as factor IIa and factor Xa inhibitors. Intraatrial septal abnormalities and defects can be repaired. Ventricular aneurysms can be resected. Valvular disease, such as from rheumatic heart disease and valvular vegetations or tumors, can be addressed by valve repair or replacement with a prosthetic. Cardiac tumors can be removed. Surgeons have operated on protruding aortic atheromas, and in the future these lesions might be attacked by endovascular techniques. Arterial lesions are often repaired surgically or using endovascular technology in the form of angioplasty and/or stenting.

Plate 9.28

Cerebrovascular Circulation and Stroke

LACUNAR INFARCTION

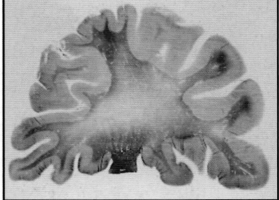

Myelin-stained brain section showing extensive demyelination

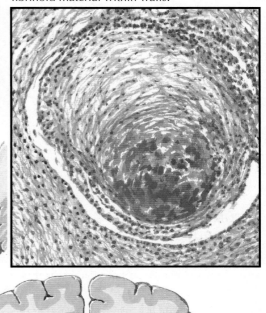

Small (100 μm) artery within brain parenchyma showing typical pathologic changes secondary to hypertension. Vessel lumen almost completely obstructed by thickened media and enlarged to about three times normal size. Pink-staining fibrinoid material within walls.

LACUNAR STROKE

Penetrating arteries are branches that supply the deeper portions of the brain. They take origin at nearly 90 degrees from their parent arteries. The most prominent of these vessels are lenticulostriate branches of the MCAs, Huebner artery branches of the ACAs, thalamogeniculate branches of the PCAs, and paramedian basilar artery branches. Occlusion of these penetrating arteries causes lacunes (small deep infarctions).

LACUNAR INFARCTIONS

Lacunar infarctions represent small, subcortical foci of encephalomalacia containing CSF and measuring less than 20 mm in diameter. They account for up to 25% of all ischemic strokes and are caused by the occlusion of a perforator of an intracranial artery. Lacunes are most often located in the lentiform nuclei, thalamus, pons, internal capsule, and cerebral white matter, and are absent in the cerebral or cerebellar cortices. Hypertension, diabetes, and smoking are particularly important risk factors for lacunar stroke development.

Several potential mechanisms have been implicated in the pathogenesis of lacunar infarctions, namely lipohyalinosis, atherosclerotic disease, cardiac embolism, and genetic causes. *Lipohyalinosis* is a concentric hyaline thickening of the cerebral small vessels that leads to occlusion of the small penetrating arteries. It is believed to originate from hypertension-related hypertrophy and fibrinoid degeneration of vessel walls, as well as subintimal foam cells obliterating the lumen of small penetrating arteries, leading to small subcortical infarctions.

Atherosclerotic disease of the parent artery may involve the ostium of perforating branches, leading to occlusion and infarction. Atheroma could originate in the parent artery, lead to luminal narrowing, and extend into the branch, or microatheroma could arise at the origin of the branch itself. The latter has been described particularly in patients with pontine lacunar stroke. Current available evidence suggests that lacunar infarctions are a rare manifestation of cardioembolic phenomena.

A number of genetic conditions are also known to predominantly affect small penetrating vessels and lead

Lacunar infarcts in base of pons interrupting some corticospinal (pyramidal) fibers. Such lesions cause mild hemiparesis.

Multiple bilateral lacunes and scars of healed lacunar infarcts in thalamus, putamen, globus pallidus, caudate nucleus, and internal capsule. Such infarcts produce diverse symptoms.

to lacunar infraction: CADASIL, CARASIL, collagen type IV alpha 2 chain, Fabry disease, and retinal vasculopathy with cerebral leukodystrophy (TREX1), among others. These conditions should be suspected in patients with absence of traditional risk factors and a positive family history.

Clinical Presentation

The most common clinical patterns of lacunar infarction are *pure motor hemiparesis* (weakness of face, arm, and leg on one side of the body with no sensory, visual, or cognitive abnormalities); *pure sensory stroke* (hemisensory loss without other signs); *dysarthria–clumsy hand* syndrome; and *ataxic hemiparesis*. Of note, up to 40% of patients with lacunar infarction experience neurologic deterioration after symptom onset, a phenomenon associated with worse functional outcomes at follow-up. Branch atheromatous disease, impaired hemodynamics, disruptions of the neurovascular units, excitotoxicity, and inflammation

Plate 9.29

Brain: PART I

RISK FACTORS FOR CARDIOVASCULAR DISEASE

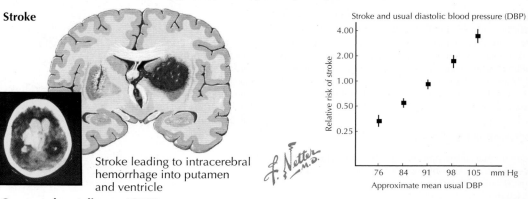

	Coronary artery disease		Stroke		Peripheral artery disease		Heart failure	
	Men	Women	Men	Women	Men	Women	Men	Women
Normal subjects	27.7	9.5	3.3	2.4	5	2	3.5	2.1
Hypertensive subjects	45.4	21.3	12.4	6.2	9.9	7.3	13.9	6.3
Risk ratio	2.0	2.2	3.8	2.6	2.0	3.7	4.0	3.0
Excess risk	22.7	11.8	9.1	3.8	4.9	5.3	10.4	4.2

(Biennial age-adjusted rate/1000)

According to hypertensive status in subjects 35–64 years of age from the Framingham Study at 36-year follow-up. *(Modified from Kannel WB. Blood pressure as a cardiovascular risk factor: prevention and treatment. JAMA. 1996;275:1571–1576.)*

Level of blood pressure is associated with cardiovascular events in a continuous, graded, and apparently independent fashion*

LACUNAR STROKE
(Continued)

have all been implicated as potential mechanisms responsible for this secondary worsening of symptoms.

Diagnostic Approach

Brain and intracranial vascular imaging are the cornerstone of diagnosis and management. Brain imaging provides information on location and possible etiology. The presence of prior lacunar strokes, white matter disease, and microhemorrhages on MRI may suggest an intrinsic vasculopathy over a cardioembolic source, for instance.

Besides demonstrating intracranial stenosis as a potential etiology for lacunar strokes, noninvasive intracranial vessel imaging, particularly vessel wall imaging using MRI techniques, has emerged as a promising tool to further characterize atherosclerotic plaques and differentiate them from other vasculopathies.

Secondary Prevention

Besides lifestyle modifications, sustained control of elevated blood pressure, tobacco use, insulin resistance, diabetes, and hyperlipidemia are the best strategies to reduce the risk of further lacunar stroke. The use of dual antiplatelet therapy, phosphodiesterase III inhibitors, IV infusion of magnesium, antiinflammatory drugs, more intensive LDL lowering, and induced hypertension during the acute phase to counteract secondary worsening of "stuttering lacunes" remain areas of active medical research.

CHRONIC SMALL VESSEL DISEASE

The accumulation of lacunar strokes over time, if severe, can lead to pseudobulbar clinical features, parkinsonism, gait disturbances, variable weakness and sensory signs, and cognitive impairment (Pierre Marie *état lacunaire,* or lacunar state). Pathologic findings include chronic white matter findings of confluent areas of soft, puckered, and granular tissue favoring the periventricular and cerebellar white matter. Also described are enlarged ventricles and small corpus callosum; on microscopic examination, islands of myelin pallor with gliosis are identified.

Stroke

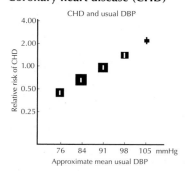

Stroke leading to intracerebral hemorrhage into putamen and ventricle

Coronary heart disease (CHD)

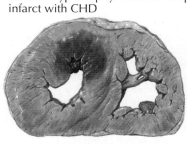

Cardiac hypertrophy and anteroseptal infarct with CHD

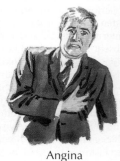

Angina

(Stroke and usual diastolic blood pressure (DBP))
Relative risk of stroke — Approximate mean usual DBP: 76, 84, 91, 98, 105 mm Hg

(CHD and usual DBP)
Relative risk of CHD — Approximate mean usual DBP: 76, 84, 91, 98, 105 mmHg

*Relative risk of stroke and CHD as a function of usual DBP in 420,000 individuals 25 years or older with a mean follow-up period of 10 years. *(Modified from MacMahon S, Peto R, Cutter S, et al. Blood pressure, stroke, and coronary heart disease: part one. Lancet. 1990;335:765-767.)*

Rarefaction of the white matter (leukoaraiosis) usually manifests as multifocal or diffuse periventricular or subcortical lesions of varying size. These white matter lesions have a predilection for the periventricular area, and their incidence increases with age. Accompanying pathologic features include axonal atrophy, gliosis, and ventricular enlargement. The main etiology is believed to be hypoxia-ischemia from diseases of small cerebral vessels attributable to common vascular risk factors.

Leukoaraiosis is strongly associated with lacunar infarctions, vascular dementia, and Alzheimer disease, and decreased elasticity of the cerebral small arteries is shared by all these conditions. The differential diagnosis is extensive, and at times the imaging characteristics can be indistinguishable. They include inflammatory and autoimmune disorders, mitochondrial abnormalities, metabolic derangements, toxic leukoencephalopathies, and certain infections.

Plate 9.30

Cerebrovascular Circulation and Stroke

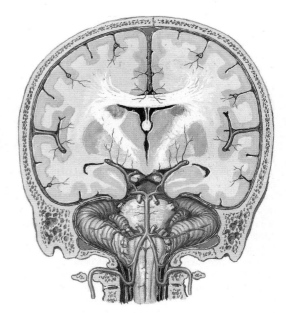

Normal brain

Hypertensive encephalopathy, with generalized constriction of cerebral arteries and their small branches

HYPERTENSIVE ENCEPHALOPATHY

Hypertensive encephalopathy refers to the consequences for brain function associated with severe and acute rises in systemic blood pressure. The effects of severe hypertension involve a variety of clinical features, including generalized tonic-clonic seizures, decreased level of consciousness, cortical blindness, and the funduscopic features of hypertensive retinopathy or malignant hypertension. This clinical picture is associated with specific correlates on imaging studies such as CT and especially MRI, characterized by abnormal signal that especially involves the white matter of the cerebral hemispheres, predominantly posteriorly. Because these changes tend to be reversible after normalization of blood pressure, these imaging findings in hypertensive encephalopathy were initially labeled *posterior reversible leukoencephalopathy syndrome* (PRES).

The MRI features of the syndrome are characterized by vasogenic edema, which corresponds to bright signal on DWI sequences and on ADC maps, the latter differentiating vasogenic edema from infarction (as infarction is expected to show decreased signal intensity on ADC maps to accompany the bright signal on DWI). These features are generally reversible, as are the clinical manifestations, including cortical blindness. However, PRES features demonstrate substantial variability, including anterior location and gray and white matter involvement. Lesions may be only partially reversible.

The occurrence of hypertensive encephalopathy is not as much a function of the absolute levels of systemic blood pressure elevation as of the percentage increase in blood pressure based on the individual's baseline blood pressure. Thus a normotensive person can present with hypertensive encephalopathy after acute blood pressure elevation (e.g., in the setting of cocaine use), whereas a patient with chronic hypertension may require a severe blood pressure elevation to trigger the syndrome. Although most patients experience clinical recovery with concomitant resolution of the imaging changes after blood pressure control, there is the potential for persistent deficits related to intracerebral bleeding into the areas of the brain affected by the encephalopathy.

There are several clinical and imaging variations in patients presenting with hypertensive encephalopathy. One variation predominantly affects the brainstem and cerebellum, presenting with headache, nausea,

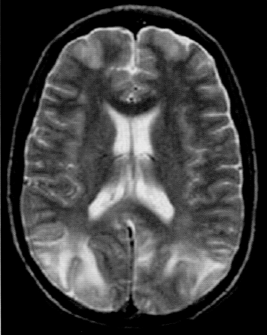

T2-weighted MRI showing bright signal predominantly in the white matter of the posterior aspect of both cerebral hemispheres in a patient with posterior reversible encephalopathy syndrome.

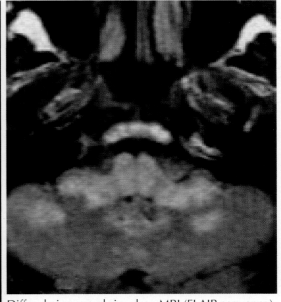

Diffusely increased signal on MRI (FLAIR sequence) in medulla and cerebellum in patient with posterior reversible encephalopathy syndrome restricted to the posterior fossa structures. *From Karakis I, MacDonald JA, Stefanidou M, Kase CS. Clinical and radiological features of brainstem variant of hypertensive encephalopathy. J Vasc Interv Neurol. 2009;2:172-176.*

vomiting, and mild or nonspecific brainstem signs such as gait disturbance, in the setting of florid vasogenic edema of the brainstem. Some patients may have no clinical signs of brainstem involvement despite florid vasogenic edema, highlighting that the imaging changes reflect vasogenic edema, not infarction.

The pathogenesis of the clinical-radiologic syndrome of hypertensive encephalopathy is thought to reflect the effects of an acute increase in blood pressure, leading to fibrinoid necrosis of the arterial wall, increase in the

permeability of the blood-brain barrier, loss of cerebral autoregulation, and subsequent formation of vasogenic edema. It remains unclear why most instances predominantly involve the posterior aspects of the cerebral hemispheres. The prevailing theory is that the posterior cerebral circulation has less sympathetic innervation than the anterior circulation, thus making it more prone to vasodilation with development of cerebral edema in the event of a sudden increase in systemic arterial pressure.

Plate 9.31

Brain: PART I

Hypoxia

The brain consumes a significant amount of energy compared with its weight and size; it is highly metabolically active and exquisitely sensitive to hypoxia and hypoperfusion. Most often, decreased brain perfusion is caused by cardiac disease. Shock and hypovolemia also decrease whole brain perfusion. Because circulatory failure usually leads to hypoventilation, and hypoxia soon causes diminished cardiac function, hypoxia and hypoperfusion are usually combined. The general term *hypoxic-ischemic encephalopathy* reflects the dual nature of the CNS stress. Pulmonary embolism is another acute disorder that causes hypotension and diminished blood oxygenation. In some patients, decreased cerebral perfusion is caused by acute blood loss, hypovolemia, or shock related to sepsis.

Globally decreased cerebral perfusion causes generalized nonfocal brain dysfunction. Dizziness, lightheadedness, confusion, and decreased concentration are common. Focal symptoms and signs, such as hemiplegia, hemianopia, and aphasia, are rarely present. At times, prior strokes or vascular occlusions may contribute to asymmetric signs. Patients with globally decreased cerebral perfusion often appear ill with sweating, tachycardia, and hypotension. Prolonged severe hypotension causes coma; initially, the patients often have no remaining brainstem reflexes (pupillary, corneal, oculovestibular).

When and if coma clears, or hypotension is less severe, abnormalities of cortical function-memory, vision, and behavior predominate.

The hippocampi are particularly vulnerable to ischemia; therefore memory loss is particularly common. The border zone of cerebral cortical perfusion located between the MCAs and the ACA and PCA is particularly vulnerable to ischemia. The posterior border zone between the MCA and the PCA territories is most often involved, possibly because these regions are farthest from the heart.

Lesions in the posterior border zones can disconnect the preserved calcarine visual cortex in the occipital lobe from the more anterior centers that control eye movements. A visual problem called *Balint syndrome* often results. Patients act as if they cannot see but sometimes surprisingly notice small objects. The features of Balint syndrome are (1) *asimultagnosia*, the inability to integrate multiple elements in the field of vision; (2) *optical ataxia*, the inability to coordinate hand and eye movements, pointing erratically at objects; and (3) *gaze apraxia*, the inability to direct gaze on command.

When hypotension is more severe, lesions can spread to the anterior border zones between the ACA and the MCA. The areas of the motor homunculus most affected are those related to the shoulder, arm, and thigh. The face territory in the central portion of the MCA territory and the foot region in the center of the ACA supply are spared. The distribution of weakness has been likened to a "man in a barrel." The frontal eye fields are also affected so that roving eye movements and hyperactive passive head movements (doll's eye reflexes) result. Stupor results from extensive bilateral border-zone ischemia.

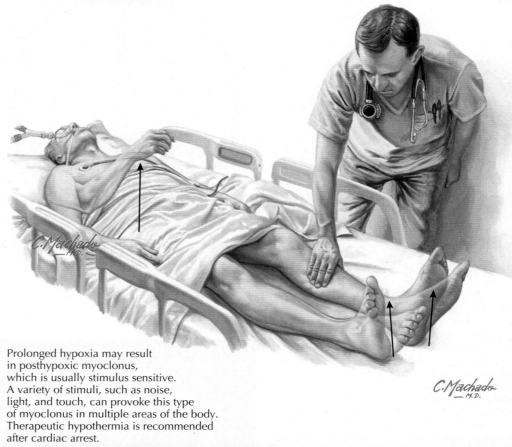

Prolonged hypoxia may result in posthypoxic myoclonus, which is usually stimulus sensitive. A variety of stimuli, such as noise, light, and touch, can provoke this type of myoclonus in multiple areas of the body. Therapeutic hypothermia is recommended after cardiac arrest.

Hypoxic-ischemic encephalopathy

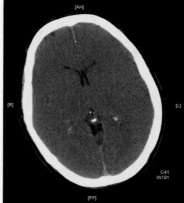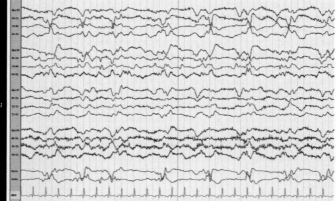

CT of the brain showing loss of normal gray-white differentiation

Electroencephalogram of the same patient showing rhythms, which are slow and disorganized

When hypoperfusion is severe and prolonged, diffuse anoxic damage to cerebral, brainstem, and cerebellar neurons occurs. The most severe damage may occur in the large cell regions of the cerebral cortex, producing a *laminar necrosis* pattern. Severe hypoxic-ischemic damage causes coma and brain death. In some patients, partial recovery leaves the patients in a minimally conscious state or a persistent vegetative state in which there is no or minimal communication.

Although hypoxic-ischemic cerebellar damage is often found at necropsy, clinical signs of cerebellar dysfunction are rare and are usually overshadowed by cerebral abnormalities. After cardiac arrest, some patients have spontaneous arrhythmic fine or coarse muscle jerking, markedly exaggerated when the limbs are used. This disorder of limb movements is referred to as *action myoclonus* or *Lance-Adams syndrome* and is often accompanied by gait ataxia.

In the setting of brain anoxia due to cardiac arrest, clinical management is focused on supportive care, treatment of the underlying cause of hypoxia, and prevention of ongoing brain injury. Targeted temperature management in comatose survivors of cardiac arrest and suspected brain hypoxia is used as the most successful neuroprotective strategy to mitigate secondary brain injury after the initial hypoxic insult.

Plate 9.32

Cerebrovascular Circulation and Stroke

ROLE OF PLATELETS IN ARTERIAL THROMBOSIS

COAGULOPATHIES

ROLE OF PLATELETS IN ARTERIAL THROMBOSIS

Normal hemostasis depends on an intricate balance between prothrombotic and antithrombotic processes, with the goal of maintaining normal blood flow and the structural integrity of the vasculature. These processes are mediated by cellular components, soluble plasma proteins, and endothelium-derived factors. Any stimulus that perturbs the normally antithrombogenic nature of the vascular system, such as the rupture of an atherosclerotic plaque, exposes subendothelial tissue elements and initiates a hemostatic response. This is a key pathophysiologic mechanism responsible not only for certain types of ischemic stroke but also for acute coronary syndromes and acute ischemia in peripheral arterial disease.

The first defense after vascular injury is known as *primary hemostasis* and consists of platelet–blood vessel interactions that lead to physiologic platelet plug formation. Platelets are produced by multinucleated megakaryocytes in the bone marrow and released into the peripheral blood, where they exist for approximately 7 to 10 days. These nonnucleated, discoid cell fragments normally circulate individually and in an unactivated state. Platelet activation and aggregation are suppressed by products of the normal endothelium, mainly nitric oxide (NO) and prostacyclin.

The exposure of subendothelial matrix leads to almost instantaneous adhesion of platelets to the site of vascular injury. Two molecules in the subendothelium are critical for this step: von Willebrand factor (vWF) and collagen. Platelets bind to vWF and collagen fibrils via the GP Ib and Ia/IIa receptors, respectively. This receptor-ligand interaction starts the process of platelet activation by which a series of intracellular signaling events leads to cytoskeletal rearrangement, shape change, and release of alpha and dense granules. These storage granules contain substances, such as ADP, serotonin, fibrinogen, and thrombospondin, that promote aggregation and recruitment of additional platelets to the growing hemostatic plug. In addition, thromboxane A_2 (TXA$_2$), formed after COX cleavage of arachidonic acid (AA) and released during platelet activation, is both a potent platelet agonist and vasoconstrictor.

The platelet receptor GP IIb/IIIa, the most abundant GP on the platelet surface, then undergoes a calcium-dependent conformational change that allows it to bind to additional vWF and circulating fibrinogen. Fibrinogen can simultaneously bind two GP IIb/IIIa receptors, thereby linking neighboring platelets. This results in platelet aggregation, formation of a fibrin network, and ultimately stabilization of the mass into a white thrombus. RBCs eventually become enmeshed in the platelet-fibrin aggregate and produce a more fully formed red thrombus. Aggregated platelets then provide cell-surface phospholipids for the assembly of coagulation factor complexes, forming a link with the processes of *secondary hemostasis* described below.

Platelets are particularly relevant in the high-pressure arterial circulation, where minor vascular damage can rapidly lead to major hemorrhage. They assume a critical role in ensuring a rapid hemostatic response, initially by containing blood loss and, as a second step, by providing an active surface for rapid fibrin and, ultimately, clot formation. In contrast, in the low-pressure

Platelets circulate individually and in an unactivated form. The intact vascular endothelium produces nitric oxide (NO), prostacyclin (PGI$_2$), and CD39, substances that inhibit platelet activation and aggregation.

If endothelial integrity is interrupted, for example by atherosclerosis or trauma, exposure of subendothelial matrix triggers a hemostatic response with rapid adhesion of platelets to the injured vessel wall. Platelets then release thromboxane A$_2$ and products of their storage granules that lead to aggregation and recruitment of additional platelets.

As more platelets aggregate, a fibrin network develops and stabilizes the mass into a white thrombus. If the thrombus develops further, red blood cells become enmeshed in the platelet-fibrin aggregate to form a red thrombus, which can grow and block the vessel lumen. Either platelet-fibrin aggregates or more fully formed clots may break off, leading to embolization in distal arteries.

Platelets attach to the injured endothelium (adhesion) and to other platelets (aggregation) via specific surface glycoproteins. During platelet activation, cyclooxygenase converts arachidonic acid into thromboxane A$_2$ (TXA$_2$), a strong platelet agonist and vasoconstrictor. The content of alpha and dense granules is released, contributing to further growth of the platelet plug.

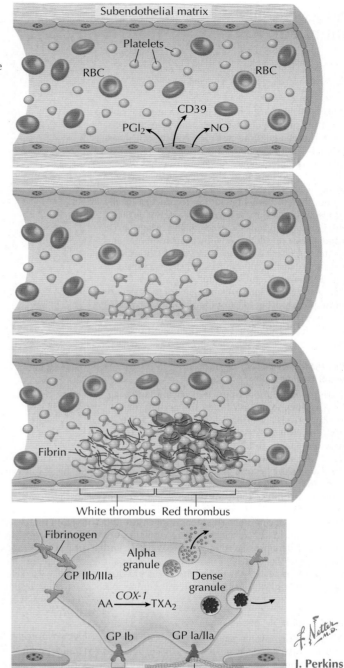

venous circulation, platelets are less relevant as the pivotal reaction controlling hemostasis is the rate of thrombin generation. Understanding the mechanism underlying a thrombotic event is critical when deciding on optimal antithrombotic management.

INHERITED THROMBOPHILIAS

Patients with unexplained arterial and venous thrombotic events require investigation for hypercoagulable states. Individuals with increased tendency to thrombosis are designated as having *thrombophilia*, either inherited because of genetic defects in protein compounds directly or indirectly involved with hemostasis, or acquired, such as APS or malignancy-associated

hypercoagulability. Clinically, inherited thrombophilia is characterized by one or more of the following: (1) thrombotic events occurring before age 45 to 50 years; (2) spontaneous, recurrent, or life-threatening events; (3) thrombosis occurring at unusual sites, including the CNS; and (4) family history of thromboembolic events.

Secondary hemostasis, or blood coagulation, is initiated by the interaction of blood with the vascular subendothelium or tissue factor exposed on cell surfaces after cellular injury. Intrinsic and extrinsic coagulation pathways converge through a series of steps to form a common pathway, ultimately leading to thrombin generation. Thrombin (factor IIa) is formed by the proteolytic cleavage of prothrombin by factor Xa. It is the final and central enzyme in the coagulation cascade as it

Plate 9.33

Brain: PART I

COAGULOPATHIES
(Continued)

generates fibrin from fibrinogen and activates not only several other procoagulant factors, but also platelets. Therefore the coagulation cascade rapidly transduces small initial stimuli into large fibrin clots.

Endogenous anticoagulant mechanisms offset the potentially explosive nature of this cascade by carefully regulating the extent of coagulation serine protease generation, thereby allowing clotting to proceed locally while preventing it from becoming a systemic process. Inherited and acquired hypercoagulable states arise when imbalance develops between prothrombotic and anticoagulant plasma activities in favor of thrombosis. In most inherited thrombophilias, genetic variations of proteins regulating hemostasis ultimately lead to increased generation, or impaired neutralization of thrombin, predisposing to thrombotic events. Hypercoagulable states are more clinically relevant as causes of venous thromboembolism (VTE) than is thrombotic arterial disease.

Antithrombin III, Protein C, and Protein S Deficiencies

These are the three most important natural anticoagulants. Antithrombin III inhibits the activity of several serine proteases of the intrinsic and common coagulation pathways, particularly thrombin. In the presence of heparin sulfate, the rate of inactivation is increased by several thousandfold. Protein C and protein S form the second regulatory system. When linked to the endothelial membrane protein thrombomodulin, thrombin activates protein C, which, in turn, cleaves factors VIIIa and Va. Protein S serves as a cofactor that accelerates this reaction. Although gene mutations in these natural anticoagulants are uncommon, when present they lead to venous and arterial thrombosis in early adulthood. If these occur in homozygosity, severe thrombogenesis occurs during infancy and childhood that is often incompatible with life.

Factor V Leiden

This is the most common genetic defect related to venous thrombosis, present in 10% to 50% of affected individuals. Worldwide carrier frequencies range from 1% to 15%, being most prevalent among White people. This point mutation in the coagulation factor V gene renders the mutant factor V resistant to proteolytic degradation by activated protein C, a feature described as *activated protein C resistance*. This leads to increased thrombin generation and a procoagulant state. FVL heterozygosity increases VTE risk threefold to eightfold; homozygosity is associated with a 50 to 100 times higher risk. The role of FVL in arterial thrombosis is debated; however, as it interacts synergistically with smoking, oral contraceptive use, and other inherited thrombophilias, it is believed to increase the risk of ischemic stroke in young patients when combined with other traditional vascular risk factors.

Prothrombin Gene Mutation

Prothrombin is a vitamin K–dependent zymogen that in its activated form (thrombin) converts fibrinogen

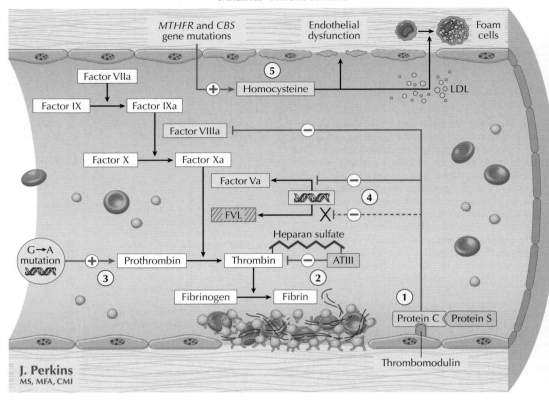

INHERITED THROMBOPHILIAS

into fibrin. A prothrombin gene G-to-A substitution in the 3′-untranslated region is associated with elevated plasma prothrombin levels and increased thrombotic risk. This is the second most common inherited thrombophilia and leads to a twofold to fivefold increased VTE risk. The prevalence of heterozygosity is 2% in White people. The relationship with arterial thrombosis and stroke remains controversial; although this mutation is associated with a moderate increase in arterial thrombotic disease, it assumes particular importance in certain subgroups, including young women taking oral contraceptives and children.

Hyperhomocysteinemia

Homocysteine is a sulfur-containing amino acid formed as an intermediary compound during methionine metabolism and metabolized by both remethylation and transsulfuration. Vitamins B_{12}, B_6, and folate are essential cofactors in these pathways. Plasma homocysteine elevations can be caused by genetic (mutations in the methylenetetrahydrofolate reductase [MTHFR] and cystathionine β-synthase [CBS] genes), nutritional (vitamin B and folate deficiencies), and acquired factors (e.g., renal failure). Deleterious effects of hyperhomocysteinemia include endothelial dysfunction, platelet activation, and arterial and venous thrombus formation. Nutritional factors and homozygosity of the MTHFR polymorphism lead to mild forms of hyperhomocysteinemia with modestly increased thrombotic risk. CBS gene mutations lead to severe hyperhomocysteinemia manifested clinically with premature severe atherosclerosis, early thromboembolic events, intellectual disability, skeletal deformities, and ectopia lentis.

ANTITHROMBOTIC AGENTS

Antithrombotic agents include both antiplatelet agents and anticoagulants. The underlying pathophysiologic mechanism defines the antithrombotic therapy used in different clinical scenarios. Antiplatelet agents are the treatment of choice in acute coronary syndromes and most types of atherothrombotic ischemic stroke. Aspirin is an irreversible inhibitor of platelet COX-1 activity, thereby blocking TXA_2 formation for the lifetime of the platelet. Clopidogrel and ticagrelor inhibit platelet activation and aggregation through the irreversible binding of its active metabolite to the $P2Y_{12}$ component of the ADP receptor on the platelet surface, preventing activation of the GP IIb/IIIa receptor complex. Eptifibatide is an IV, high-affinity, GP IIb/IIIa inhibitor with a rapidly reversible antiplatelet effect. Dipyridamole inhibits platelet phosphodiesterase, thereby raising cyclic adenosine monophosphate levels and interfering with platelet aggregation. Nonsteroidal antiinflammatory drugs bind to COX-1 reversibly and competitively, and, unlike aspirin, their effects are therefore dependent on plasma levels of the drug.

Anticoagulants act on the coagulation cascade and ultimately reduce the generation of thrombin. They are used for the prophylaxis and treatment of systemic and cerebral venous thrombosis, as well as arterial embolic events. Warfarin interferes with the synthesis of vitamin K–dependent clotting factors (factors II, VII, IX, and X) and therefore has a slow onset of action. Heparin binds with antithrombin III and promotes its inhibitory effect on thrombin and factor Xa. Anticoagulants that directly inhibit the enzymatic activity of thrombin (e.g., argatroban and dabigatran) and factor Xa (e.g., rivaroxaban, apixaban, and edoxaban) have been developed. These drugs have been shown to have a safe side effect profile

Plate 9.34

Cerebrovascular Circulation and Stroke

COAGULOPATHIES
(Continued)

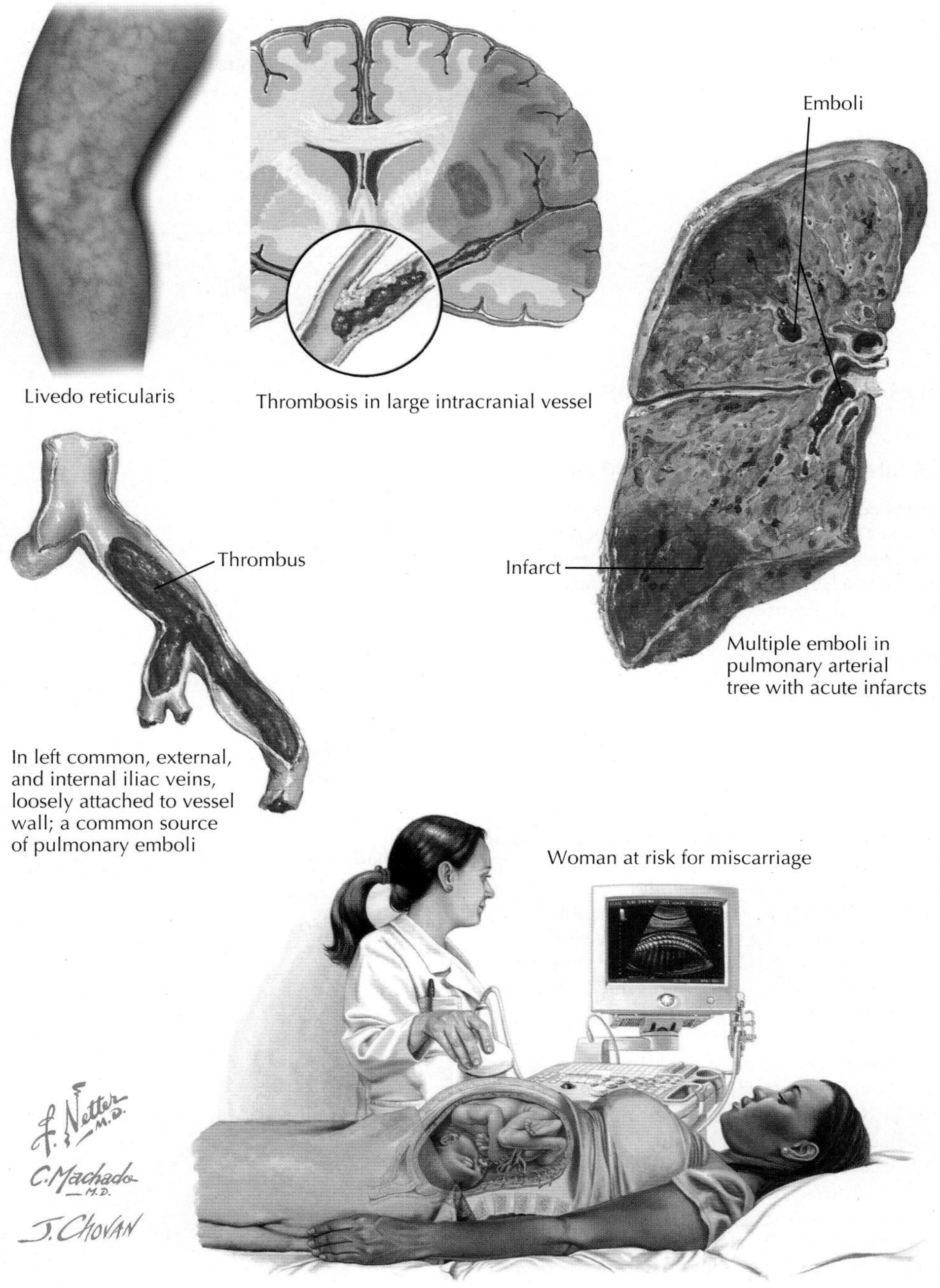

and are currently the drugs of choice in the prevention of embolic events in atrial fibrillation.

ANTIPHOSPHOLIPID ANTIBODY SYNDROME

APS, also known as Hughes syndrome, is an acquired autoimmune prothrombotic condition characterized clinically by venous or arterial thrombosis and/or recurrent fetal loss associated with persistent laboratory evidence of antibodies directed against phospholipids or phospholipid-binding proteins. The most commonly detected subgroups of aPL are LA, anticardiolipin antibodies (aCL), and anti–β2-GP I. The disorder can be primary or secondary to another major autoimmune disease, most commonly SLE. This is one of few conditions that can manifest with both arterial thromboembolism and VTE, and it can affect both large and small vessels. Increasingly, microthrombotic disease is being recognized as a manifestation of APS, particularly in the form of renal thrombotic microangiopathy.

The cardinal features of APS include thrombotic manifestations, recurrent fetal loss, and thrombocytopenia. Cardiac valvular abnormalities, livedo reticularis, and hemolytic anemia are additional common findings. Patients are typically 35 to 45 years old when they experience their first thrombotic event. Males and females are equally affected. Almost two-thirds of patients have thrombi limited to the venous system, 20% to 30% are arterial, and in 10% to 15% of individuals both circulations are affected. Most patients present with deep vein thrombosis of the lower extremities, up to half of whom subsequently develop pulmonary emboli. Thrombosis can also affect the superficial and deep cerebral venous system, and it typically does so at a young age with relatively more extensive involvement.

Ischemic stroke and TIAs are the most common neurologic presentation of APS. They occur in approximately one-fifth of patients, followed by myocardial infarction at about half this frequency. Most of these events are clinically indistinguishable from atherosclerotic or small vessel strokes; they therefore require a high level of suspicion. The syndrome should be suspected in young patients with ischemic stroke whenever other atypical vascular beds are involved, particularly the subclavian, renal, or retinal arteries, or when a patient experiences recurrent thromboembolic events with no defined etiology. Of note, not all arterial episodes are thrombotic in origin. Emboli, especially from mitral valve or aortic valve vegetations, can lead to cerebral events. Paradoxical embolization through a patent foramen ovale may also occur. The association of livedo reticularis with cerebral thrombosis characterizes Sneddon syndrome. The most severe and fortunately least frequent form of APS is catastrophic APS characterized by multiorgan failure due to widespread thrombotic disease, typically microvascular in nature. The mortality rate of this devastating condition is greater than 50%.

The mechanisms by which aPL induce thrombosis are not entirely appreciated. It is postulated that these antibodies interfere with endogenous anticoagulant pathways, bind and activate platelets, and lead to activation of the complement cascade. Thrombosis in APS may occur

ANTIPHOSPHOLIPID ANTIBODY SYNDROME

Livedo reticularis

Thrombosis in large intracranial vessel

Emboli

Infarct

Multiple emboli in pulmonary arterial tree with acute infarcts

Thrombus

In left common, external, and internal iliac veins, loosely attached to vessel wall; a common source of pulmonary emboli

Woman at risk for miscarriage

spontaneously or in the setting of predisposing factors, including smoking, oral contraceptive use, vascular stasis, surgery, or trauma. Women are at particularly high risk for VTE during pregnancy and the postpartum period. Some patients, most commonly those with venous rather than arterial thrombotic events, may have concurrent genetic thrombophilic conditions. There is no definitive association between specific clinical manifestations and particular subgroups of aPL. However, the risk for recurrence after a first episode of VTE in the presence of aCL is particularly high (approximately 30%), which correlates with the antibody titer.

The diagnosis of APS is made by combining clinical features with laboratory evidence of medium- or high-titer circulating aPL that are identified on two or more occasions at least 12 weeks apart. The antibodies can be of either IgG or IgM subtypes and are measured by a standard enzyme-linked immunosorbent. The term *lupus anticoagulant* is a misnomer that resulted from the early observation that its presence can prolong the PTT. An abnormal PTT should not be used as a screening test for APS. However, patients with APS need to be investigated for possible underlying SLE.

Given the high risk of recurrent thromboembolism that characterizes this condition, the mainstay of treatment in patients with APS is anticoagulant therapy, often lifelong. Warfarin continues to be the drug of choice, and a higher INR (3.0–4.0) may have to be achieved in patients with recurrent thrombotic events. The addition of aspirin may also be considered, taking into consideration the higher bleeding risk in patients with thrombocytopenia as a manifestation of their disease. In addition, immunomodulation may be required in patients with thrombotic microangiopathy or catastrophic APS.

Plate 9.35

Brain: PART I

MENINGES AND SUPERFICIAL CEREBRAL VEINS

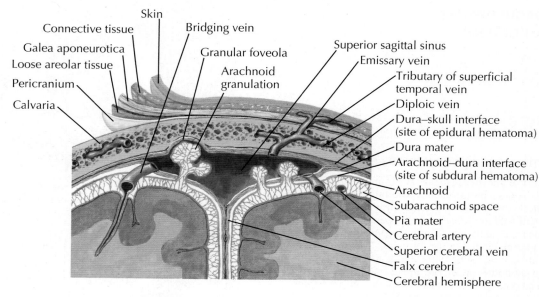

Skin
Connective tissue
Bridging vein
Galea aponeurotica
Granular foveola
Superior sagittal sinus
Loose areolar tissue
Emissary vein
Arachnoid granulation
Tributary of superficial temporal vein
Pericranium
Diploic vein
Calvaria
Dura–skull interface (site of epidural hematoma)
Dura mater
Arachnoid–dura interface (site of subdural hematoma)
Arachnoid
Subarachnoid space
Pia mater
Cerebral artery
Superior cerebral vein
Falx cerebri
Cerebral hemisphere

Branches of middle meningeal artery
Superior cerebral veins (bridging veins) (penetrating arachnoid and dura mater to enter superior sagittal sinus)
Superior sagittal sinus
Dura mater
Superior cerebral veins (beneath arachnoid)
Superior anastomotic vein (of Trolard)
Inferior anastomotic vein (of Labbé)
Superficial middle cerebral vein
Inferior cerebral veins (beneath arachnoid)
Middle meningeal artery and veins
Temporalis muscle

VENOUS SINUS THROMBOSIS

VENOUS SINUSES OF THE DURA MATER

Located between the two layers of the dura mater, the venous sinuses are divided into a posterosuperior group within the upper and posterior skull and an anteroinferior group situated at the base of the skull, consisting of paired sinuses and plexuses.

Posterosuperior Group

Superior Sagittal Sinus. The SSS traverses the superior margin of the falx cerebri, gradually increasing in dimension as it passes posteriorly, receiving superior cerebral veins and veins from the pericranium, the diploe, and dura mater. Its anterior portion is occasionally absent, replaced by two veins converging behind the coronal suture. The SSS terminates near the occipital protuberance and joins the straight sinus to form the *confluence of sinuses (torcular herophili).*

Inferior Sagittal Sinus. The inferior sagittal sinus (ISS) traverses the posterior two-thirds of the lower falx cerebri margin; this becomes larger as it receives veins from the falx and cerebral hemisphere's medial surfaces to join the *great cerebral vein of Galen,* forming the straight sinus.

Straight Sinus. The straight sinus is located at the falx cerebri junction with the tentorium cerebelli, receiving superior cerebellar veins to terminate and join the confluence of sinuses. It is usually a single channel, although occasionally doubled or tripled.

Transverse Sinuses. The transverse sinuses (bilateral, usually of unequal size) are at the internal occipital protuberance, where usually the right side is the direct SSS continuation, whereas the other derives from the *straight sinus.* Each becomes larger running anterolaterally within the tentorium cerebelli margin, receiving the *superior petrosal sinuses,* and inferior cerebral, cerebellar, diploic, condyloid, and mastoid veins. These leave the tentorium, entering the jugular foramen as the *sigmoid sinus.*

Sigmoid Sinuses. Sigmoid sinuses are continuations of the transverse sinuses situated over the temporal mastoid bones. These terminate at the jugular foramens, draining into the internal jugular veins.

Occipital Sinus. The occipital sinus is the smallest, usually single, sinus. It originataes from small venous channels at the foramen magnum, communicates with the transverse sinus, and terminates at the confluence of the sinuses.

Anteroinferior Group

Cavernous Sinuses. Cavernous sinuses are irregular networks of communicating venous channels beginning at the superior orbital fissures and extending to the petrous apex of the temporal bones. The ICA, carotid plexus, and abducens nerve lie on the medial wall, whereas oculomotor, trochlear, and ophthalmic/maxillary divisions of trigeminal nerves traverse the lateral wall. Each sinus receives ophthalmic (superior and inferior) and middle cerebral veins and the small *sphenoparietal sinus,* and it communicates via the *intercavernous sinuses.* These drain into the *transverse sinuses* via the *superior petrosal sinuses,* the *internal jugular veins* via the *inferior petrosal sinuses,* the plexus of veins on the ICA, and the *pterygoid venous plexus.*

Intercavernous Sinuses. Anterior and posterior sinuses connect the two cavernous sinuses, forming a venous circle around the pituitary stalk.

Sphenoparietal Sinuses. They course along the undersurface of the lesser wing of the sphenoid bone and drain into the cavernous sinuses.

Petrosal Sinuses. Superior petrosal sinuses receive blood from cerebellar, inferior cerebral, and tympanic cavity veins; traverse the tentorium cerebelli; and connect

Plate 9.36

Cerebrovascular Circulation and Stroke

VENOUS SINUS THROMBOSIS (Continued)

the cavernous and transverse sinuses. *Inferior petrosal sinuses* originate within the inferior petrosal sulcus at the junction of the petrous temporal and basilar occipital bones and the jugular foramen. These receive blood from the internal auditory veins, medulla, pons, and cerebellum and connect the cavernous sinus with the *internal jugular vein* bulb.

Basilar Plexus. The basilar plexus consists of interlacing venous channels over the basilar occipital bone; it connects the *inferior petrosal sinuses* while also draining the anterior vertebral venous plexus.

CEREBRAL VENOUS SYSTEM

The cerebral veins are best considered as being related to either superficial or deep brain structures.

Superficial Group

These veins drain the cerebral cortex and subcortical white matter into the SSS and the straight, transverse, and cavernous sinuses. These include (1) the *great anastomotic vein of Trolard,* connecting the middle cerebral veins to the SSS; (2) the *vein of Labbé,* connecting the middle cerebral veins with the transverse sinuses; and (3) the *middle cerebral veins,* receiving communicating branches from the veins of Trolard and Labbé and draining into cavernous sinuses.

Veins of the posterior fossa, draining the cerebellum and brainstem, are divided into (1) the superior vein (of Galen), including precentral, superior cerebellar, superior vermian, posterior mesencephalic, lateral mesencephalic, quadrigeminal, and anterior pontomesencephalic veins that drain the superior portion of the cerebellum and upper brainstem into the vein of Galen; (2) the anterior (petrosal) vein, including petrosal, anterior medullary, cerebellar hemispheric, and lateral medullary veins, each draining into the petrosal sinuses; and (3) the posterior (tentorial) vein, including the inferior vermian and some cerebellar bihemispheric veins, which drain into the confluence of the sinuses and neighboring transverse sinuses.

Deep Group

These veins drain the deep central white matter and basal ganglia to empty into the subependymal veins of the lateral ventricles. The major subependymal veins include (1) *septal veins* draining frontal horns of the lateral ventricles near the septum pellucidum, the corpus callosum, and deep frontal white matter; uniting with (2) the *thalamostriate veins* formed by the anterior caudate and terminal veins. These run in the floor of the

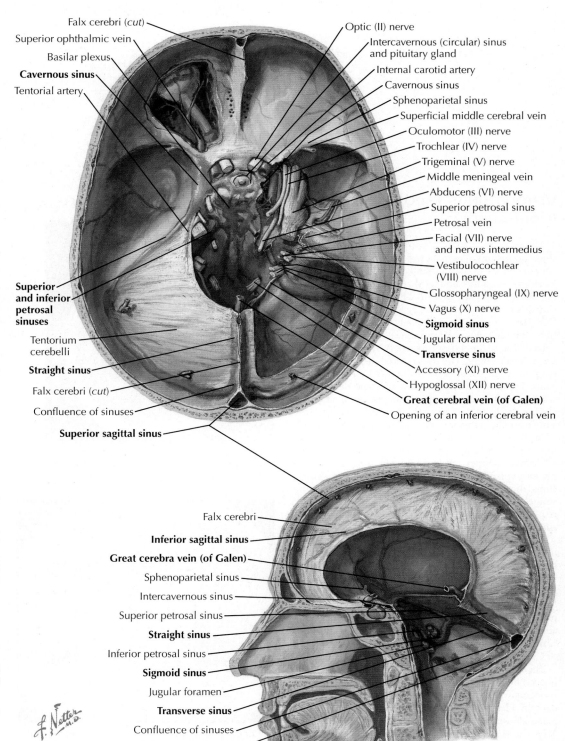

INTRACRANIAL VENOUS SINUSES

Falx cerebri (*cut*)
Superior ophthalmic vein
Basilar plexus
Cavernous sinus
Tentorial artery
Superior and inferior petrosal sinuses
Tentorium cerebelli
Straight sinus
Falx cerebri (*cut*)
Confluence of sinuses
Superior sagittal sinus

Optic (II) nerve
Intercavernous (circular) sinus and pituitary gland
Internal carotid artery
Cavernous sinus
Sphenoparietal sinus
Superficial middle cerebral vein
Oculomotor (III) nerve
Trochlear (IV) nerve
Trigeminal (V) nerve
Middle meningeal vein
Abducens (VI) nerve
Superior petrosal sinus
Petrosal vein
Facial (VII) nerve and nervus intermedius
Vestibulocochlear (VIII) nerve
Glossopharyngeal (IX) nerve
Vagus (X) nerve
Sigmoid sinus
Jugular foramen
Transverse sinus
Accessory (XI) nerve
Hypoglossal (XII) nerve
Great cerebral vein (of Galen)
Opening of an inferior cerebral vein

Falx cerebri
Inferior sagittal sinus
Great cerebra vein (of Galen)
Sphenoparietal sinus
Intercavernous sinus
Superior petrosal sinus
Straight sinus
Inferior petrosal sinus
Sigmoid sinus
Jugular foramen
Transverse sinus
Confluence of sinuses
Occipital sinus

lateral ventricle and drain into (3) the *internal cerebral veins,* each receiving blood from the thalamostriate, choroidal, septal, epithalamic, and lateral ventricular veins and situated within the roof of the third ventricle. Both internal cerebral veins unite beneath the splenium of the corpus callosum to merge with (4) the *basal veins of Rosenthal* arising within the sylvian fissure. These receive blood from the anterior cerebral, deep middle cerebral, and inferior striate veins and then course around the cerebral peduncles and midbrain tectum to

form the *great cerebral vein of Galen.* This curves around the splenium in the quadrigeminal cistern, terminating near the tentorial apex, where it joins the ISS to form the *straight sinus.*

DIAGNOSIS AND TREATMENT OF CEREBRAL VENOUS SINUS THROMBOSIS

Hypercoagulability, whether genetic or acquired, and infections are the main causes of dural and venous

Plate 9.37

Brain: PART I

DIAGNOSIS OF VENOUS SINUS THROMBOSIS

Causes of venous sinus thrombosis

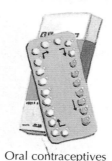
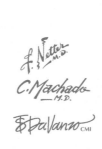
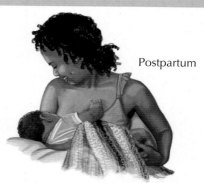

Postpartum

Oral contraceptives

VENOUS SINUS THROMBOSIS (Continued)

sinus occlusions. Pregnancy, puerperium, use of oral contraceptives, cancer, and infections in parameningeal locations (ear, sinus, and face) are important predisposing factors. Recently several cases of cerebral venous sinus thrombosis have been reported in patients with COVID-19 infections and after COVID-19 vaccination. The sagittal and lateral sinuses are most often involved. The main and at times only symptom is headache. Brain edema, infarction, and hemorrhage can develop in the brain regions drained by the occluded veins. In these patients, focal neurologic deficits and seizures often occur. In some patients, dural sinus occlusion leads to increased ICP with a presentation similar to idiopathic intracranial hypertension.

In most patients, the D-dimer level in the blood is increased, reflecting increased blood clotting. However, a normal D-dimer level should not preclude further evaluation if the clinical suspicion for cerebral venous sinus thrombosis is high. Radiologic brain imaging studies visualizing the thrombosed sinus or vein are required to confirm the diagnosis of cerebral venous sinus thrombosis.

MRI is superior to CT scanning and is the imaging modality of choice. Plain CT may show evidence of brain swelling and edema, or venous infarctions, which tend to be hemorrhagic with large surrounding edema not conforming to well-defined arterial vascular territories (see Plates 9.15 and 9.23–9.25). However, plain CT scan may only show subtle and nonspecific abnormalities in the absence of venous infarction. Contrast administration may increase the sensitivity of CT imaging.

The major cerebral sinuses and veins can be reliably imaged by magnetic resonance venography (MRV), CT venography (CTV), or conventional catheter-based angiography. Plate 9.37, *D* depicts a normal MRV showing all major sinuses and veins, whereas Plate 9.37, *B* depicts an MRV showing absence of flow in the posterior portion of the *SSS* and some of the neighboring cortical veins. It is noteworthy that two-dimensional (2D) time-of-flight MRV is subject to flow-related image artifacts because it uses blood flow for contrast generation. The use of gadolinium-enhanced MRV is less likely to be affected by flow artifact, and when combined with 3D magnetization-prepared rapid gradient echo, it is superior to 2D MRV, particularly in complicated cases with anatomic variants. Conventional angiography with a prolonged venous phase is the gold standard for diagnosing cerebral sinus or vein thrombosis (see Plate 9.37, *C*), and its use is usually reserved for cases with high suspicion when MRV and CTV are negative or equivocal.

Diagnosis of sinus thrombosis

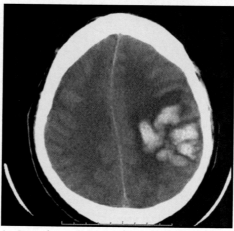

A. CT 2 days after admission showing left posterior frontal parietal patchy hemorrhage within the ischemic region.

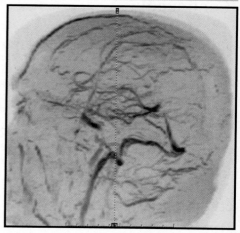

B. Magnetic resonance venography (MRV) demonstrates absence of flow in posterior sagittal sinus and some cortical veins.

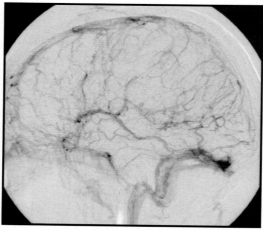

C. Digital angiogram, venous phase confirms the MRV findings.

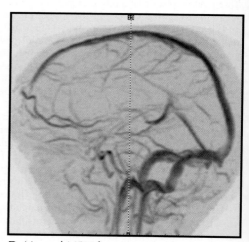

D. Normal MRV for comparison.

The specific treatment of cerebral venous sinus thrombosis depends on the underlying etiology. Most patients without contraindications for anticoagulation are initially treated either with body weight–adjusted subcutaneous low-molecular-weight heparin or dose-adjusted IV heparin and transitioned to oral anticoagulation, to avoid thrombus extension and to prevent pulmonary embolism. Emerging data suggest that DOACs may be acceptable alternatives to warfarin. The optimal duration of oral anticoagulation is uncertain and varies from 3 to 12 months in idiopathic cases or those provoked by thrombogenic drugs. Lifelong anticoagulation may be necessary in those with thrombophilia.

Local thrombolysis may be occasionally used in patients who deteriorate despite anticoagulation and in whom other causes of deterioration have been excluded. Symptomatic treatment includes the management of increased ICP, antiepileptic drugs if seizures develop, and analgesics for headache.

Plate 9.38

Cerebrovascular Circulation and Stroke

INTRACEREBRAL HEMORRHAGE

ICH represents 10% to 15% of strokes. Its relative importance derives from the associated high mortality (35%–50% at 6 months) and the severity of the permanent sequelae in survivors: only 20% are independent at 6 months compared with 60% after ischemic stroke. The mortality and morbidity related to ICH are primarily dependent on location and hematoma size; the latter is known to increase substantially soon after ICH onset in almost 40% of patients. Hemorrhages less than 30 cm³ generally have a good prognosis; hemorrhages of 30 to 60 cm³ may be more amenable to surgery and have a better outlook, whereas those greater than 60 cm³ have a very poor outlook, particularly when associated with a diminished level of consciousness. In contrast, hemorrhages due to rupture of small arteriovenous malformations may have a substantially better outcome.

The risk factors for ICH include hypertension, advancing age, vascular malformations, cerebral amyloid angiopathy, anticoagulant and fibrinolytic agents, brain tumors, sympathomimetic agents, and vasculitis. Hypertension is the primary risk factor across all ages, with the highest representation in those aged 40 to 69 years, whereas cerebral amyloid angiopathy is a more common risk factor in patients older than 70 years. In younger persons, sympathomimetic agents, especially cocaine, and vascular malformations are dominant factors. Brain tumors associated with ICH are typically the malignant varieties, either primary (particularly glioblastoma multiforme) or metastatic, including melanoma, choriocarcinoma, bronchogenic, renal cell, and thyroid carcinoma.

Warfarin-related ICH is an important group, particularly in senior or middle-aged individuals who are more likely to be taking this medication because of underlying atrial fibrillation. Here a leading risk factor is excessively increased INR. This variety of ICH is associated with a particularly high mortality because of the generally large hematoma volumes that develop because of frequent enlargement of the hematoma within the initial hours after onset of symptoms. The ICHs that occur after treatment of acute ischemic stroke with thrombolytics are also generally of large size, tending to occur within hours of completion of the thrombolytic treatment, and typically are near the manifesting cerebral infarction.

The locations of ICH and their approximate frequency are putaminal (35%), lobar (25%), thalamic (20%), cerebellar (10%), pontine (5%), and caudate (5%) (see Plate 9.39). The predominant location of ICH in deep subcortical and brainstem locations reflects the anatomic distribution of chronic changes within the wall of deep, small penetrating arteries subjected to chronic hypertension. In contrast, the more superficially located lobar ICHs reflect the classic pathoanatomy related to cerebral amyloid angiopathy.

The clinical presentation of an ICH has several general features that are frequent with all topographic varieties and particularly reflect the clinical symptomatology that results from a rapidly expanding intracranial mass lesion. These include headache, vomiting, and depressed level of consciousness. Although these are not constant features, their presence is virtually diagnostic of an ICH, particularly if a gradual decline in the level of consciousness occurs in parallel with a gradual increase in the severity of the presenting focal neurologic deficits. The specific findings on neurologic examination are related to the location of the ICH within the brain.

INTRACEREBRAL HEMORRHAGE: PATHOGENESIS AND TYPES

Pathogenesis

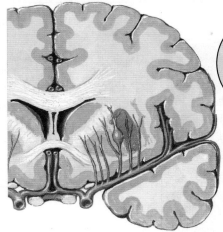
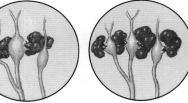
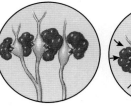
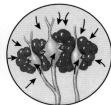

B. Microaneurysm ruptures, causing pressure on adjacent (satellite) vessels.

C. Satellite vessels rupture.

D. Amount of blood extravasated into brain tissue depends on tissue turgor opposed to intravascular blood pressure.

A. Microaneurysm formed in parenchymal artery of brain as result of hypertension. Lenticulostriate vessels (shown) most commonly involved, but similar process may occur in other parts of brain, especially the lobar white matter, thalamus, pons, and cerebellum.

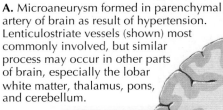
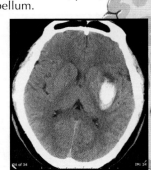
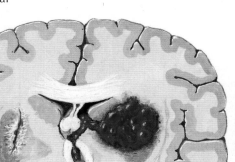

Moderate-sized intracerebral hemorrhage involving left putamen, with rupture into lateral ventricle; brain displaced to opposite side; scar of healed hemorrhage on right side.

CT scan showing large putaminal hemorrhage

Types

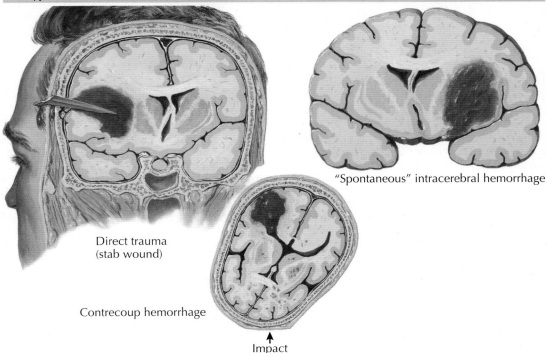

Direct trauma (stab wound)

Contrecoup hemorrhage

Impact

"Spontaneous" intracerebral hemorrhage

Plate 9.39

Brain: PART I

CLINICAL MANIFESTATIONS OF INTRACEREBRAL HEMORRHAGE RELATED TO SITE

Pathology	CT scan	Pupils	Eye movements	Motor and sensory deficits	Other
Caudate nucleus (blood in ventricle)		Sometimes ipsilaterally constricted	Conjugate deviation to side of lesion; slight ptosis	Contralateral hemiparesis, often transient	Headache, confusion
Putamen (small hemorrhage)		Normal	Conjugate deviation to side of lesion	Contralateral hemiparesis and hemisensory loss	Aphasia (if lesion on left side)
Putamen (large hemorrhage)		In presence of herniation, pupil dilated on side of lesion	Conjugate deviation to side of lesion	Contralateral hemiparesis and hemisensory loss	Decreased consciousness
Thalamus		Constricted, poorly reactive to light bilaterally	Both lids retracted; eyes positioned downward and medially; cannot look upward	Contralateral hemiparesis, but greater hemisensory loss	Aphasia (if lesion on left side)
Occipital lobar white matter		Normal	Normal	Mild, transient hemiparesis	Contralateral hemianopsia
Pons		Constricted, reactive to light	No horizontal movements; vertical movements preserved	Quadriplegia	Coma
Cerebellum		Slight constriction on side of lesion	Slight deviation to opposite side; movements toward side of lesion impaired, or sixth cranial nerve palsy	Ipsilateral limb ataxia; no hemiparesis	Gait ataxia, vomiting

INTRACEREBRAL HEMORRHAGE
(Continued)

The tendency of the hematoma to expand in the initial hours after symptom onset is a very important feature of ICH. This is common to all locations of ICH. More than one-third of patients will have an increase in the ICH size within the first 3 hours, and most all who eventually develop mass effect will do so within 6 hours from symptom onset. This hematoma expansion is typically associated with deteriorating neurologic function. The risk factors for this occurrence are still not clearly identified, although uncontrolled hypertension is suggested by some; this underlies the need to stress the potential value of maintaining blood pressure control within the early hours after ICH onset. Another factor associated with a high frequency of early hematoma expansion is the occurrence of ICH in patients taking oral anticoagulants such as warfarin or the DOACs dabigatran, rivaroxaban, apixaban, and

edoxaban. In either situation, urgent reversal of the anticoagulation is mandatory, with correction of the elevated INR with the combination of vitamin K and prothrombin complex concentrate in cases related to warfarin. Reversal of a DOAC requires antidotes such as idarucizumab for dabigatran, and andexanet alpha for rivaroxaban, apixaban, and edoxaban. In the event of unavailability of such antidotes, prothrombin complex concentrate is the recommended reversal agent. The risk for hematoma expansion is correlated with the finding of the "spot sign" in CTA at presentation with ICH. This finding on CTA consists of the presence of a dot of contrast within the hematoma, reflecting active bleeding at the time of the IV contrast infusion during CTA. The presence of the spot sign shows high correlation with subsequent hematoma enlargement.

CEREBELLAR HEMORRHAGE

Cerebellar hemorrhage represents about 5% to 10% of ICH cases, and despite its relatively low frequency, it is of great clinical importance because prompt diagnosis may lead to lifesaving emergency surgical intervention. The clinical presentation typically includes abrupt onset of vertigo, vomiting, headache, and inability to stand and walk. In patients who are alert enough to undergo full neurologic examination, the classic findings include ipsilateral cerebellar ataxia, horizontal gaze palsy, and peripheral facial palsy as a triad that is highly suggestive of the diagnosis. Other signs of ipsilateral pontine tegmental involvement can be present, including trigeminal sensory loss and Horner syndrome, findings that occur in the absence of contralateral hemiplegia because the pressure effects of the cerebellar hematoma are exerted on the dorsal portion of the pons, sparing the basis pontis and the corticospinal tracts.

Plate 9.40

Cerebrovascular Circulation and Stroke

VASCULAR MALFORMATIONS

Arteriovenous malformations.
On surface of brain, covered by arachnoid.

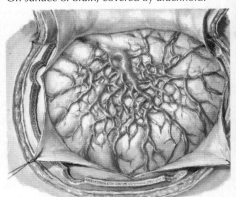

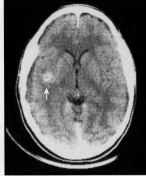

CT scan without contrast medium. Does not clearly demonstrate arteriovenous malformation (AVM).

CT scan with contrast medium. Demonstrates enhancement corresponding to AVM *(arrow)*.

INTRACEREBRAL HEMORRHAGE
(Continued)

The clinical course in cerebellar hemorrhage is notoriously unpredictable because patients who are alert and responsive at presentation can suddenly deteriorate due to brainstem compression rapidly leading to coma, respiratory depression, and death. This sudden change can occur without stepwise progression. From a clinical standpoint, the presence of signs of compression of the pontine tegmentum at presentation (ipsilateral horizontal gaze palsy, facial palsy) calls for strong consideration of surgical evacuation of the hematoma, especially if associated with imaging features that have been found to correlate with potential for neurologic deterioration, including hematoma diameter greater than 3 cm, supratentorial hydrocephalus, obliteration of the ipsilateral quadrigeminal cistern, and deformation/compression of the fourth ventricle. These imaging features have been correlated with high frequency of sudden neurologic deterioration requiring emergency surgical treatment, whereas their absence may predict a more benign clinical course without need for surgical removal of the hematoma.

For these reasons, it is imperative that patients with cerebellar hemorrhage be assessed at presentation with the specific purpose of determining whether they should have surgical intervention in the early course of their illness before neurologic deterioration. These considerations are based on the correlation between preoperative level of consciousness and surgical outcome; patients who are alert or lethargic preoperatively have a surgical mortality of approximately 15%, whereas those who have reached the stage of stupor or coma have a surgical mortality of at least 75%. Once the decision has been made to subject the patient to surgery, an initial consideration is whether an emergency ventriculostomy is required before performing the more definitive suboccipital craniectomy for hematoma evacuation. This procedure is indicated in patients with massive hydrocephalus whose level of consciousness has suddenly deteriorated, and it is used as an emergency temporizing procedure while arrangements are being made for surgical suboccipital craniectomy. Despite an initially severely compromised neurologic condition, successful removal of the cerebellar hematoma is generally followed by an adequate functional outcome with limb and gait ataxia gradually improving, potentially leaving no long-term motor disability.

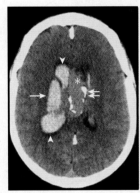

CT scan with acute hemorrhage in right hemisphere *(arrow)* and right lateral ventricle *(arrowheads)*, caused by ruptured AVM *(asterisk)*, surrounded by calcifications *(double arrows)*.

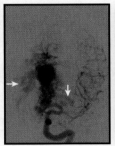

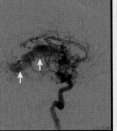

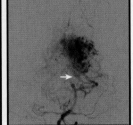

Contrast angiogram showing large midline AVM with arterial supply from left anterior cerebral artery branches (anteroposterior view; lateral view) and left posterior cerebral artery branches (anteroposterior view of vertebral artery injection). All views show, in addition to multivessel arterial supply of the AVM, prominent dilated draining veins *(arrows)*.

f. Netter M.D.

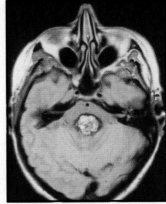

Large pontine cavernous angioma with central portion with mixed high and low signals and irregular margins ("popcorn" aspect), surrounded by black halo corresponding to old hemosiderin deposits.

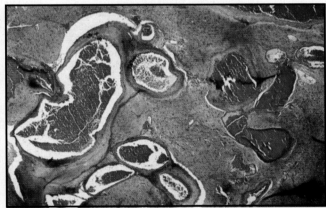

Hematoxylin and eosin–stained cavernous angioma showing characteristic aggregate of vascular structures of thin walls, without arterial or venous morphology, in a background of sclerotic tissue, without areas of intervening brain parenchyma among the vascular channels. Areas of calcification are visible in the lower right corner.

Hemorrhage into the cerebellar vermis is a type of cerebellar hemorrhage that differs from the classic unilateral hemispheric type described above. This type of hemorrhage tends to be more severe in its initial manifestations with less potential for benefit from surgery because of the early bilateral compression of the tegmentum of the pons. This often results in severe compromise in the level of consciousness and bilateral oculomotor deficits at onset, progressing to coma and bilateral ophthalmoplegia with miosis, resembling primary pontine hemorrhage. Because of the midline cerebellar location and early bilateral compromise of the pontine tegmentum, the surgical evacuation is generally less successful than with hemispheric cerebellar hemorrhage. Therefore most patients are only treated with ventriculostomy to address prominent supratentorial hydrocephalus because of fourth ventricular compression.

Plate 9.41

Brain: PART I

INTRACRANIAL ANEURYSMS AND SUBARACHNOID HEMORRHAGE

Intracranial aneurysm rupture is the most common cause of nontraumatic SAH. SAH accounts for only 5% of all cases of stroke but is associated with particularly high morbidity and mortality. The total loss of quality-adjusted life years from SAH is similar to that of ischemic stroke. Approximately 30,000 Americans are admitted annually for SAH. Prehospital mortality rates may reach 10% to 15%, and many patients who survive the initial rupture require intensive care, are at high risk for medical complications, and have permanent neurologic sequelae. The 1-month mortality rate approaches 50%. Hence SAH imparts a significant public health burden. Promisingly, the incidence of SAH may be decreasing globally along with declining tobacco use and improved blood pressure management, although considerable regional and demographic variation persists.

The incidence of aneurysmal SAH is higher in women than men and peaks during the sixth decade of life. The frequency of SAH is low in children. The most important risk factors are smoking, hypertension, and heavy alcohol use; although these exposures are less common in females, they may be more hazardous for this group. The mechanisms by which female hormones and reproductive functioning influence cerebral aneurysm formation and rupture are unclear, although the condition is known to increase after menopause. Sympathomimetic drugs, emotional stress, sexual intercourse, and physical activity may all incite aneurysm rupture, likely via a spike in blood pressure.

Saccular (berry) aneurysms are found at sites with a predilection for hemodynamic stress, namely at the bifurcations of major intracranial arteries (see Plate 9.41). Approximately 85% arise adjacent to the circle of Willis, with the most common locations including the anterior communicating artery, the MCA bifurcation, and the junction of the ICA and posterior communicating artery. Beyond saccular aneurysms, the differential for nontraumatic SAH includes other aneurysmal pathologies

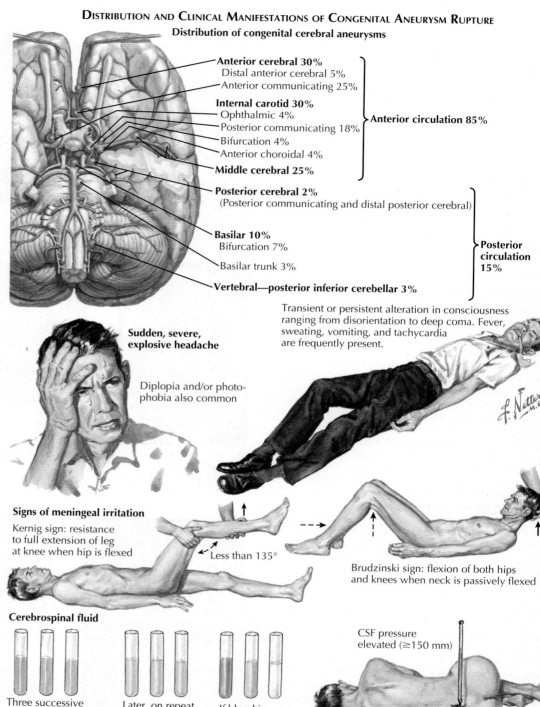

DISTRIBUTION AND CLINICAL MANIFESTATIONS OF CONGENITAL ANEURYSM RUPTURE

Distribution of congenital cerebral aneurysms

Anterior cerebral 30%
Distal anterior cerebral 5%
Anterior communicating 25%

Internal carotid 30%
Ophthalmic 4%
Posterior communicating 18%
Bifurcation 4%
Anterior choroidal 4%

Middle cerebral 25%

} Anterior circulation 85%

Posterior cerebral 2%
(Posterior communicating and distal posterior cerebral)

Basilar 10%
Bifurcation 7%
Basilar trunk 3%

Vertebral—posterior inferior cerebellar 3%

} Posterior circulation 15%

Sudden, severe, explosive headache

Diplopia and/or photophobia also common

Transient or persistent alteration in consciousness ranging from disorientation to deep coma. Fever, sweating, vomiting, and tachycardia are frequently present.

Signs of meningeal irritation

Kernig sign: resistance to full extension of leg at knee when hip is flexed

Less than 135°

Brudzinski sign: flexion of both hips and knees when neck is passively flexed

Cerebrospinal fluid

Three successive fluid samples collected shortly after subarachnoid hemorrhage show frank blood or are orange tinged in color.

Later, on repeat tap, all 3 samples are xanthochromic (yellow) as a result of hemoglobin release or bilirubin formation.

If blood is due to traumatic tap, fluid clears progressively in successive samples.

CSF pressure elevated (≥150 mm)

(dolichoectatic, mycotic, neoplastic), intracranial arterial dissection, RCVS, PRES, vasculitis, cerebral amyloid angiopathy with superficial siderosis, nonaneurysmal vascular malformations (dural AVF, arteriovenous malformation), and coagulopathy. Dolichoectatic and dissecting aneurysms often affect the posterior circulation, and neoplastic and mycotic (infection secondary to endocarditis) aneurysms usually affect distal arterial branches, resulting in cortical hemorrhages. Perimesencephalic SAH is an entity in which bleeding is located near the brainstem and is generally nonaneurysmal, with the likely cause thought to be venous bleeding. Additionally, some neurologic entities, including meningitis, leptomeningeal disease, and imaging artifacts, may mimic the radiographic appearance of SAH.

PATHOPHYSIOLOGY

The unique architecture of intracranial arterial walls, which lack a second layer of elastic lamina, likely

Plate 9.42

Cerebrovascular Circulation and Stroke

GIANT CONGENITAL ANEURYSMS

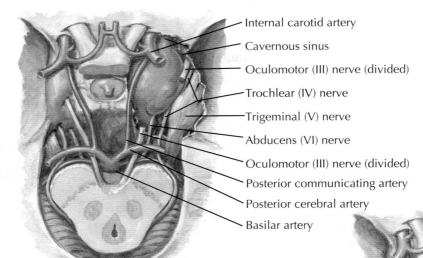

Internal carotid artery
Cavernous sinus
Oculomotor (III) nerve (divided)
Trochlear (IV) nerve
Trigeminal (V) nerve
Abducens (VI) nerve
Oculomotor (III) nerve (divided)
Posterior communicating artery
Posterior cerebral artery
Basilar artery

A. Intracavernous (infraclinoid) internal carotid aneurysm compressing abducens (VI) nerve. Oculomotor (III), trochlear (IV), and trigeminal (V) nerves may also be affected. Trigeminal involvement may cause facial pain.

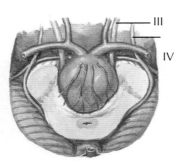

III
IV

B. Aneurysm of supraclinoid segment of internal carotid artery elevating optic chiasm, distorting infundibulum, and compressing oculomotor (III) nerve.

INTRACRANIAL ANEURYSMS AND SUBARACHNOID HEMORRHAGE (Continued)

contributes to the formation and rupture of intracranial aneurysms. Internal elastic lamina damage allows for outpouching of the vessel wall. The wall of a saccular aneurysm contains intima, media, and adventitia but it may be quite thin, particularly at the dome. The risk of rupture positively correlates with aneurysm size. Lesions greater than 25 mm in diameter are considered giant aneurysms (see Plate 9.42). In addition to lesion size, female sex, and tobacco use, irregular shape and interval growth also increase risk of rupture. The PHASES Score is a tool predicting rupture risk that may guide clinical decision-making regarding continued observation versus intervention of unruptured intracranial aneurysms.

Individuals with diseases affecting connective tissue, including Ehlers-Danlos syndrome, Marfan syndrome, fibromuscular dysplasia, coarctation of the aorta, moyamoya disease, and polycystic kidney disease, are at heightened risk for intracranial aneurysms. Approximately 25% of patients with an intracranial aneurysm will have more than one aneurysm. Family members of patients with an intracranial aneurysm have a greater risk, which suggests a genetic linkage; however, only a small proportion have an identifiable hereditary syndrome. As yet, no specific genetic locus associated with saccular aneurysms has been identified. Offering noninvasive vascular screening for patients with a family history of two or more first-degree relatives with intracranial aneurysms may be considered, although individuals should be counseled regarding the significance of identifying an asymptomatic intracranial aneurysm.

PRESENTATION AND DIAGNOSIS

An incidental unruptured intracranial aneurysm may be discovered when vessel imaging is performed for another indication. Unruptured aneurysms may compress adjacent neurologic structures. A new-onset

C. Aneurysm of basilar bifurcation projecting posteriorly, invading peduncles and compressing cerebral aqueduct. Corticospinal tracts may be affected, resulting in paralysis or paresis.

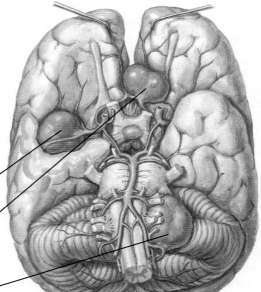

D. Aneurysm of middle cerebral artery

E. Aneurysm of anterior cerebral-anterior communicating arteries

F. Aneurysm of posterior inferior cerebellar artery

cranial nerve palsy, particularly of the oculomotor (CN III) nerve, given its proximity to the posterior communicating artery, may require intracranial vessel imaging as rapidly growing intracranial aneurysms may warrant intervention to prevent rupture (see Plate 9.43). Rarely, giant aneurysms may irritate the cortex and lead to seizures, or aneurysms may be a source of thrombi due to stasis and nonlaminar blood flow, leading to embolism and TIA or ischemic stroke.

In contrast, rupture of an intracranial aneurysm is a very dramatic event. The cardinal symptom is a thunderclap headache, often described as the worst headache of one's life. Focal neurologic deficits may occur depending on the location of the blood. Patients may experience nausea, vomiting, photophobia, and phonophobia or altered mental status, loss of consciousness, or seizures. Blood is an irritant in the subarachnoid space and leads to meningeal symptoms, which may include

Plate 9.43

Brain: PART I

OPHTHALMOLOGIC MANIFESTATIONS OF CEREBRAL ANEURYSMS

A. Cranial neuropathies

Abducens nerve palsy: affected eye turns medially. May be first manifestation of intracavernous carotid aneurysm. Pain above eye or on side of face may be secondary to trigeminal (V) nerve involvement.

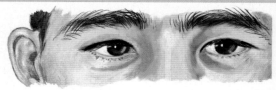

Oculomotor nerve palsy: ptosis, eye turns laterally and inferiorly, pupil dilated. Common finding with cerebral aneurysms, especially carotid-posterior communicating aneurysms.

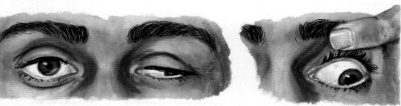

B. Visual field disturbances

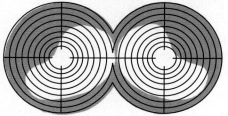

Superior bitemporal quadrantanopia caused by supraclinoid carotid aneurysm compressing optic chiasm from below

Inferior bitemporal quadrantanopia caused by compression of optic chiasm from above

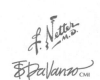

Right (or left) homonymous hemianopsia caused by compression of optic tract. Unilateral amaurosis may occur if optic (II) nerve is compressed.

C. Retinal changes

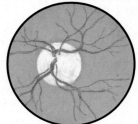

Optic atrophy may develop as a result of pressure on optic (II) nerve from a supraclinoid carotid, ophthalmic, or anterior cerebral aneurysm.

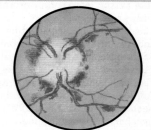

Hemorrhage into optic (II) nerve sheath after rupture of aneurysm may result in subhyaloid hemorrhage, with blood around disc.

INTRACRANIAL ANEURYSMS AND SUBARACHNOID HEMORRHAGE (Continued)

neck pain and stiffness and nuchal rigidity. Ophthalmologic exam may reveal intraocular (subhyaloid, intraretinal, or subretinal) hemorrhages, also known as Terson syndrome, which most commonly occur in critically ill patients. Several grading systems are used clinically in aneurysmal SAH, including the Hunt and Hess Classification, which provides an initial clinical grade (from 1 for asymptomatic/minimal headache to 5 for deep coma) as an index of surgical risk and prognosis.

Noncontrast head CT is the initial step in evaluation for SAH. Modern CT scanners have a sensitivity approaching 100% for detecting SAH when performed within 6 hours of headache onset and interpreted by qualified neuroradiologists. A ruptured intracranial aneurysm may also lead to intraparenchymal and/or intraventricular hemorrhage, in addition to SAH. The role for lumbar puncture (LP) has declined; however, if the CT scan is unremarkable or is performed after 6 hours from headache onset and clinical suspicion for SAH persists, an LP should be performed. In the presence of SAH, CSF appears xanthochromic after centrifugation and RBC count does not clear across collection tubes, in contrast to a bloody, traumatic LP. Additional diagnostic studies including electrocardiogram, complete blood count, comprehensive metabolic panel, and coagulation studies should be performed to screen for comorbidities and early medical complications of SAH.

CTA or MRA may identify an underlying aneurysm and guide the approach for securing the aneurysm. If no lesion is identified in a suspected aneurysmal SAH, DSA should be performed to identify and potentially allow endovascular treatment of the aneurysm. DSA is the standard for diagnosis of intracranial aneurysm, but even this study may need to be repeated to detect occult aneurysms when a high suspicion persists after DSA is performed.

Aneurysmal SAH is a medical emergency that is frequently unrecognized. Prompt diagnosis of SAH is imperative for timely and successful management. Common alternative diagnoses include migraine and other primary headache etiologies, sinusitis, meningitis, ischemic stroke, and cervical pathology. Misdiagnosis increases the risk of recurrent hemorrhage, vasospasm, delayed cerebral ischemia, hydrocephalus, seizures, and poor prognosis.

TREATMENT AND PROGNOSIS

After the identification of a suspected or confirmed SAH, a multidisciplinary team of neurosurgeons, neurointerventionalists, neurologists, and intensive care clinicians are usually involved in the care of the patient. As with all medical emergencies, initial steps should focus on ensuring adequate circulation, airway, and breathing. Patients may require intubation and hemodynamic support. If the patient's condition allows, the aneurysm should be secured with either surgical clipping (see Plate 9.44) or endovascular coiling within 24 hours of onset to improve outcome. Historically,

Plate 9.44

Cerebrovascular Circulation and Stroke

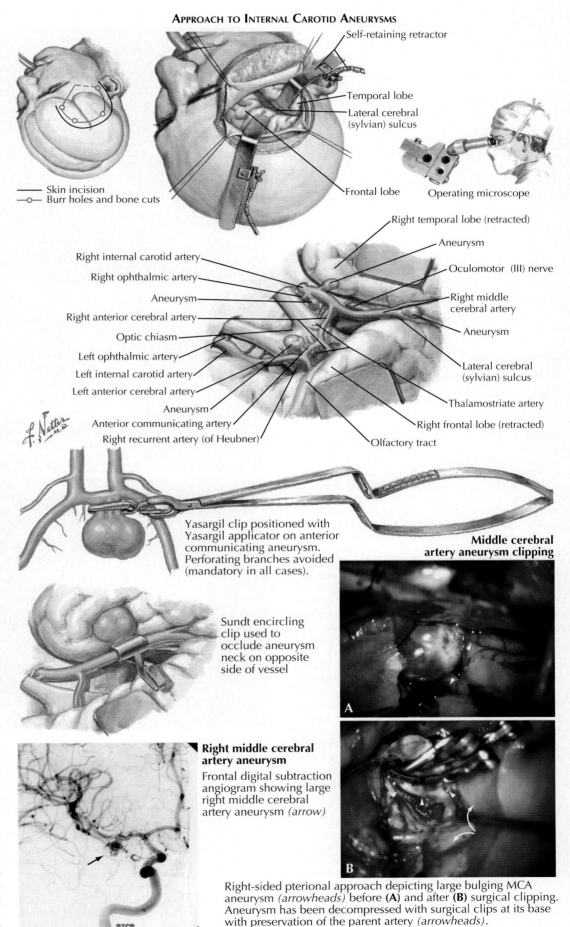

APPROACH TO INTERNAL CAROTID ANEURYSMS

Self-retaining retractor

Temporal lobe

Lateral cerebral (sylvian) sulcus

Frontal lobe

Operating microscope

— Skin incision
—o— Burr holes and bone cuts

Right temporal lobe (retracted)

Aneurysm

Right internal carotid artery

Right ophthalmic artery

Aneurysm

Right anterior cerebral artery

Optic chiasm

Left ophthalmic artery

Left internal carotid artery

Left anterior cerebral artery

Aneurysm

Anterior communicating artery

Right recurrent artery (of Heubner)

Oculomotor (III) nerve

Right middle cerebral artery

Aneurysm

Lateral cerebral (sylvian) sulcus

Thalamostriate artery

Right frontal lobe (retracted)

Olfactory tract

Yasargil clip positioned with Yasargil applicator on anterior communicating aneurysm. Perforating branches avoided (mandatory in all cases).

Middle cerebral artery aneurysm clipping

Sundt encircling clip used to occlude aneurysm neck on opposite side of vessel

Right middle cerebral artery aneurysm

Frontal digital subtraction angiogram showing large right middle cerebral artery aneurysm *(arrow)*

A

B

Right-sided pterional approach depicting large bulging MCA aneurysm *(arrowheads)* before **(A)** and after **(B)** surgical clipping. Aneurysm has been decompressed with surgical clips at its base with preservation of the parent artery *(arrowheads)*.

INTRACRANIAL ANEURYSMS AND SUBARACHNOID HEMORRHAGE (Continued)

surgical management was the primary approach, but after the International Subarachnoid Aneurysm Trial, which showed lower morbidity and mortality at 1-year follow-up but higher risk of incomplete occlusion and rebleeding in the endovascular group compared with the surgical arm, the endovascular approach gained popularity and continues to evolve. Advanced techniques, such as stent- and balloon-assisted coiling, flow diverters (see Plate 9.45), and embolic agents, can target complex aneurysms that are not amenable to clipping or coiling. Aneurysm location and morphology, hematoma size, patient age, comorbidities, clinical status, and operator experience may factor into the decision regarding clipping versus coiling. The goal of both surgical and endovascular intervention is to prevent recurrent hemorrhage. The risk of rebleeding is highest in the first 24 hours, particularly if the aneurysm is unsecured, and is associated with a poor prognosis. Short-term antifibrinolytic therapy (tranexamic acid or aminocaproic acid) may be considered in patients with unavoidable delays in aneurysm treatment; however, it may increase thrombosis risk, and routine use of antifibrinolytic therapy is not recommended.

During the ensuing 10 to 21 days, patients with SAH are closely monitored to identify, prevent, and treat complications. Frequent neurologic complications include seizures, vasospasm with delayed cerebral ischemia, hydrocephalus, and elevated ICP. Common medical issues include hyperglycemia, hyponatremia, other electrolyte disturbances, cardiac arrhythmias, pulmonary edema, VTE, fevers, and infection.

Vasospasm involves constriction of the large- and medium-sized intracranial arteries, which peaks approximately 1 week after aneurysm rupture, often affects intracranial arteries adjacent to the aneurysm, and may cause secondary cerebral infarction. The modified Fisher scale is a grading system to evaluate vasospasm risk based on the hemorrhage pattern on the initial CT scan. Prophylactic nimodipine is an established neuroprotective

Plate 9.45

Brain: PART I

FLOW DIVERSION STENT FOR TREATMENT OF UNRUPTURED INTRACRANIAL ANEURYSM

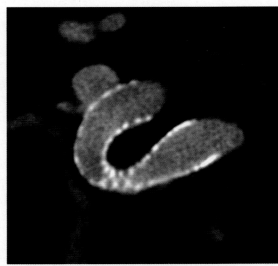

Dyna-CT image showing a right supraclinoid internal carotid artery aneurysm with flow diverter stent covering the neck of the aneurysm

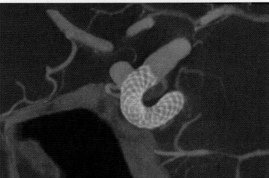

Digital subtraction angiography (DSA) image of the flow diverter stent across the neck of the aneurysm

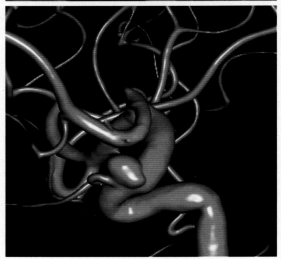

Three-dimensional reconstruction

Images courtesy Dr. Edgar Samaniego, University of Iowa Hospitals and Clinics, Department of Neurology.

INTRACRANIAL ANEURYSMS AND SUBARACHNOID HEMORRHAGE (Continued)

therapy in SAH, although the primary mechanism is debated. Once an aneurysm is secured, blood pressure goals may be liberalized. Once-popular "triple H" therapy with hypervolemia, hemodilution, and hypertension does not prevent vasospasm and may lead to complications from pulmonary and cerebral edema. Instead, maintaining euvolemia is recommended. TCDs, CT perfusion, continuous electroencephalogram (EEG), and other monitoring, in concert with frequent neurologic exams, may allow early identification of developing vasospasm and delayed ischemia. In the setting of cerebral vasospasm, inducing hypertension and ensuring euvolemia or catheter-based angiography with intraarterial vasodilators and/or angioplasty may be used to help avoid cerebral infarction. Use of other agents to prevent or treat vasospasm and delayed cerebral ischemia, such as magnesium, steroids, vasodilators, and other calcium channel blockers, require further investigation.

Hydrocephalus may develop after SAH because of obstruction of normal CSF flow and reduction of CSF absorption at the arachnoid granulations secondary to blood products in the subarachnoid space. An external ventricular drain can monitor ICP and help alleviate hydrocephalus. Hyperosmotic therapy, head-of-bed positioning, and symptom management (addressing pain, nausea, vomiting, agitation, and fever) can also help reduce elevated ICP. In severe cases, surgical decompression may be required. Some patients with SAH develop chronic hydrocephalus and require shunt placement for long-term CSF drainage.

Seizures may occur at the onset, during hospitalization, or posthospitalization for SAH and are associated with poor outcomes. Abnormal posturing may be mistaken for seizures at presentation, but its frequency is unclear. In general, routine seizure prophylaxis is not known to be beneficial in the absence of clinical or electrographic seizures. Standard prophylactic antiseizure dosing and duration may be insufficient to adequately prevent seizures, and antiseizure medications may have adverse side

effects. However, a subset of patients at higher risk of early seizures (based on presentation, blood volume and location, and medical history, for example) may benefit from seizure prophylaxis after SAH, but the ideal drug, dosing, and duration of treatment are unknown. EEG monitoring should be considered, particularly for patients with neurologic deficits. In addition to seizures, EEG may detect early changes associated with delayed cerebral ischemia.

The syndrome of inappropriate secretion of antidiuretic hormone and cerebral salt wasting are potential mechanisms of hyponatremia, which may be an independent predictor of poor outcome in patients with SAH.

Electrolyte and volume status should be closely monitored and managed. Hypertonic saline and corticosteroids may have a role in the management of hyponatremia after SAH. A potential cardiac complication of SAH is takotsubo cardiomyopathy, which is associated with high levels of catecholamines at the time of the hemorrhage.

Aneurysmal SAH is a significant public health issue. Intracranial aneurysm rupture yields high morbidity and mortality and requires coordinated management by multiple specialties to prevent and treat neurologic and medical complications. Many unknowns persist regarding the optimal management of this condition.

Plate 9.46

Cerebrovascular Circulation and Stroke

PEDIATRIC CEREBROVASCULAR DISEASE

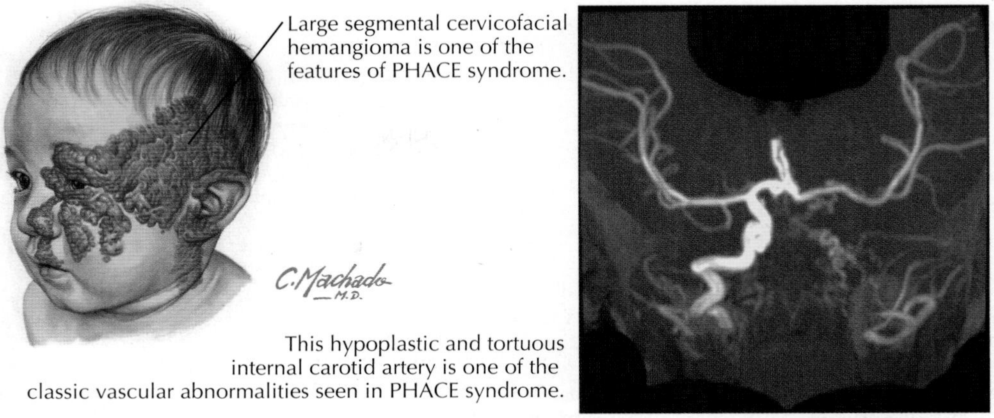

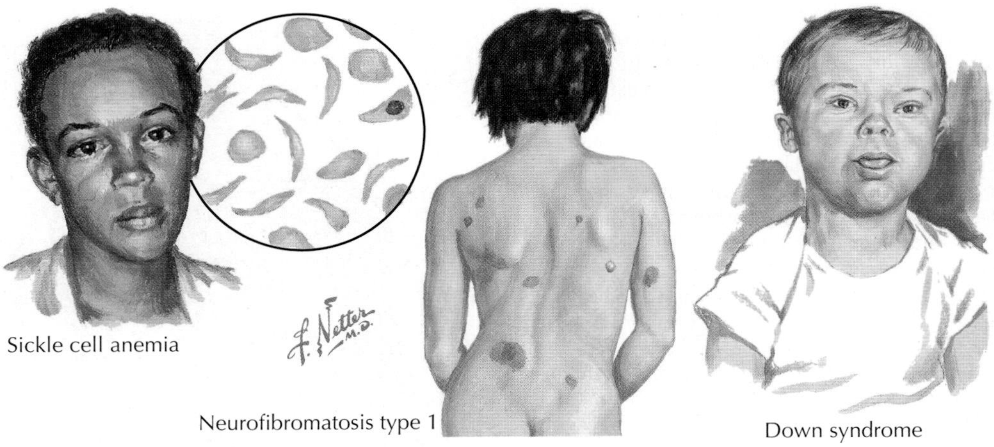

Every year in the United States, at least 5000 children have a stroke; half of these strokes are hemorrhagic (ICH or SAH). The causes of childhood stroke are diverse and heterogenous. Four related diseases are particularly unique to childhood.

MOYAMOYA

Moyamoya is a chronic progressive occlusive arteriopathy of the distal ICAs. The idiopathic form, also known as primary moyamoya or *moyamoya disease,* occurs more commonly in children of Japanese or Korean descent, although it has been observed in all ethnicities. Secondary moyamoya, or *moyamoya syndrome,* can develop after brain radiation for the treatment of childhood cancers, most commonly retinoblastoma, or can occur in genetic conditions, such as sickle cell disease, Down syndrome, neurofibromatosis type 1, and a rare form of primordial dwarfism. The name *moyamoya* (Japanese for "haze" or "puff of smoke") comes from small collateral blood vessels that form near the site of occlusion and give a hazy appearance on conventional angiography. Moyamoya typically manifests with ischemic strokes or TIAs in early to mid-childhood. However, if a child develops enough collateral blood flow to preclude ischemic events, they may not present until young adulthood with a hemorrhagic stroke, typically due to rupture of the abnormal moyamoya collaterals. Surgical treatment of moyamoya includes a variety of revascularization procedures intended to bypass the internal carotid circulation and improve cerebral perfusion.

FOCAL CEREBRAL ARTERIOPATHY

Focal cerebral arteriopathy of childhood (FCA) is an acute arteriopathy thought to have a postinfectious inflammatory mechanism. One of the most common causes of arterial ischemic stroke in a previously healthy child, it causes irregularity and stenosis of the distal ICA and its proximal branches, the MCA and ACA. Children typically present with an acute onset hemiparesis from an infarction in the distribution of the lenticulostriate arteries, the small branches arising from the distal ICA and proximal MCA. FCA can follow chickenpox, an acute infection with varicella-zoster virus (VZV). VZV remains latent in the trigeminal ganglion, which innervates the walls the same arteries affected in FCA. Hence the leading hypothesis for FCA pathogenesis is a pathologic immune response to viruses in the trigeminal nerve resulting in collateral injury to the nearby arteries. Children with FCA after COVID-19 have also been reported. Treatment trials of corticosteroids for FCA are commencing.

PHACE SYNDROME

PHACE is a neurocutaneous syndrome that includes *p*osterior fossa abnormalities, such as cerebellar hypoplasia or Dandy-Walker malformation; large, segmental cervicofacial *h*emangiomas; cervical and/or cerebral *a*rterial anomalies; *c*ardiac anomalies, such as coarctation of the aorta; and *e*ye abnormalities, such as optic nerve atrophy, congenital cataracts, and retinal vascular abnormalities. The skin hemangiomas seen in PHACE are considered infantile hemangiomas, defined as benign neoplasms of the vascular endothelium that display a characteristic natural history of being absent or minimally apparent at birth, growing rapidly during

Large segmental cervicofacial hemangioma is one of the features of PHACE syndrome.

This hypoplastic and tortuous internal carotid artery is one of the classic vascular abnormalities seen in PHACE syndrome.

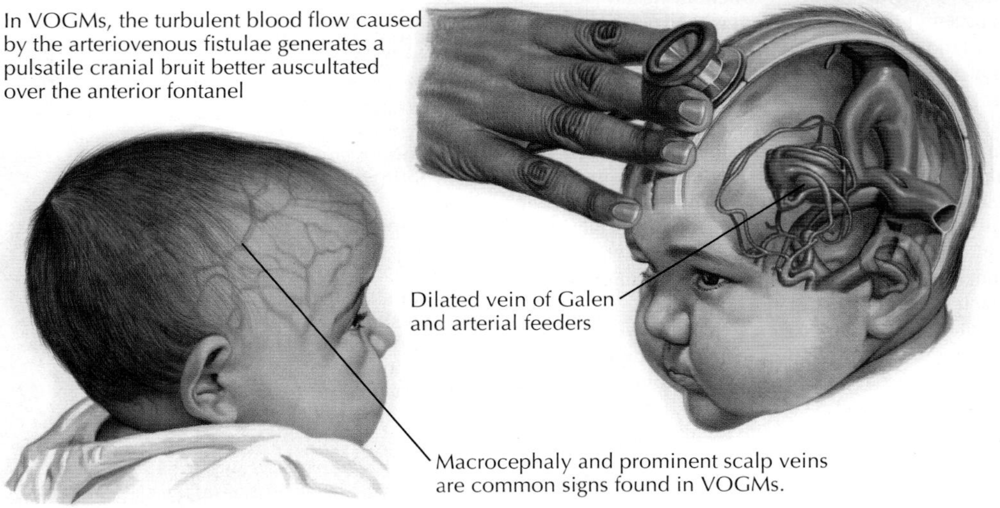

In VOGMs, the turbulent blood flow caused by the arteriovenous fistulae generates a pulsatile cranial bruit better auscultated over the anterior fontanel

Dilated vein of Galen and arterial feeders

Macrocephaly and prominent scalp veins are common signs found in VOGMs.

Children at risk for moyamoya syndrome

Sickle cell anemia

Neurofibromatosis type 1

Down syndrome

infancy, and then slowly regressing. The cerebrovascular anomalies vary widely from clinically insignificant normal variants, such as a duplicated vessel or persistent fetal vessel, to severe hypoplasia of the ICA that can lead to ischemic stroke.

VEIN OF GALEN MALFORMATIONS

Vein of Galen malformations (VOGMs) are congenital AVFs, or direct connections between arteries and veins, that drain into the developmental precursor of the vein of Galen, a midline vein that is part of the deep venous drainage system of the brain. VOGMs are easily detected on head imaging, even prenatal ultrasounds, as a large midline vascular structure. VOGMs can present in the neonatal period with high-output congestive heart failure, often with pulmonary hypertension. If the flow is not sufficient to lead to heart failure, they will often present later in infancy with symptoms of hydrocephalus. VOGMs can injure the brain by causing venous ischemia (poor perfusion due to local high venous pressures), or, rarely, intraventricular hemorrhage or ICH. Findings on exam will include a pulsatile cranial bruit, macrocephaly, and prominent scalp veins. These lesions are treated with embolization, that is, endovascular placement of embolic material to close off the abnormal artery to vein connections. Although presentation during the neonatal period with congestive heart failure portends a poor prognosis, children whose VOGMs can be cured before the brain is injured can have a normal outcome.

Plate 9.47

Brain: PART I

TRANSFER TRAINING AND SEATED POSITIONING

INTRODUCTION AND INITIAL STROKE REHABILITATION

Very few clinical events provide such a major challenge to the previously healthy and physically vigorous individual than the precipitous, unexpected, and emotionally devastating loss of focal neurologic function that occurs with a stroke. Rehabilitation is the primary mechanism by which individuals regain function, ideally administered by a multidisciplinary team with expertise in stroke rehabilitation. The core multidisciplinary rehabilitation team includes physical medicine and rehabilitation clinicians (i.e., physiatrists), advanced practice providers, physical therapists, occupational therapists, speech and language pathologists, and rehabilitation nurses, with multiple other disciplines contributing based on an individual's specific needs. In the acute care setting, rehabilitation is initiated once the individual is medically stable and is characterized by early mobilization to prevent secondary complications such as pressure injuries, joint contractures, and aspiration pneumonia.

Positioning after stroke is carried out with goals of preventing joint contractures, edema of the paretic extremity, pressure injuries over bony prominences, and aspiration. As it relates to the upper limb, supporting the weight of the arm in individuals presenting with glenohumeral subluxation remains critical; however, there is inadequate evidence to support the use of slings or resting hand splints, as they may restrict and deincentivize the recovery of volitional movement and have not been shown effective in reducing the incidence of pain. Furthermore, the use of slings may contribute to adhesive capsulitis and further restrict full shoulder range of motion. Passive range-of-motion exercises can be administered with caution to help avoid injury to the fragile and complex shoulder joint. Individuals who remain bedridden or nonambulatory are also at risk for ankle plantar flexion contractures. A resting ankle splint in which heels are kept off the bed for pressure relief is useful in maintaining ankle range of motion. Alternatively, passive weight-bearing activities including the use of a tilt table have been shown to be beneficial in preventing contractures and promoting upright posture.

Early mobilization involves sitting, standing, and gait training relatively early after stroke once the individual is medically stable. Although the precise timing to initiate early mobilization is not well understood, field experts agree that prolonged bed rest can have harmful effects on the cardiopulmonary, musculoskeletal, and immune systems. Furthermore, immobility can lead to serious complications including deep vein thrombosis, decubitus ulcers, and the formation of contractures. Clinical trials have shown that mobilization approximately 24 to 48 hours after stroke onset is safe and can lead to favorable outcomes as it relates to reducing long-term disability.

Transfer training begins early in rehabilitation of the individual with hemiplegia. Assisted transfers can be performed using a sliding board, lateral scoot technique, or a stand-pivot technique, where the clinician may need to block the knee and provide significant physical assistance to move the person from one sitting surface to another. As the patient recovers, the degree

The therapist or nurse can use a stand-pivot transfer in the early poststroke period to assist the individual out of bed to a wheelchair. Transferring toward the nonparetic side is easier for the patient, allowing transitioning weight onto the stronger lower limb and reaching for the armrest of the wheelchair with the nonparetic arm. Blocking just beneath the paretic knee can serve to facilitate weight acceptance on the hemiparetic lower limb while simultaneously preventing the limb from buckling. As the patient progresses, stepping, rather than pivoting, is encouraged, and transfers toward the paretic side are taught, with the goal of facilitating motor recovery and restoring normal movement patterns.

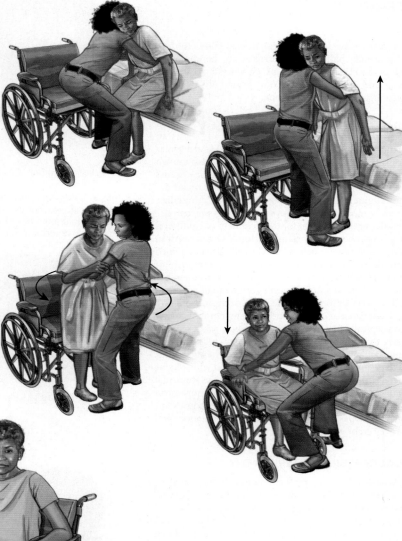

Early mobilization is encouraged as soon as the patient is medically stable, most commonly within 24–48 hours poststroke. Positioning in a chair with adequate support for the pelvis, trunk, and hemiplegic limbs is necessary to optimize alignment and upright postural control. The hemiplegic upper extremity should be supported in a neutral position, with the humerus in slight abduction. Elevating the distal upper extremity can be considered for edema management.

of assistance provided decreases, and normal movement patterns are encouraged, including standing and stepping rather than pivoting or sliding, with the goal of full independence.

Depression is an expected complication of any major stroke, due not only to an emotional reaction to the sudden change in functional abilities but also to the brain damage itself. It is important to keep this possibility under consideration at all phases of rehabilitation therapy. Initial family support and encouragement are essential if available. The clinician must be alert to loss of interest in pursuing rehabilitation efforts, as functional recovery is a long and arduous process that requires sustained engagement and participation. Antidepressant agents, including selective serotonin and serotonin-epinephrine reuptake inhibitors, and psychotherapeutic interventions, such as cognitive-behavioral therapy, are recommended alone or in combination. Exercise has been shown to help improve depressive symptoms in some studies.

Plate 9.48

Cerebrovascular Circulation and Stroke

CLINICAL SYNDROMES RELATED TO SITE OF LEGION

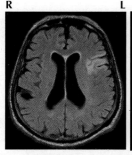 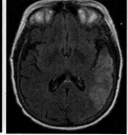 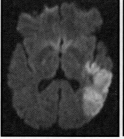 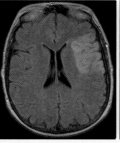 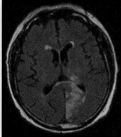

Broca aphasia MRI-FLAIR	Wernicke aphasia	Angular gyrus-posterior temporal, inferior parietal	Global aphasia-T2 FLAIR	Alexia without agraphia

	Broca aphasia	Wernicke aphasia	Angular gyrus	Global aphasia	Alexia without agraphia
Pronunciation, speech rhythm	Dysarthria, stuttering, effortful	Normal, fluent, loquacious	Normal	Very abnormal	Normal
Speech content	Missed syllables, agrammatical, telegraphic	Use of wrong or nonexistent words	Often normal	Very abnormal	Normal
Repetition of speech	Abnormal but better than spontaneous	Abnormal	Normal	Very abnormal	Normal
Comprehension of spoken language	Normal	Very abnormal	Normal	Very abnormal	Normal
Comprehension of written language	Not as good as for spoken language	Abnormal but better than for spoken	Very abnormal	Very abnormal	Normal
Writing	Clumsy, agrammatical, misspelled	Penmanship OK but misspelled and inaccurate	Very abnormal, spelling errors	Very abnormal	Normal
Naming	Better than spontaneous speech	Wrong names	Often abnormal	Very abnormal	Normal
Other	Hemiplegia, apraxia	Sometimes hemianopsia and apraxia	Slight hemiparesis, trouble calculating, finger agnosia, hemianopsia	Hemiplegia	Abnormal reading

APHASIA REHABILITATION

Aphasia is an acquired neurogenic language disorder resulting from an injury to one or more areas of the brain, specifically in the left hemisphere, and is present in 25% to 40% of individuals with stroke. Impairments can affect expressive and receptive language abilities, word retrieval, reading comprehension, and functional reading and writing skills. The speech-language pathologist's goal in assessment and treatment of aphasia is to identify the underlying impairments in written, expressive, and receptive language skills and the effects this has on the individual's quality of life, functional limitations relative to their premorbid activities, and their life in the community. Associated impairments that may affect communication are dysarthria, apraxia, concurrent cognitive deficits, and visual perceptual deficits.

Broca aphasia is an expressive language impairment of the dominant hemisphere in the inferior frontal lobe. Individuals with Broca aphasia often have intact comprehension but nonfluent, effortful, slow, halting speech with impaired naming. Utterances can range from single words to phrases, often with loss of normal grammatical structure. The ability to repeat words or phrases is compromised. These individuals often have associated apraxia (buccofacial, speech, and of the nonparalyzed limb) and right-sided weakness of the face and hand.

Wernicke aphasia is a language dysfunction occurring within the left superior temporal gyrus, often secondary to a left MCA embolus. Typically, comprehension of language is impaired, but fluent spontaneous speech with appropriate length, intonation, and rate is spared. Speech can consist of phonemic (mixed articulation) and paraphasic errors (word substitutions). Naming and repetition skills are impaired, and individuals may have associated deficits in reading and writing. Sometimes they have poor awareness of their language deficit. Pure word deafness, also known as auditory verbal agnosia, is the inability to comprehend speech and language, repeat words, and write from dictation. Individuals describe hearing speech as meaningless noise or as people speaking in a foreign language. Hearing acuity is normal, and they are usually able to recognize nonverbal sounds such as a dog barking or a telephone ringing.

Global aphasia, the most severe of the aphasias, is a result of damage to the language processing centers of both the Broca and Wernicke areas. Individuals have severely impaired receptive and expressive language and communication skills, as well as deficits in reading and writing. As symptoms improve, damage may remain more pronounced in the frontal or temporal parietal cortex, with either a Broca- or Wernicke-type residual language impairment.

Prognosis for aphasia recovery depends on the severity and location of the lesion, age, premorbid status, and overall health of the individual. Most patients improve to some extent, with the greatest gains within the first few months, although continued improvement with intervention can occur for a year or more. Rehabilitation of aphasia involves a multimodal approach with goals of improving an individual's maximum level of functional communication skills. Intervention focuses on patient-centered goals while using the individual's residual communication skills to provide skilled services to improve communication of safety, medical, and environmental needs. Treatment may consist of reading and writing tasks, word-retrieval exercises, comprehension activities, melodic intonation therapy (mostly with Broca aphasia), teaching effective gestures and written communication, creating a customized picture communication book to help supplement verbal expression, and interactive Internet-based aphasia applications for home programs. An alternative communication device can be considered for those with more severe communication challenges.

Plate 9.49

Brain: PART I

OTHER REHABILITATIVE ISSUES: GAIT TRAINING, UPPER LIMB DYSFUNCTION, LOCKED-IN SYNDROME

GAIT DISORDERS

Residual deficits in walking and mobility affect approximately two-thirds of stroke survivors, contributing to long-term disability and decreased community reintegration. Task-specific training that applies motor learning principles has been shown to be most effective in improving locomotor function and walking capacity poststroke. Task-specific training involves repeatedly practicing whole or parts of a specific task to improve motor control and thereby task proficiency. As it relates to the recovery of walking, considerable evidence exists supporting the use of overground gait training in addition to technology-assisted approaches, including treadmill training, body weight–supported treadmill training, functional electric stimulation-assisted gait training, virtual reality training, and robotic-assisted gait training. Cardiovascular exercise has also been shown to have a therapeutic benefit, with high-quality evidence demonstrating its effectiveness. Therefore aerobic intensity should be an important consideration when prescribing exercise, with high-intensity interval training and aerobic cycling resulting in improved walking speed, endurance, walking capacity, and gait symmetry. Strategies in the acute setting to improve upright mobility and function involve assisted standing to retrain standing balance and stability. Physical assistance is often needed for individuals with dense hemiplegia or poor trunk control and can include the use of assistive devices such as parallel bars, a cane, walker, or harness systems to provide partial body weight support. Task-specific training principles are applied to improve hemiplegic stance stability and swing phase efficiency while simultaneously facilitating trunk stability to improve upright postural control. *Ankle-foot orthoses* can be used to improve swing phase efficiency and compensate for foot drop. A *functional electric stimulation orthosis* is a recent advance that programmatically stimulates the peroneal nerve during swing phase to improve gait biomechanics.

UPPER LIMB DYSFUNCTION

Residual upper limb dysfunction due to hemiparesis, spasticity, or loss of sensorimotor function is prevalent poststroke. Similar to techniques used for the recovery of gait, task-specific training using motor learning–based approaches has been found most effective in the recovery of upper limb function. Functional tasks that require a combination of reaching, grasping, manipulating and/or moving, and releasing an object are practiced repeatedly and graded to challenge an individual's abilities. Tasks are graded to increase difficulty by requiring movement out of synergy, increasing movement requirements, incorporating increasingly difficult grasp types, increasing force requirements, varying the size and shapes of the objects, and varying the use of adaptive equipment. Functional electric stimulation and dynamic splinting to improve joint alignment and the use of robotics may be considered in the context of task-specific practice. Constraint-induced movement therapy in which the nonparetic upper limb is restrained to force use of the paretic

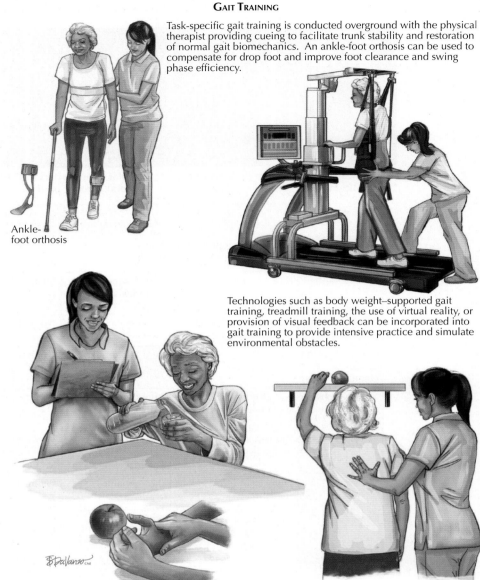

GAIT TRAINING

Task-specific gait training is conducted overground with the physical therapist providing cueing to facilitate trunk stability and restoration of normal gait biomechanics. An ankle-foot orthosis can be used to compensate for drop foot and improve foot clearance and swing phase efficiency.

Ankle-foot orthosis

Technologies such as body weight–supported gait training, treadmill training, the use of virtual reality, or provision of visual feedback can be incorporated into gait training to provide intensive practice and simulate environmental obstacles.

Tasks relevant to the individual's daily function are graded to accommodate to the individual's abilities and practiced repeatedly to facilitate sensorimotor recovery. The therapist breaks down components of the task as necessary to practice gross movement patterns in addition to fine motor coordination. A variety of power and precision grasps are incorporated into task practice to allow for transfer of training in alignment with motor learning principles. Dynamic splinting can be used to improve joint alignment, and technologies such as functional electrical stimulation are effective when incorporated into functional task-based training.

limb has been effective for a small percentage of patients who present with minimal movement requirements.

The management of symptoms that may interfere with rehabilitation and the performance of daily activities should not be neglected. For instance, central neuropathic pain may benefit from pharmacologic treatment with medications such as gabapentin and tricyclic antidepressants. Spasticity can be addressed with treatment modalities including stretching, oral medications such as baclofen or tizanidine, local injections with botulinum toxin or phenol, and intrathecal baclofen therapy in cases not responsive to other modalities. The potential for detrimental side effects, and the fact that spasticity may help preserve function and posture, should be weighed against the potential benefits, and careful monitoring is needed. It is also important to note that direct improvement of motor control from spasticity management is limited by other neurologic deficits.

LOCKED-IN SYNDROME

Patients with locked-in syndrome, often resulting from basilar thrombosis (see Plate 9.23), benefit from early intensive rehabilitation. Although most patients remain locked in, survival has improved, and some can regain motor function over time. Even in the absence of motor recovery, rehabilitation is essential to help prevent complications such as contractures and pressure injuries, and to maximize the person's ability to interact with the environment. For example, augmentative communication devices triggered by sensitive switches or eye tracking systems can allow individuals to communicate and to control their environment. The involvement of a multidisciplinary rehabilitation team is essential, given the multiple affected areas, such as communication, dysphagia, respiratory function, vision seating, mobility, mood, cognitive impairment in some patients, and, when applicable, activities of daily living.

Plate 9.50

Cerebrovascular Circulation and Stroke

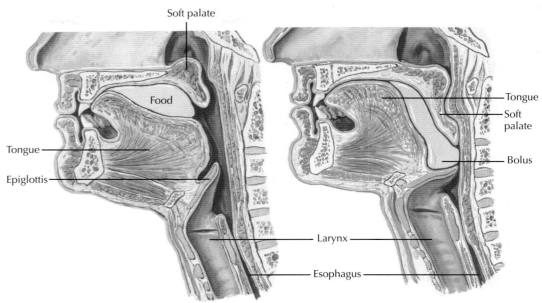

Bolus (food) pushed backward toward palate by tongue

Bolus reaches epiglottis while larynx moves upward and forward. Soft palate closes off nasopharynx.

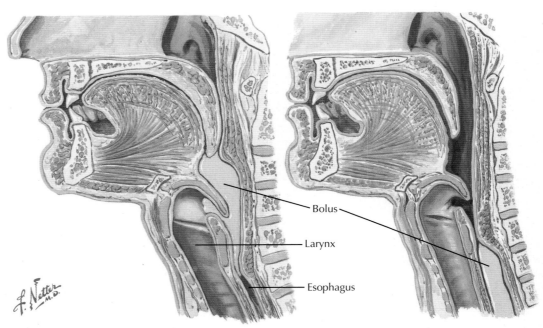

Pharyngeal constrictors contract and knead bolus into the esophagus. Epiglottis prevents bolus from entering the larynx. Trickle of food shown here entering esophagus, but is prevented from going farther by closure of ventricular folds.

Peristaltic contraction of esophagus moves bolus toward stomach, and epiglottis begins to return to resting position.

OTHER REHABILITATIVE ISSUES: DYSPHAGIA

Dysphagia, defined as difficulty swallowing, occurs in 30% to 65% of stroke survivors. Impairments are typically seen in the oral and pharyngeal phases of swallowing function and place the individual at high risk of aspiration, including silent aspiration. Complications of dysphagia can lead to pneumonia, weight loss, compromised respiratory status, malnutrition, mortality, dehydration, and increased length of stay. A dysphagia screen, such as the 3-oz water test, is a safe, quick, and efficient method that can be used to identify patients at a high risk of aspiration. If signs of aspiration or dysphagia are recognized, patients should be referred for a comprehensive assessment by a speech pathologist. The speech pathologist will conduct an oral peripheral examination and presentation of foods and liquids. If further instrumental assessment is required to evaluate oral-pharyngeal swallow function and rule out aspiration, a modified barium swallow or fiberoptic endoscopic evaluation of swallow function can be completed. During these assessments, the speech pathologist determines the safety of various textures and assesses compensatory strategies such as a chin tuck, head rotation to the weaker side, and alternating solids and liquids to determine any improvements in swallow function and various swallow strategies that may decrease risk of aspiration.

Dysphagia treatment is multidisciplinary and often involves the patient, family/caregivers, nurses, dietitians, physicians, speech pathologists, and gastroenterologists if alternative nutrition is required. Results and recommendations, including specific diet modifications, safe swallow techniques, pacing and feeding strategies, and the importance of oral care, are discussed to ensure patient safety. Examples of treatments can include oral-pharyngeal range-of-motion and strengthening exercises, diaphragmatic breathing exercises, deep pharyngeal neuromuscular stimulation, and neuromuscular electric stimulation.

Prognosis depends on the nature and severity of the swallowing disorder and the patient's cognitive and medical status. With intervention, improvements can occur within a few weeks or up to 6 months or longer with more severe impairments.

MULTIPLE SCLEROSIS AND OTHER CENTRAL NERVOUS SYSTEM AUTOIMMUNE DISORDERS

Plate 10.1

Brain: PART I

MULTIPLE SCLEROSIS: OVERVIEW

Multiple sclerosis (MS) is one of the most common disabling neurologic illness of early adult years. Clinical manifestations often begin with optic nerve (optic neuritis), spinal cord (myelitis), or brainstem inflammatory demyelination, presenting with a subacute time course and improvement or resolution over weeks to months. Subacute attacks are characterized by periodic and focal loss of central nervous system (CNS) myelin within focal lesions that are visible on brain magnetic resonance imaging (MRI) and clinically manifest as focal symptoms and corresponding findings on neurologic examination. As episodes (termed *relapses*) recur, disability accumulates. More insidious progression of disability likely occurs in many patients subclinically, and in some patients this insidious progression of disability is the dominant clinical manifestation in the absence of relapses, likely owing to CNS-resident immune and degenerative processes that remain poorly understood.

MS is thought to be primarily an autoimmune disease, although no single antigen has been identified with certainty, against which a disease-relevant autoimmune response may be directed. As with other autoimmune entities, there is a genetically determined propensity to develop the illness. The strongest single contributor to the risk of developing MS is the class II major histocompatibility complex (MHC) antigen; that is, the human leukocyte antigen (HLA)-DRB1*15:01. HLA-DR alleles present antigenic peptides to CD4+ T cells, pointing to a major disease-promoting role for CD4+ T cells in MS. In contrast, HLA-A*02:01 expression is reduced in MS, indicating a protective role for the most commonly expressed class I allele in humans. The less prevalent HLA-A*03:01 class I allele doubles risk for developing MS. HLA-A alleles present antigenic peptides to CD8+ T cells, indicating that CD8+ T-cell–mediated protection is suboptimal in MS. HLA-A*03:01 and HLA-DRB1*15:01 are independent risk factors. Genome-wide studies have identified some 50 additional minor genetic associations. Most have a role in immune system function with a major enrichment in cell surface receptor genes implicated in T-cell activation and proliferation. One-third of identified genomic loci overlap with regions associated with one or more other autoimmune diseases.

The prevalence of MS can be as high as 1 in 400 in the overall population. Twenty percent of patients have a blood relative with the disease. In siblings and in children of an affected parent, concordance for MS is 1% to 3%, ruling out simple dominant, recessive, or sex-linked inheritance. Siblings share half their genes, yet even among identical twins sharing all of their genes, MS concordance is only 25%, indicating that environmental factors have a major role in determining risk for MS.

Epstein-Barr virus (EBV) is acquired in adolescence or early adult years in developed countries, where MS is encountered frequently and where EBV often causes infectious mononucleosis. In less-developed countries, where MS is uncommon, EBV is usually acquired asymptomatically in early childhood. Unlike controls, at diagnosis all MS patients test positive for prior contact with EBV, and a history of frank infectious mononucleosis (always before disease onset) is increased threefold over the general population. EBV is at present the leading environmental trigger candidate for propensity to develop MS. The presence of subnormal vitamin D levels is a possible additional putative environmental factor in MS. This vitamin is an inflammatory response inhibitor and an enhancer of regulatory T-cell function. Of note, MS is uncommon in regions with high sunlight

exposure, the chief inducer of vitamin D synthesis. Other major risk factors may include cigarette smoking and obesity, common to other autoimmune conditions.

CLINICAL COURSE

MS usually begins in young adults, and the peak age at first attack is 30 years, but onset can occur before age 10 years or after age 50 years. MS is two to three times more common in females. Eighty-five percent of patients present with a clinically isolated syndrome characterized by subacute loss of neurologic function that will usually worsen over a week or more, stabilize for a time, and eventually recover partially or, quite often, completely. Subsequently, after highly variable intervals, relapses develop. These relapses, having finite spans of a few weeks, are followed by recovery of variable extent and duration. Periods of seeming disease

quiescence occur with remissions lasting months or years. These patients are referred to as having *relapsing-remitting MS* (RRMS). Symptoms and signs vary from one relapse to the next as additional sites of myelin loss accumulate within the CNS white matter (WM). Sites of myelin loss are called *plaques;* their locations determine symptoms.

After some years, the character of MS can change. Relapses diminish in frequency, ultimately cease, and are replaced by slow but steady worsening of nervous system impairment referred to as *secondary progressive MS* (SPMS), distinguishing it from the 15% of cases in which a primary progressive course is present from first symptom onset. Primary progressive MS (PPMS) usually begins later in life than RRMS, and female preponderance is less evident. The usual presentation is a slowly progressive myelopathy evolving into paraparesis or paraplegia.

Visual manifestations

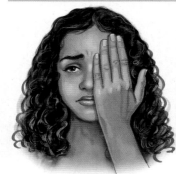

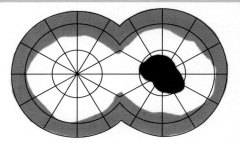

Subacute, usually painful, self-limited monocular vision loss lasting 2–4 weeks before improvement. Patient covering one eye realizes other eye is partially or totally blind, often with color desaturation.

Visual fields reveal central scotoma due to acute retrobulbar neuritis.

Brainstem and/or cerebellar manifestations

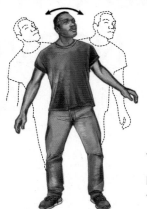

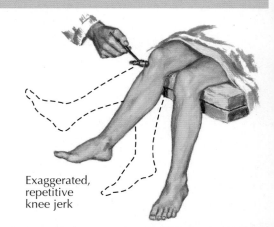

Wide-based gait. Patient teeters back and forth and sideways.

Exaggerated, repetitive knee jerk

Spinal cord manifestations

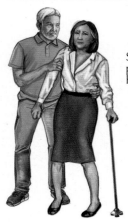

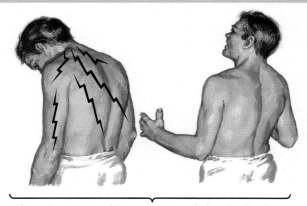

Spastic gait; patient needs help walking

Lhermitte sign: sudden sensation of electric shock down spine and along arms when patient flexes neck

Multiple Sclerosis: Clinical Manifestations

Signs and symptoms of MS vary with the locations of the plaques in the CNS and can occur in adults and less often in children.

OPTIC NERVE LESIONS

Optic neuritis causes relatively abrupt unilateral decrease in central or paracentral vision with pain on movement of the globe. MRI may show a lesion in the affected optic nerve, and other lesions indicative of earlier clinically silent MS activity are seen on brain and spinal cord MRI. Optic disc pallor often develops during recovery.

BRAINSTEM LESIONS

Brainstem lesions are common and tend to occur early in the course of MS. *Diplopia* is usually caused by a lesion affecting the abducens (VI) nerve. *Nystagmus* is usually asymptomatic and is a particularly useful localizing sign when it is pronounced in degree and especially when the primary component is vertical. *Internuclear ophthalmoplegia* is a classic MS sign indicating involvement of the medial longitudinal fasciculus. Examination reveals paresis of adduction on lateral gaze and associated nystagmus in the abducting eye. Despite the unilateral loss of adduction on lateral gaze, the ability to converge (i.e., bilateral adduction) may be preserved. *Vertigo* may be difficult to differentiate from a benign labyrinthitis, although a finding of vertical nystagmus points to a CNS rather than a peripheral cause. *Trigeminal neuralgia* is common in MS, and when it occurs in young adults or is bilateral, it is highly suggestive of MS. Similarly, facial weakness in the young may be mistaken for *Bell palsy* when MS should be considered.

CEREBELLAR LESIONS

Cerebellar symptoms can be severely disabling and occur often in MS. Symptoms can include loss of balance, intention tremor, dysarthria, ataxia, and titubation.

SPINAL CORD LESIONS

Paresthesias and dysesthesias are often described as constricting or swollen sensations; these symptoms indicate posterior column demyelination in the spinal cord. A hemi-circumferential band-like patch of numbness or pressure, usually mid-trunk, is frequently seen with transverse myelitis but can also be seen with spinal cord mass lesions. Patients may also report Lhermitte sign, which is typified by momentary electric shock–like sensations radiating down the arms, back, or legs precipitated by neck flexion. Examination often reveals diminished vibration and position sense.

Corticospinal tract dysfunction results in hyperreflexia, spasticity, weakness, and clonus, and the Babinski sign is frequently elicited.

OTHER SYMPTOMS

Inordinate fatigability is common and is related to lesions in multiple locations. Demyelinated axons require more energy to conduct nerve impulses than properly insulated axons; thus conduction may fail with continued activation. For example, a limp may replace a seemingly normal

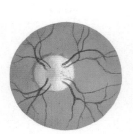

Temporal pallor in optic disc, caused by delayed recovery of temporal side of optic (II) nerve

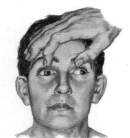

Eyes turned to left, right eye lags

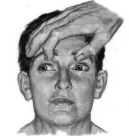

Eyes turned to right, left eye lags (to lesser degree)

——— Internuclear ophthalmoplegia ———

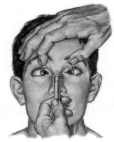

Convergence unimpaired

Pain and depression can be seen

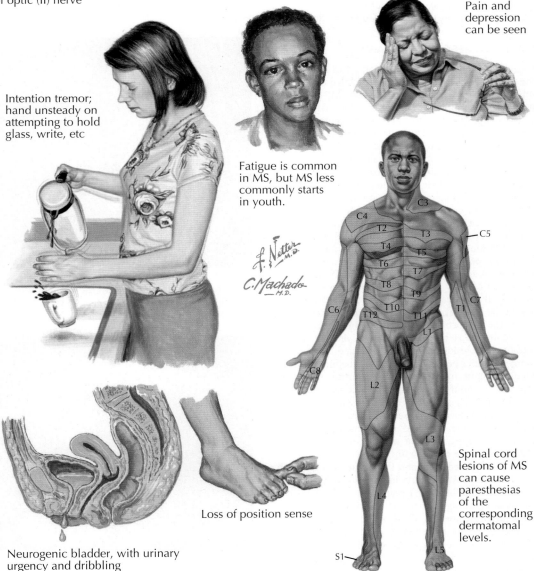

Intention tremor; hand unsteady on attempting to hold glass, write, etc

Fatigue is common in MS, but MS less commonly starts in youth.

Loss of position sense

Neurogenic bladder, with urinary urgency and dribbling

Spinal cord lesions of MS can cause paresthesias of the corresponding dermatomal levels.

gait after walking some distance and then resolve after a rest period. The inefficiency of demyelinated axons worsens as body temperature rises; thus short-lived symptoms can be provoked by summer heat, a hot shower, fever, or during the modest diurnal upward body temperature that normally occurs in the afternoon.

A number of other conditions occur in the course of MS. Urinary frequency and urgency suggest a hyperreflexic bladder. Constipation, bowel and bladder incontinence, and sexual dysfunction can also develop. Pain can occur, sometimes on a neuropathic basis, but requires investigation for possible unrelated causes. Autonomic nervous system dysfunction can manifest as gastric dysmotility, orthostatic hypotension, sexual dysfunction, and sweating dysregulation. The incidence of depression is significantly higher in patients with MS. Cognitive dysfunction may develop early in the course of MS and worsen over years.

Plate 10.3

Brain: PART I

TYPICAL **MRI** FINDINGS IN **MS**: BRAIN

MULTIPLE SCLEROSIS: DIAGNOSIS

The diagnosis of MS is made using clinical, imaging, and laboratory evidence. The diagnostic criteria require the demonstration of injury to the CNS that is disseminated in time and space. Formal criteria for the diagnosis of MS are codified and regularly updated, the most recent of which was the 2017 McDonald criteria.

MAGNETIC RESONANCE IMAGING

MRI plays a central role in the diagnosis of MS. In 1983 the diagnostic criteria already included MRI, and through several iterations and updates MRI has been used to allow a more accurate and earlier diagnosis.

The diagnosis of relapsing MS, the most common form of the disease, rests on the demonstration of CNS lesions disseminated in time (DIT) and in space (DIS). DIS and DIT can be demonstrated by objective clinical evidence of lesions using the neurologic examination or by MRI. On MRI, MS lesions must display certain characteristics, including ovoid or round shape and a size of at least 3 mm in their long axis. MS lesions may also show contrast enhancement, which typically indicates that they have developed in the past 4 to 8 weeks. Typical MS lesions can be seen on MRI in four key areas, including periventricular, cortical/juxtacortical, infratentorial, and spinal cord structures. DIS criteria can be met on MRI by demonstration of lesions in two or more of these locations. Cortical lesions are located within the cerebral cortex, and juxtacortical lesions are within the subcortical WM abutting the cortex without intervening WM between the lesion and the cortex. Infratentorial lesions are typically located in the brainstem, cerebellar peduncles, or the cerebellum. Periventricular lesions involve the WM abutting the lateral ventricles without intervening WM between the lesion and the ventricle. MRI can also be used to meet DIT criteria, established by presence of both simultaneous gadolinium-enhancing and nonenhancing lesions at any time or appearance of new lesions on follow-up MRI, irrespective of follow-up timing.

MRI can be used to support the diagnosis of PPMS. To fulfill the diagnostic criteria in addition to progressive increase in disability over 1 year, there should be two of the three following criteria: (1) one or more lesions in periventricular, cortical, juxtacortical, or infratentorial lesions; (2) two or more lesions in the spinal cord; and (3) presence of unmatched oligoclonal bands (OCBs) in cerebrospinal fluid (CSF).

If the typical MRI findings for MS are found incidentally in a patient without typical signs or symptoms of MS, these findings are referred to as a *radiologically isolated syndrome* (RIS). These individuals have been shown to be at increased risk for developing MS in the future.

Given the significant variability in MRI techniques and sequences, international consensus recommendations on the use of MRI have been developed. MRI should include axial T2-weighted, axial and sagittal T2-weighted fluid-attenuated inversion recovery (FLAIR), and contrast-enhanced axial T1-weighted sequences, ideally at 3.0 Tesla, and with three-dimensional acquisition.

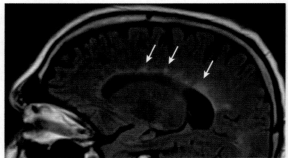

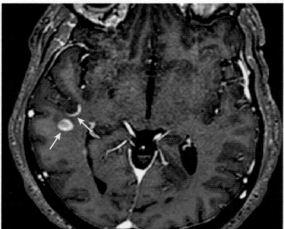

Periventricular lesions involving the corpus callosum located perpendicular to the ventricle on T2-weighted sagittal FLAIR imaging

Typical open ring enhancement pattern in a juxtacortical lesion and nodular enhancement in a subcortical white matter lesion seen on axial post-contrast T1-weighted imaging

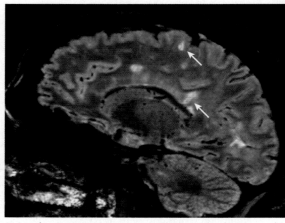

Central vein sign seen in a periventricular lesion and a juxtacortical lesion on sagittal FLAIR* imaging

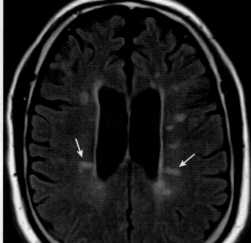

Periventricular lesions involving the corpus callosum located perpendicular to the ventricle on axial T2-weighted FLAIR imaging

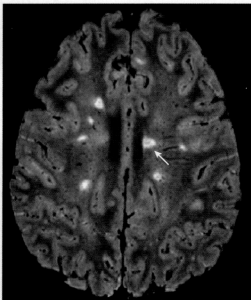

Central vein sign seen in a periventricular lesion on axial combined T2*-weighted and FLAIR* imaging

FLAIR sequences are more useful in evaluating supratentorial lesions, while T2-weighted images may be more sensitive for evaluating infratentorial lesions. For spinal cord imaging the recommendation is sagittal T1-weighted postcontrast sequences plus at least two of the following: sagittal T2-weighted, proton density–weighted, or short tau inversion recovery (STIR) sequences.

Periventricular lesions are common in MS, and their presence is often used to meet MRI criteria for MS;

however, periventricular capping and hyperintensities could also be seen with aging and in healthy individuals. It is important to emphasize that lesions must be in physical contact with the ventricle to be called truly periventricular. Similarly, juxtacortical WM lesions must touch the cortex, not just occur in the vicinity of the cortex, to be classified as such. Corpus callosum lesions, particularly those perpendicular to the ventricles, are more specific for MS, whereas rounded lesions within the body of the corpus callosum are commonly

MULTIPLE SCLEROSIS: DIAGNOSIS (Continued)

seen in Susac syndrome. Periaqueductal and periependymal lesions can be seen in neuromyelitis optica spectrum disorder (NMOSD) but are less common in MS. On T1-weighted imaging, MS lesions may appear hypointense; when this is a persistent finding, they are referred to as "T1 black holes" and are thought to be lesions with significant axonal loss. Acute lesions may also at times demonstrate diffusion restriction; this is true especially when imaging is acquired soon after lesion onset and is more commonly seen around the lesion edge.

The enhancement pattern in MS lesions is typically transient (4–8 weeks) and has been described as nodular or open ring; patchy, multiple closed-ring, punctate, miliary, or persistently enhancing lesions could point to alternate diagnoses. Leptomeningeal enhancement is relatively rare in MS and should be interpreted cautiously because this pattern of enhancement is more commonly seen in other demyelinating, infectious, and infiltrative disorders.

It is important to recognize that the McDonald criteria are meant to be used in the appropriate clinical setting (typical clinical attack); a key criterion is the absence of any better explanation of the clinical picture. McDonald criteria therefore are not designed to be applied outside typical clinical attacks, and misinterpretation of MRI criteria may result in misdiagnosis. The specificity for the McDonald 2017 criteria is around 61% when applied to patients at the time of a first demyelinating attack, and misdiagnosis can occur in roughly 20% of patients referred to an MS center with a prior diagnosis of MS. Disease characteristics and particularly MRI should be carefully evaluated to rule out other mimickers when applying these criteria.

MRI identification of central veins in MS lesions has been the focus of research to improve MRI diagnostic specificity. Susceptibility weighted and T2*-weighted images can be used to detect a central vein sign (CVS). Typical MS lesions are thought to occur around venules, and the CVS refers to presence of a thin hypointense line or small hypointense dot that can be visualized in at least two perpendicular planes running centrally through the entire or part of the lesion. The presence of this sign may increase diagnostic accuracy. Another possible finding is the presence of a hypointense susceptibility rim around the periphery of a lesion, termed a *paramagnetic rim lesion*. Thought to be due to accumulation of iron-enriched macrophages, its presence may offer increased diagnostic specificity.

Cortical lesions are difficult to detect with conventional imaging techniques in patients with MS. Ultrahigh-field 7.0 Tesla MRI can double the detection rate for cortical lesions. However, even at ultrahigh field, the majority of cortical lesions are still not detected.

In the spinal cord, MS lesions are typically focal and wedge-shaped and span less than three vertebral segments in longitudinal extension. Spinal cord lesions affect the cervical cord most commonly but also the thoracic cord, typically with sparing of the central gray matter (GM). Longitudinally extensive transverse myelitis

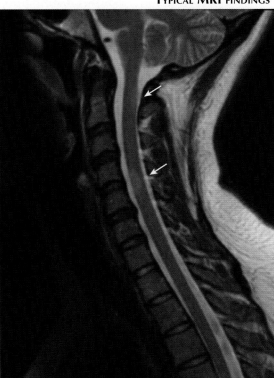

Spinal cord lesions in the upper and mid cervical spine on sagittal T2-weighted imaging

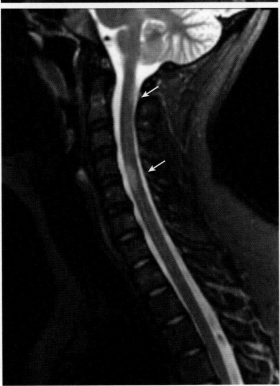

Spinal cord lesions in the upper and mid cervical spine on sagittal STIR imaging

affecting three or more vertebral segments is more commonly seen in NMOSD or myelin oligodendrocyte glycoprotein antibody-associated disease (MOGAD). Leptomeningeal and root enhancement in the spinal cord could indicate neurosarcoidosis, MOGAD, or infectious or infiltrative processes.

MS can frequently affect the optic nerves with optic neuritis. Although not routinely required, optic nerve MRI can be used to identify these lesions. Axial and coronal fat-suppressed T2-weighted and postcontrast

T1-weighted sequences are ideally used to detect hyperintensities or enhancement in the optic nerve. Newer iterations of the diagnostic criteria may allow evidence of optic nerve involvement on paraclinical testing to support the diagnosis of MS.

CEREBROSPINAL FLUID

Although evaluation of CSF is not always necessary to establish the diagnosis, it can frequently be helpful and

Plate 10.5

Brain: PART I

VISUAL EVOKED POTENTIAL AND SPINAL FLUID ANALYSIS

MULTIPLE SCLEROSIS: DIAGNOSIS (Continued)

aid in the diagnosis. DIT criteria for relapsing MS can be established based on MRI alone, but the McDonald criteria allow establishing DIT through presence of OCBs in the CSF when not found in serum (unmatched). Furthermore, unmatched OCBs can help fulfill criteria for PPMS and indicate an increased risk of developing MS after a first clinical event or RIS.

OCBs are measured through protein gel electrophoresis of serum and CSF simultaneously. This is ideally done through isoelectric focusing followed by immunofixation. Presence of two or more discrete bands in the CSF but not the serum indicates presence of intrathecal antibody production and forms part of the diagnostic criteria. Although not unique to MS, OCBs are thought to be more specific for MS compared with NMOSD and MOGAD. Immunoglobulin G (IgG) index and intrathecal antibody synthesis are other tests that help indicate intrathecal antibody synthesis.

CSF studies can be useful in the assessment of atypical clinical presentations when other diagnoses must be explored. Findings against the diagnosis of MS include significant pleocytosis (>50 cells/mm³), pleocytosis with neutrophilic or eosinophilic predominance, elevated protein (>100 mg/dL), or presence of atypical cells on cytologic examination. Several novel biomarkers in the CSF are under investigation to improve diagnosis or predict outcomes. Neurofilament light (NfL) chain, a unique marker of neuronal cells, when found in excess in CSF, is thought to be due to neuronal injury and could possibly correlate with MS disease activity.

EVOKED POTENTIALS

Neurophysiologic studies permit an objective analysis of the integrity of neuronal pathways in the CNS. Before the ready availability of MRI, evoked potentials (EPs) were widely used to identify subclinical CNS disease. Testing is easily performed and requires minimal patient cooperation, particularly when testing the visual pathways by means of visual evoked potentials (VEPs). In centers where MRI is at hand, brainstem and somatosensory EPs are less frequently required today to confirm a tentative diagnosis of MS.

Today the primary value of EP testing is in establishing whether a specific symptom (limb numbness, blurred vision) that occurred in the past may have been due to a demyelinating lesion to provide objective supportive evidence of dissemination of lesions in space and time. EP testing may establish support for the disease in patients who have had subclinical optic neuritis or who have forgotten or ignored prior neurologic events.

With VEPs as an example, a retinal stimulus, typically a reversing high-contrast checkerboard pattern, provides a means to study the integrity of the visual system. Response latencies provide objective data regarding the ability of the nervous system to transmit impulses efficiently from the optic nerve to the occipital cortex. If

absence or delay of conduction is unilateral, one can conclude that there is slowed conduction between the retina and the optic chiasm typical for unilateral optic neuritis. VEPs are most helpful when patients have fully regained their vision. Remyelination is never perfect, so VEP-documented slowing of conduction velocity provides an indelible marker of prior damage. When delayed latencies, attenuated potentials, or conduction block are bilateral, the lesion cannot be localized

precisely because it could be situated anywhere along the visual pathway.

EP testing is often used as second-line of testing in cases where preferred sensitive anatomic imaging such as MRI or optical coherence tomography cannot be obtained because of limited healthcare resource access or patient factors such as embedded metal fragments or implanted devices that preclude MRI studies.

Visual evoked potential (VEP)

Patient undergoing test for visual evoked responses. The patient is asked to concentrate on the yellow dot in the middle of the screen while the checkerboard pattern moves. Usually a patch is placed over one eye at a time. The room is darkened for the actual procedure.
From MacDonald S, Pagana K, Pagana T. Mosby's Canadian Manual of Diagnostic and Laboratory Tests. 2nd ed. Elsevier; 2019.

Cerebrospinal fluid electrophoresis

MULTIPLE SCLEROSIS: PATHOPHYSIOLOGY

PERIPHERAL EVENTS THAT PRECEDE A MULTIPLE SCLEROSIS RELAPSE

There is no known cause of MS, and it remains unclear whether the underlying etiology is an intrinsic or extrinsic CNS defect. A variety of environmental and genetic factors have been identified that may play a role in the complex immune process leading to the development of MS. One potential trigger is viral illness that results in immune system activation and development of pathogenic antigens. Immune responses to viruses involve drainage of pathogenic antigens and antigen-presenting cells (APCs) along lymphatic channels to a regional lymph node (LN). Upper respiratory viruses and viral antigens drain via nasal lymphatic channels into the subcapsular sinuses of the deep cervical LNs. Immature dendritic cells (DCs) and monocytes lie beneath the subcapsular sinus and protrude processes into it, permitting them to sample newly arrived lymph and capture viral antigens. Drainage of CSF and brain parenchymal interstitial fluid occurs through the cribriform plate located below the olfactory bulb into nasal lymphatics and then into these very same deep cervical LNs.

Immature DCs in the CNS subarachnoid space ingest myelin elements; after that, they may mature in situ. Mature DCs express the cell surface molecule C-C chemokine receptor 7 (CCR7), whereas endothelial cells in afferent lymphatic channels express chemokine ligand 21 (CCL21) counterligand. Ligation of CCR7 permits mature self-antigen–bearing DCs to migrate via afferent lymphatics to deep cervical LNs. Mature DCs are short lived and have lost their capacity to sample newly presented viral or other antigenic material, whereas long-lived immature DCs or macrophages can do so.

Extracellular debris, including myelin and its peptides, flows from a damaged CNS to deep cervical LNs where subcapsular macrophages and immature DCs capture it. Unlike controls, deep cervical LNs of patients with MS with inactive disease contain numerous immature DCs and macrophages with ingested myelin and myelin proteins that can, under appropriate circumstances, be presented to T cells. Immature DCs and macrophages retain the capacity to respond to subsequently encountered viral antigens.

Naïve CD4+ T cells (Tn) move swiftly through LNs, making serial brief contacts with antigen-loaded DCs draped atop the fibroblastic reticular cells that enwrap the collagen fiber structural backbone of the LN. Lymph is transferred from the subcapsular sinus to the medulla via the collagen-containing channels of the conduit network. DCs insert processes into the

conduit channels to capture peptide elements contained therein, which they can then process and present to T cells. Tn cells seek that rare DC expressing the cognate antigen they are programmed to recognize. When a CD4+ Tn cell fails in its quest, as usually occurs, it migrates to the LN medulla and exits via efferent lymph. Exit requires expression of the sphingosine-1-phosphate receptor-1 (S1PR1) by migrating CD4+ Tn cells. This requirement has been exploited in MS therapy. CD4+ Tn cells pass from the efferent

lymph into the circulation and move on via the blood to sample another LN. They do not enter the tissues.

Circulating CD4+ Tn cells express CCR7 and low levels of the adhesion molecule leukocyte function–associated antigen-1 (LFA-1). CCL21 and intercellular adhesion molecule-1 (ICAM-1), counterligands for CCR7 and LFA-1, respectively, are expressed by the high endothelial cells of venules sited in LN T-cell–dependent areas with a nearby cortical ridge that is enriched in DCs. CCR7 binding to CCL21 and LFA-1

Deep Cervical Lymph Node: Multiple Sclerosis in Remission

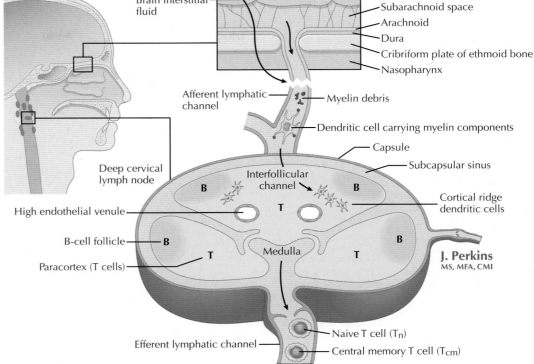

J. Perkins
MS, MFA, CMI

Interfollicular Channel (IFC)

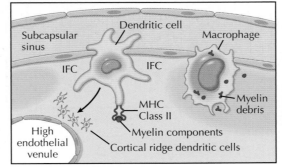

Cortical Ridge and Conduit Network

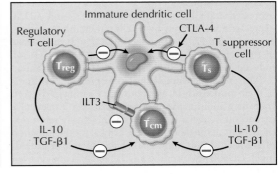

High Endothelial Venule

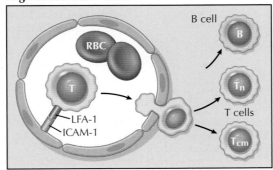

Tolerizing Signals

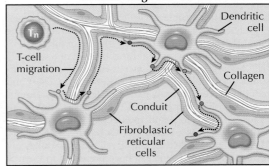

Plate 10.7

Brain: PART I

Deep Cervical Lymph Node: Immunostimulatory Events That Lead to a Relapse

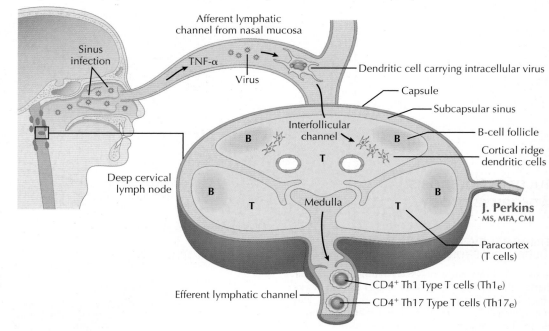

MULTIPLE SCLEROSIS: PATHOPHYSIOLOGY (Continued)

binding to ICAM-1 enable CD4$^+$ T$_n$ cells to cross from the blood via these venules into LNs passing either between LN endothelial cells or, intriguingly, as illustrated, through them.

When a CD4$^+$ T$_n$ cell finally contacts a cognate antigen–expressing DC, it is either activated or tolerized. Both outcomes are germane to MS. Both require contact between the CD4$^+$ T$_n$-cell receptor and an MS-relevant small peptide fragment cleaved from an ingested protein and inserted into a cleft in an HLA molecule that then is expressed on the DC surface. Cognate antigen contact lasts longer than contact with DCs expressing irrelevant peptides, and contact is of even longer duration if the CD4$^+$ T$_n$ cell is being activated rather than tolerized.

DC maturation is critical for activation of a CD4$^+$ T$_n$ cell. Maturation involves increased expression of costimulatory molecules (e.g., CD80/86 and CD40) and reduced expression of tolerizing molecules (e.g., immunoglobulin-like transcript 3 [ILT3], transforming growth factor-β1 [TGF-β1], and interleukin-10 [IL-10]). Full activation of CD4$^+$ T cells by DCs requires two signals. The first signal is delivered by T-cell receptors following contact with their cognate antigen presented to them at an immunologic synapse by an MHC class II molecule. The second set of signals is delivered by a network of interactive costimulatory molecule pairs with CD80/86, expressed initially at low level by DCs, and CD28, expressed constitutively by T cells, providing one prototypic pair, and CD40 expressed by DCs in the early stage of their activation and CD40 ligand (CD40L/CD154), induced on T cells in the early hours of their activation.

Both cross-communicating pairs upregulate synthesis of their counterligand, and both pairs, acting in concert, transduce additional activating signals via intracellular second messengers. Each pair synergistically reinforces the actions of the other. CD28 is critical for the initiation of T-cell activation, and CD40L has a key role in sustaining it. CD40L also promotes a Th1 cell bias and an even more marked Th17 cell bias. T cells, once activated, proliferate within the LN to generate an up to 10^4-fold increase of CD4$^+$ effector T cells (T$_e$ cells).

Cytotoxic T lymphocyte antigen-4 (CTLA-4), a homologue of CD28, has a critical role in the prevention of autoimmunity. CTLA-4 is expressed by activated T cells and by regulatory T cells. CTLA-4 is focused at the immunologic synapse where it opposes CD28. Both CD28 and CTLA-4 bind CD80/86, but because of its higher affinity, CTLA-4 can outcompete CD28 and reverse or blunt the T-cell–activating actions of CD28. DCs downregulate their expression of CD80/86 in

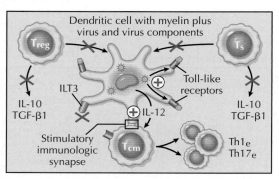

Cortical Ridge: Stimulation and Loss of Inhibitory Signals

Simplified Stimulatory Immunologic Synapse

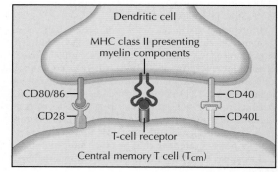

response to the potent negative signal provided by CTLA-4 when it binds to CD80/86. In this way, CTLA-4 promotes tolerance.

CTLA-4 is not expressed by resting T cells but comes to be expressed by activated T cells as an immune response evolves. CTLA-4 tempers what would otherwise be an excessive T-cell expansion. CTLA-4 is constitutively expressed, and highly so, on the surface of regulatory T cells and, additionally, as a released biologically active soluble splice variant. Regulatory T cells have a major role in autoimmunity prevention. Even when prevention fails, as in MS, regulatory T cells can lessen MS relapse frequency and the severity of those relapses that do occur. Regulatory T cells also participate in the processes that end a relapse (see later). Agents that duplicate actions of CTLA-4 are of interest as MS treatments.

CD4$^+$ T$_e$ cells are divided into subtypes known as Th1, Th17 cells, and Th2 cells. Broadly viewed, Th1 cells protect against intracellular organisms and Th17 cells protect against fungi, whereas Th2 cells protect against helminths, certain other extracellular pathogens, and allergens. DCs, over the course of their activation of naive T cells, can polarize T-cell development along paths that lead to the preferential expansion of a single Th-cell subset. Th-cell subsets interact; Th2 cells inhibit Th1 cells and vice versa. Th1 cells and Th17 cells cause damage in MS, whereas Th2 cells protect because they inhibit Th1 and Th17 cells. Thus any drug (e.g., glatiramer acetate, teriflunomide) or mechanism that shifts polarization from a Th1 to Th2 dominance might be expected to prove beneficial in MS.

Plate 10.7 continued on next page

MULTIPLE SCLEROSIS: PATHOPHYSIOLOGY (Continued)

The CD4$^+$ T$_e$-cell population in MS contains both interferon-γ (IFN-γ)–secreting Th1 cells and interleukin-17–secreting Th17 cells. Deep cervical LN-generated MS-relevant CD4$^+$ T$_e$ cells migrate to the LN medulla, express S1PR1, and move via efferent lymph into the blood and then to the CNS to participate in an MS relapse (see later).

As a relapse ends, most CNS-infiltrating Th1 and Th17 T$_e$ cells die in situ by apoptosis, but perhaps 5% survive as T-effector memory (T$_{em}$) cells that remain in the periphery to provide a prompt defense against a subsequent challenge. An additional 5% to 10% remain as CD4$^+$ T central memory (T$_{cm}$) cells that express the same adhesion molecules as T$_n$ cells so that they too reenter LNs via high endothelial venules, sample DCs, and recirculate via efferent lymph and then the blood to other LNs. Unlike T$_n$ cells, MS-relevant T$_{cm}$ cells also survey the tissues and other body compartments, including the CSF, seeking an APC loaded with the MS-relevant peptide they are programmed to recognize. T$_{cm}$ cells outnumber T$_n$ cells with the same specificity so that a secondary CD4$^+$ T$_{cm}$-cell response in a LN is usually more rapid and robust than a CD4$^+$ T$_n$-cell response. Activation of CD4$^+$ T$_n$ cells requires peptide presentation by mature DCs, but requirements for CD4$^+$ T$_{cm}$-cell reactivation are less stringent; they can respond to some extent to antigenic peptide–presenting macrophages and to immature DCs. CD4$^+$ T$_{cm}$-cell reactivation leads to generation of a new CD4$^+$ T$_e$-cell population that again migrates to the circulation and then to the CNS.

Throughout MS remissions, myelin debris–laden immature DCs and macrophages in the cervical LNs of patients with MS are thought to promote tolerance. Deep cervical LNs are favored sites for tolerance induction because they are continuously bathed with products released by the commensal biota of the nasal mucosa. The immune system is programmed to tolerate commensal organisms and to eliminate pathogens. Tolerance is mediated primarily by antigen-specific regulatory (suppressor) T cells that powerfully inhibit T-cell activation. For this reason, when antigen-specific regulatory T cells are deleted, overly robust T$_e$-cell responses ensue. The finding points to a ceaseless positive versus negative competition for control of DC function.

Multiple types of regulatory T cells are described. CD4$^+$CD25$^+$ T regulatory cells (T$_{reg}$) and CD8$^+$CD28$^-$ T suppressor cells (T$_s$) are the most studied in MS. The role of CD4$^+$CD25$^+$ T$_{reg}$ cells in MS remains unresolved. CD8$^+$CD28$^-$ T$_s$-cell function is grossly defective during MS relapses. CD8$^+$CD28$^-$ T$_s$-cell function reverts toward normal as relapses end and is restored, although not always fully, during remissions. Agents that augment CD8$^+$CD28$^-$ T$_s$-cell function would be expected to be beneficial in MS.

CD8$^+$CD28$^-$ T$_s$ cells are antigen specific. The CD8$^+$CD28$^-$ T$_s$-cell receptor makes direct contact with its cognate antigen presented by an HLA class I allele expressed on a DC. Contact between them shunts the DC into a tolerizing mode with costimulatory molecule (e.g., CD86) expression reduced and tolerance-inducing molecule (e.g., ILT3) expression increased. In the obverse, when DC expression of ILT3 is silenced, proinflammatory cytokine synthesis upregulates, and generation of disease-provoking T$_e$ cells soars. ILT3 expression and CD8$^+$CD28$^-$ T$_s$-cell function are reduced during MS relapses. Blood levels of type 1 interferons (IFN-α and IFN-β) are low in MS. IFN-β, widely used to treat MS, increases ILT3 expression and augments CD8$^+$CD28$^-$ T$_s$-cell function.

A single DC can present multiple peptides to CD4$^+$ and CD8$^+$ T cells and can interact with up to 10 T cells, each with a different specificity, at any point in time. Likewise, a CD8$^+$CD28$^-$ T$_s$ cell can interact sequentially with several DCs, provided that each expresses the antigenic peptide specific for that CD8$^+$CD28$^-$ T$_s$ cell. It follows that several CD4$^+$ T cells with different specificities can be tolerized in a cascade by a single CD8$^+$CD28$^-$ T$_s$ cell. Further, as relapses recur and additional DCs are driven to maturity, new immune responses to recently captured self-antigens may be generated. This process is known as *epitope spreading*.

Multiple factors released during viral infections can drive immature tolerance-inducing DCs to maturity and convert them into immune system activators. Reinforcing actions of several factors may be required to ramp up costimulatory molecule expression and ramp down tolerogenic molecule expression to extents that permit an override of CD8$^+$CD28$^-$ T$_s$-cell–mediated tolerance. Included are proinflammatory cytokines, such as tumor necrosis factor-α (TNF-α) released at sites of inflammation and swept into LNs plus binding of virus components to toll-like receptors expressed by DCs and macrophages. Viral infections commonly shunt MS-relevant peptide-loaded immature DCs and macrophages into a CD4$^+$ T-cell–activating mode. This disease-enhancing action of viruses is probably facilitated by an unmasking in MS of a defect in CD8$^+$CD28$^-$ T$_s$-cell function that is at least in part genetically determined.

Mature DCs present antigen to T cells at the onset of an immune response, but their life span is short (only 3 days in mice). During the later stages of an immune response, B cells often assume the dominant APC role. The role of B cells has been supported by presence of antimyelin antibodies within MS lesions and the successful use of B-cell–depleting agents as disease-modifying treatments. Like DCs, B cells have been shown to traffic freely across the blood-brain barrier, but the majority of the B-cell maturation occurs outside of the CNS. B cells are thought to be exposed to antigens in the lymph nodes, primarily deep cervical LNs that drain brain tissue. B-cell receptors bind unprocessed antigen rather than the short peptide sequences recognized by T-cell receptors. Nonetheless, once an unprocessed antigen bound to a B-cell receptor has been internalized, B cells can process internalized antigenic material into small peptides, insert them into the clefts of MHC class II molecules, and transfer MHC class II–processed peptide complexes to the cell surface for presentation to CD4$^+$ T cells.

B cells enter LNs via high endothelial venules in T-cell–dependent areas. Most B cells move quickly from the T-cell–rich paracortex into B-cell zones called *follicles*. Follicle entry occurs because follicle-destined B cells express the chemokine CXCR5 that binds to its CXCL13 counterligand expressed by follicular dendritic cells (FDCs), a distinct population of follicle-confined stromal cells. Follicle-infringing subcapsular macrophages transport particulate material into the follicle and pass it along to FDCs that can then present it to B cells. In addition, soluble antigens percolate into the follicle, are captured by FDCs, and are presented to B cells. Antigen-pulsed B cells next leave the follicle to form monogamous immunologic synapses with DC-primed CD4$^+$ T cells at the T-cell–B-cell boundary. Each B cell drags its T-cell partner along the border for a time, but the B cell then separates from its T-cell partner with the B cell moving back into the follicle, only to be followed much of the time by its prior partner T cell that has now come to express the CXCR5 chemokine, a marker for so-called follicular helper T cells (T$_{fh}$).

Bidirectional interactions between CD4$^+$ T$_{fh}$ cells and B cells are important for (1) germinal center formation, (2) expansion of both populations, (3) hypermutation of B cells that diversifies their antigen receptors and permits affinity-driven clonal selection, (4) differentiation of B cells into long-lived plasma cells that secrete high-affinity antibody and confer long-lasting protection from secondary challenge, and (5) development of memory B cells.

Importantly, T cells can shift lineages. Antigen-presenting B cells may shift CD4$^+$ T$_{fh}$ cells into CD4$^+$ T$_{cm}$ cells, CD4$^+$ IFN-γ–secreting Th1 T$_e$ cells, and CD4$^+$ Th17 T$_e$ cells in response to low doses of autoantigens. B cells can also express proinflammatory cytokines including interleukin-6, interleukin-12, and tumor necrosis factor. Thus B cells can contribute in a major way to MS.

Plate 10.8

Brain: PART I

INFLAMMATORY EVENTS IN THE NERVOUS SYSTEM DURING A RELAPSE

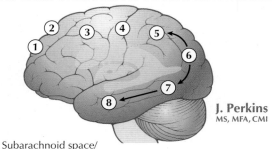

J. Perkins
MS, MFA, CMI

MULTIPLE SCLEROSIS: RELAPSES

The initiation of an MS relapse is thought to involve sequential CNS-restricted steps. Much of the evidence to support this concept derives from study of experimental autoimmune encephalomyelitis (EAE), an inducible animal model of MS. The validity of extrapolating findings from EAE to human disease is questionable, but fundamental mechanisms, such as antigen recognition, are likely to be similar, if not identical.

STEP 1

Step 1 is clinically silent and takes place in the subarachnoid space (SAS) and within the cerebral ventricles. Between 10^5 and 5×10^5 lymphoid cells are present in the noninflamed CSF of humans at any point in time. Eighty percent of these are $CD4^+$ T_{cm} cells in search of their cognate antigen, with lesser representations of $CD8^+$ T_{cm} cells and of $CD4^+$ T_e cells, which are probably derived from $CD4^+$ T_{cm} cells that have found their cognate antigen.

Postcapillary venules on the pial surface and within the choroid plexuses express C-C motif CCL21 and ICAM-1, whereas $CD4^+$ T_{cm} cells express C-C motif CCR7, the counterligand for CCL21, and richly express lymphocyte function–associated antigen-1 (LFA-1), the counterligand for ICAM-1. CCR7-CCL21 and LFA-1–ICAM-1 interactions permit $CD4^+$ T_{cm} cells to pass from postcapillary venules into the SAS and from choroid plexus venules into the ventricles. $CD4^+$ T_{cm} cells, once in the SAS, move first along the outer surface of meningeal vessels and then along the pial surface, searching for their cognate antigen. If they encounter their cognate antigen, offered to them in processed form by an APC, a local immune response is initiated. If surveillance of the SAS proves fruitless, $CD4^+$ T_{cm} cells return to the blood.

In humans, MHC class II–expressing DCs with up-regulated costimulatory molecule expression are present in the CSF compartment. They are situated on the surface of meningeal microvessels and on pial and ependymal surfaces. Their numbers appear to be enriched in MS. Abundant myelin debris with contained protein antigens, residua of prior MS relapses, follows the established drainage paths of interstitial fluid through the ependyma into the ventricular CSF and via the foramen of Luschka and the foramen of Magendie into the SAS. Residual myelin particles are mostly extracellular but are also detected within DCs and macrophages. Myelin debris is not found in controls.

$CD4^+$ T_{cm} cells prepare the terrain for the subsequent entry of T_e cells into the CNS parenchyma and the onset of the clinically evident component of a relapse. Adhesion molecules are not expressed by resting brain parenchymal endothelial cells, nor do meningeal vessels ordinarily express vascular cell adhesion molecule-1 (VCAM-1), the adhesion molecule required for $CD4^+$ T_e cell exit from the blood. $CD4^+$ T_{cm} cells, having been reactivated by an APC, may undergo several cycles of division, still within the meninges or the ventricles, to generate a small locally restricted $CD4^+$ T_e cell cohort. Some members of this cohort cross the pia or ependyma to enter the subjacent CNS parenchyma. These pioneer $CD4^+$ T_e cells secrete IFN-γ and TNF-α, as

1. Surveillance

2. T-Cell–Mediated Microglial Activation

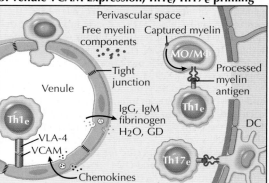

3. Venule VCAM Expression; Th1e, Th17e priming

4. Perivenular Inflammatory Cell Infiltrate

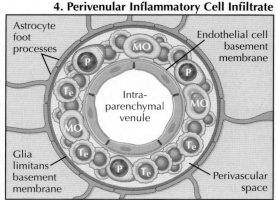

5. Glia Limitans Disruption

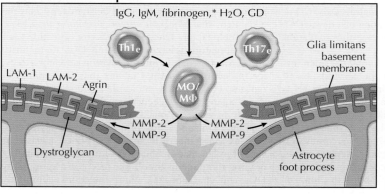

*Fibrinogen in solution has no effect on immune responses but fibrinogen immobilized on CNS tissues and fibrin, its insoluble downstream product, activate microglia, monocytes, and macrophages by a mechanism distinct from their procoagulant properties.

does a subpopulation of still SAS-confined $CD4^+$ T_{cm} cells that may transition into T_e cells.

Released IFN-γ diffuses from the pial and ventricular ependymal surfaces and from the immediately subjacent CNS parenchyma to a considerable depth in the CNS parenchyma, oozing preferentially along fiber tracts. In addition, the released IFN-γ increases the expression of MHC molecules and activates intraparenchymal microglia as evidenced morphologically by

retraction and thickening of their processes. Microglial activation is essential for the subsequent invasion of the CNS parenchyma by T_e cells and by blood monocytes destined to become macrophages. Activated microglia secrete cytokines and, notably, TNF-α, which activates nearby parenchymal postcapillary venules. These venules quickly come to resemble the high endothelial venules of LNs and, most important, now begin to express the adhesion molecules ICAM-1 and VCAM-1.

MULTIPLE SCLEROSIS: RELAPSES (Continued)

STEP 2

Expression of microglial-driven ICAM-1 and VCAM-1 by parenchymal venular endothelial cells modulates blood-brain barrier permeability and permits very late antigen-4 (VLA-4)–expressing $CCR7^-$ $CD4^+$ Th1-type T_e cells and $CCR7^-$ $CD4^+$ Th17-type T_e cells to traverse CNS parenchymal venules and form perivascular inflammatory cuffs (an accumulation of leukocytes in the perivascular space before infiltration into the CNS parenchyma). Monocytes also express VLA-4, and interactions between VLA-4 and VCAM-1 are critical for their cotransmigration into perivascular cuffs and their subsequent disease-promoting activities. The tight junctions that join CNS endothelial cells to create the blood-brain barrier are not disrupted during MS relapses. The perivascular space is bounded by an inner endothelial cell and a laminin-containing basement membrane in which pericytes and vascular smooth muscle cells are embedded. This endothelial cell basement membrane is permissive for T-cell and monocyte transmigration into the perivascular space and the formation of perivascular inflammatory cell cuffs. At this stage, the perivascular cuffs remain clinically silent.

STEP 3

Perivascular cuff monocytes function as APCs. They capture local antigenic material, process it, and present processed antigen in the context of surface-expressed MHC class II molecules to prime abutting $CD4^+$ T_e cells for full effector function. In addition, microglial-derived DCs, resident in the juxtavascular CNS parenchyma, extend processes between astrocyte foot processes and through the basement membrane of the glia limitans that express MHC class II alleles and likewise present antigen to perivascular T_e cells, further priming them in anticipation of their movement into the CNS parenchyma.

STEP 4

Plasma proteins leak into the CNS parenchyma at sites of acute MS disease activity. Plasma proteins, including fibrinogen and high-molecular-weight IgM, are carried across endothelial cells by an energy-requiring intracytoplasmic vesicular transport mechanism. Gadolinium is transported into the CNS parenchyma in the same fashion, at least in guinea pigs with EAE. Transport is maximal across capillaries rather than across the postcapillary venules that CNS-invading immune system cells traverse. Gadolinium-enhancing lesions are often clinically silent, indicating that breakdown of the blood-brain barrier can occur without symptoms of an MS relapse.

STEP 5

Perivascular cuff T cells and monocytes must next cross the glia limitans (GL). The GL is composed of astrocytic end-foot processes and a basement membrane. It covers the entire surface of the brain and spinal cord, where it faces the SAS. Internally, the GL forms the

outer barrier of the extravascular space. The laminins of this outer basement membrane (LAM-1, LAM-2) differ from those of the vascular basement membrane. The GL blocks T-cell transmigration. However, monocytes, comigrants with T cells into perivascular spaces, secrete matrix metalloproteinase (MMP)-2 and MMP-9 in response to the VLA-4–VCAM-1 interaction that permitted their diapedesis into a perivascular cuff. Acting together, these proteases cleave the dystroglycan that

anchors astrocyte end feet to the GL basement membrane so that dystroglycan no longer binds to LAM-1 and LAM-2 or to agrin, a laminin stabilizer. As astrocyte foot processes retract, the GL opens. Products released from perivascular cells can now freely percolate into the CNS parenchyma, and T cells and macrophages can migrate into the CNS parenchyma and induce the neurologic deficits that characterize an MS relapse.

INFLAMMATORY EVENTS IN THE NERVOUS SYSTEM DURING A RELAPSE (CONTINUED)

6a. Healthy Myelinated Axon

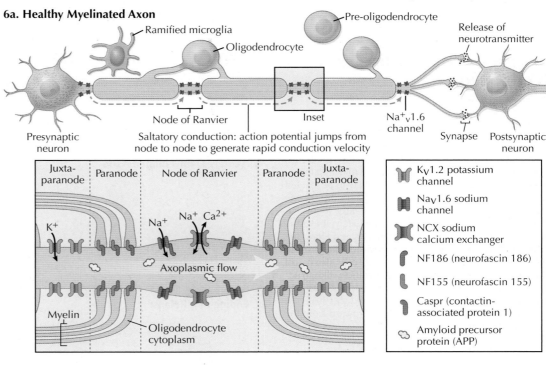

6b. Events That Lead to Conduction Block at Onset of MS Relapse

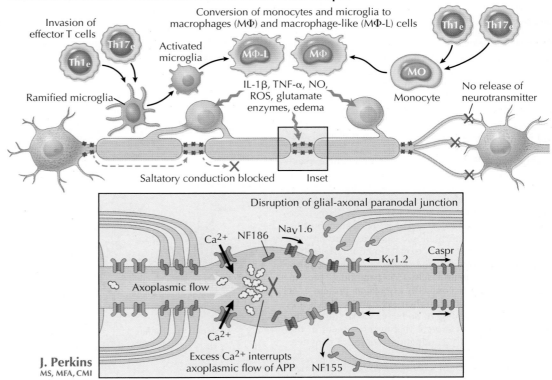

J. Perkins
MS, MFA, CMI

Plate 10.10

Brain: PART I

INFLAMMATORY EVENTS IN THE NERVOUS SYSTEM DURING A RELAPSE (CONTINUED)

MULTIPLE SCLEROSIS: RELAPSES (Continued)

The preferred locations of MS plaques are probably largely determined by these events. CD4$^+$ T$_{cm}$ cells patrolling within the ventricles are likely to be attracted preferentially to nearby CCL21 chemokine gradients. For this reason, areas of intraparenchymal inflammation and maximal tissue damage are likely to be located close to the choroid plexuses, thus accounting for the frequency with which MS plaques are found in the corpus callosum, which sits immediately above the choroid plexuses of the lateral ventricles and along the floor of the fourth ventricle just beneath the choroid plexus of the fourth ventricle. CD4$^+$ T$_{cm}$ cells also patrol the SAS. This may explain why B-cell follicle–like structures are found in the meninges of patients with MS and why plaques are often located juxtacortically in proximity to the meninges with spread inward from the meningeal surface.

Clinical Features of an MS Relapse

Events during the clinically apparent phase of a relapse, as with its prelude, involve a series of steps.

STEP 6

Conduction Block

The symptoms of a relapse begin as CD4$^+$ T$_e$ cells and macrophages move across the GL into the CNS parenchyma. MS relapses include inflammation, demyelination, and reactive changes in astrocytes within MS plaques. The inflammatory infiltrate that was formerly purely perivascular now becomes largely intraparenchymal. Tissue-invading T cells, macrophages, and newly activated CNS-resident microglial cells release multiple proinflammatory cytokines, glutamate, reactive oxygen and nitric oxide intermediates, other free radicals, and proteolytic enzymes, including MMPs. Collectively, these elements damage axons as the initial clinically relevant event of an MS relapse. Early toxic damage is centered on nodes of Ranvier and abutting paranodes, with morphologic changes that provide markers of compromised axonal function. The initial event is a disruption of the coupling of oligodendrocyte end foot neurofascin-155 paranodal protein (NF155) to axonal contactin-associated protein 1 at the paranode, resulting in their separation. This is followed by an uncoupling of nodal Na$_v$1.6 sodium channels from NF186, a protein that anchors them in the membrane. Saltatory conduction requires a complete separation of nodal sodium channels from juxtaparanodal potassium channels. As these channels intermingle, nerve impulse conduction fails. Calcium entry at the node causes nodal swelling, and axonal transport ceases. Immunohistochemistry for amyloid precursor protein (APP), which is synthesized in the cell body and then transported to synapses, can be used to visualize interruption of axonal transport through the development of APP-containing spheroids. Such spheroids are seen at sites of irreversible axonal severing, but only some axons that develop spheroids are doomed. As axonal transport recovers, spheroids may regress and axonal conduction of nerve impulses may resume.

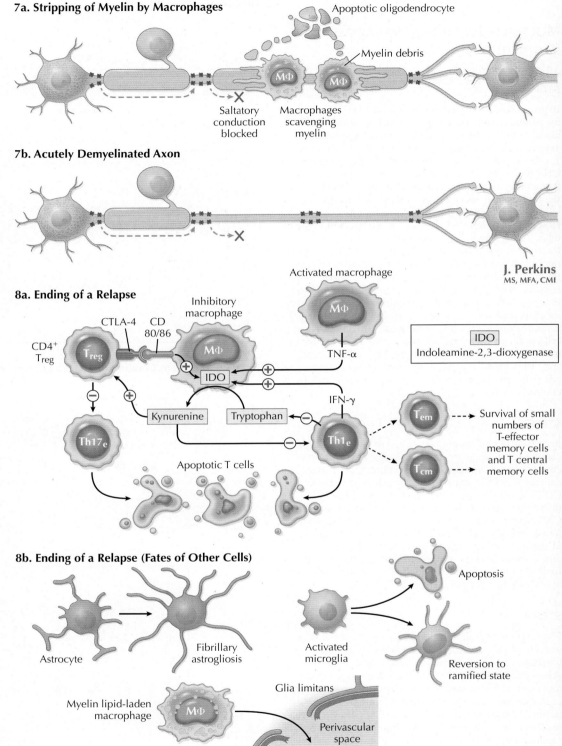

7a. Stripping of Myelin by Macrophages

Apoptotic oligodendrocyte

Myelin debris

Saltatory conduction blocked

Macrophages scavenging myelin

7b. Acutely Demyelinated Axon

J. Perkins
MS, MFA, CMI

8a. Ending of a Relapse

Activated macrophage

Inhibitory macrophage

CTLA-4 CD 80/86

CD4$^+$ T$_{reg}$

T$_{reg}$

MΦ

TNF-α

IDO
Indoleamine-2,3-dioxygenase

IDO

Kynurenine   Tryptophan

IFN-γ

Th17$_e$

Th1$_e$

T$_{em}$

T$_{cm}$

Survival of small numbers of T-effector memory cells and T central memory cells

Apoptotic T cells

8b. Ending of a Relapse (Fates of Other Cells)

Apoptosis

Astrocyte

Fibrillary astrogliosis

Activated microglia

Reversion to ramified state

Myelin lipid-laden macrophage

MΦ

Glia limitans

Perivascular space

STEP 7

Demyelination

Macrophages remove damaged myelin. They may derive from infiltrating monocytes and perhaps from CNS-resident activated microglia. Macrophage processes insinuate themselves between compromised myelin lamellae, physically remove myelin fragments, ingest them, and degrade them. So-called foamy macrophages, present in active plaques, contain the myelin degradation products and are stuffed with lipid droplets. Naked or transected axons are left behind.

As noted, in myelinated axons sodium channels cluster at nodes of Ranvier. This ensures saltatory axonal conduction that jumps from one node of Ranvier to the next. Nerve impulse conduction across acutely demyelinated axonal segments fails. Compensation for demyelination and resumption of nerve impulse conduction require a redistribution of sodium channels

MULTIPLE SCLEROSIS: RELAPSES (Continued)

along myelin-denuded axonal segments to permit the slower and less efficient cable conduction that is normal for unmyelinated axons. Channel redistribution takes a week or two, sometimes longer. Until this occurs, conduction along a demyelinated segment cannot resume. Notably, redistribution of ion channels can eventually become maladaptive and lead to neurodegeneration.

STEP 8

End of the Relapse

MS relapses have a finite duration and are terminated by a classic feedback loop in which the end product eliminates the originator. Most CNS-invading Th1 and Th17 T_e cells apoptose in situ. Apoptosis is facilitated by a cytokine-mediated induction of the macrophage/microglial enzyme indoleamine-2,3-dioxygenase (IDO). IFN-γ released by invading Th1 cells activates IDO, with synergistic support provided by macrophage-secreted TNF-α. IDO shunts tryptophan, an amino acid essential for cell growth and functioning, along a pathway that leads to kynurenine. Quinolinic acid, a product of the kynurenine metabolic pathway, is toxic to both neurons and oligodendrocytes. IDO-mediated tryptophan starvation compromises immune cell function and initiates stress-induced apoptosis, chiefly of Th1 effector cells. In addition, catabolites derived from the kynurenine metabolic pathway are directly cytotoxic to Th1 effector cells.

Th17 effector cells are relatively insensitive to tryptophan starvation and kynurenine toxicity. However, CD4$^+$ regulatory T cells, now evident in the inflammatory infiltrates, further activate IDO-mediated production of kynurenine via an interaction of cytotoxic T-lymphocyte–associated protein 4 and CD80 or CD86. Kynurenine back-signals to the regulatory CD4$^+$ T cells, instructing them to send a proapoptotic message to Th17 effector cells. In addition, regulatory T cells upregulate protective cytokines, including IL-10. All three mechanisms contribute to the termination of a relapse.

As a relapse concludes, some of the amplified activated microglia are culled by apoptosis and others revert to a ramified state. Astrocytes become gliotic, whereas lipid-laden macrophages make their way to the perivascular space and are thought to slowly exit the CNS.

STEP 9

Repair

Demyelinated segments may be remyelinated by preoligodendrocytes that enter demyelinated plaques from surrounding areas. Remyelinated segments are readily recognized because internodal distances are shorter and the myelin sheaths are thinner than their predecessors. Areas of remyelination are known as shadow plaques. Remyelination is spotty at best and becomes minimal as disease evolves. Remyelinated areas are seldom protected from demyelination in subsequent relapses. Therapies with a variety of mechanisms have been or are being investigated for promotion of

Irreversible Axonal Interruption

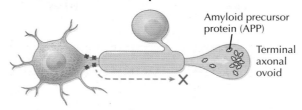

Resumption of Conduction, Often Imperfect, Through Demyelinated Internodes

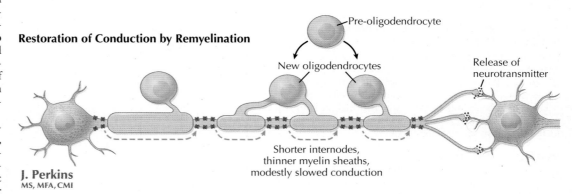

*Na$_V$1.6 sodium channels are usually confined to nodes of Ranvier, and Na$_V$1.2 channels to unmyelinated axons. Both are present in demyelinated axonal segments.

Restoration of Conduction by Remyelination

J. Perkins
MS, MFA, CMI

remyelination. These include antihistamines, a monoclonal antibody to leucine-rich repeat and immunoglobulin-like domain containing protein-1, and gold nanocrystals to promote oligodendrocyte differentiation and maturation.

EVOLUTION OF THE MS PLAQUE

Pathologists have classified MS plaques in numerous ways. Perhaps the simplest has been to judge them as acute, chronic active, or chronic silent. Acute plaques are likely to be responsible for new exacerbations. They manifest as regions of active demyelination with ill-defined boundaries, extensive inflammatory cell infiltrates throughout, perivascular cuffs, and macrophages engaged in myelin stripping and removal. Diffuse MHC class II–positive macrophages and microglia are also present, which express surface-bound costimulatory

molecules. Additionally, they release cytokines including IL-1β and TNF-α, as well as lymphotoxin, free radicals like nitric oxide, and proteolytic enzymes such as MMPs.

Chronic active plaques show recent disease along their periphery, or parts of it, but chronic changes centrally. Ongoing demyelination is restricted to the plaque edge and extends into the adjacent parenchyma in a centrifugal fashion with a border of MHC class II positivity. Chronic silent plaques have a marked downregulation of MHC class II expression throughout, an absence of further demyelinating activity, and a sharp border. Astrocytes take on a fibrillary morphology and express the sinuous processes of chronic gliosis. There may be clusters of demyelinated axons in a chronic silent plaque, but axonal loss is also evident, especially centrally. Oligodendrocytes are absent.

Plate 10.12

Brain: PART I

ENIGMA OF PROGRESSIVE MULTIPLE SCLEROSIS

Progressive MS manifests as gradual disability worsening independent of MRI activity or clinical relapses. Plate 10.12 reviews potential mechanisms that occur independent of peripherally driven immune infiltration: glial and meningeal inflammation, reactive oxygen and nitrogen species, ion channel and mitochondrial dysfunction, and impaired axonal transport. Together, these processes promote a clinically insidious neurodegenerative phenotype due to neuroaxonal dysfunction and loss, although their relative contribution in progressive MS is unknown.

MECHANISMS OF NEUROAXONAL INJURY

Glial-Mediated Inflammation

Activated microglia have distinct populations and can either produce detrimental proinflammatory cytokines, reactive oxygen and nitrogen species, and proteolytic enzymes or beneficially promote repair, clear debris, prune synapses to protect the soma, and play an antiinflammatory role. They are present in active lesions, chronic active lesion borders, and otherwise normal-appearing WM and GM. Glia are not homogenous because interactions with their environment influence their morphology, development, and function and also influence the same in other cell types.

Reactive Species, Ionic Channel Imbalance, and Energy Dysfunction

Neuronal and axonal function requires an operational axolemmal ionic gradient and functional mitochondria for energy. Proinflammatory conditions can directly injure axons from reactive oxygen and nitrogen species released by glia and inflammatory cells, which in turn cause axonal conductional blockade and impaired mitochondrial respiratory chain function.

Meningeal Inflammation

Leptomeningeal lymphoid follicle–like structures composed of inflamed vessels in arachnoid trabeculae with proliferating lymphocytes (plasma and CD4[+] T cells) and FDCs have been found adjacent to subpial cortical demyelination and axonal loss. This compartmentalized inflammation may propagate chronic injury by ectopic expression of proinflammatory cytokines, intrathecal immunoglobulin production, and molecules promoting B-cell activity. Meningeal inflammation is associated with neuronal loss and greater clinical disability and is detected in the deep forebrain and cerebellar sulci as well as spinal cord meninges.

IMAGING BIOMARKERS

MS lesion topography influences clinical phenotype. Lesions involving the corticospinal tract in the brainstem and spinal cord (Plate 5.12, B) are associated with motor progression. Intracortical and sulcal lesions are independently associated with disability progression, and cortical lesions are more common in progressive MS. Cortical lesions with persistent leptomeningeal enhancement, a possible marker of meningeal inflammation, are associated with focal cortical atrophy, suggesting a link between this chronic inflammation and neuronal injury.

A crude sequela of neuroaxonal loss is identified with volumetric measurements as global or regional brain and spinal cord atrophy. Axonal loss can result from direct injury or remote lesions because distant demyelination can cause injury along the axon. Atrophy is particularly apparent in the upper cervical cord because it contains axons traveling the length of the cord, in regions with great connectivity such as the thalamus; this can vary by race and sex.

Iron is readily detected on MRI due to its high magnetic susceptibility. Some chronic active lesion borders have paramagnetic rims with iron-laden microglia/macrophages. These are more common in patients with progressive versus relapsing MS and are associated with greater destruction within the lesions and greater Wallerian degeneration in the periplaque regions. Greater iron in deep GM structures, possibly secondary to greater Wallerian degeneration due to their prominent connectivity, is observed in progressive MS.

CONCLUSIONS

Whereas the pathophysiology and clinical manifestations of relapsing MS are relatively well understood, correlates of the insidious neurologic decline in progressive MS are more enigmatic. Glial pathology, metabolic derangement, and meningeal inflammation appear to play a role, although the relative contribution of each in driving clinical progression remains unclear. MRI and histopathologic studies will continue to tease apart underlying mechanisms to identify potential therapeutic opportunities.

A. Functional mitochondria (*green*) are increased in number, size, activity, and migration as a response to damaged neuroaxonal injury. **B.** Ongoing injury can damage mitochondria (*red*) and lead to mitochondrial dysfunction and energy deficiency in neurons/axons. **C.** Continued environmental stressors and mitochondrial injury lead to displacement of abnormal mitochondria from the neuronal cell body to the site of axonal damage, leading to energy failure and continued production of reactive oxygen species. *From Mahad DH, Trapp BD, Lassmann H. Pathological mechanisms in progressive multiple sclerosis. Lancet Neurol. 2015;14(2):183-93.*

MULTIPLE SCLEROSIS: PATHOLOGY

MS is characterized by inflammation, neurodegeneration, and widespread pathology throughout the CNS, involving brain and spinal cord WM and GM. In addition to demyelination, neuroaxonal injury/loss, glial activation, and peripheral immune infiltration occur throughout the disease course.

LESIONAL PATHOLOGY

Myelin sheaths provide trophic support to axons and promote rapid conduction; their loss is striking within focal lesions. On gross examination, demyelinated lesions are hyperpigmented and are small, discrete ovoid lesions that can coalesce to larger confluent lesions. Hyperpigmented discolorations are also apparent along the surface of the spinal cord, in juxtacortical (but not subpial or intracortical) lesions, in deep GM, and in WM/GM within the brainstem and spinal cord.

Myelin is composed of lipids (70%–85% by weight) and proteins (e.g., myelin basic, proteolipid, myelin oligodendrocyte glycoprotein), and its loss is detected by histologic lipid (Luxol fast blue) and immunohistologic (antibodies to protein antigens) stains. Using immunohistochemistry, lesions can be subclassified and occur around venules (perivenular) and tissue adjacent to CSF (subpial and subependymal).

Cortical lesions are subclassified as type I (leukocortical or juxtacortical), spanning the GM/WM interface; type II (intracortical), limited within the cortex; type III (subpial), involving the superficial cortical layers; and type IV, infrequently encountered subpial lesions involving the entirety of the cortical layers. Type III lesions commonly occur in deep sulci, can involve entire gyri, often have clear borders with a line of activated microglia halting at layers III/IV, and have been reported to associate with meningeal follicle–like structures containing B cells.

Neuronal injury and loss are variable and include neurite transection, synaptic stripping, and reduced soma size. Axonal loss in chronic lesions can be as high as 80%, disproportionally affect smaller caliber diameter axons, and include transection and proximal spheroids. Activated microglia/macrophages and granules from cytotoxic T cells can release proteases and reactive oxygen/nitrogen species directly mediating tissue injury within lesions.

T2*-weighted MRI can detect a central vein sign in MS lesions, which are absent in non-MS (e.g., microvascular) lesions. Fifty-five percent of T2-only lesions in patients with MS are demyelinated, whereas 83% of demyelinated lesions are T2 hyperintense, T1 hypointense, and have a low magnetization transfer ratio. Regions of persistent leptomeningeal enhancement with B-cell aggregates are found in proximity to subpial demyelination and cortical atrophy and correlate with greater clinical disability, suggesting alternative mechanisms for cortical demyelination. Patients with "myelocortical MS" have spinal cord and cortical demyelination with relatively sparse cerebral demyelinating lesions but cerebral hyperintensities on T2-weighted MRI. The lower specificity for detecting demyelination demonstrates the need for improved imaging modalities.

NEURODEGENERATIVE CHANGES

Inflammatory conditions cause neuroaxonal degeneration by axoplasmic membrane ionic imbalance, impaired transport, and energy failure. Elevated levels of NfL chain may be a potential biomarker for neuroaxonal injury in chronic active lesions with active gadolinium-enhancing lesions.

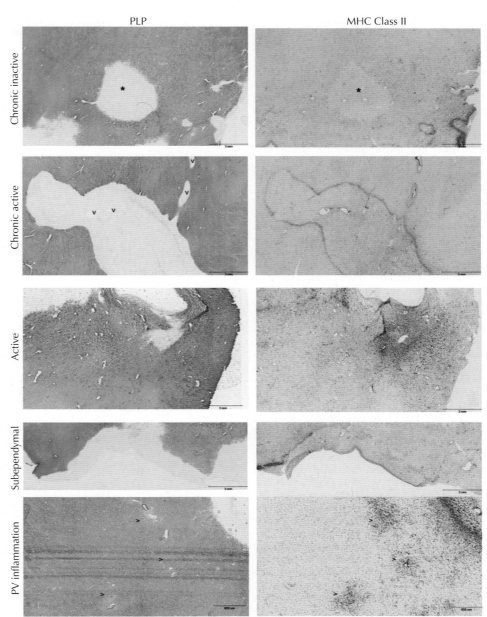

Staining for myelin with proteolipid protein (PLP) and activated microglia/macrophages with MHC class II depicted. Perivascular (PV) lesions include chronic inactive–hypocellular, chronic active–hypocellular centrally with a rim of hypercellularity, and active–hypercellular. An area of subependymal demyelination is shown in the thalamus abutting the third ventricle with a thin line at a portion of its border. Regions of PV inflammation without demyelination termed "pre-active" are also depicted. *From Mahajan KR, Nakamura K, Cohen JA, Trapp BD, Ontaneda D. Intrinsic and extrinsic mechanisms of thalamic pathology in multiple sclerosis. Ann Neurol. 2020;88(1):81-92.*

Neuronal, axonal, and synaptic loss occur within focal inflammatory lesions and can propagate along tracts far from the injury epicenter. Clinically, such focal lesions, particularly involving eloquent tracts (e.g., corticospinal) in the brainstem and spinal cord, can lead to gradual worsening of ambulatory function even years later in the absence of new MRI disease activity or clinical exacerbations.

Loss of myelin, axons, and neurons throughout the CNS collectively contributes to atrophy visible on MRI (greater annualized rate of whole brain atrophy) and on gross pathology (ventriculomegaly and widened sulci in the brain and lateral scalloping of the spinal cord at the site of lesions). The sequela of focal WM lesions contributing to GM/WM loss is exemplified in the thalamus with its extensive connectivity, because lower thalamic volumes correlate with global WM lesion burden. Likewise, the upper cervical cord area reflects lesion burden (and axonal loss) throughout the cord. These changes can occur early in life; children with MS can fail to reach age-expected brain and thalamic growth. Although WM lesion burden tends to be a focus of clinical attention in early stages of illness, collectively these less conspicuous neurodegenerative changes better correlate with clinical disability over time.

CONCLUSION

Ongoing MRI and pathology correlation studies demonstrate extensive changes beyond simple demyelinating lesions. Because no two individuals have the same distribution of lesions or extent of tissue injury, determining the pathologic correlates of disability, developing new MRI techniques, and linking these changes with neurologic function and quality of life measures drive the future direction of MS research and treatment.

Plate 10.14

Brain: PART I

MULTIPLE SCLEROSIS: TREATMENT

The current paradigm of MS treatment involves comprehensive multidisciplinary care aimed at ameliorating symptoms, addressing medical and psychological co-morbidities, rehabilitating patients, and using disease-modifying therapies (DMTs) to reduce the number and severity of relapses and prevent disability accumulation. Over the past several decades, outcomes in MS have improved because of earlier diagnosis, increasing number of DMT options, early initiation of disease therapy, and recognition of the importance of management of comorbidities and health behaviors.

The available DMTs with regulatory approval to treat relapsing MS represent a range of mechanisms of action, routes of administration and dosing schedules, levels of efficacy, and safety and tolerability. Mechanisms of action include immune modulation (interferon betas, glatiramer acetate, fumarates), altered immune cell migration (natalizumab, S1PR modulators), inhibition of immune cell division (mitoxantrone, teriflunomide), and immune cell depletion (cladribine, anti-CD20 monoclonal antibodies, and alemtuzumab). Based on head-to-head clinical trials and observational studies comparing DMTs, the relative levels of efficacy are generally thought to be as follows: low efficacy (interferon betas, glatiramer acetate, teriflunomide), moderate efficacy (fumarates, S1PR modulators), and high efficacy (mitoxantrone, cladribine, natalizumab, anti-CD20 monoclonal antibodies, and alemtuzumab). Selection of the appropriate DMT for an individual with MS involves consideration of disease characteristics and risk of future disability, efficacy and risk of adverse effects of the DMTs, and other factors such as anticipated pregnancy, comorbidities, and individual preferences and priorities of the person with MS. DMT selection is best made as a shared decision by the person with MS and treatment team. After therapy is commenced, monitoring for incomplete disease control, side effects, safety issues, and pregnancy is necessary. Several ongoing clinical trials are investigating the optimal overall treatment approach; that is, comparing the traditional escalation approach (initiating therapy with a safe medication with modest efficacy and then switching therapy as needed to achieve disease control) versus initiating therapy with a highly efficacious treatment (greater likelihood of disease control but with potential safety concerns).

Despite the increasing availability of DMTs, relapses requiring treatment still occur. Management of acute relapses includes laboratory testing to identify a potential trigger (most often an infection), a short course of high-dose corticosteroids, symptomatic management, and rehabilitation.

The available DMTs are effective in reducing relapses, MRI lesion activity, and accumulation of disability in relapsing MS. Although some have benefit in progressive MS, efficacy is modest and largely limited to patients with recent relapses or active MRI. Efficacious therapies for progressive MS, including therapies that promote repair and restore function in the damaged CNS, represent important unmet needs.

IMMUNE MODULATION

Interferon beta preparations, which include interferon β-1b, two preparations of interferon β-1a, and PEGylated interferon β-1a, are administered by subcutaneous or intramuscular injections. Beneficial biologic actions in MS include induction of a large number of genes in immune cells, inhibition of lymphocyte

Augmented Tolerizing Signals

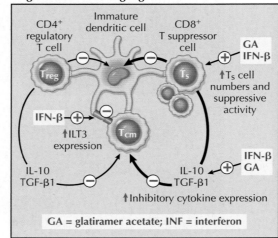

GA = glatiramer acetate; INF = interferon

Immunologic Synapse Modulation

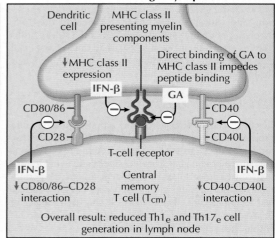

Overall result: reduced Th1$_e$ and Th17$_e$ cell generation in lymph node

Reduced CSF Surveillance

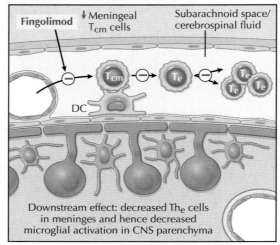

Downstream effect: decreased Th$_e$ cells in meninges and hence decreased microglial activation in CNS parenchyma

J. Perkins
MS, MFA, CMI

Intraparenchymal Venules and Perivascular Space

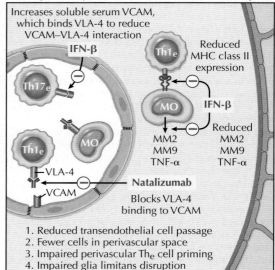

Natalizumab
Blocks VLA-4 binding to VCAM

1. Reduced transendothelial cell passage
2. Fewer cells in perivascular space
3. Impaired perivascular Th$_e$ cell priming
4. Impaired glia limitans disruption

Lymph Node Entrapment

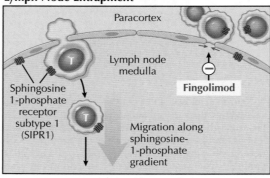

CNS Effects of Fingolimod Possibly Relevant to MS

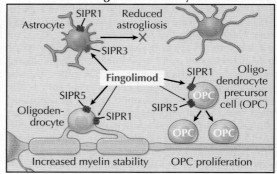

proliferation, a shift from a Th1 to Th2 immune phenotype, altered cytokine production, reduced expression of MHC class II molecules and costimulatory molecules on APCs, inhibition of blood-brain barrier leakage, and inhibition of immune cell migration into the CNS. Interferon betas were among the initial DMTs approved for MS, and there is substantial experience with their use. As a group, they have modest efficacy. The most common side effects are injection site

reactions, constitutional flu-like symptoms, and accentuation of preexisting MS symptoms such as spasticity, headache, and depression. Periodic complete blood count and liver function tests are recommended. Up to one-third of patients receiving some interferon beta preparations develop neutralizing antibodies, requiring a change of therapy.

Glatiramer acetate is a complex mixture of synthetic random polypeptides containing glutamic acid, lysine,

Plate 10.14 continued on next page

MULTIPLE SCLEROSIS: TREATMENT (Continued)

alanine, and tyrosine, thought to mimic the structure of myelin basic protein, a putative autoantigen in MS. Glatiramer acetate is administered by subcutaneous injection and competitively binds to major histocompatibility molecules on APCs and functions as an altered peptide ligand with inhibition of activation of antigen-specific T lymphocytes, induction of immune tolerance, and augmented production of neurotrophic factors. Like the interferon betas, glatiramer acetate was one of the first medications approved to treat MS. It also has relatively modest efficacy, but some patients do quite well. The main side effects include injection site reactions, lipoatrophy of injection sites with chronic treatment, and rare systemic postinjection reaction. Both interferon beta and glatiramer acetate are typically used in patients who are risk averse because newer medications are more efficacious and are easier to administer. Some older patients with MS were started on these medications when they became available and have done well. In these patients there is no need to change therapy without a clear indication.

Fumarates (dimethyl fumarate, monomethyl fumarate, diroximel fumarate) have several immunomodulatory and tissue-protective actions through activation of nuclear factor E2–related factor-2 and inhibition of nuclear factor-κB transcription pathways. Fumarates are administered orally and have moderate efficacy in MS. The most common side effects are skin flushing and gastrointestinal (GI) symptoms, which are most bothersome with initiation of therapy and tend to decrease over time. Complete blood count and liver function tests are tested prior to therapy and periodically to monitor for lymphopenia and hepatotoxicity, which are uncommon. Rare cases of progressive multifocal leukoencephalopathy have been reported in patients with persistent lymphopenia. Fumarates are often used as initial therapy in patients newly diagnosed, especially those who prefer an oral therapy or are concerned about the potential risks of the high-efficacy therapies.

ALTERED IMMUNE CELL MIGRATION

Natalizumab is a humanized monoclonal antibody directed against α4-integrin expressed on the surface of T lymphocytes, B lymphocytes, and macrophages. By blocking the binding of α4-integrin to VCAM-1 expressed by endothelial cells, natalizumab inhibits migration of immune cells into the CNS, markedly reducing parenchymal inflammation. Natalizumab is administered by monthly intravenous infusion, which can be accompanied by mild infusion-related side effects. The most significant adverse effects of natalizumab are rare hepatotoxicity, herpes simplex encephalitis, and progressive multifocal leukoencephalopathy, an opportunistic infection that almost exclusively occurs in patients with serologic evidence of prior infection with John Cunningham virus (JCV). In common with other DMTs that work via altering lymphocyte trafficking, increased, sometimes fulminant, rebound disease activity after stopping natalizumab has been reported. Natalizumab is typically used as a second-line medication, but in selected patients with highly active MS and negative JCV antibodies, natalizumab is sometimes used as initial therapy.

Fingolimod, an S1PR modulator, was the first oral medication approved to treat MS. In addition to being a component of cell membranes, sphingosine-1-phosphate functions as a soluble regulator of a large number of biologic processes during development and in the adult through interaction with a five-member family of G-protein–coupled cell surface receptors, which are widely expressed in various tissues. Through interaction with S1PR subtype 1 on T and B lymphocytes, fingolimod inhibits their egress from lymph nodes and inflammatory infiltration of the CNS. Direct effects on cells in the CNS also possibly contribute to clinical benefit. Fingolimod usually is well tolerated. However, in addition to increased risk of certain infections (herpes infections, cryptococcal meningitis, rare progressive multifocal leukoencephalopathy), interaction of fingolimod with S1PR subtypes 1, 3, 4, and 5 in other tissues leads to a range of potential off-target adverse effects, which are uncommon but can include bradycardia and slowed atrioventricular conduction with initiation of treatment, macular edema, hypertension, hepatotoxicity, and increased airway resistance. Selective S1PR modulators (siponimod, ozanimod, and ponesimod) have been developed that preserve the efficacy of fingolimod and lessen off-target adverse effects. In addition to receptor selectivity, dose uptitration with treatment initiation contributes to the attenuation of cardiac effects. As with natalizumab, rebound disease activity, sometimes marked, can occur after discontinuation of S1PR modulator therapy. SIPR modulators are favored for patients who prefer an oral medication and are concerned about the immunosuppressant effects of other medications.

INHIBITION OF IMMUNE CELL DIVISION

Mitoxantrone, an anthracenedione antineoplastic agent, intercalates into DNA and interferes with synthesis and repair. Immunologic effects include inhibition of cellular and humoral immune mechanisms. Mitoxantrone is approved to treat SPMS and worsening RRMS. Administered intravenously, adverse effects include infusion-associated nausea, myelosuppression, cardiotoxicity, secondary hematologic malignancies, and infertility. Mitoxantrone is no longer commonly used in clinical practice because of safety concerns and availability of other high-efficacy therapies.

Teriflunomide is the active moiety of leflunomide used to treat rheumatoid arthritis. It blocks dihydroorotate dehydrogenase, the rate-limiting enzyme in de novo pyrimidine synthesis required for T- and B-lymphocyte proliferation. It is administered orally. Principal adverse effects include GI symptoms, alopecia, hepatotoxicity, bone marrow suppression, hypertension, and peripheral neuropathy. Because teriflunomide is teratogenic and secreted in semen, effective contraception is needed when either the female or male partner is treated. Teriflunomide is eliminated mainly through biliary excretion and has a long half-life due to prominent enterohepatic recirculation. If needed because of planned change in MS DMT or pregnancy, clearance can be accelerated with oral administration of cholestyramine or activated charcoal. Teriflunomide is generally used in patients with mild disease who prefer an oral medication.

IMMUNE CELL DEPLETION

Cladribine (2-chloro-deoxyadenosine) undergoes intracellular phosphorylation leading to the incorporation of 2-chloro-deoxyadenosine triphosphate into DNA, inhibiting DNA repair. It is relatively specific for proliferating and resting lymphocytes. It is administered orally as two 4- to 5-day cycles separated by 1 month repeated after 1 year. Treatment leads to profound lymphocyte depletion followed by reconstitution and prominent and long-lasting clinical efficacy in MS. The principal adverse effects include nausea, headache, prolonged lymphopenia, infection, hepatotoxicity, myocarditis, and potential increased risk of malignancy. Although highly effective, it is often used only after patients have not responded to treatment with other DMTs because of potential risks.

Ocrelizumab is a humanized monoclonal antibody specific for the surface marker CD20. It is administered by intravenous infusion every 6 months and leads to rapid and potent depletion of circulating B lymphocytes. *Ofatumumab* is a fully human anti-CD20 monoclonal antibody administered by monthly subcutaneous injection. The two antibodies bind to somewhat different CD20 antigenic sites and have some different specific mechanisms of B-lymphocyte killing. Both are highly efficacious treatments for RRMS. Ocrelizumab is the only medication with regulatory approval to treat PPMS. The principal adverse effects of anti-CD20 monoclonal antibody therapy are cell lysis syndrome (potentially including fever, rash, laryngeal edema, hypotension) with initiation of therapy, risk of infection, and potential risk of malignancy, particularly breast cancer. Hypogammaglobulinemia with prolonged therapy is increasingly recognized. Both medications are used in patients who have not responded to other therapies or as initial therapy in the absence of contraindications.

Alemtuzumab is a humanized monoclonal antibody targeting CD52 expressed on the surface of T and B lymphocytes, monocytes, and eosinophils. It is administered intravenously as a 5-day course followed by a 3-day course 1 year later. It produces rapid and profound lymphocyte depletion. The reconstituted lymphocyte populations have an altered profile and function leading to long-lasting clinical benefit. Adverse effects include infusion reactions, risk of infections, vasculitis, and potential increased risk of malignancy. Stroke (both hemorrhagic and ischemic) after infusion has been reported. The most noteworthy adverse effects are secondary autoimmune conditions, including thyroid disease, immune thrombocytopenia purpura, neutropenia, and renal glomerular basement membrane disease. Autoimmunity is thought to result from more rapid B-lymphocyte reconstitution prior to restoration of T-lymphocyte regulatory mechanisms. Because of safety concerns, alemtuzumab generally is reserved for patients who have inadequate disease control with other DMTs.

Plate 10.15

Brain: PART I

NEUROMYELITIS OPTICA SPECTRUM DISORDER, MOGAD, AND ACUTE DISSEMINATED ENCEPHALOMYELITIS

NEUROMYELITIS OPTICA SPECTRUM DISORDER

Neuromyelitis optica spectrum disorder (NMOSD) is an inflammatory demyelinating disease of the CNS predominantly affecting the optic nerves, brainstem, and spinal cord. Although initially considered an MS variant, it is now known to be a distinct clinical and pathophysiologic entity. Approximately 80% of patients have autoantibodies to aquaporin-4 (AQP4), a water channel present on astrocytic foot processes. AQP4 antibodies activate complement- and cell-mediated astrocytic damage, causing secondary oligodendrocyte damage and demyelination.

The prevalence of NMOSD is similar across the world and rarely exceeds 5 per 100,000 persons. It typically presents in the fourth decade of life, and there is a 9:1 female predominance. Clinically, NMOSD is characterized by relapses, which often evolve rapidly and are characterized by incomplete recovery despite treatment. There are four cardinal manifestations: optic neuritis, acute myelitis, area postrema syndrome, and acute brainstem syndrome, some of which have features that help differentiate them from MS. Optic neuritis is more likely to be bilateral, to recur, and to have worse long-term visual outcomes. Acute myelitis is more often disabling. Area postrema syndrome, characterized by intractable nausea and vomiting, is rarely seen in MS.

NMOSD is also commonly associated with other antibody-mediated autoimmune diseases, including systemic lupus erythematosus, Sjögren syndrome, and antiphospholipid antibody syndrome. The presence of any cardinal manifestations of NMOSD in people with these diseases should prompt testing for AQP4 antibodies.

On MRI, lesions most commonly occur at regions with high AQP4 expression, including the periaqueductal gray, hypothalamic, and periventricular regions of the brain. Lesions can also involve the subcortical and deep WM. Optic neuritis commonly involves both optic nerves and predominantly affects the posterior optic pathway. Myelitis is typically longitudinally extensive, spanning three or more contiguous vertebral segments, often with involvement of the central cord and cord edema (see Plate 10.15).

As a biomarker, AQP4 IgG is highly specific for NMOSD. Testing for AQP4-IgG should be done in serum because CSF is less sensitive. CSF findings in NMOSD often include a mixed pleocytosis and elevated protein. Positive OCBs are found in fewer than 30% of people with AQP4-IgG.

The diagnostic criteria for NMOSD are based on six core clinical characteristics: (1) optic neuritis, (2) acute myelitis, (3) area postrema syndrome, (4) acute brainstem syndrome, (5) symptomatic narcolepsy or acute diencephalic clinical syndrome with NMOSD-typical diencephalic MRI lesions, and (6) symptomatic cerebral syndrome with NMOSD-typical brain lesions. NMOSD with AQP4-IgG requires at least one core clinical characteristic, a positive test for AQP4-IgG, and exclusion of alternative diagnoses. NMOSD without AQP4-IgG or NMOSD with unknown AQP4-IgG status requires two different core clinical characteristics (at least one of which is optic neuritis, longitudinally extensive transverse myelitis, or area postrema syndrome), additional

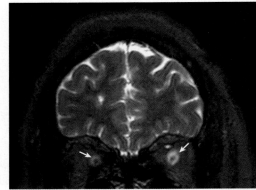

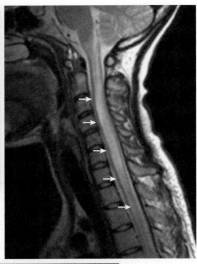

Coronal *(above)* and sagittal *(right)* T2 MRI photomicrographs showing bilateral optic neuritis and longitudinally extensive transverse myelitis seen in neuromyelitis optica

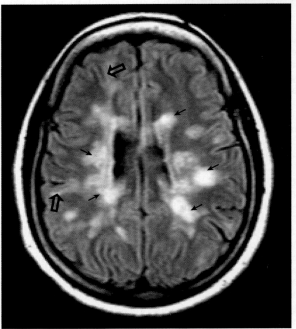

Axial FLAIR T2 MRI photomicrograph showing extensive lesions in the deep white matter *(solid arrows)* and juxtacortical regions *(open arrows)* seen in ADEM

MRI requirements demonstrating findings typical of the core clinical syndrome, and exclusion of alternative diagnoses.

Intravenous corticosteroids are the initial treatment for an acute attack, typically 1 g methylprednisolone daily for 3 to 5 days, followed by an oral prednisone taper. Oral prednisone should be tapered slowly and continued until maintenance therapy has been established. Plasmapheresis is a second-line therapy for those with minimal to no response to corticosteroids. Intravenous immunoglobulin (IVIg) has also been used as a second-line therapy, but the evidence to support its use is not as strong.

Until 2019, there was no approved maintenance therapy. The US Food and Drug Administration (FDA) has now approved eculizumab, inebilizumab, and satralizumab for adult patients who are AQP4-IgG seropositive. Although not FDA approved, rituximab has been widely used off-label, supported by robust effects in

several retrospective studies and a small randomized controlled trial. Azathioprine and mycophenolate mofetil have been used historically, although systematic literature suggests that rituximab has better efficacy.

MYELIN OLIGODENDROCYTE GLYCOPROTEIN ANTIBODY-ASSOCIATED DISEASE

Myelin oligodendrocyte glycoprotein antibody disorder (MOGAD) is an idiopathic inflammatory CNS demyelinating disease. Originally identified in NMOSD antibody–negative patients, it shares many features with NMOSD but has distinct clinical and pathophysiologic features.

Although rare, the precise prevalence of MOGAD is still being defined. It can occur at any age, but children and young adults are more commonly affected, and it has a roughly equal distribution among females and males. It most commonly presents as recurrent episodes

Neuromyelitis Optica Spectrum Disorder, MOGAD, and Acute Disseminated Encephalomyelitis (Continued)

of optic neuritis, myelitis, or both, but may be monophasic. In younger people, it can also present as acute disseminated encephalomyelitis (ADEM). Compared with people with AQP4-positive NMOSD, people with MOGAD are typically younger and more likely to present with a monophasic course or with ADEM. Long-term prognosis is better in MOGAD.

To meet the diagnostic criteria for MOGAD, individuals must have serum-positive MOG-IgG and one of the following clinical presentations: ADEM, optic neuritis, short or long segment transverse myelitis, or a brain or brainstem syndrome compatible with demyelination. There should also be a work-up for and exclusion of alternative diagnoses.

For an acute attack, the treatment approach is the same as that for NMOSD: an initial course of high-dose IV steroids followed by a prolonged steroid taper. Most reported cases show excellent response to steroid treatment with full recovery. There are limited data on long-term management of recurrent MOGAD, although the treatment approach is often similar to NMOSD maintenance therapy.

ACUTE DISSEMINATED ENCEPHALOMYELITIS

ADEM is an acute inflammatory disorder of the CNS characterized by widespread demyelination involving the brain and spinal cord. Infection or vaccination often precedes its development, and animal models suggest that ADEM may result from an autoimmune attack triggered by molecular mimicry or direct CNS infection with a secondary inflammatory cascade.

In children, the estimated incidence of hospitalization is 0.5 per 100,000 per year in the United States. Incidence in adults is lower but not well quantified. ADEM typically presents as a rapidly progressive encephalopathy associated with multifocal neurologic deficits. Most cases follow an infectious illness or vaccination, usually within 4 weeks. A wide variety of infectious agents have been associated with ADEM, mainly viral or bacterial, and often involving the upper respiratory tract. Association with vaccination is less common.

Altered level of consciousness, ataxia, and brainstem symptoms are frequently reported in both children and adults. In children, long-lasting fever and headaches occur more frequently. In adults, motor and sensory deficits are more common. Seizures occur in up to one-third of children but rarely occur in adults. Recurrent attacks are rare.

Brain MRI shows patchy, poorly marginated areas of T2 hyperintensity involving the subcortical and central WM and cortical gray-white junction (see Plate 10.15). Lesions are typically large, multifocal, and asymmetric. The GM of the thalami and basal ganglia may also be involved, typically in a symmetric pattern, and can help distinguish ADEM from MS. Spinal cord involvement has been described in up to one-third of patients, often showing large confluent lesions spanning multiple segments, sometimes associated with cord swelling. Most lesions resolve on follow-up imaging studies.

HISTOPATHOLOGIC FINDINGS

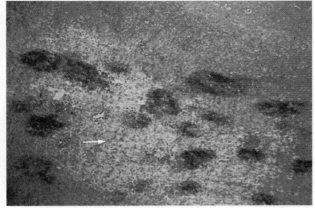

Cingulate gyrus white matter showing area of perivenous demyelination (Luxol fast blue Holmes, ×100)

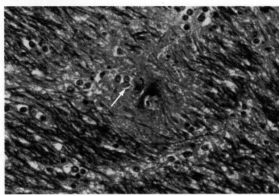

Cerebral white matter with scattered deep hemorrhages in pale, edematous areas (H&E stain, ×10)

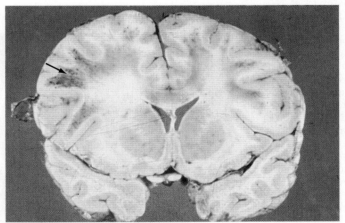

Coronal section of cerebral hemispheres at level of corpus striatum showing punctate hemorrhagic lesions in subcortical white matter

CSF may show lymphocytic pleocytosis and an elevated CSF albumin-to–serum albumin ratio. The presence of OCBs is less common than in MS, especially in children, and, unlike other neuroinflammatory disorders, may be present transiently.

Consensus diagnostic criteria require all of the following: (1) a first polyfocal, clinical CNS event with presumed inflammatory demyelinating cause; (2) encephalopathy that cannot be explained by fever; (3) no new clinical and MRI findings emerging 3 months or more after the onset; (4) abnormal brain MRI during the acute (3-month) phase; and (5) typical MRI findings. Multiphasic ADEM is defined as two episodes consistent with ADEM separated by at least 3 months. Although designed for the pediatric population, these criteria are often applied to adults as well.

High-dose IV steroids are the first-line therapy for management of an acute attack and are followed by an oral steroid taper for 4 to 6 weeks. IVIg and plasmapheresis have been used in refractory cases with some success.

Because the majority of ADEM is monophasic, only acute treatment is indicated in most cases. With early initiation of steroids, the majority of children with ADEM are reported to have good outcomes, with a return to baseline in weeks to months. However, mortality rates of 1% to 3% have been reported, and there are conflicting reports regarding long-term neuropsychological impairment.

Initially thought to be a variant of ADEM, acute hemorrhagic leukoencephalitis (AHL) is characterized by a fulminant clinical presentation, high mortality, and hemorrhage into demyelinating lesions. There is now debate about whether AHL represents a separate disease entity due to differences in pathology, including increased neutrophils, small vessel destruction with fibrin deposition, and hemorrhage (Plate 10.16). Lesions on MRI tend to be large, with perilesional edema and mass effect, and death from brain edema is common early in the disease course. However, favorable neurologic outcomes have been reported with early and aggressive treatment.

Plate 10.17

Brain: PART I

Introduction to Autoimmune Neurologic Syndromes

There is an ever-increasing recognition of the role of immunologic mechanisms underlying many neurologic diseases. Traditionally, only a few neurologic disorders were thought to have an autoimmune mechanism. Over the past few decades, there has been tremendous growth in the understanding and treatment of autoimmune neurologic disorders. In particular, the discovery of neural-specific autoantibody markers has provided invaluable insight into this class of disorders.

Starting in the 1960s, many autoimmune neurologic disorders were associated with systemic malignancies such as small cell lung carcinoma and various gynecologic tumors. These disorders were termed paraneoplastic neurologic syndromes (PNSs) and included Lambert-Eaton myasthenic syndrome (LEMS) associated with anti-P/Q type voltage-gated calcium channel antibodies and the rapidly progressive cerebellar syndrome associated with Yo (also known as PCA1) autoantibodies. In many cases, neurologic symptoms precede the diagnosis of cancer, and identification of one these antibodies can help focus the oncologic evaluation, thus improving outcomes. These high-risk autoantibodies associated with PNS usually target intracellular antigens.

Other autoimmune neurologic disorders may be caused by parainfectious triggers or adverse events related to various immunotherapies, yet in many cases the exact trigger is unknown. The discovery of N-methyl-D-aspartate receptor (NMDA-R) autoantibodies has helped expand our understanding of autoimmune neurologic disorders with antibodies directed against extracellular domains of neuronal proteins (i.e., synaptic receptors or other proteins located on the neuronal cell surface membrane). It is now recognized that the overall burden of neurologic disease associated with these autoantibodies not only outweighs those disorders associated with antibodies directed against intracellular antigens but is also more common than viral encephalitis.

Autoimmune diseases can affect any part of the nervous system, including the peripheral and autonomic nervous systems. Guillain-Barré syndrome (GBS), a group of heterogeneous conditions that share a similar clinical phenotype, is a prototypic immune-mediated peripheral nervous system disorder. Infections of the GI tract and upper respiratory tract are common triggers for GBS, with *Campylobacter jejuni* being the most common causative agent. Although there is a wide range of clinical phenotypes associated with GBS, all of the variants share similar pathophysiology, including endoneural inflammation mediated by both the innate and adaptive immune system.

Diagnosing and managing autoimmune neurologic diseases can be challenging. Symptoms can be multifocal and involve any combination of central, peripheral, and autonomic nervous system functions. It is vital to seek objective evidence of neurologic dysfunction to anchor the diagnosis of an autoimmune neurologic disorder. Potential diagnostic clues include a subacute clinical course that progresses over weeks to months, inflammatory CSF (e.g., pleocytosis, increased CSF immunoglobulins, unique OCBs), and MRI abnormalities (e.g., temporal lobe T2-weighted hyperintensity or cerebellar degeneration). When possible, serum and CSF should be screened for autoantibodies because of differences in the sensitivity of commercially available assays.

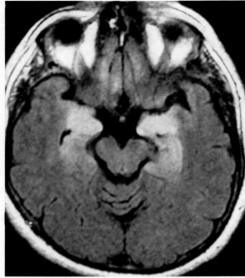

Axial FLAIR MRI of a patient with paraneoplastic limbic encephalopathy. There is marked hyperintensity in the medial temporal lobes bilaterally. In addition, there is slight dilation of the temporal horns, suggesting atrophy. *From Irani SR. Paraneoplastic and nonparaneoplastic autoimmune syndromes of the nervous system. In: Aminoff MS, Josephson A. Aminoff's Neurology and General Medicine. 6th ed. Elsevier; 2021:499-520.*

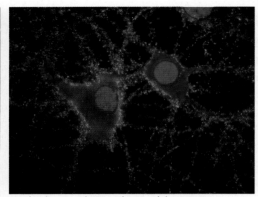

Antibodies to GluN1 subunit of the NMDA receptor in a patient with anti-NMDA-R encephalitis. Live rat hippocampal neurons incubated with the patient's CSF are immunolabeled with antibodies against cell surface antigens; subsequent characterization demonstrated that the antigen is the GluN1 subunit of the NMDA-R. *From Rosenfeld MR, Dalmau J. Autoimmune encephalitis with antibodies to cell surface antigens. In: Jankovic J. Bradley and Daroff's Neurology in Clinical Practice. 8th ed. Elsevier; 2022:1263-1268.*

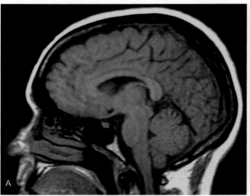 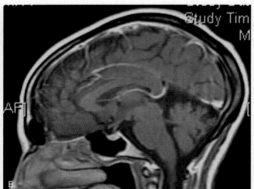

(**A**) Normal sagittal MRI of the brain. (**B**) T1 contrast-enhanced sagittal MRI of the brain in a patient with paraneoplastic cerebellar degeneration. The cerebellum is atrophic, but the rest of the brain is normal. *From Irani SR. Paraneoplastic and nonparaneoplastic autoimmune syndromes of the nervous system. In: Aminoff MS, Josephson A. Aminoff's Neurology and General Medicine. 6th ed. Elsevier; 2021:499-520.*

Patients with autoimmune neurologic syndromes and neural autoantibodies with high risk of cancer association should undergo malignancy evaluation including computed tomography of the chest, abdomen, and pelvis. Depending on a patient's age, sex, smoking history, and whether autoantibody is detected, additional tests may be required, including mammography, testicular ultrasound, and positron emission tomography of the body. If malignancy is not detected, further surveillance over time may be advised.

In PNS with an identified cancer, the primary goal is treatment of the underlying malignancy, but adjunct therapy with immunomodulation may improve the neurologic clinical course. In general, patients with autoantibodies to intracellular antigens respond less well to therapeutic interventions. For nonparaneoplastic autoimmune neurologic disorders, immunomodulation is the mainstay of treatment. Typical immunomodulatory therapies include corticosteroids, IVIg, plasma exchange, rituximab, azathioprine, mycophenolate mofetil, and cyclophosphamide, as well as other options. The choice of immunotherapy is dictated by the type of neural autoantibody, severity of the underlying neurologic disorder, possible cancer treatment, and the patient's medical comorbidities. The consensus from retrospective studies is that early initiation of immunotherapy leads to improved disease outcomes.

The following plates explore in more detail the growing spectrum of autoimmune neurologic disorders. Recognition of characteristic clinical syndromes is critical given the potential reversibility of these disorders.

STIFF PERSON SYNDROME SPECTRUM DISORDER

Stiff person syndrome (SPS) (previously termed *stiff man syndrome*) was originally described in 1956 by Moersch and Woltman. SPS was found later to have a strong association with glutamic acid decarboxylase 65 (GAD65) autoantibody production, but over time the spectrum of clinical presentations has expanded; patients are now recognized with less typical presentations such as focal symptoms or progressive encephalopathy. Given this broad clinical phenotype, these disorders have now been collectively termed stiff person syndrome spectrum disorder (SPSD). Recognition of a broader clinical spectrum has occurred in parallel with discovery of novel autoantibody associations, most of which are targeting antigens on inhibitory neuronal synapses. Patients with GAD65 autoantibodies may have a variety of neurologic manifestations, including cerebellar ataxia, epilepsy, encephalitis, and brainstem dysfunction.

CLINICAL PRESENTATION

Generalized Stiff Person Syndrome

Generalized SPS is characterized by paraspinal, abdominal, and lower extremity rigidity, leading to significant gait impairment. Patients can experience superimposed spasms precipitated by a variety of stimuli, including noise, anxiety, or touch. The spasms can be painful and abrupt, leading to precipitous falls and inhibiting socializing in large groups and events.

On neurologic examination, patients often display paraspinal and abdominal musculature contractions along with lower extremity rigidity. Touching the patient may cause a generalized opisthotonic spasm mimicking tetanus. Muscle stretch reflexes are usually exaggerated and associated with upper motor neuron signs. Lumbar hyperlordosis can occur, and the gait may appear rigid with a "wooden man" or "tin soldier" pattern.

Stiff Limb Syndrome

The variant of stiff limb syndrome presents focally in one or more limbs with rigidity and spasms; axial involvement is less common. Patients may progress to a more classic SPS phenotype with abdominal and truncal involvement. Diagnosis is challenging due to a presentation that can mimic focal dystonia and the absence of GAD65 autoantibody in some cases.

Progressive Encephalomyelitis With Rigidity and Myoclonus

This group of patients can experience broad neurologic involvement with a more fulminant onset. Axial and limb rigidity can be associated with cognitive impairment, disorders of consciousness, epilepsy, brainstem and cranial nerve dysfunction, and dysautonomia. Patients with progressive encephalomyelitis with rigidity and myoclonus (PERM) can have a rapidly progressive course requiring intensive care unit monitoring and, despite appropriate treatment, may be left with severe disability.

PARACLINICAL EVALUATION

Approximately 60% to 80% of patients with SPS are GAD65 autoantibody seropositive with titers 100- to 500-fold higher than those found in type 1 diabetes. There is some evidence to suggest that the presence of intrathecal GAD antibody is a more specific finding

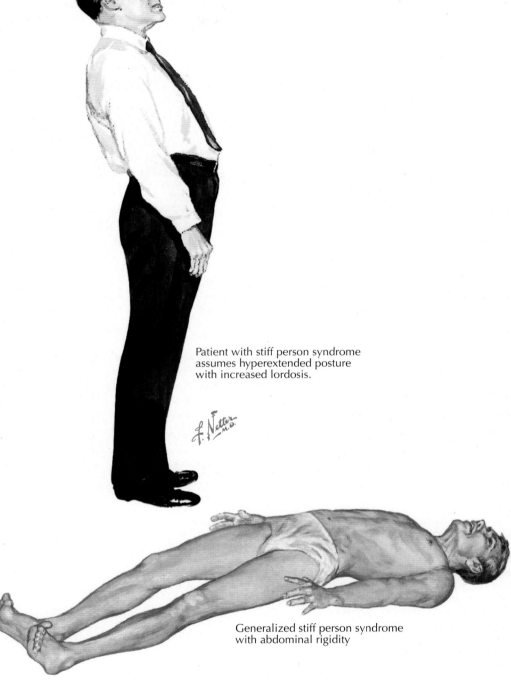

Patient with stiff person syndrome assumes hyperextended posture with increased lordosis.

Generalized stiff person syndrome with abdominal rigidity

than elevated serum titers. Other antibodies that have been associated in SPS include autoantibodies against amphiphysin, glycine receptor (GlyR), γ-aminobutyric acid (GABA)$_A$ receptor, gephyrin, and dipeptidyl peptidase-like protein 6 (DPPX). Amphiphysin-related SPSD is associated with breast cancer, so appropriate malignancy screening should be completed in those patients. Electromyography (EMG) can help support a diagnosis of SPSD, though GABAergic treatments (i.e., benzodiazepines, baclofen) can attenuate the abnormalities. Findings include continuous motor unit activity within agonist-antagonist muscle pairs and exaggerated startle reflexes.

TREATMENT

Diazepam is first-line symptomatic therapy. Benzodiazepines are GABA$_A$ receptor agonists and inhibit excessive motor unit firing and thus improve painful muscle contraction. Baclofen, a GABA$_B$ receptor agonist, can also be effective, especially when paired with a benzodiazepine. Potential immunotherapies can be used, including high-dose corticosteroids, IVIg, plasma exchange, and other steroid-sparing medications. Up to 20% to 30% of patients have a refractory course despite multiple treatment approaches.

Plate 10.19   Brain: PART I

Tumorigenesis
- Carcinogens
- Radiation
- Viruses
- Inflammation
- Inherited mutations

Intrinsic Tumor Suppression
- Repair
- Senescence
- Apoptosis

Innate and Adaptive Immunity
- Repair
- Senescence
- Apoptosis

- Perforin
- IFN-α/β
- IFN-γ
- TRAIL
- NGK2D
- IL-12

Elimination
Cancer immuno-surveillance

Equilibrium
Cancer persistence/dormancy

Escape
Cancer progression

J. Perkins
MS, MFA, CMI

AUTOIMMUNE AND PARANEOPLASTIC NEUROLOGIC SYNDROMES

Autoimmune neurologic syndromes are subacute, progressive syndromes with associated neural autoantibodies that serve as diagnostic biomarkers and in some circumstances are pathogenic. The neurologic manifestations can involve the central and peripheral nervous systems, muscle, and neuromuscular junction. Some of these autoimmune neurologic disorders occur because of the body's immune response to a neoplasm and are therefore referred to as *paraneoplastic neurologic syndromes* (PNSs) and can precede initial tumor recognition or recurrence by months to years.

A neoplasm arises through a complex set of germline variations, tissue-specific genetic mutations, and environmental interactions, resulting in a process of tissue transformation. The immune response to a tumor is a complex interaction that evolves during tumor development and varies with tumor type, organ involvement, and the individual. This can be conceptualized as immunoediting with three phases: elimination, equilibrium and escape.

Elimination occurs when senescence, apoptosis, and innate and adaptive immune responses combine to restore the tissue to health, eliminating the neoplasm. Equilibrium is when the neoplasm fails to progress without any clinical effort (surgery, radiotherapy, chemotherapy) to suppress or remove it due to a competent immune response. Clinically, such neoplasms may be undetectable, occult, or detectable, yet at limited early-stage disease. Escape is when the neoplasm undergoes further genetic and epigenetic mutations and modifications to become less immunogenic and/or more locally immunosuppressive and escapes immune control. Clinically, such neoplasms may be undetectable, occult, or

Immune Effectors	Immune Dysregulation
- Macrophages	- Th17/IL-17, IL-22
- CD8 T cells	- B10/IL-10
- CD4 T cells	- CD4 CD25 FoxP3 Treg
- Treg	- STAT 4 vs. STAT 6
- Killer T cells	- Genetic/epigenetic
- B cells	variation
- Antibodies	- CTLA4
- Cytokines	- PD-1/B7-H1 (PD-L1)

Nervous System Immune-Mediated Injury
- Mechanisms of immune effector access to specific nervous system targets largely unknown
- Specificity of nervous system targets likely related to molecular mimicry between nervous system antigens and tumor antigens processed via antigen-presenting cells
- Multiple levels of the nervous system may be affected simultaneously or at different points in time
- Multiple autoantibody markers present simultaneously
- In some cases may be associated with better tumor prognosis
- In some instances autoantibodies may be directly involved in pathogenesis; better prognosis for immunotherapy compared to intracellular
- Non-antibody immune-mediated tissue injury likely irreversible; early identification and intervention critical

detectable, yet at limited early-stage disease at any of these stages of immune response.

Paraneoplastic autoimmunity occurs when the immune system is activated against proteins (antigens) expressed on both cancer cells and neural tissue (onconeural antigens). Local tissue DCs and other APCs process these antigens and present them to naive T cells that are then activated and differentiate and proliferate. This subsequently leads to the activation of cytotoxic T cells and CD4 helper cells that differentiate into plasma cells and produce autoantibodies. The pattern of immune activation toward Th1, Th2, Th17, and T regulatory cells (Treg), governed by the cytokine

milieu, dictates the effects of the immune response. The paraneoplastic autoantibodies available for clinical measurement only represent a subset of those generated by the body's immune response to the neoplasm.

The development of autoimmunity is also regulated by immune effector access across the blood-brain or peripheral nerve barrier and multiple immune checkpoints. These include but are not limited to the status of regional and systemic Treg, Th17 mediators, regulatory B cells (B10 via IL-10), relative activation of STAT 4 versus STAT 6 transcription factors, genetic and epigenetic variation regulating any given individual's immune response and generation of tolerance, the

Autoantibody	Antigen Location	Commonly Associated Symptoms/Syndromes	Commonly Associated Neoplasms	Neoplasm Found (%)
ANNA-1 (anti-Hu)	Intracellular	Sensory neuronopathies, gastrointestinal pseudo-obstruction, encephalomyelitis, subacute cerebellar degeneration, limbic encephalitis	Small cell lung cancer, thymoma, neuroblastoma	~87
ANNA-2 (anti-Ri)	Intracellular	Brainstem/cerebellar syndrome (including opsoclonus myoclonus), movement disorders (e.g., jaw opening dystonia)	Breast carcinoma, small and non–small cell lung cancer	~86
ANNA-3	Intracellular	Myelopathy, brainstem and limbic encephalitis, neuropathies	Small cell lung cancer	90
PCA-1 (anti-Yo)	Intracellular	Cerebellar ataxia	Breast, fallopian tube, endometrial and ovarian carcinoma	>90
PCA-2	Intracellular	Encephalomyelitis, cerebellar ataxia, sensorimotor neuropathy	Small and non–small cell lung cancer, breast cancer	80
PCA-Tr	Intracellular	Cerebellar/brainstem syndrome	Hodgkin lymphoma	90
Ma-1 (anti-Ma)	Intracellular	Diencephalitis, limbic or brainstem encephalitis, cerebellar dysfunction, ophthalmoplegia	Lung, breast, colon, and renal cancer; non-Hodgkin lymphoma	>75
Ma-2 (anti-Ma2/Ta)	Intracellular		Testicular, breast, ovarian, and lung cancer; non-Hodgkin lymphoma	>75
Amphiphysin	Intracellular	Stiff person syndrome, polyradiculoneuropathy, encephalomyelitis, sensory neuronopathy	Breast carcinoma, small cell lung cancer	>80
CRMP-5 (anti-CV2)	Intracellular	Encephalomyelitis, sensory neuronopathy, myelopathy, cerebellar degeneration, movement disorders (e.g., chorea), optic neuropathy	Small cell lung cancer, thymoma, thyroid carcinoma	>80
KLHL11	Intracellular	Brainstem/cerebellar syndrome	Testicular cancer (e.g., seminoma), teratoma	80
GAD65	Intracellular	Stiff person syndrome, cerebellar ataxia, temporal lobe epilepsy, limbic encephalitis	Small cell lung cancer, thymoma	<15
NMDA-R	Extracellular	Limbic encephalitis, cortical encephalitis, striatal encephalitis	Ovarian teratoma	25-50
LGI1	Extracellular	Limbic encephalitis, seizures (particularly faciobrachial dystonic seizures)	Thymoma	<5-10
CASPR2	Extracellular	Limbic encephalitis, Morvan syndrome (neuromyotonia, memory and sleep disturbances, autonomic instability), neuropathic pain	Thymoma, lung cancer, endometrial adenocarcinoma	<5 overall, but 40–50 with Morvan syndrome
Glycine-R	Extracellular	PERM, stiff person syndrome	Thymoma, Hodgkin lymphoma, metastatic breast cancer	10
GABA$_A$-R	Extracellular	Cortical encephalitis with high seizure burden (including status epilepticus)	Thymoma, non-Hodgkin lymphoma, small cell lung cancer, rectal cancer	~20
GABA$_B$-R	Extracellular	Limbic encephalitis with high seizure burden (including status epilepticus)	Small cell lung cancer	50
AMPAR	Extracellular	Limbic encephalitis	Small cell lung cancer, breast cancer, thymic cancer, ovarian cancer	~50
mGluR1	Extracellular	Cerebellar ataxia	Hodgkin lymphoma	30
mGluR5	Extracellular	Encephalitis	Hodgkin lymphoma, small cell lung cancer	~50
DPPX	Extracellular	PERM, encephalitis, hyperekplexia	B-cell neoplasms (e.g., GI follicular lymphoma and chronic lymphocytic leukemia)	<10
IgLON5	Extracellular	Extrapyramidal features, parasomnias, bulbar dysfunction	—	Unknown

ANNA = antineuronal nuclear autoantibody; PCA = Purkinje cell cytoplasmic autoantibody; CRMP-5 = collapsin-response mediator protein 5; KLHL11 = Kelch-like protein 11; GAD65 = glutamic acid decarboxylase 65; NMDA-R = anti-N-methyl-D-aspartate receptor; LGI1 = anti-leucine-rich glioma inactivated 1; CASPR2 = contactin-associated protein-like 2; Glycine-R = glycine receptor; GABA-R = gamma-aminobutyric acid receptor; AMPAR = α-amino-3-hydroxy-5-methylisoxazole-4-proprionic acid receptor; mGluR = metabotropic glutamate receptor; DPPX = dipeptidyl peptidase-like protein 6; IgLON5 = immunoglobulin-like cell adhesion molecule 5; PERM = progressive encephalomyelitis with rigidity and myoclonus.

AUTOIMMUNE AND PARANEOPLASTIC NEUROLOGIC SYNDROMES (Continued)

status of important negative regulators of immune activation such as CTLA-4, and programmed cell death 1 (PD-1) and its ligand B7-H1 (or PD-L1).

New cancer treatments—such as *immune checkpoint inhibitors* (ICIs)—take advantage of these immune checkpoint molecules (PD-1/PD-L1, CTLA-4) by blocking their expression in T lymphocytes and tumor cells in an effort to enhance the immune system's ability to fight neoplasms. These therapies have led to improved remission rates and survival because of this augmentation of the immune system; however, they are also associated with a risk of developing immune-related adverse events and PNSs.

Paraneoplastic autoantibodies against intracellular neural antigens (nuclear or cytoplasmic components) are biomarkers of the antitumor immune response and are not necessarily directly pathogenic. Some paraneoplastic autoantibodies can be associated with specific syndromic presentations, but can vary from one patient to another despite the presence of the same autoantibody profile. Therefore paraneoplastic autoantibodies are often more predictive of a cancer type versus a neurologic syndrome.

Autoimmune neurologic syndromes also occur in the setting of autoantibodies against extracellular antigens (cell surface proteins, neurotransmitter receptors). These extracellular autoantibodies cause neuronal dysfunction via functional blocking of a receptor, internalization of receptors, and disruption of interactions between proteins, leading to receptor dysfunction. Although some extracellular autoantibodies have paraneoplastic associations (e.g., anti-NMDA-R-IgG encephalitis associated with ovarian teratoma and

anti-GABA$_B$-R and anti-AMPAR encephalitis and AMPA-R-IgG encephalitis associated with small cell lung cancer), many autoimmune neurologic disorders with extracellular autoantibodies are not associated with tumors. Some extracellular autoantibodies without paraneoplastic associations occur in the postinfectious setting. An example of this is anti-NMDA-R encephalitis that can develop after herpes simplex virus (HSV) infection. It is postulated that NMDA-R autoantibodies develop via molecular mimicry between HSV proteins and the NMDA-R or that viral-induced neuronal destruction leads to antigen release, followed by B- and T-lymphocyte exposure to these processed antigens in

regional lymph nodes and, ultimately, the development of autoantibodies (see Plates 10.21 and 10.22).

Some extracellular autoantibodies also have a component of genetic susceptibility. For instance, associations between leucine-rich glioma-inactivated 1 (LGI1-IgG) and the HLA-DRB1*07:01 allele, contactin-associated protein-like 2 (CASPR2-IgG) and HLA allele DRB1*11:01, and immunoglobulin-like cell adhesion molecule 5 (IgLON5-IgG) and the HLA-DRB1*-DQB1*05:01 allele have been identified. These HLA associations suggest an interplay between genetics and possibly other environmental triggers in autoimmune neurologic disorders.

Plate 10.21

Brain: PART I

AUTOIMMUNE NEUROLOGIC SYNDROMES: CENTRAL AND PERIPHERAL NERVOUS SYSTEM MANIFESTATIONS

CEREBRAL CORTEX AND LIMBIC SYSTEM

Limbic encephalitis is a clinical syndrome characterized by cognitive impairment, seizures, and behavioral abnormalities and may occur as a primary autoimmune or paraneoplastic condition. The most commonly associated neoplasm is small cell lung cancer (SCLC). Several autoantibody biomarkers are associated with this syndrome, including NMDA-R-IgG, LGI1-IgG, AMPA-R-IgG, GABA$_B$-R-IgG, CASPR2-IgG, GAD65-IgG, antineuronal nuclear antibody type 1 (ANNA-1/Hu-IgG), Ma2-IgG, anti-DPPX-IgG, and metabotropic glutamate receptor 5 (mGluR5-IgG). Other levels of the neuroaxis are frequently clinically involved when associated with a paraneoplastic autoantibody. *Cortical encephalitis* is less common but can occur with GABA$_A$-R-IgG and with MOG-IgG.

One of the most frequently encountered examples of limbic encephalitis is anti-NMDA-R encephalitis. In this condition, autoantibodies bind to the NR1 subunit of the NMDA receptor, causing neuronal dysfunction. This disorder is characterized by a subacute onset neuropsychiatric presentation with agitation, psychosis, hallucinations, and delusions. Females are more commonly affected, primarily in the first 3 decades of life. Manifestations can also include dyskinesias (particularly orofacial), echolalia, and periods of catatonia-like akinesis. Patients often develop seizures and may have a characteristic extreme delta brush pattern on an electroencephalogram with generalized rhythmic slowing and overriding fast activity. Autonomic instability and central hypoventilation requiring prolonged ventilatory support are common and, in combination with ongoing seizure activity, can result in a decreased level of consciousness or coma within weeks. Anti-NMDA-R encephalitis is associated with ovarian teratoma in women of childbearing age and in some cases post-HSV encephalitis.

Anti-leucine glioma-inactivated 1 encephalitis is another frequently encountered limbic encephalitis. This disorder typically presents with subacute cognitive decline, seizures, and hyponatremia, particularly in older males. The typical seizure phenotype is faciobrachial dystonic seizures with brief dystonic contractions of the face and arm lasting seconds. MRI brain may show T2/FLAIR hyperintensities of the temporal lobe(s). It is associated with thymoma in approximately 5% to 10% of cases.

DIENCEPHALON

Diencephalitis can present with excessive daytime sleepiness and cataplexy secondary to hypothalamic dysfunction, in addition to hyperthermia and hyperphagia. It is a feature of an anti-Ma2 PNS and typically occurs in males with underlying testicular germ cell tumors. CSF hypocretin levels may be low or undetectable. Patients can have concurrent limbic and brainstem encephalitis, resulting in seizures, ophthalmoplegia, and ataxia.

BASAL GANGLIA AND EXTRAPYRAMIDAL SYSTEM

Patients with autoimmune neurologic syndromes may present with movement disorders as part of a multifocal

CENTRAL NERVOUS SYSTEM: PARANEOPLASTIC

NMDA anti-NMDA-R encephalitis, young woman with ovarian teratoma

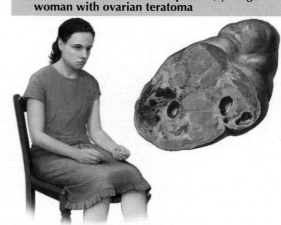

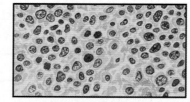

Limbic encephalitis with small cell lung cancer

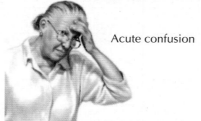

Acute confusion

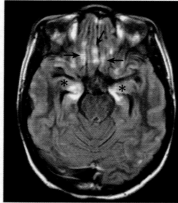

Axial FLAIR T2 MRI photomicrograph showing lesions in the bilateral hippocampus (*stars*) and orbitofrontal cortex (*arrows*) seen in limbic encephalitis

Ataxic man with small cell lung cancer

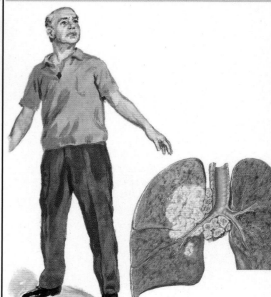

SPS in a women with breast cancer

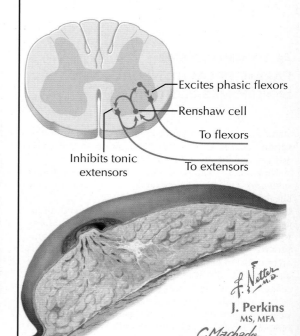

Excites phasic flexors
Renshaw cell
To flexors
Inhibits tonic extensors
To extensors

J. Perkins
MS, MFA

CNS disorder involving the extrapyramidal system. Choreiform movements can occur with collapsin response-mediator protein (CRMP-5-IgG) often in association with SCLC or thymoma. Less frequently, choreiform movements can be seen in patients with anti-LGI1, CASPR2, and GAD65 autoimmune neurologic disorders. Anti-NMDA-R encephalitis is associated with orofacial dyskinesias, although various parts of the body may be involved, as well as dystonia and chorea.

IgLON5-IgG may present with extrapyramidal features, including gait instability and supranuclear gaze palsy resembling progressive supranuclear palsy. Other features include sleep disorders such as parasomnia and sleep-disordered breathing (sleep apnea, stridor), as well as bulbar symptoms (dysphagia, dysarthria).

AUTOIMMUNE NEUROLOGIC SYNDROMES: CENTRAL AND PERIPHERAL NERVOUS SYSTEM MANIFESTATIONS (Continued)

Autopsy studies have demonstrated a tauopathy, suggestive of a neurodegenerative process.

CEREBELLUM

Subacute cerebellar ataxia can present with double vision, nystagmus, dysarthria, and limb and gait ataxia. This is the most common manifestation in patients seropositive for anti-PCA/anti-Yo. This PNS is associated with female malignancies such as breast and gynecologic cancers. Patients develop global cerebellar degeneration, resulting in a severe axial and appendicular ataxia, with a subset of patients developing bulbar symptoms because of concurrent brainstem involvement.

Kelch-like protein 11 (KLHL11-IgG), CRMP-5-IgG, ANNA-1/Hu-IgG, ANNA-2/Ri-IgG, PCA-Tr-IgG, Ma2-IgG, and mGluR1-IgG have also been associated with paraneoplastic cerebellar degeneration, and CASPR2-IgG can cause an episodic ataxia syndrome.

BRAINSTEM

Autoimmune brainstem encephalitis or *rhombencephalitis* can be seen with PNS including KLHL11-IgG, ANNA-1-IgG, ANNA-2-IgG, and Ma2-IgG and may present with subacute onset of ophthalmoplegia, vertigo, ataxia, and bulbar palsy. Opsoclonus-myoclonus-ataxia syndrome is a feature of rhombencephalitis and manifests as involuntary multidirectional saccades in addition to ataxic gait, myoclonus, and tremor. It is commonly associated with SCLC in adults. PNS with ANNA-1/Hu-IgG can present with lower brainstem symptoms including dysphagia, dysarthria, cranial nerve palsies, and central hypoventilation from medullary involvement.

Cochleovestibulopathy with rapid-onset sensorineural hearing loss and vestibular dysfunction, as well as other brainstem symptoms, including vertigo, tinnitus, dysarthria, and gaze palsy, can be observed in PNS with KLHL11-IgG, commonly associated with testicular seminoma.

OPTIC NERVES

Paraneoplastic *optic neuropathy* can be observed in CRMP-5-IgG in association with SCLC. Patients present with subacute vision loss that is painless and insidious, at times bilateral, and often without evidence of optic nerve enhancement on MRI. Most patients have an associated iritis, retinitis, or vitritis in addition to their optic neuropathy. Glial fibrillary acidic protein (GFAP-IgG) autoimmunity can present with a painless optic neuropathy with bilaterally symmetric optic disc edema, often with concurrent meningoencephalitis and/or myelitis.

SPINAL CORD

Subacute onset myelopathy is associated with several different cancers and cancer-specific autoantibodies. It typically presents symmetrically, with longitudinally extensive long-tract or GM–specific MRI changes. Motor involvement can be severe, especially the necrotizing variant, and a distinct cord level is often found on

clinical exam. This is observed with CRMP-5-IgG and SCLC and less commonly with amphiphysin-IgG and ANNA-1-IgG.

GFAP-IgG autoimmunity can present with myelitis as part of a multifocal *meningoencephalomyelitis.* Patients often present with a prodromal flu-like illness followed by signs of meningeal irritation (neck stiffness, headache, vomiting), ataxia, and myelitis. GFAP-IgG autoimmune myelitis can be longitudinally extensive, and CSF may show marked inflammation with a

lymphocyte-predominant pleocytosis and elevated protein. In many patients, MRI of the brain classically demonstrates radial perivascular enhancement extending out from the ventricles.

SPSD occurs with GAD65-IgG and GlyR-IgG. The mechanism of SPSD likely involves dysfunction of the GABAergic and glycinergic inhibitory interneurons in the spinal cord and brainstem. Patients can present with truncal and limb stiffness, spasms, and an exaggerated startle. They often have hyperactive

PERIPHERAL MOTOR SENSORY UNIT: PARANEOPLASTIC

Subacute sensory neuropathy

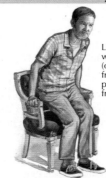

Gray matter
White matter
Filaments of dorsal root
Dorsal root of spinal n.
Filaments of ventral root
Spinal sensory (dorsal root) ganglion
Ventral root of spinal n.
Ventral ramus of spinal n.

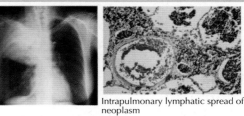

Intrapulmonary lymphatic spread of neoplasm

Lambert-Eaton myasthenic syndrome in bronchogenic small cell carcinoma

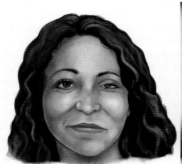

Lambert-Eaton myasthenic syndrome; weakness of proximal muscle groups (often manifested by difficulty in rising from chair); compound muscle action potential facilitation with high frequency motor nerve stimulation

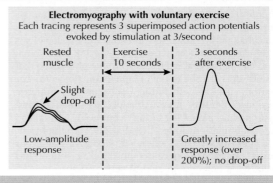

Electromyography with voluntary exercise
Each tracing represents 3 superimposed action potentials evoked by stimulation at 3/second

Rested muscle | Exercise 10 seconds | 3 seconds after exercise

Slight drop-off

Low-amplitude response | Greatly increased response (over 200%); no drop-off

Myasthenia gravis thymoma

Thymus gland abnormality in myasthenia gravis

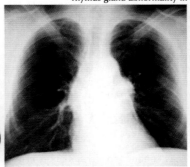

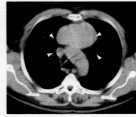

CT scan clearly demonstrates same large tumor anterior to aortic arch *(arrowheads).*

Radiograph showing large mediastinal tumor, which localized to anterior compartment (not shown)

Dermatomyositis and typical rash

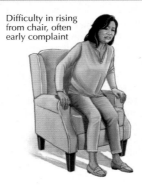

Difficulty in rising from chair, often early complaint

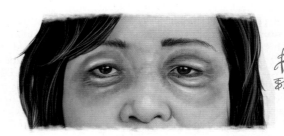

Edema and heliotrope discoloration around eyes a classic sign; more widespread erythematous rash may also be present

AUTOIMMUNE NEUROLOGIC SYNDROMES: CENTRAL AND PERIPHERAL NERVOUS SYSTEM MANIFESTATIONS
(Continued)

abdominal and paraspinal muscles and a loss of lumbar lordosis. PERM is a more widespread disorder with encephalopathy, bulbar dysfunction, and myelopathy.

Myeloneuropathy, a syndrome involving both spinal cord and peripheral nerves, is a unique phenotype that results in a combination of upper and lower motor neuron features, including subacute asymmetric weakness, sensory ataxia, bladder dysfunction, and neuropathic pain. The most commonly associated autoantibodies include CRMP5-IgG, amphiphysin-IgG, and ANNA-1-IgG, often with underlying SCLC or breast cancer. MRI may demonstrate T2 spinal cord lesions and nerve root enhancement.

PERIPHERAL NERVES

Motor neuronopathies rarely occur, most often in the context of lymphoma and as part of multifocal PNS. These paraneoplastic neuronopathies tend to be subacute in onset, with a lower motor neuron predominance and an inflammatory CSF profile. Concurrent nonmotor manifestations and specific autoantibody profiles distinguish these motor neuronopathies from amyotrophic lateral sclerosis.

Multifocal motor neuropathy presents with painless, progressive asymmetric weakness and fasciculations in the setting of GM1 ganglioside autoantibodies. The electrophysiologic hallmark of this disorder is conduction block at noncompressible sites.

Paranodal and nodal autoantibodies have been observed in demyelinating polyradiculoneuropathy, also referred to as *nodo-paranodopathies.* These disorders have clinical features similar to chronic inflammatory demyelinating polyradiculopathy (CIDP). Patients with NF155-IgG4 present with chronic distal greater than proximal weakness predominantly affecting the lower limbs. Other clinical features include painful paresthesias, cranial neuropathies, cerebellar ataxia, and action tremor, as well as autonomic dysfunction. MRI may reveal symmetric enlargement of the lumbosacral roots. Contactin-1-IgG is a more rapidly progressive demyelinating paraneoplastic nodopathy, occurring within weeks, with a sensory-predominant presentation, ataxia, and neuropathic pain.

Subacute sensory neuronopathy affecting the dorsal root and autonomic ganglia is distinguished clinically by the involvement of the face, trunk, and extremities, in contrast to a classic distal-predominant sensory peripheral neuropathy. Patients develop widespread sensory ataxia with loss of proprioception, pseudoathetosis, and diffuse hyporeflexia. They may also report severe pain and hyperalgesia. EMG demonstrates the widespread absence of peripheral sensory nerve action potentials. Subacute sensory neuronopathy is a classical presentation of ANNA-1/Hu-IgG PNS in the setting of SCLC.

Sensory neuropathy is a common paraneoplastic accompaniment. However, polyneuropathy can sometimes be multifactorial in the setting of metastatic disease, radiotherapy and chemotherapy effects, and metabolic disorders. Axonal neuropathy/polyradiculopathy can be seen with various autoantibodies including CRMP5-IgG, ANNA-1-IgG, amphiphysin-IgG, ANNA-2/Ri-IgG, and PCA-2/MAP1B-IgG.

Peripheral nervous syndrome hyperexcitability may present with neuromyotonia or spontaneous and continuous muscle fiber activity, as well as a painful polyneuropathy. Peripheral nerve hyperexcitability can occur with CASPR2-IgG, and a subgroup of patients have Morvan syndrome with concurrent sleep disorders (insomnia, rapid eye movement sleep behaviors) and encephalopathy.

ICIs such as anti-PD-1 (nivolumab, pembrolizumab) and anti-CTLA-4 (ipilimumab) may augment autoimmune neurologic disorders and result in immune-related neurologic adverse events including peripheral neuropathy, polyradiculoneuropathy, and cranial neuropathy.

Several other immune-mediated neuropathies are covered in other chapters, including monoclonal protein-associated neuropathies, vasculitic neuropathies, neuropathies associated with connective tissue disorders, Guillain-Barré syndrome, and CIDP.

AUTONOMIC NERVOUS SYSTEM

Autonomic neuropathy or ganglionopathy can occur as a paraneoplastic or primary autoimmune disorder. Orthostatic hypotension, anhidrosis, dry mouth, erectile dysfunction, heart rate irregularity, and GI dysmotility are variably present. Cancer-attributed symptoms, including cachexia, anorexia, early satiety, postprandial abdominal pain, and vomiting, may also contribute to gastroparesis or severe constipation.

Autoimmune autonomic ganglionopathy can be associated with high titers for ganglionic nicotinic acetylcholine receptor (gAChR-IgG) and is often severe and disabling. It presents in a subacute progressive and monophasic pattern, with orthostasis and lower GI dysfunction being the most commonly reported symptoms.

Chronic intestinal pseudo-obstruction is a paraneoplastic enteric neuropathy that presents with symptoms of large bowel obstruction (abdominal pain, nausea, vomiting, and constipation) and radiologic evidence of large bowel dilatation despite the absence of a true anatomic obstruction. This syndrome is associated with gAChR-IgG or ANNA-1/anti-Hu-IgG.

NEUROMUSCULAR JUNCTION

LEMS is a disorder of presynaptic cholinergic neuromuscular junction transmission classically resulting in proximal limb weakness and sometimes bulbar and extraocular muscle dysfunction. Typically, weakness briefly improves within seconds of forceful voluntary muscle activation, and symptoms initially may exceed physical examination findings. Electromyographic characteristics and seropositivity for neuronal calcium (Ca^{2+}) channel autoantibodies distinguish presynaptic LEMS from postsynaptic myasthenia gravis. High-titer P/Q-type Ca^{2+} channel autoantibody is a specifically pathogenic, mediating presynaptic surface channel alteration that distinguishes LEMS from other paraneoplastic disorders.

SCLC is found in 60% of patients with LEMS, and LEMS clinically affects 1% to 2% of patients with SCLC, despite the frequency of P/Q-type Ca^{2+} channel autoantibody positivity being higher. Profound dysautonomia, especially if gastrointestinal motility is impaired, may indicate a coexistent ANNA-1-IgG.

Myasthenia gravis (MG) is a postsynaptic disorder of nicotinic acetylcholine receptor function at the neuromuscular junction. Fatigable ptosis, diplopia, and motor weakness are characteristic. Thymoma occurs in 10% to 15% of cases. Autoantibodies directed at the extracellular muscle AChR domain are pathogenic in MG. Autoantibodies modulating the AChR, as well as autoantibodies directed against muscle-specific tyrosine kinase IgG, may be present in patients with ocular and bulbar predominant symptoms.

MUSCLE

Inflammatory myopathy can present with subacute proximal limb weakness, muscle pain, and elevated serum creatine kinase. EMG demonstrates small-amplitude, short-duration polyphasic motor units and abnormal spontaneous electrical activity. Cancer coexists in ~15% of patients with dermatomyositis and less frequently in polymyositis. Symptoms and signs are indistinguishable in paraneoplastic and nonparaneoplastic forms, although skin lesions (Gottron papules, heliotrope rash, photodistributed poikiloderma), rapid onset, and older age provide clues to paraneoplastic dermatomyositis. Multiple dermatomyositis-related autoantibodies exist, with anti-Mi-2 being the most classically associated, whereas anti-TIF-1γ is most highly correlated with malignancy. Antisynthetase syndrome can result in an antibody-mediated inflammatory myopathy, often associated with severe interstitial lung disease and anti-Jo-1. Polymyositis and dermatomyositis are covered in further detail in their respective chapters.

Acute necrotizing myopathy presents with a severe inflammatory myopathy with rare extramuscular involvement. It is rarely associated with cancer. Autoantibodies associated with this disorder include autoantibodies to signal recognition particle, as well as anti-HMG-CoA. Coincidental association with statin use is important to recognize, because some but not all patients will have been exposed to statin medication.

ICIs used in cancer treatment are associated with immune-mediated myopathies, including necrotizing myopathy, polymyositis, dermatomyositis, granulomatous myositis, necrotizing myopathy, and nonspecific myopathy.

INFECTIONS OF THE NERVOUS SYSTEM

Plate 11.1

Brain: PART I

BACTERIAL MENINGITIS

Most common causative organisms

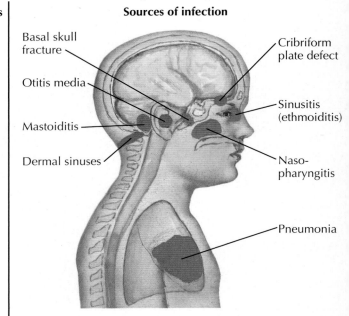

Sources of infection

Basal skull fracture

Otitis media

Mastoiditis

Dermal sinuses

Cribriform plate defect

Sinusitis (ethmoiditis)

Naso-pharyngitis

Pneumonia

Infection of leptomeninges is usually hematogenous but may be direct from the paranasal sinuses, middle ear, mastoid cells, or CSF leak from cribriform plate defect or via dermal sinuses.

In neonates

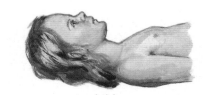
Gram-negative bacilli
(*E. coli, Klebsiella pneumoniae*, etc.)

Group B streptococci

Other (*S. aureus, Listeria monocytogenes, H. influenzae*, etc.)

In children

N. meningitidis
S. pneumoniae

Other (*Listeria* spp., etc.)

In adults

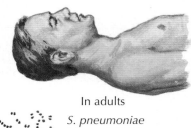
S. pneumoniae
N. meningitidis

Gram-negative bacilli

Other (*Listeria* spp., etc.)

Diagnosis

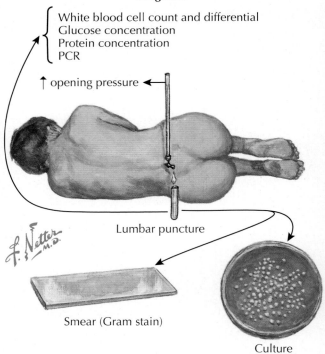

White blood cell count and differential
Glucose concentration
Protein concentration
PCR

↑ opening pressure

Lumbar puncture

Smear (Gram stain)

Culture

BACTERIAL MENINGITIS

PATHOPHYSIOLOGY

Bacterial meningitis is initially an acute purulent infection of the meninges and subarachnoid space that is followed by an inflammatory reaction in the subarachnoid space, the brain parenchyma, and the cerebral arteries (arteritis) and veins (dural sinus thrombosis and thrombophlebitis). Meningitis is most often the result of bacterial invasion of the subarachnoid space from hematogenous dissemination. Bacterial meningitis may be preceded by colonization of the nasopharynx by the organism or develop as a complication of pneumonia, acute otitis media, acute sinusitis, endocarditis, skull fracture, a neurosurgical procedure, or the use of a catheter to decrease intracranial pressure or administer chemotherapeutic or antimicrobial agents.

The meningeal pathogen can be predicted by the patient's age. In neonates, the most common pathogens are group B streptococci (*Streptococcus agalactiae),* gram-negative bacilli, and *Listeria monocytogenes*. In children, adolescents, and adults, the most common causative organisms of community-acquired bacterial meningitis are *Neisseria meningitidis* and *Streptococcus pneumoniae*. *L. monocytogenes* is a causative organism of meningitis in individuals with impaired cell-mediated immunity due to organ transplantation, chronic illness, pregnancy, acquired immunodeficiency syndrome (AIDS), malignancy, immunosuppressive therapy, or age. When meningitis complicates acute otitis media, mastoiditis, or sinusitis, the causative organisms are *Streptococci* spp., gram-negative anaerobes, *S. aureus, Haemophilus* sp., or Enterobacteriaceae. Meningitis in the postneurosurgical patient and the patient with a ventriculostomy or other indwelling catheter may be due to staphylococci, gram-negative bacilli, or anaerobes.

Clinical Manifestations. The signs and symptoms of meningitis in the neonate include irritability, lethargy, poor feeding, vomiting, diarrhea, temperature instability, respiratory distress, apnea, seizures, and a bulging fontanel. The signs and symptoms of bacterial meningitis in children, adolescents, and adults include fever, vomiting, photophobia, headache, nuchal rigidity (meningismus), and a decreased level of consciousness ranging from lethargy to stupor, obtundation, or coma.

On physical examination, the classic sign of bacterial meningitis is meningismus, but this sign is not invariably present. The neck resists passive flexion. Kernig sign and Brudzinski sign are also signs of meningeal irritation (see Plate 11.2). Both signs are elicited with

the patient in the supine position. To elicit the Kernig sign, the thigh is flexed on the abdomen with the knee flexed. Attempts to passively extend the leg elicit pain and are met with resistance when meningeal irritation is present. The Brudzinski sign is positive when passive flexion of the neck results in spontaneous flexion of the hips and knees. The presence of a petechial rash on the trunk and lower extremities, in the mucous membranes and conjunctiva, and occasionally on the palms and

soles is typical of the rash of meningococcemia. A petechial rash is not seen in all cases of meningococcal meningitis, and a petechial rash is rarely seen in *H. influenzae,* pneumococcal, and staphylococcal meningitis. Patients with enteroviral meningitis may also have a rash, but this is an erythematous maculopapular rash that involves the face and neck early in infection.

Diagnosis. The gold standard for the diagnosis of bacterial meningitis is analysis of the cerebrospinal

Plate 11.2

Infections of the Nervous System

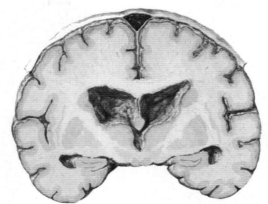

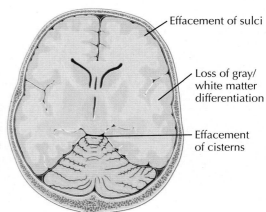

Effacement of sulci

Loss of gray/
white matter
differentiation

Effacement
of cisterns

Thrombophlebitis of superior sagittal sinus and
suppurative ependymitis, with beginning
hydrocephalus

Diffuse cerebral edema

BACTERIAL MENINGITIS
(Continued)

fluid (CSF). A computed tomography (CT) scan should
be obtained in the patient with any of the following: an
altered level of consciousness, papilledema, a focal neurologic deficit, new-onset seizure activity, immunocompromised state, a dilated or poorly reactive pupil,
signs of a posterior fossa mass lesion (cranial nerve
[CN] abnormalities, cerebellar deficit, and a wide-
based ataxic gait), or a risk for neurocysticercosis. The
classic abnormalities in bacterial meningitis on examination of the CSF are the following: (1) an opening
pressure greater than 180 mm H$_2$O, (2) an increased
white blood cell count with a predominance of polymorphonuclear leukocytes, (3) a decreased glucose
concentration (<40 mg/dL), (4) an increased protein
concentration, and (5) a positive Gram stain and bacterial culture. Gram stain is positive in identifying the
organism in 60% to 90% of cases of bacterial meningitis. The probability of detecting bacteria on a Gram-
stained specimen depends on the number of organisms
present. The CSF bacterial polymerase chain reaction
(PCR) detects bacterial nucleic acid in CSF. The CSF
meningitis pathogen panel that is most commonly used
detects the nucleic acid of *S. pneumoniae, N. meningitidis, L. monocytogenes, E.coli, H. influenzae,* and *S. agalactiae.* The sensitivity and specificity of the CSF meningitis pathogen panel has not been defined. The PCR
assay is most useful in rapidly distinguishing between
bacterial and viral meningitis because the panel also
tests for the nucleic acid of enteroviruses and herpes
simplex virus 2 (HSV-2). The PCR assay will not replace bacterial culture because culture is essential for
antimicrobial sensitivity testing.

The classic CSF abnormalities in viral meningitis are
(1) normal opening pressure, (2) lymphocytic pleocytosis, (3) normal glucose concentration, and (4) normal
or slightly elevated protein concentration. Enteroviruses can either be isolated in CSF culture or detected
in CSF by the reverse-transcriptase (RT) PCR. HSV-2
DNA can be detected in CSF by PCR. Human immunodeficiency virus-1 (HIV-1) RNA can be detected and
measured in CSF, and the virus can be cultured from
CSF. Viral immunoglobulin M (IgM) antibodies can be
detected in CSF.

In patients with a clinical presentation of meningitis and a CSF lymphocytic pleocytosis with a decreased glucose concentration, fungal infections,
Mycobacterium tuberculosis infection, sarcoidosis,

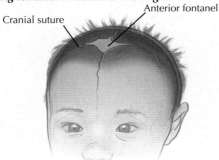

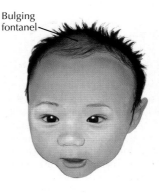

Kernig sign. Patient supine, with
hip flexed 90 degrees. Knee cannot be
fully extended.

**Neck rigidity (Brudzinski
neck sign).** Passive flexion
of neck causes flexion of
both legs and thighs.

Bulging fontanel in bacterial meningitis

Anterior fontanel

Cranial suture

Bulging
fontanel

and lymphoma/leptomeningeal metastases are in the
differential diagnosis. A subarachnoid hemorrhage
manifests with headache and a sudden transient loss
of consciousness. Examination of the spinal fluid will
reveal red blood cells and xanthochromia, although
it may take several hours for xanthochromia to
appear.

Treatment. When bacterial meningitis is suspected,
dexamethasone and empiric antimicrobial therapy are
begun immediately. The choice of empiric antimicrobial therapy depends on the suspected meningeal
pathogen, which is determined by the age of the patient

and predisposing or associated conditions. Once the
organism is identified and the results of antimicrobial
sensitivity testing are known, antimicrobial therapy is
modified accordingly.

Complications. The major complications of bacterial meningitis are focal and diffuse brain edema, hydrocephalus, arterial cerebrovascular complications
(ischemic and/or hemorrhagic stroke), septic sinus
thrombosis with thrombophlebitis, hearing loss and
vestibulopathy, and seizures. The complications of bacterial meningitis are the cause of the acute and chronic
neurologic deficits.

Plate 11.3   Brain: PART I

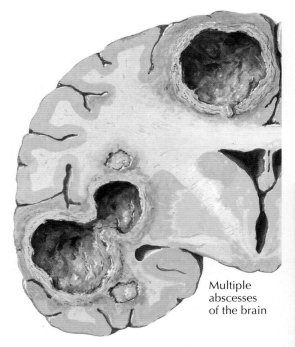

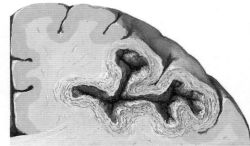

Scar of healed brain abscess, with
collapse of brain tissue into cavity

Multiple
abscesses
of the brain

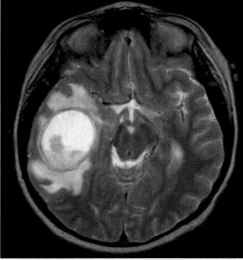

Axial T2 MRI showing large right temporal lobe
intracranial abscess (central T2 hyperintense
internal debris and peripheral T2 hypointense
capsule), with surrounding vagogenic edema

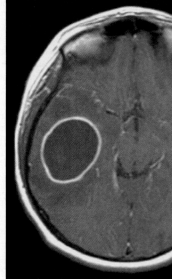

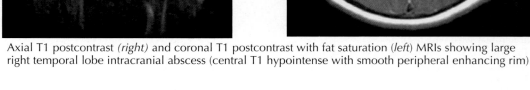

Axial T1 postcontrast *(right)* and coronal T1 postcontrast with fat saturation *(left)* MRIs showing large
right temporal lobe intracranial abscess (central T1 hypointense with smooth peripheral enhancing rim)

Brain Abscess

A brain abscess is a focal suppurative process that develops in the brain parenchyma in one of the following ways: (1) by direct spread from a contiguous cranial site of infection (paranasal sinusitis, mastoiditis, otitis media, or dental infections), (2) after cranial trauma, or (3) as a result of hematogenous spread from a remote site of infection (cyanotic congenital heart disease, endocarditis, lung abscess, intraabdominal infection). The most common etiologic organisms of a brain abscess are streptococci, *Bacteroides* spp., staphylococci (after trauma or craniotomy), *Fusobacterium* spp., *Haemophilus* spp., Enterobacteriaceae, and *Pseudomonas aeruginosa.* A brain abscess manifests with fever, headache, and a focal neurologic deficit. Headache is the most common symptom, but fever is not invariably present. As the area of cerebral edema surrounding the brain abscess increases, signs of increased intracranial pressure develop.

Magnetic resonance imaging (MRI) with contrast administration is the neuroimaging procedure of choice because MRI better demonstrates an abscess that is in the cerebritis stage than a cranial CT scan does. On T1-weighted MRI after the administration of

intravenous gadolinium, the abscess appears as a central area of hypointensity with a smooth peripheral enhancing rim. On T2-weighted MRI, the abscess appears as a hyperintense lesion surrounded by a hypointense capsule. A lumbar puncture is contraindicated. Aerobic and anaerobic blood cultures can be obtained, and a careful physical examination may identify the source of infection. Definitive diagnosis is made by CT- or MRI-guided stereotactic aspiration of the abscess for Gram staining and culture. Empiric antimicrobial therapy is typically started before the

results of Gram stain and culture are known and is based on the possible causative organism if the source of infection is known. Empiric therapy is modified once the results of Gram stain and bacterial culture and antimicrobial sensitivity testing are known. Corticosteroids are recommended in patients with significant edema but only for a short period of time because they decrease antibiotic penetration into the abscess cavity. Prophylactic antiepileptic medications are recommended because a brain abscess is an epileptogenic focus.

Plate 11.4

Infections of the Nervous System

Subdural abscess

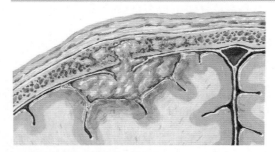

Osteomyelitis of skull, with penetration of dura to form subdural "collar button" abscess

Epidural abscess

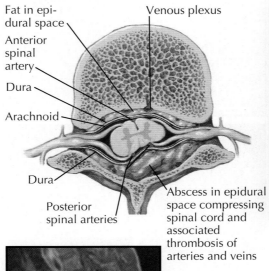

Fat in epidural space
Venous plexus
Anterior spinal artery
Dura
Arachnoid
Dura
Posterior spinal arteries
Abscess in epidural space compressing spinal cord and associated thrombosis of arteries and veins

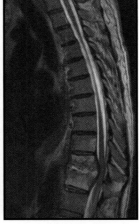

Sagittal T2 MRI showing extensive marrow edema, intervertebral disk space collapse, and cortical erosion at the T10–11 level, compatible with diskitis-osteomyelitis and associated ventral epidural abscess. Note marked resultant mass effect and compression of the mildly edematous distal thoracic spinal cord. Abnormal edema is also present within the T9 vertebral body.

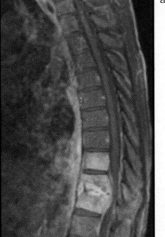

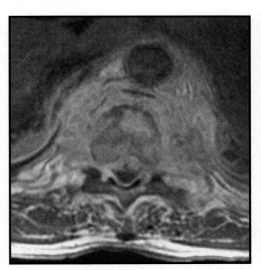

Sagittal T1 postcontrast with fat saturation *(left)* and axial T1 postcontrast *(right)* MRIs showing extensive abnormal enhancement within the bone marrow, intervertebral disk space, and anterior epidural space at the T10–11 level, compatible with diskitis-osteomyelitis and associated ventral epidural abscess. Note the marked resultant mass effect and compression of the distal thoracic spinal cord. The sagittal view shows abnormal enhancement also present within the T9 vertebral body. The axial view shows significant associated paravertebral phlegmon.

Parameningeal Infections

SUBDURAL EMPYEMA

A subdural empyema is a collection of pus in the space between the dura and the arachnoid. Paranasal sinusitis is the most common predisposing condition associated with a subdural empyema, but otitis media, mastoiditis, and a neurosurgical procedure may also be complicated by a subdural empyema. A subdural empyema that is a complication of sinusitis, otitis media, or mastoiditis is usually due to aerobic, microaerophilic, or anaerobic streptococci. Subdural empyemas that are a complication of a neurosurgical procedure are often due to staphylococci. The initial signs and symptoms of a subdural empyema are due to increased intracranial pressure from an expanding infectious mass lesion. Headache and fever are the initial symptoms, followed by focal neurologic deficits, seizures, and a decrease in the level of consciousness. A subdural empyema is a life-threatening infection because patients may have a rapid progression of neurologic deficits and altered level of consciousness. A subdural empyema is readily imaged by CT scan or MRI with contrast administration. The definitive step in the management of subdural empyema is surgical drainage and antimicrobial therapy. Empiric therapy with a combination of a third- or fourth-generation cephalosporin plus vancomycin and metronidazole is begun and then modified when the results of Gram stain and bacterial cultures and sensitivities are known.

SPINAL EPIDURAL ABSCESS

A spinal epidural abscess develops in the space outside the dura mater but within the spinal canal as a result of the hematogenous spread of infection from a remote site of infection or by direct extension from a contiguous infection, such as vertebral osteomyelitis, decubitus ulcers, or infected abdominal wounds. Neurologic deficits are the result of direct mechanical compression of the spinal cord and/or inflammatory thrombosis of the intraspinal vessels with subsequent ischemia and infarction. The initial symptom is back pain. Fever may be present. Back pain is followed by radicular pain, then weakness, then paralysis of appendicular musculature, loss of sensation below the level of the lesion, and loss of bowel and bladder control. MRI is the procedure of choice to demonstrate a spinal epidural abscess and a contiguous area of infection when present. If there is evidence of compression of the spinal cord from the epidural abscess, an emergency decompression with evacuation of pus and granulation tissue is performed. This also allows for identification of the causative organism and guides antimicrobial therapy. Empiric antimicrobial therapy is directed at the most common causative organisms, which are staphylococci (*S. aureus* and coagulase-negative staphylococci) and gram-negative bacilli.

Plate 11.5

Brain: PART I

PROGRESSIVE MULTIFOCAL LEUKOENCEPHALOPATHY AND NOCARDIOSIS

Progressive multifocal leukoencephalopathy (PML)

Coronal section of brain showing many minute demyelinating lesions in white matter, which have coalesced in some areas to form irregular cavitations

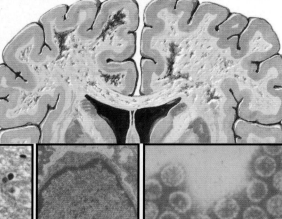

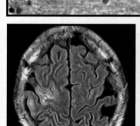

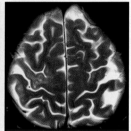

Abnormal oligodendro-cytes *(left)* with large hyper-chromatic nuclei, section from edge of demyelinated focus (hematoxylin and eosin stain)
Giant glial nucleus *(middle)* with inclusion bodies, electron micrograph
Polyomavirus virions *(right)* isolated from brain, electron micrograph

Axial FLAIR *(left)* and axial T2 *(right)* MRIs showing patchy abnormal hyperintense signal within the subcortical white matter of both (right > left) posterior frontal lobes (precentral gyri) and anterior right parietal lobe (post-central gyrus), with characteristic sparing of the subcortical U fibers

Nocardiosis

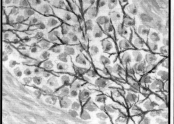

Multiple nocardial abscesses in brain

Branching hyphae of *Nocardia asteroides* in brain abscess (methenamine-silver stain)

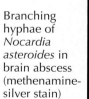

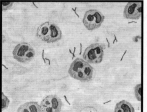

Modified acid-fast organisms as they may appear in pus, sputum, or tissues. They may be mistaken for tubercle bacilli but are actually fragmented nocardial hyphae.

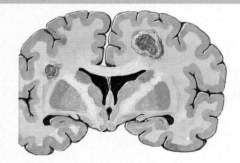

INFECTIONS IN THE IMMUNOCOMPROMISED HOST

Four central nervous system (CNS) infections are unique to the immunocompromised host: progressive multifocal leukoencephalopathy, brain abscess due to *Nocardia asteroides,* meningitis due to *L. monocytogenes,* and toxoplasmosis.

PROGRESSIVE MULTIFOCAL LEUKOENCEPHALOPATHY

Progressive multifocal leukoencephalopathy (PML) is a disease caused by the John Cunningham (JC) virus, a polyomavirus that is acquired in childhood. PML establishes latent infection in the kidneys and lymphoid organs, and it reactivates in the setting of cellular immunosuppression. Individuals at risk for PML are those with HIV infection, those with hematologic malignancies, and those treated with immunomodulatory therapy for relapsing-remitting multiple sclerosis. Because PML is a viral infection of oligodendrocytes causing focal areas of demyelination, the clinical presentation is that of focal or multifocal neurologic deficits, including hemianopsia, hemiparesis, or aphasia. On neuroimaging, the lesions are located in the subcortical hemispheric white matter, sparing the U fibers, and are typically not contrast enhancing and not surrounded by edema. The spinal fluid is similarly noninflammatory. There may be a slight increase in the white blood cell count and a mild elevation in the protein concentration. The diagnosis is made by demonstration of JC virus DNA by PCR of CSF or by brain biopsy. There is no specific antiviral therapy, and treatment is directed at reversing the immunosuppression, so-called *immune reconstitution.*

NOCARDIOSIS

N. asteroides is a gram-positive bacterium found in soil and decaying vegetables. This bacterium is a causative

organism of a brain abscess in individuals with impaired cell-mediated immunity. Risk factors include organ transplantation, immunosuppressive therapy, pulmonary alveolar proteinosis, sarcoidosis, and pregnancy. Unlike the primary management of the majority of bacterial brain abscesses by stereotactic aspiration guided by CT or MRI, a brain abscess due to *N. asteroides* requires surgical excision through a craniotomy. These are thick-walled multiloculated brain abscesses. The infection is treated with trimethoprim-sulfamethoxazole

or sulfonamide. Nocardial brain abscesses are relatively rare in individuals who are HIV positive because many of these individuals take trimethoprim-sulfamethoxazole to prevent *Pneumocystis carinii.*

LISTERIOSIS

L. monocytogenes is a gram-positive bacterium that causes meningitis in individuals who are immunocompromised from organ transplantation, malignancies,

Plate 11.6

Infections of the Nervous System

LISTERIOSIS AND TOXOPLASMOSIS

Listeriosis

Smear of CSF showing white blood cells and *Listeria* organisms, which appear as gram-positive rods. They may be very short, resemble cocci, and often orient in palisades suggestive of Chinese characters. They cause severe purulent meningitis, most commonly in immuno-compromised patients or newborns.

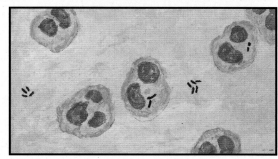

Toxoplasmosis

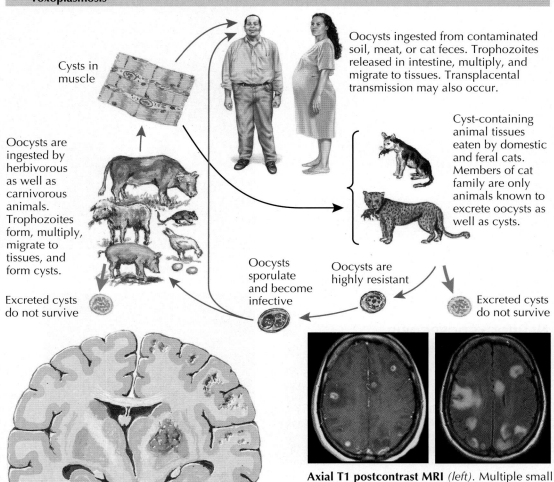

Cysts in muscle

Oocysts are ingested by herbivorous as well as carnivorous animals. Trophozoites form, multiply, migrate to tissues, and form cysts.

Oocysts ingested from contaminated soil, meat, or cat feces. Trophozoites released in intestine, multiply, and migrate to tissues. Transplacental transmission may also occur.

Cyst-containing animal tissues eaten by domestic and feral cats. Members of cat family are only animals known to excrete oocysts as well as cysts.

Excreted cysts do not survive

Oocysts sporulate and become infective

Oocysts are highly resistant

Excreted cysts do not survive

Brain section with nodule of *Toxoplasma gondii* in basal ganglia and necrotizing encephalitis in left frontal and temporal corticomedullary zones

Axial T1 postcontrast MRI *(left)*. Multiple small ring-enhancing cystic lesions within the bilateral frontal and bilateral parietal juxtacortical white matter. **Axial FLAIR MRI** *(right)*. Significant vasogenic edema surrounding the multiple cystic lesions within the bilateral frontal and bilateral parietal juxtacortical white matter.

INFECTIONS IN THE IMMUNOCOMPROMISED HOST (Continued)

chronic corticosteroid therapy, immunosuppressive therapy, diabetes mellitus, or pregnancy. Increasing age is also a risk factor for *L. monocytogenes* meningitis due to the natural decrease in cell-mediated immunity. Infection is acquired from soft cheeses, unpasteurized milk, hot dogs, deli meats, and coleslaw. In addition to meningitis, *L. monocytogenes* is one of the causative organisms of a brainstem encephalitis (rhombencephalitis). Patients typically have headache, nausea, vomiting, and fever, followed by brainstem symptoms and signs, the most common of which is a unilateral facial nerve palsy. This is followed by dysarthria, vertigo, dysphagia, and hemiataxia. Spinal fluid analysis demonstrates CSF pleocytosis with a predominance of neutrophils but also a mixture of lymphocytes and monocytes. The spinal fluid may also show a predominance of lymphocytes or monocytes. The glucose concentration may be decreased or normal. The organism can be grown in culture of CSF. In rhombencephalitis, a lesion of increased signal intensity on T2-weighted and fluid-attenuated inversion recovery (FLAIR) imaging can be seen in the pons and medulla. Therapy for meningitis due to *L. monocytogenes* is with ampicillin. In patients who are obtunded, gentamicin is added. Rhombencephalitis is treated with a combination of ampicillin and gentamicin.

TOXOPLASMOSIS

Toxoplasma gondii is a parasite that is acquired by ingesting the oocysts from contaminated soil, meat, or cat feces; however, *Toxoplasma* encephalitis is the result of reactivation of latent infection. Individuals with HIV and patients receiving immunosuppressive therapy for lymphoproliferative disorders are at greatest risk for this infection. Patients present with headache, fever, an altered level of consciousness, focal neurologic deficits, and/or seizures. Neuroimaging demonstrates one or more focal or multifocal ring-enhancing lesions with edema. Diagnosis begins with serology for anti-*Toxoplasma* immunoglobulin G (IgG). In an individual with HIV with multiple enhancing lesions with edema and a positive anti-*Toxoplasma* IgG, a treatment trial is often initiated with a combination of pyrimethamine and sulfadiazine. If clinical and radiographic improvement occurs with treatment, a presumptive diagnosis of *Toxoplasma* encephalitis is made. Clinical improvement is expected in 90% of patients by day 7 of therapy; if this does not occur, additional diagnostic studies are warranted because primary CNS lymphoma and tuberculous abscesses may have a similar clinical and radiographic appearance in individuals with HIV. Because primary CNS lymphoma is the leading disease in the differential diagnosis, CSF can be sent for the detection of Epstein-Barr virus (EBV) DNA by PCR. If spinal fluid analysis is not safe because of the degree of edema, a stereotactic CT-guided brain biopsy is recommended.

Plate 11.7

Brain: PART I

Ovum of *Taenia solium* (pork tapeworm)

Cysticercus (larval stage) of pork tapeworm. Fluid-filled sac (bladder) containing scolex (head) of worm.

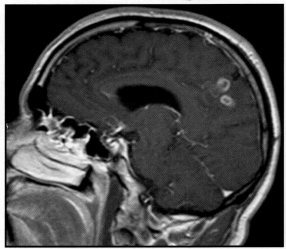

T. solium may produce a single cyst or multiple cysts in the brain.

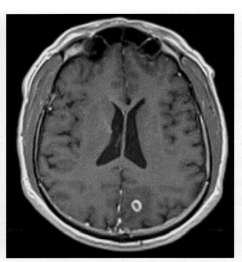

Sagittal T1 postcontrast MRI. Two subjacent small ring-enhancing cystic lesions within the left parietal juxtacortical white matter.

Axial T1 postcontrast MRI. Small ring-enhancing cystic lesion within the left parietal juxtacortical white matter.

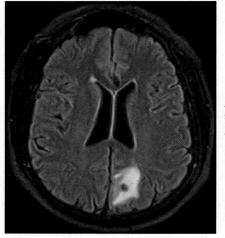

Axial FLAIR MRI. Significant vasogenic edema surrounding the cystic lesion within the left parietal juxtacortical white matter.

NEUROCYSTICERCOSIS

Neurocysticercosis is a parasitic infection of the CNS acquired by either fecal-oral transmission of the eggs of the tapeworm *Taenia solium* as a result of exposure to feces of asymptomatic *Taenia* carriers or by the ingestion of undercooked pork contaminated by larva of the tapeworm *T. solium*. The embryos of the eggs develop and hatch in the intestine and then enter the bloodstream. Larvae migrate to the CNS. The most common clinical manifestation is a seizure, and neurocysticercosis is the most common cause of acquired epilepsy in the developing world. The clinical presentation is affected by the number and location of cysts in the brain parenchyma, the basilar or perimesencephalic cisterns, and the subarachnoid space. Cysts may also be attached to the choroid plexus or the ventricular wall. As such, the presentation may be that of headache, signs of increased intracranial pressure, or focal neurologic deficits. Cysticercal cysts evolve through four stages: the vesicular stage, the colloidal stage, the granular stage, and the stage of calcification. The appearance of the cyst on CT and MRI depends on the stage. In the vesicular stage, the cyst contains living larvae and has the appearance of a nonenhancing cystic lesion without edema. In the colloidal stage, the larva is degenerating, and a CT scan demonstrates a ring-enhancing lesion with edema. On CT scan, but better demonstrated on

MRI, cysts in the vesicular stage and those in the colloidal stage contain live active cysts that have the appearance of a nodule, which is the invaginated scolex. In the granular stage, the larva continues to degenerate and the cyst develops a ring enhancement. Finally, a calcified lesion is seen on neuroimaging. The most definitive neuroimaging evidence of neurocysticercosis is a cystic lesion showing the scolex. The diagnosis is supported by a serum immunoblot assay that detects anticysticercal antibodies. In every stage, with the exception of the vesicular stage, the parasite is in the process of dying. Patients often become

symptomatic from cysts in the colloidal and vesicular stages, when the parasite elicits an inflammatory response and the lesion becomes surrounded by edema. In addition, during therapy with anticysticidal agents, there is a risk of a strong inflammatory reaction, with an increase in cerebral edema. Prednisone is started either before or with the first dose of anticysticidal therapy and continued throughout the course of treatment. Patients may also become symptomatic with a seizure when the cyst has evolved to a calcified lesion, but this stage and the granular stage do not require anticysticidal therapy.

Plate 11.8

Infections of the Nervous System

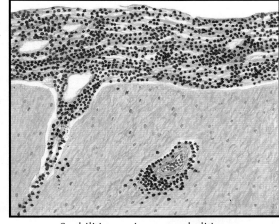

Syphilitic meningoencephalitis
with perivascular infiltration

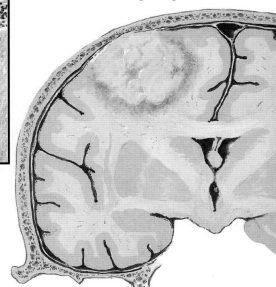

Gumma with beginning erosion of skull

SPIROCHETAL INFECTIONS: NEUROSYPHILIS

Neurosyphilis is the result of infection of the CNS by the bacterium *Treponema pallidum*. There are several different forms of neurosyphilis, which can be divided into early and late neurosyphilis. Early neurosyphilis includes asymptomatic neurosyphilis, syphilitic meningitis, and meningovascular syphilis. The late forms of neurosyphilis are tabes dorsalis and general paresis (dementia paralytica).

Asymptomatic neurosyphilis is defined by the presence of spinal fluid abnormalities in the absence of neurologic signs and symptoms.

Syphilitic meningitis is defined by the appearance of meningeal signs and symptoms, including headache, nausea, vomiting, stiff neck, and cranial nerve abnormalities. Spinal fluid analysis in syphilitic meningitis reveals an increased opening pressure, a lymphocytic pleocytosis, a normal or slightly decreased glucose concentration, and an elevated protein concentration. The serum rapid plasma reagin (RPR) is usually positive.

Meningovascular syphilis is defined by the appearance of focal neurologic signs due to an inflammatory arteritis involving small and medium-size arteries in association with signs of meningeal inflammation. Vascular syphilis may also involve the arterial blood supply to the spinal cord.

General paresis (dementia paralytica) is a chronic progressive meningoencephalitis with a peak incidence 10 to 20 years after primary infection. Initially, there is a slow deterioration in cognitive functioning and personality changes, but as the disease progresses there is loss of appendicular strength, abnormality of the pupils, dysarthria, tremor, and loss of bowel and bladder control. *Tabes dorsalis* develops 10 to 20 years after primary infection and is characterized at onset by episodic lancinating pain in the lower extremities. As the disease progresses, there is loss of proprioceptive and vibratory sensation due to neuronal degeneration and infiltration of inflammatory cells in the dorsal column and posterior spinal nerve roots of the spinal cord. *Tabes dorsalis* is also characterized by loss of the pupillary reaction to light, with preservation of pupillary

Section of thoracic spinal
cord in tabes dorsalis

General paresis: astrocytosis in cortex in reaction to loss
of nerve cells. Inset shows spirochetes in brain.

constriction to accommodation—the Argyll Robertson pupillary abnormality. Because of lumbosacral nerve root dysfunction, lower extremity areflexia, impotence, and loss of urinary continence may develop.

Gummatous neurosyphilis is a rare manifestation, but when it occurs CNS gummas present as space-occupying lesions.

Diagnosis. The diagnosis of neurosyphilis is made by a combination of serologic tests and spinal fluid analysis.

The serologic tests are typically the Venereal Disease Research Laboratory (VDRL) or the RPR, although the *T. pallidum* hemagglutination assay is more specific. A diagnosis of neurosyphilis is made by the detection of a reactive CSF VDRL. When the CSF VDRL is nonreactive but there is a positive serologic test and an elevated CSF white blood cell count and protein concentration, treatment for neurosyphilis is recommended. Neurosyphilis is treated with intravenous aqueous penicillin G.

Plate 11.9

Brain: PART I

LYME DISEASE

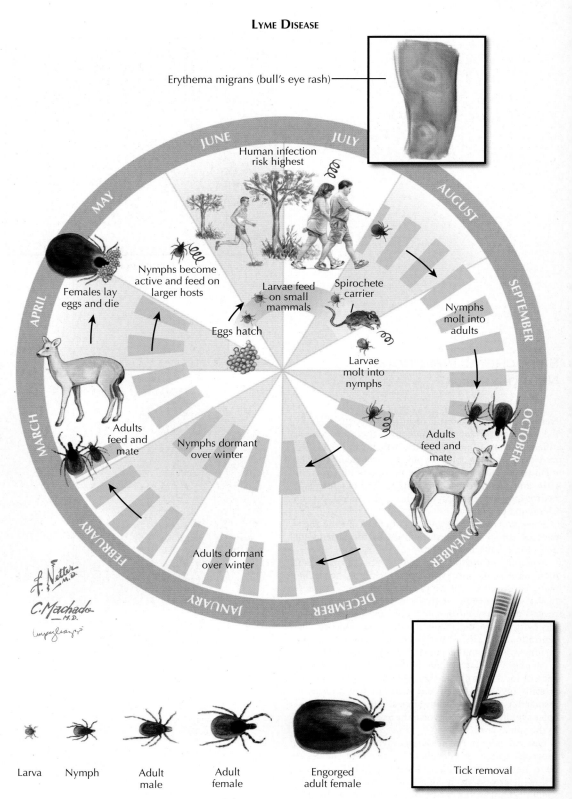

Erythema migrans (bull's eye rash)

Human infection risk highest

Nymphs become active and feed on larger hosts

Larvae feed on small mammals

Spirochete carrier

Females lay eggs and die

Eggs hatch

Nymphs molt into adults

Larvae molt into nymphs

Adults feed and mate

Nymphs dormant over winter

Adults feed and mate

Adults dormant over winter

JUNE · JULY · AUGUST · SEPTEMBER · OCTOBER · NOVEMBER · DECEMBER · JANUARY · FEBRUARY · MARCH · APRIL · MAY

Larva   Nymph   Adult male   Adult female   Engorged adult female

Tick removal

SPIROCHETAL INFECTIONS: LYME DISEASE

In North America, Lyme disease is caused by the spirochete *Borrelia burgdorferi*. The endemic regions for Lyme disease in the United States are the East Coast from Maine to Virginia, Pennsylvania, Minnesota and Wisconsin, and areas of Northern California. The infection can also be acquired in areas in Europe and Asia. Patients with meningitis due to *B. burgdorferi* report headache and fatigue. A unilateral or bilateral facial nerve palsy or a painful radiculopathy may be present. For patients with cranial neuritis or radiculoneuritis who reside in or who have traveled to a Lyme-endemic area, inquire about the lesion of erythema migrans. This is an erythematous lesion that, as it expands, develops central clearing so that it has the appearance of a target lesion. Diagnosis begins with a serum enzyme-linked immunosorbent assay to measure antibody to *B. burgdorferi*. A positive result is confirmed with a Western blot. Examination of the CSF demonstrates a lymphocytic pleocytosis with a normal glucose concentration and a mild to moderately elevated protein concentration. The demonstration of anti-*Borrelia* antibodies in CSF should not be regarded as definitive evidence of neurologic Lyme disease because antibodies can be passively transferred from serum to CSF, and Lyme antibodies may persist in the CSF for years. To detect the intrathecal production of antibodies, an antibody index is recommended. The antibody index is the ratio of (anti–*Borrelia* IgG in CSF/anti–*Borrelia* IgG in serum) to (total IgG in CSF/total IgG in serum). The antibody index is considered positive when the result is greater than 1.3 to 1.5. Lyme meningitis, cranial neuritis, and radiculitis are treated with intravenous ceftriaxone, intravenous cefotaxime, intravenous penicillin G, or oral doxycycline for 2 to 4 weeks.

Plate 11.10

Infections of the Nervous System

TUBERCULOSIS OF BRAIN AND SPINE

Mycobacterium tuberculosis CNS infections take a variety of forms, including acute fulminant meningoencephalitis, subacute meningitis, tuberculoma, and vertebral tuberculosis (Pott disease). Infection with *M. tuberculosis* is acquired by inhalation of aerosolized droplet nuclei. Tuberculous meningitis does not develop acutely from hematogenous spread of tubercle bacilli to the meninges. Rather, isolated miliary tubercles form in the brain parenchyma or the meninges during hematogenous dissemination of bacilli and subsequently enlarge and are usually caseating. Subependymal caseous foci may remain quiescent for months or years but then may discharge bacilli and tuberculous antigens into the subarachnoid space, causing meningitis. The neurologic complications of tuberculous meningitis are initiated by the intense inflammatory reaction to the discharge of tubercle bacilli and tuberculous antigens into the subarachnoid space. The inflammatory reaction leads to the production of a thick exudate that fills the basilar cisterns, obstructing the flow of CSF and surrounding the cranial nerves. Vasculitis typically involves the major blood vessels at the base of the brain, resulting in cerebral ischemia and infarction. Tuberculous meningitis may manifest as a subacute meningitis or as a fulminant meningitis, resembling bacterial meningitis. When the presentation is that of a subacute meningitis, headache, fever, and lethargy are often present for 4 weeks or longer before the patient presents for evaluation. Patients present for evaluation of unrelenting headache, night sweats, stiff neck, and lethargy. Cranial nerve abnormalities occur in approximately one-fourth of patients.

The diagnosis of tuberculous meningitis is made by examination of the spinal fluid. The classic spinal fluid abnormalities in tuberculous meningitis are as follows: (1) elevated opening pressure, (2) lymphocytic pleocytosis, (3) elevated protein concentration in the range of 100 to 500 mg/dL, and (4) decreased glucose concentration. A CSF glucose concentration between 45 and 35 mg/dL in combination with a lymphocytic pleocytosis and an unrelenting headache, stiff neck, fatigue, night sweats, and fever is highly suspicious for tuberculous meningitis. At an early stage in the clinical illness, polymorphonuclear leukocytes may predominate in the spinal fluid, but typically lymphocytes become the predominant cell type within 48 hours. The CSF glucose concentration is only mildly decreased. The last tube of fluid collected at lumbar puncture is the best tube to send for smear for acid-fast bacilli. Culture of CSF takes 4 to 8 weeks to identify the organism, except in cases of fulminant tuberculous meningitis where culture is often positive in 1 to 2 weeks. A PCR is available for *M. tuberculosis* ribosomal RNA. Neuroimaging abnormalities are nonspecific and include enhancement of the meninges after contrast administration, communicating and/or obstructive hydrocephalus, and infarctions typically in the basal ganglia. Patients should undergo chest radiography and an intradermal tuberculin skin test. The tuberculin skin test may be negative because patients with CNS tuberculosis are immunosuppressed. With treatment, the skin test may become positive. Treatment of tuberculous meningitis includes a combination of isoniazid, rifampin, pyrazinamide, ethambutol, and pyridoxine. Dexamethasone therapy is recommended for patients who develop hydrocephalus. This

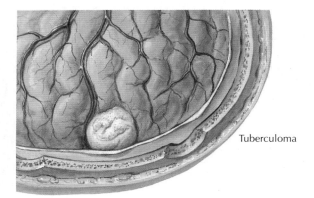
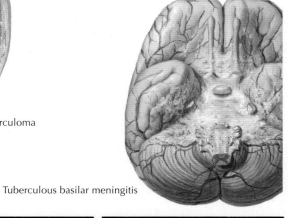

Tuberculoma

Tuberculous basilar meningitis

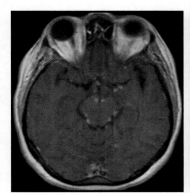
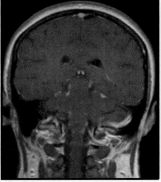
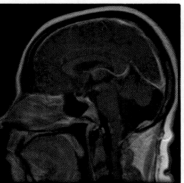

Axial T1 postcontrast MRI showing nodular leptomeningeal enhancement along the basifrontal lobes, perimesencephalic cisterns, interpeduncular cistern, and medial left temporal lobe.

Coronal T1 postcontrast MRI showing nodular leptomeningeal enhancement along the perimesencephalic cisterns, medial temporal lobes, and lateral thecal sac at the craniocervical junction.

Sagittal T1 postcontrast MRI showing nodular leptomeningeal enhancement extending along the basifrontal lobes, interpeduncular cistern, and ventral and dorsal thecal sac surrounding the lower brainstem and cervical cord. Note presence of incidental Dandy-Walker malformation.

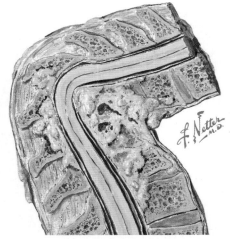

Tuberculosis of the spine. Pott disease with marked kyphosis.

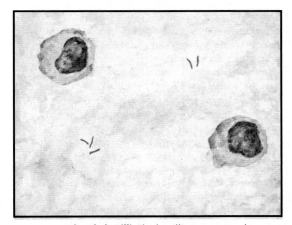

Tubercle bacilli. The bacilli appear as red rods in smear of CSF (Ziehl-Neelsen stain).

complication may also require a ventriculostomy or a ventriculoperitoneal shunt.

Tuberculomas manifest as space-occupying lesions. On CT scan, they often have the appearance of a central nidus of calcification surrounded by a ring of enhancement and/or edema. Tuberculomas may develop during the course of therapy for tuberculous meningitis. The treatment of tuberculomas includes a three- or four-drug regimen similar to the treatment of tuberculous meningitis. Superficial tuberculomas can be surgically excised if they do not respond to antituberculous chemotherapy.

Pott disease refers to vertebral tuberculosis or tuberculous spondylitis. Two or more adjacent vertebral bodies are often involved, and infection can spread to the disk and/or the epidural space. The thoracic and lumbar spine are the most commonly affected areas; thus the clinical presentation includes back pain in the thoracic or lumbar area and fever. When the epidural space is involved, signs and symptoms of progressive spinal cord compression can develop. Diagnosis is made by stereotactic aspiration of the lesion. Treatment includes antituberculous chemotherapy and surgical decompression if spinal cord compression is present.

Plate 11.11

Brain: PART I

TETANUS

The bacterium *Clostridium tetani* produces a neuro-toxin tetanospasmin (tetanus toxin) in wounds it con-taminates. Tetanus toxin enters the CNS by retrograde axonal transport in motor neurons from its site of for-mation in a wound to its site of action—the motor neuron cell bodies in the ventral gray of the spinal cord and brainstem.

Tetanus toxin produces spasticity by blocking the release of the inhibitory neurotransmitters glycine and glutamic acid decarboxylase from presynaptic nerve terminals that synapse on alpha motor neurons in the spinal cord and brainstem. With the loss of inhibitory input, the uninhibited lower motor neuron increases resting muscle tone, producing rigidity. Tetanus is di-vided into four clinical forms: localized, generalized, cephalic, and neonatal. The *incubation period* is defined as the time from inoculation with *C. tetani* spores to the appearance of the first symptom. The incubation period is followed by *the period of onset of tetanus*, which is defined as the interval from the first symptom to the first reflex spasm. Localized tetanus is limited to the extremity in which there is a contaminated wound, blister, or burn. The patient's initial complaint is stiff-ness of the muscles in the extremity with voluntary movement. This is followed by the development of a continuous spasm or rigidity in the group of muscles in close proximity to the wound. Local tetanus may re-main restricted to the limb or may become generalized. In generalized tetanus, the usual manifesting sign is trismus (lockjaw), which is a rigidity of the masseter muscles causing an inability to open the mouth to speak or to chew. Another early sign is risus sardonicus due to increased tone in the orbicularis oris, causing a sneering grin. The generalized spasm consists of opis-thotonic posturing with flexion and adduction of the arms, clenching of the fists, and extension of the lower extremities. The spasms are often precipitated by exter-nal stimuli and are extremely painful. Sudden spasms of the muscles of respiration may stop respiration for 10 to 20 seconds, and laryngeal or pharyngeal spasms may obstruct the airway, compromising respiration. Cephalic tetanus involves the muscles supplied by one or more cranial nerves and almost always follows a head wound. The facial nerve is affected most often. Neonatal tetanus typically develops as a result of infection of the umbili-cal stump, and the usual manifesting symptom is poor feeding. The infant cannot suck, and, when a finger is put into its mouth, the baby's jaw clamps tightly. This is followed by involvement of the muscles of facial expression, risus sardonicus, and then opisthotonos.

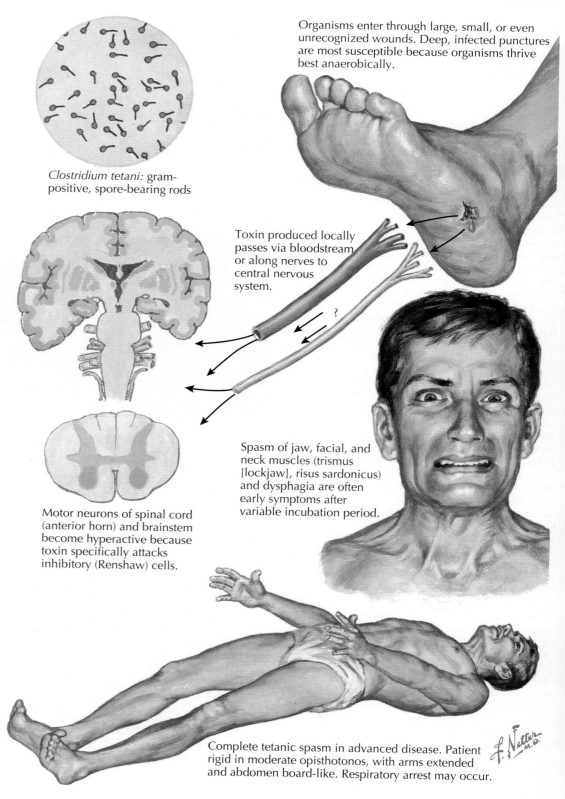

Clostridium tetani: gram-positive, spore-bearing rods

Organisms enter through large, small, or even unrecognized wounds. Deep, infected punctures are most susceptible because organisms thrive best anaerobically.

Toxin produced locally passes via bloodstream or along nerves to central nervous system.

Motor neurons of spinal cord (anterior horn) and brainstem become hyperactive because toxin specifically attacks inhibitory (Renshaw) cells.

Spasm of jaw, facial, and neck muscles (trismus [lockjaw], risus sardonicus) and dysphagia are often early symptoms after variable incubation period.

Complete tetanic spasm in advanced disease. Patient rigid in moderate opisthotonos, with arms extended and abdomen board-like. Respiratory arrest may occur.

Tetanus is a clinical diagnosis. When tetanus is sus-pected, a careful immunization history should be ob-tained because tetanus is unlikely if the patient has received a complete primary series of toxoid injec-tions with booster doses every 10 years. Diagnosis is dependent on ruling out the diseases that have an appearance similar to tetanus, including strychnine poisoning, a dystonic reaction secondary to a neuro-leptic agent or a dopamine-blocking agent, and rabies.

Dystonic reactions are quickly reversed with intrave-nous benztropine or diphenhydramine.

There are three goals of treatment in tetanus: (1) securing the airway and treating generalized spasms with benzodiazepines, (2) stopping production of the toxin by surgical debridement of the wound and anti-microbial therapy (the most frequently recommended antibiotic is metronidazole), and (3) passive immuniza-tion with human tetanus immunoglobulin.

Plate 11.12

Infections of the Nervous System

ASEPTIC MENINGITIS AND SELECT ARTHROPOD-BORNE VIRUS INFECTIONS

ASEPTIC MENINGITIS

Aseptic meningitis is a disorder in which the characteristic symptoms and findings of meningeal irritation are present, and CSF analysis is suggestive of meningitis but without evidence of bacterial infection. In many instances the cause is viral; less often, mycobacterial, spirochetal, parasitic, or fungal infection is responsible. A similar syndrome can arise with sarcoidosis, various connective tissue diseases, neoplastic leptomeningeal involvement, or as a medication-induced complication. Sterile CSF with an increased cell count may also be found with parameningeal infections and partially treated bacterial meningitis. In addition to a spinal tap (with CSF analysis), Gram and other stains, culture, serology, cytology, and PCR, other investigations may include complete blood count, MRI of the brain and spine, chest radiography, blood cultures, and other studies depending on the clinical evaluation. Treatment depends on the cause.

SELECT ARTHROPOD-BORNE VIRUS INFECTIONS

Various mosquito-borne viruses may cause infectious encephalitis. Treatment is primarily symptomatic, making preventive strategies important, especially for arthropod-borne viruses (arboviruses) such as eastern equine encephalitis virus and West Nile virus (WNV). The related St. Louis encephalitis virus is transmitted mainly in North America during late summer or early autumn and typically causes mild nonspecific symptoms but occasionally an encephalitic illness.

Eastern equine encephalitis virus, found in the Caribbean and Eastern United States, infects humans, horses, and some bird species. Other variants of the virus occur in Central and South America, where they cause equine disease. Most infected persons are asymptomatic. When symptoms do occur, they may consist solely of a mild nonspecific flu-like systemic illness, with headache, fever, malaise, aching pains, and vomiting, with complete recovery occurring in 7 to 10 days in the absence of cerebral involvement. In uncommon instances, however, fulminating encephalitic illness occurs after an incubation period of 3 to 10 days that is characterized by confusion, delirium, irritability, restlessness, seizures and, eventually, loss of consciousness. The encephalitic illness is associated with a 33% mortality rate, and about half of survivors have residual cognitive or other neurologic deficits. There is a pleocytosis in the CSF, with an increased neutrophil count and an elevated protein concentration; glucose level is normal. Serologic diagnosis depends on IgM testing of serum and CSF and antibody testing of acute- and convalescent-phase serum. MRI most often shows unilateral or bilateral abnormalities (increased T2 signal intensity) of the basal ganglia; the internal capsule, thalamus, brainstem, periventricular white matter, and cerebral cortex may also be involved. There is no specific therapy, and treatment is purely supportive. No vaccine is available, and prevention therefore depends on reducing exposure to mosquitoes.

West Nile virus, a flavivirus usually found in Africa, West Asia, and the Middle East, was not documented in

the Western Hemisphere until 1999. Reservoirs for the virus include humans, horses, certain other mammals, birds, and mosquitoes. In humans, infection may be asymptomatic or lead to mild disease (West Nile fever) with flu-like symptoms (sometimes accompanied by a skin rash) that develop within 2 weeks after the bite of an infected mosquito and usually last for only a few days. However, encephalitis, meningitis, or meningoencephalitis sometimes develops, as may a poliomyelitic illness, and sometimes leads to a fatal outcome.

The CSF shows a lymphocytic pleocytosis with elevated protein and normal glucose concentrations. PCR may be diagnostic, but false-negative results are common. Thus the diagnosis is usually established by serologic assays of blood and CSF (IgM). Treatment is supportive; no specific drug therapy is available. Prevention depends on avoidance of infected mosquitoes because no vaccine is available. Residual deficits, such as cognitive changes or muscle weakness, may occur in survivors.

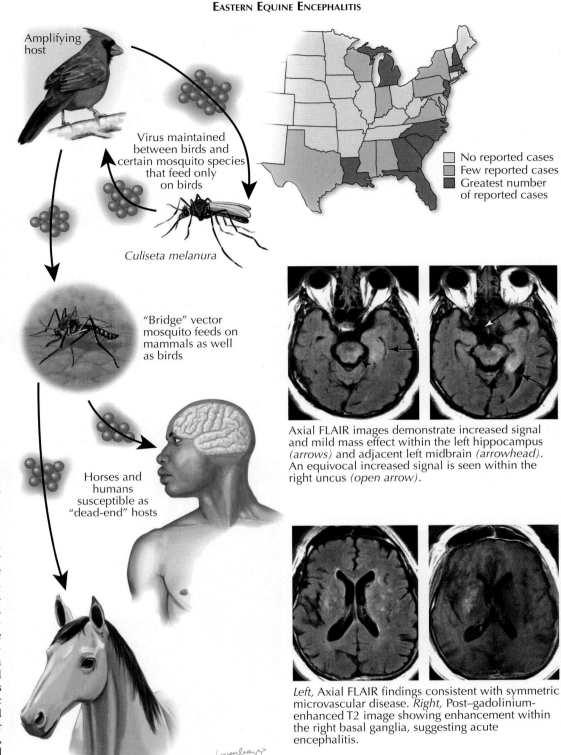

EASTERN EQUINE ENCEPHALITIS

Amplifying host

Virus maintained between birds and certain mosquito species that feed only on birds

Culiseta melanura

"Bridge" vector mosquito feeds on mammals as well as birds

Horses and humans susceptible as "dead-end" hosts

No reported cases
Few reported cases
Greatest number of reported cases

Axial FLAIR images demonstrate increased signal and mild mass effect within the left hippocampus (arrows) and adjacent left midbrain (arrowhead). An equivocal increased signal is seen within the right uncus (open arrow).

Left, Axial FLAIR findings consistent with symmetric microvascular disease. *Right,* Post–gadolinium-enhanced T2 image showing enhancement within the right basal ganglia, suggesting acute encephalitis.

Plate 11.13

Brain: PART I

PRIMARY HIV INFECTION OF THE NERVOUS SYSTEM

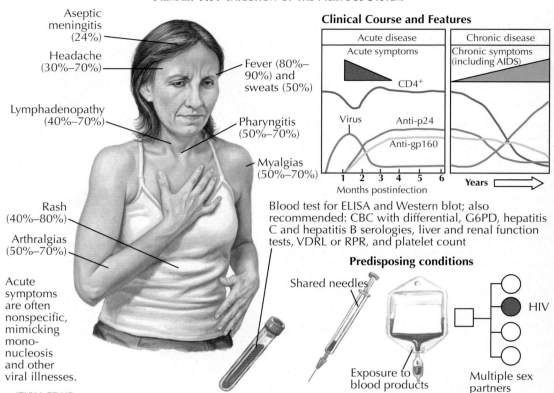

Aseptic meningitis (24%)

Headache (30%–70%)

Lymphadenopathy (40%–70%)

Fever (80%–90%) and sweats (50%)

Pharyngitis (50%–70%)

Myalgias (50%–70%)

Rash (40%–80%)

Arthralgias (50%–70%)

Acute symptoms are often nonspecific, mimicking mononucleosis and other viral illnesses.

Clinical Course and Features

Acute disease	Chronic disease
Acute symptoms	Chronic symptoms (including AIDS)

CD4+

Virus — Anti-p24

Anti-gp160

1 2 3 4 5 6 Months postinfection

Years

Blood test for ELISA and Western blot; also recommended: CBC with differential, G6PD, hepatitis C and hepatitis B serologies, liver and renal function tests, VDRL or RPR, and platelet count

Predisposing conditions

Shared needles

Exposure to blood products

HIV

Multiple sex partners

JOHN A.CRAIG_MD
with
E. Hatton

C.Machado
M.D.

HUMAN IMMUNODEFICIENCY VIRUS

Human immunodeficiency virus (HIV) is a retrovirus that causes acquired immunodeficiency syndrome (AIDS), which is a progressive failure of the immune system with a declining CD4+ cell count. Infection occurs by the transfer of blood, semen or vaginal fluid, or breast milk containing the virus. If this occurs, for example, by unprotected sex or blood transfusion, patients with HIV may remain asymptomatic for years. Two types of HIV are recognized, with HIV-1 being the more virulent and responsible for most infections worldwide. An acute systemic infection is followed by a variable latent period and then by the development of AIDS. A fatal outcome may follow opportunistic infection or the development of malignancies, such as Epstein-Barr virus (EBV)-associated Hodgkin and non-Hodgkin lymphomas. Primary CNS lymphoma is a B-cell lymphoma associated with EBV in individuals with HIV and can involve the entire neuroaxis and cranial nerves. Treatment of HIV infection is with antiretroviral drugs, which improve the prognosis but do not cure HIV infection. Preventive measures include the use of latex condoms. Depending on the CD4+ count, prophylaxis against opportunistic infection is also indicated.

Acute aseptic meningitis is a common manifestation in patients with primary neurologic HIV-1 infection and leads to headache and meningismus. Other less common neurologic presentations at the time of initial HIV infection include acute disseminated encephalomyelitis, myelopathy, meningoradiculitis, and peripheral neuropathy, including Guillain-Barré syndrome (GBS). Systemic abnormalities are commonly also present. Laboratory studies may reveal leukopenia, thrombocytopenia, and elevated transaminases. An HIV antibody study may initially be negative even if serum HIV viral load is positive. Once seroconversion occurs, patients are at risk for many neurologic complications.

HIV-associated neurocognitive disorders are a complication of chronic HIV infection. Over time, patients

AIDS encephalopathy in a 39-year-old male with gait difficulties and cognitive decline. Brain MRI was normal 2 years ago.

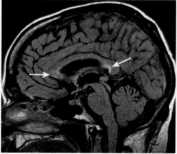

A. Axial T2 fast spin echo demonstrates ill-defined area of augmented T2 signal in upper left pons *(arrow)*.

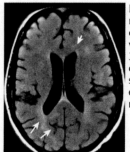

B. Axial FLAIR shows moderate sulcal and ventricular enlargement consistent with diffuse atrophy for age 39, in addition to paraventricular augmentation of T2 signal, which in some regions extends to subcortical white matter and cortex *(arrows)*.

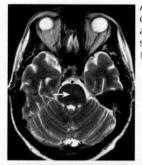

C. Midsagittal FLAIR with ill-defined augmentation in both genu and splenium of corpus callosum *(arrows)*.

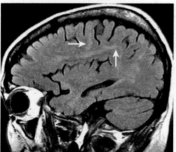

D. FLAIR imaging more laterally again demonstrates paraventricular involvement extending to subcortical white matter *(arrows)*.

develop cognitive impairment and behavioral disturbances, with a marked change in personality, apathy, inattention, memory disturbances, and language dysfunction. Motor deficits (slowness, clumsiness, ataxia, weakness) also occur.

Milder HIV-associated neurocognitive disorders have a high prevalence, even in patients who are HIV-positive with a long-standing aviremia, but usually do not limit daily activities. Clinically asymptomatic individuals with

HIV-1 may have abnormal brain MRIs with white matter (demyelination) and gray matter (atrophy) changes.

Opportunistic infection with bacteria, viruses (Epstein-Barr, cytomegalovirus [CMV], and hepatitis B), fungi *(Cryptococcus neoformans),* or parasites *(Toxoplasma gondii)* may involve the CNS directly. Toxoplasmosis (see Plate 11.6) may manifest with seizures and cryptococcal meningitis with a subacute alteration of mental function. Such infections can lead also to vasculopathy. Other,

Plate 11.14

Infections of the Nervous System

HIV LIFE CYCLE AND ANTIRETROVIRAL MEDICATIONS

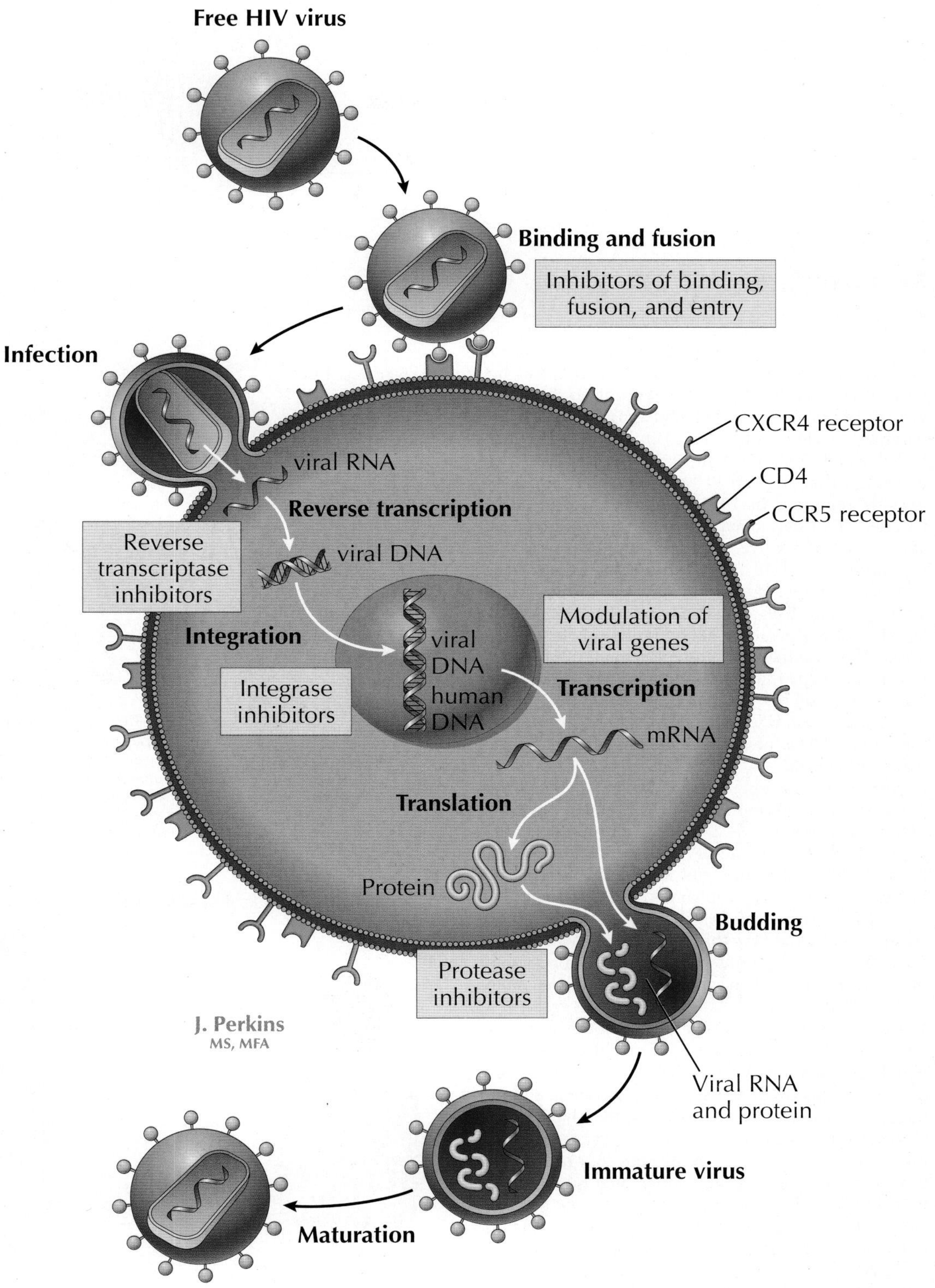

Free HIV virus

Binding and fusion

Inhibitors of binding, fusion, and entry

Infection

CXCR4 receptor

CD4

CCR5 receptor

viral RNA

Reverse transcription

Reverse transcriptase inhibitors

viral DNA

Integration

viral DNA human DNA

Modulation of viral genes

Transcription

Integrase inhibitors

mRNA

Translation

Protein

Budding

Protease inhibitors

J. Perkins
MS, MFA

Viral RNA and protein

Immature virus

Maturation

HUMAN IMMUNODEFICIENCY VIRUS (Continued)

rarer causes of a CNS vasculitis in this context include neoplastic disease or recreational drug abuse.

A primary vacuolar and inflammatory myelopathy may occur in AIDS and may mimic the myelopathy of vitamin B_{12} or copper deficiency, with predominant involvement of the posterior columns. There is no effective treatment.

Symptomatic neuropathies are common in patients with HIV-1, becoming more common as the immunodeficiency worsens. Distal symmetric sensory polyneuropathy is the most frequent, is progressive, and presents with symmetric distal pain, paresthesias, and numbness in the feet. A similar neuropathy is associated with several of the nucleoside reverse-transcriptase inhibitor drugs (zalcitabine, didanosine, and stavudine) used for treating HIV infection. Acute inflammatory demyelinating polyradiculopathy sometimes occurs at the time of seroconversion, but polyradiculopathy may also occur at more advanced stages of HIV-1 infection. The CSF in patients with polyradiculopathy typically contains lymphocytosis (10–50 cells/mm³). Mononeuritis multiplex is an infrequent complication of HIV-1 infection.

Patients coinfected with CMV may develop mononeuritis multiplex, polyradiculoneuropathy, or polyradiculopathy. The CSF may show a polymorphonuclear pleocytosis, and CMV PCR in CSF is positive in 90% of cases.

Various myopathies may occur in patients with HIV-1 and may require biopsy for their distinction. In rare instances, rhabdomyolysis occurs. Some patients appear to have a disorder resembling polymyositis that is steroid responsive; others develop inclusion body myositis. Various muscle-wasting syndromes have been described, as is vasculitic myopathy. Rod body myopathy is characterized by the presence of rod-shaped bodies and loss of thick filaments and may respond to corticosteroids. Opportunistic infections of muscle sometimes occur, as in muscle toxoplasmosis, and

treatment is of the offending organism. Nucleoside reverse transcriptase inhibitors can cause neuromuscular weakness. The presumed mechanism is mitochondrial toxicity.

Significant advancements have been made, but patients continue to present with opportunistic infections as the first indication of HIV infection. The initiation of antiretroviral therapy in association with treatment for an opportunistic infection can

lead to a clinical worsening as the immune system reconstitutes. This is referred to as *immune reconstitution inflammatory syndrome*. Testing for opportunistic infections is recommended for all patients with HIV seroconversion, and antiretroviral therapy should be delayed for a week or two after initiation of therapy for the infection. If immune reconstitution inflammatory syndrome occurs, corticosteroids are the treatment of choice.

Plate 11.15

Brain: PART I

Poliomyelitis

Poliomyelitis became an epidemic disease at the beginning of the 20th century, and the poliovirus was first isolated in 1908. By 1941 it was recognized that poliovirus infection begins as an acute gastroenteritis, and paralysis develops in less than 1 in 100 individuals infected with the poliovirus. In 1952 the epidemic reached its peak, with more than 20,000 cases of paralytic poliomyelitis reported. In 1955 an inactivated, injectable vaccine (IPV) developed by Jonas Salk became available, followed by a live, attenuated monovalent oral virus vaccine (OPV) in 1961, developed by Albert Sabin. With the widespread use of the oral poliovirus vaccine, which contains live, attenuated poliovirus strains, vaccine-associated paralytic poliomyelitis was first recognized. This eventually led to replacement of OPV with IPV in developed countries. Infants and children receive a dose of IPV at 2 months, 4 months, 6 to 18 months, and 4 to 6 years of age. Outbreaks of polio in the United States now occur mostly among unvaccinated individuals.

Poliovirus is a single-stranded RNA enterovirus. There are three immunologically defined serotypes of poliovirus (serotypes 1, 2, and 3), all of which cause paralytic disease. Natural polio infection occurs through ingestion of the virus, which initially replicates in the mucosa of the oropharynx and gastrointestinal tract. The virus enters the CNS via either the bloodstream or alternatively through afferent neural pathways into motor neurons of the anterior horn, motor nuclei of the brainstem, and Betz cells of the motor cortex.

The earliest cellular change in the motor neurons is dissolution of the cytoplasmic Nissl substance (chromatolysis). Infected neurons that have only a mild degree of chromatolysis survive and continue to support motor units. In contrast, neurons that have severe chromatolysis become necrotic and cannot support motor units. As a result, permanent loss of function occurs in the muscle groups innervated by the motor unit. Historically, poliovirus infections have been divided into a minor illness and a major illness. The minor illness is characterized by fever, myalgias, nausea, and diarrhea. A major illness can be associated with the minor illness or follow the minor illness by a few afebrile days and is characterized by increasing signs of meningeal irritation, headache, and stiff neck. When the illness progresses to the paralytic form, muscle soreness is prominent, particularly in the back and neck. Patients who develop paralysis usually do so on the second to fifth day after meningeal signs and fever develop. The weakness is generally an asymmetric flaccid muscle weakness, and the legs are involved more often than the arms.

During the polio epidemic in the past century, the diagnosis was based on the clinical syndrome of fever with paralysis and lower motor neuron weakness. Today, poliovirus is the least common cause of an asymmetric flaccid lower extremity weakness. The other enteroviruses (coxsackieviruses, echoviruses, and numbered enteroviruses) and the flaviviruses, most notably WNV, are much more common etiologic agents of flaccid paralysis.

When poliovirus infection is suspected, at least two stool specimens and two throat swabs should be obtained 24 hours apart. As with all suspected enteroviral infections, acute and convalescent serology should be sent 4 weeks apart to detect a fourfold increase in IgG. Spinal fluid analysis demonstrates lymphocytic pleocytosis, normal glucose concentration, and enteroviral RNA by PCR.

The treatment of poliovirus infection is primarily supportive, and prevention with mass vaccination of all children is essential.

Hypothesis of pathogenesis of poliomyelitis

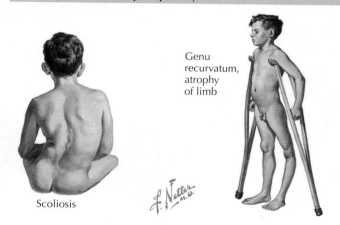

A. Virus is ingested by mouth.

B. Only if amount of ingested virus is very large is there primary infection of oropharyngeal mucosa.

C. In most instances, virus is swallowed and passes through stomach into intestine, where it multiplies rapidly and invades aggregated lymph nodules of intestinal wall (Peyer patches).

D. Varying amounts of virus enter bloodstream.

E. Other susceptible extraneural tissues, including oropharynx, are then frequently secondarily infected via bloodstream, where the virus also multiplies.

Other susceptible extraneural tissues

Medulla oblongata

Spinal cord

G. Virus is excreted in feces, by which it is disseminated.

F. From sites of multiplication in intestine, oropharynx, and other extraneural tissues, virus reaches CNS, probably via regional afferent neural pathways, first into motor neurons of spinal cord (primary spinal paralysis) or medulla (primary bulbar paralysis). Further axonal spread of virus then occurs along tracts to distal neurons elsewhere in the CNS, and also by contiguity to adjacent motor neurons.

Stages in destruction of a motor neuron by poliovirus

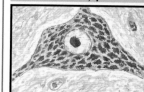

A. Normal motor neuron

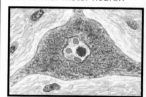

B. Diffuse chromatolysis; three acidophilic nuclear inclusions around nucleolus

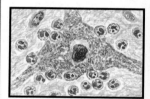

C. Polymorphonuclear cells invading necrotic neuron

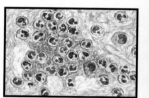

D. Complete neuronophagia

Paralytic residual of spinal poliomyelitis

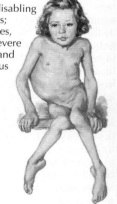

Scoliosis

Genu recurvatum, atrophy of limb

Multiple disabling deformities; contractures, atrophy, severe scoliosis, and equinovarus

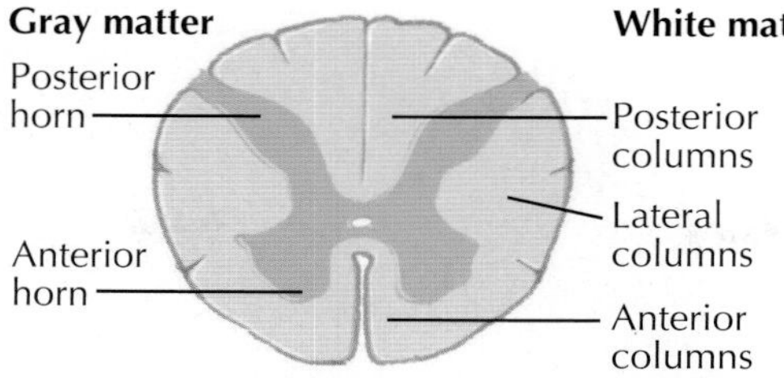

Plate 11.16

Infections of the Nervous System

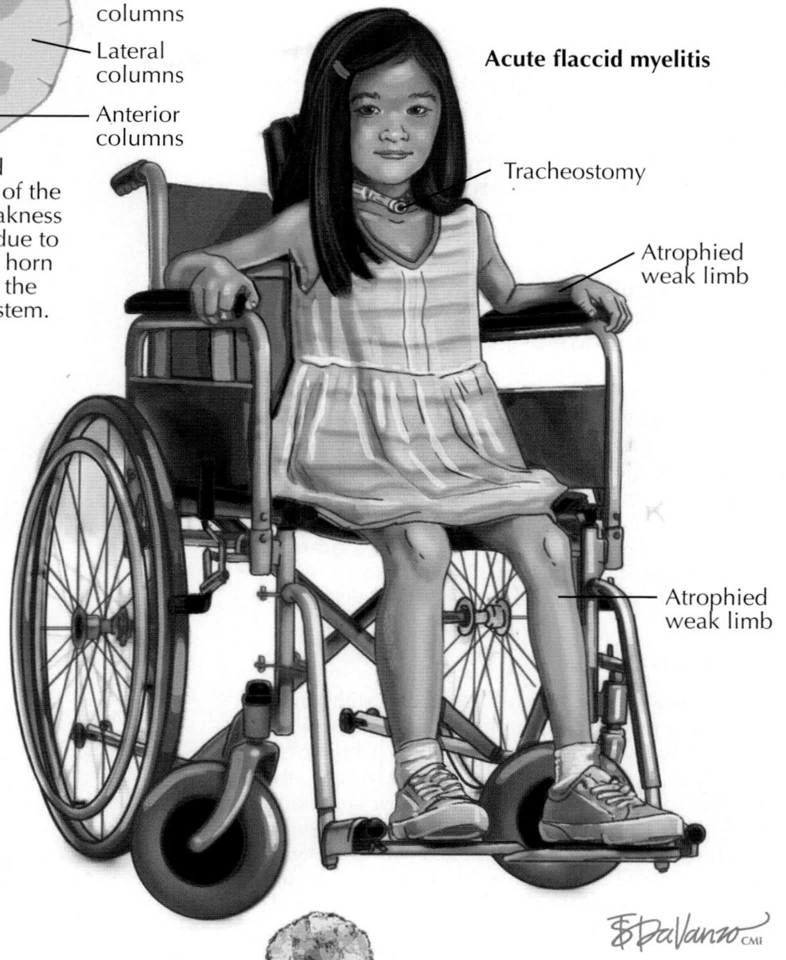

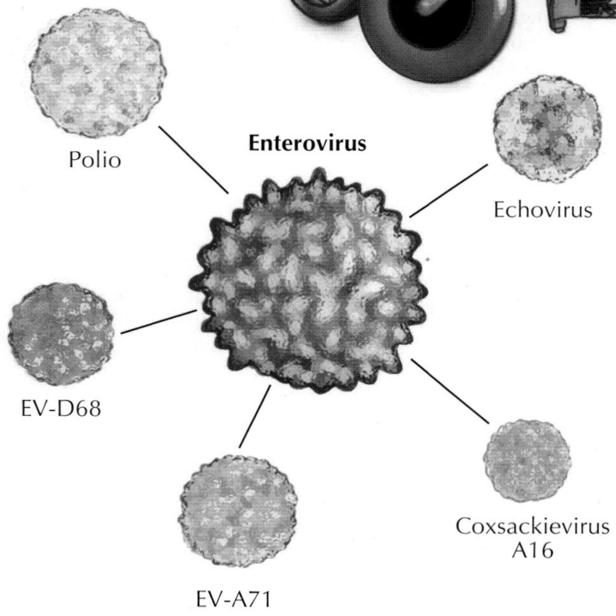

ACUTE FLACCID PARALYSIS

There are striking and worrisome similarities between the 1918–1919 pandemic and polio and the 2020–2023 severe acute respiratory syndrome coronavirus-2 (SARS-CoV-2) pandemic and acute flaccid myelitis (AFM). In 1916 there were 27,000 cases of polio in the United States and 6000 deaths. This was followed by the 1918–1919 flu pandemic that killed tens of millions of people worldwide, followed in turn by further outbreaks of polio, one of which affected future president Franklin Roosevelt. Every 2 years since 2012, there have been outbreaks of acute flaccid myelitis in the United States. Polio and acute flaccid myelitis are both characterized by acute flaccid limb weakness and associated with a prodromal viral infection. If history repeats itself, it is possible that a pandemic of acute flaccid myelitis, like the polio pandemic, will follow the SARS-CoV-2 pandemic as polio followed the influenza pandemic.

Acute flaccid myelitis is an illness that begins with acute flaccid asymmetric weakness due to involvement of the anterior horn cells of the spinal cord and the motor neurons of the brainstem. The majority of cases occur in children between August and October. This is reminiscent of the "polio summers." There is often a prodromal viral-like syndrome, either respiratory or gastrointestinal. The prodromal syndrome is followed by the development of asymmetric flaccid limb weakness. There may be cranial nerve involvement and respiratory failure. Testing of CSF and respiratory (nasopharyngeal swabs) and gastrointestinal specimens by the Centers for Disease Control and Prevention (CDC) has revealed enterovirus-A71, enterovirus-D68, coxsackievirus A16, and echovirus. An enterovirus is the suspected etiologic agent of acute flaccid myelitis. Enteroviruses can be isolated from throat and stool cultures but not be the causative pathogen of the CNS infection. An enterovirus identified in a CSF sample is definitive evidence that the enterovirus is the etiologic agent of a CNS infection. Acute and convalescent serology demonstrating a fourfold increase in IgG to a specific enterovirus is definitive evidence of a recent enteroviral infection.

In acute flaccid myelitis, a hyperintensity lesion largely restricted to gray matter and spanning one or more vertebral segments is seen on T2-weighted MRI of the spinal cord, although it may take longer than 72 hours to develop. The cervical cord is often involved, and the brainstem may also demonstrate a hyperintensity lesion on T2-weighted imaging. Examination of the CSF demonstrates a lymphocytic pleocytosis with a normal glucose concentration. Because the flaviviruses WNV and St. Louis encephalitis virus may also cause acute asymmetric flaccid weakness, CSF should be sent for PCR testing for enteroviruses and WNV as well as WNV IgM. Acute and convalescent serology (obtained 4 weeks later) is especially helpful to identify a specific enterovirus or arthropod-borne virus as the etiologic agent.

The most recent Summary of Clinical Guidance from the CDC states the following: (1) there is no indication that intravenous immunoglobulin should be either preferred or avoided in the treatment of AFM, (2) there is no indication that corticosteroids should be either preferred or avoided in the treatment of AFM, (3) there is no indication that therapeutic plasma exchange should be either preferred or avoided in the treatment of AFM, and (4) there is no indication that fluoxetine, currently available antiviral medications, interferon, or biologic modifiers should be used for the treatment of AFM.

The lesson to be learned from the SARS-CoV-2 pandemic is that both vaccines and therapeutics are critical.

Because acute flaccid myelitis appears to be of either a parainfectious or postinfectious etiology, antiviral and immunomodulating therapies are both critical to decreasing morbidity and mortality. Until an enterovirus or viruses have definitively been identified as the pathogen associated with acute flaccid myelitis, therapeutics should be the priority, with the development of a vaccine subsequently.

Gray matter — Posterior horn, Anterior horn

White matter — Posterior columns, Lateral columns, Anterior columns

Cross section of spinal cord demonstrating the location of the anterior horn cells. The weakness of acute flaccid myelitis is due to involvement of the anterior horn cells of the spinal cord and the motor neurons of the brainstem.

Acute flaccid myelitis — Tracheostomy, Atrophied weak limb, Atrophied weak limb

Polio, **Enterovirus**, Echovirus, EV-D68, Coxsackievirus A16, EV-A71

Plate 11.17

Brain: PART I

HERPES ZOSTER

Varicella-zoster virus (VZV) is the etiologic agent of chickenpox (varicella) and shingles (zoster). VZV is a double-stranded DNA virus. Initial infection occurs in the upper respiratory tract, followed by a viremia and the appearance of the characteristic vesicular lesions of chickenpox. VZV establishes latency in the cranial nerve ganglia and dorsal root ganglia along the neuraxis. Reactivation of the virus causes shingles, which presents with severe localized pain followed within 3 to 4 days by the appearance of a vesicular rash on an erythematous base in one to three dermatomes. Zoster has a predilection for the mid- to lower thoracic, upper lumbar, and ophthalmic (V_1) dermatomes. The neurologic complications of varicella, or chickenpox, include encephalitis (which most often manifests as an acute cerebellar ataxia), aseptic meningitis, polyneuritis, multiple cranial neuropathies, and Reye syndrome. The neurologic complications of zoster include meningitis, encephalitis, vasculopathy, cerebellitis, Ramsay Hunt syndrome, postherpetic neuralgia, myelopathy, and chronic radicular pain without rash (zoster sine herpete).

ENCEPHALITIS

VZV encephalitis can develop associated with zoster, follow zoster by days to months, or may develop without any history of a vesicular rash. The symptoms of encephalitis include fever, headache, seizures, focal neurologic deficits, and an altered level of consciousness. VZV encephalitis is due to ischemic and hemorrhagic infarctions in both cortical and subcortical gray matter and white matter. Small demyelinative lesions have been attributed to a small-vessel vasculopathy. Neuroimaging in patients with VZV encephalitis may demonstrate ischemic and hemorrhagic infarctions and demyelinative lesions. Zoster reactivation may also cause ventriculitis and periventriculitis with hydrocephalus, altered mental status, and gait abnormalities.

OPHTHALMIC HERPES ZOSTER

Patients with reactivation of VZV in the trigeminal ganglion develop vesicular lesions in the ophthalmic division of the trigeminal nerve and are at risk for infarction in the distribution of the carotid, anterior, or middle cerebral arteries due to VZV vasculopathy. There is also a risk of corneal scarring.

CEREBELLITIS

An acute cerebellar ataxia can complicate childhood varicella but may also occur in adulthood.

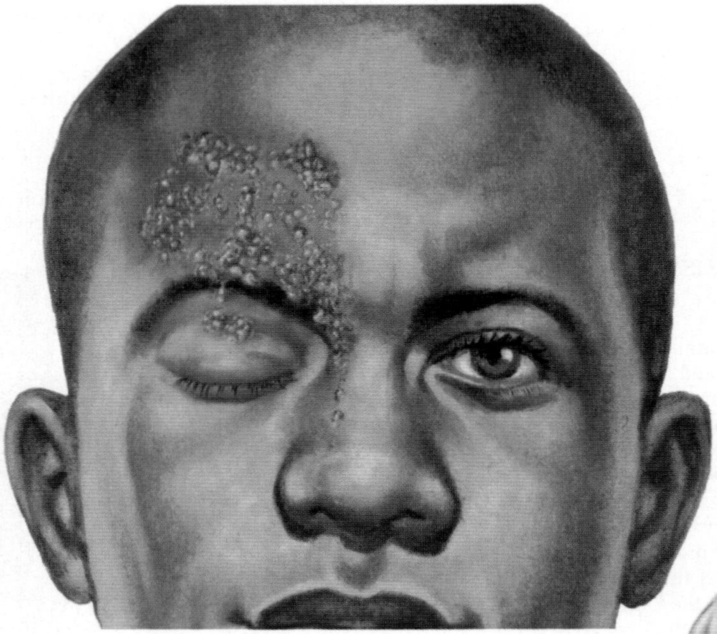

RAMSAY HUNT SYNDROME

Ramsay Hunt syndrome is due to the reactivation of VZV in the geniculate ganglion, resulting in a peripheral facial nerve palsy. Vesicular lesions may be found on the pinna or in the mouth.

POSTHERPETIC NEURALGIA

Postherpetic neuralgia is the most common neurologic complication of VZV. The pain of zoster tends to resolve as the lesions heal but may be associated with or followed by postherpetic neuralgia. Postherpetic neuralgia

Herpes zoster. Painful vesicles, erosions with an erythematous base.

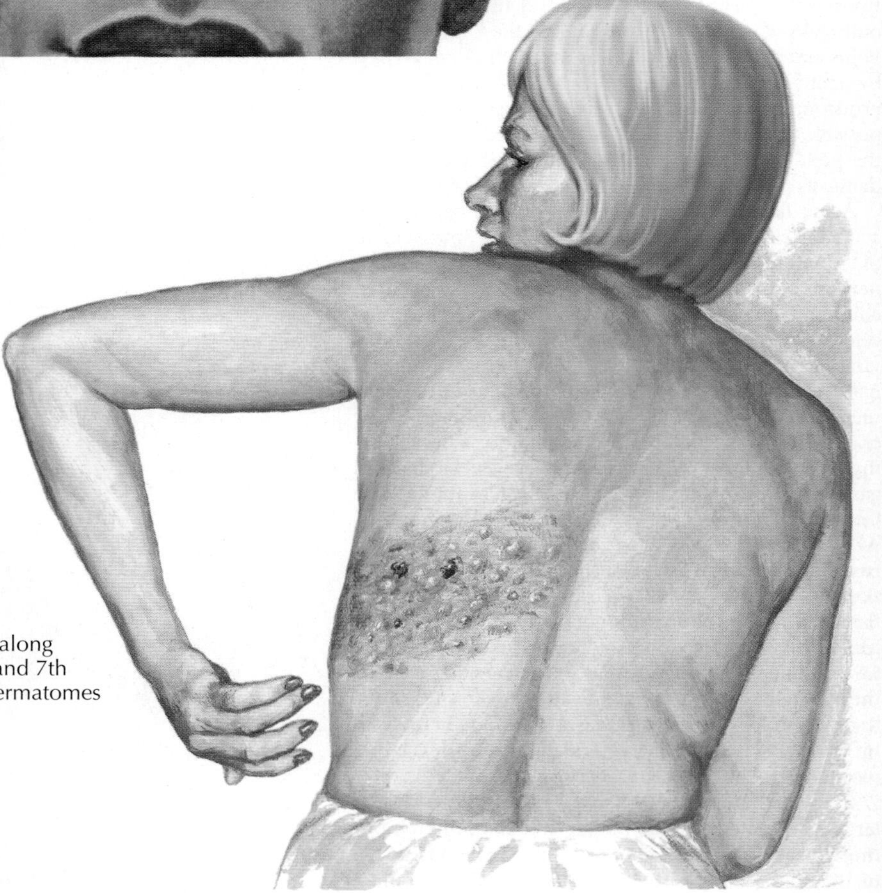

Herpes zoster along course of 6th and 7th left thoracic dermatomes

is defined as the presence of pain in the dermatomal distribution of the vesicular rash for more than 1 month after the onset of zoster, after the lesions have healed.

ZOSTER SINE HERPETE

Zoster sine herpete is pain in a dermatomal distribution without the appearance of a vesicular rash. It is diagnosed by either a fourfold increase in serum antibodies to VZV between acute and convalescent serology obtained 4 weeks later or by the demonstration of VZV IgM in CSF and/or VZV DNA in CSF by PCR.

The best diagnostic test for VZV encephalitis is the detection of VZV IgM antibodies in CSF. VZV DNA can also be detected in CSF by PCR, but this is less sensitive than the antibody.

VZV encephalitis is treated with intravenous acyclovir. Zoster is treated with oral valacyclovir, famciclovir, or acyclovir. Postherpetic neuralgia is treated with a combination of amitriptyline and gabapentin. The routine use of the varicella vaccine in childhood has decreased the incidence of chickenpox. Effectiveness declines with time, and a booster immunization is required. There is also a zoster vaccine that decreases the risk of zoster.

Plate 11.18

Infections of the Nervous System

Herpes simplex encephalitis

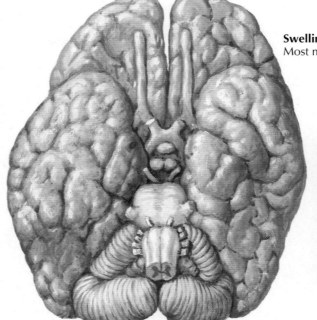

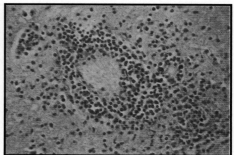

Swelling and patchy hemorrhagic areas. Most marked in right temporal lobe.

Perivascular infiltration, with mononuclear cells in disrupted brain tissue.

HERPES SIMPLEX VIRUS ENCEPHALITIS AND RABIES

Herpes simplex virus 1 (HSV-1) is acquired in childhood by contact with oral secretions. First exposure is usually asymptomatic, but in some individuals vesicular lesions develop in the mouth. The virus spreads by retrograde and anterograde transport to the trigeminal ganglion, where it establishes latent infection. HSV encephalitis is due to reactivation of latent HSV infection and presents with a subacute progression of fever, hemicranial headache, behavioral abnormalities, focal seizure activity, and focal neurologic deficits, most often dysphasia or hemiparesis. In 90% of adult patients with HSV encephalitis, FLAIR and T2- and diffusion-weighted MRI sequences demonstrate an abnormal lesion of increased signal intensity in the temporal lobe at 48 hours from symptom onset. Spinal fluid analysis demonstrates a lymphocytic pleocytosis with a normal or rarely mildly decreased glucose concentration. There may be red blood cells or xanthochromia in the CSF because this is a necrotizing encephalitis. A PCR assay for HSV-1 has a sensitivity and specificity of more than 95%. The CSF HSV PCR may be negative in the first 72 hours of symptoms of HSV encephalitis. If the clinical suspicion is high, spinal fluid should be reexamined for HSV-1 DNA. HSV antibodies can be detected in the CSF approximately 8 to 12 days after symptom onset and for as long as 3 months. A serum-to-CSF ratio of less than 20:1 is considered diagnostic of HSV encephalitis. HSV encephalitis is treated with intravenous acyclovir for 3 weeks.

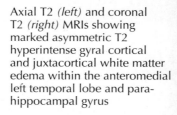

Axial T2 *(left)* and coronal T2 *(right)* MRIs showing marked asymmetric T2 hyperintense gyral cortical and juxtacortical white matter edema within the anteromedial left temporal lobe and parahippocampal gyrus

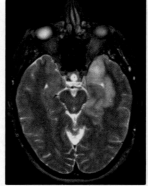

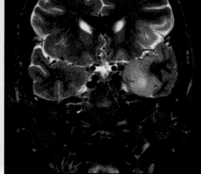

Rabies

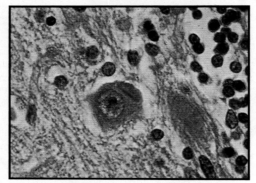

Negri inclusion body. In Purkinje cell of brain.

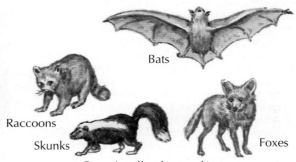

Bats

Raccoons

Skunks

Foxes

Occasionally, dogs and cats

Common animal disseminators

RABIES

Humans acquire rabies from the bite of a rabid animal or from inhalation from aerosolized virus in caves inhabited by rapid bats. Two forms of classic rabies are recognized: furious rabies, which is characterized by fever, fluctuating consciousness, phobic spasms, and autonomic dysfunction and paralytic rabies, which resembles GBS. Patients with bat rabies have different clinical features than those with classic rabies. Rabies acquired by the bite of a bat manifests with focal neurologic deficits, choreiform movements, myoclonus, seizures, and hallucinations. Phobic spasms are not a cardinal feature of bat rabies.

The diagnosis of rabies can be made by performing the reverse transcriptase PCR on saliva, nuchal skin biopsy specimens, or CSF for rabies RNA detection. Classically, the diagnosis was made by biopsy and demonstration of cytoplasmic Negri inclusion bodies. Treatment begins with an immediate washing and flushing of the wound with soap and water and disinfecting with iodine. Rabies immunoglobulin should be infiltrated into and around the wound, and rabies vaccine is administered either intramuscularly or intradermally. Postexposure prophylaxis should not await the results of laboratory confirmation of the diagnosis.

Plate 11.19

Brain: PART I

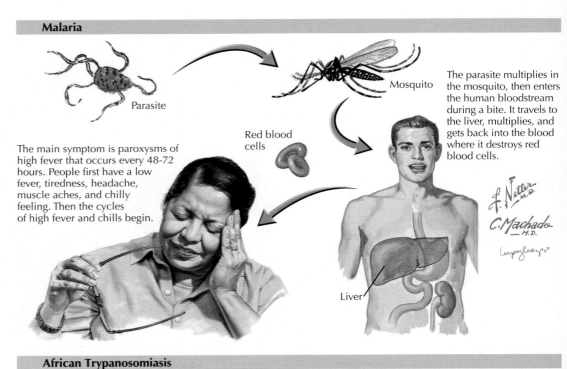

Malaria

Parasite

Mosquito

The parasite multiplies in the mosquito, then enters the human bloodstream during a bite. It travels to the liver, multiplies, and gets back into the blood where it destroys red blood cells.

Red blood cells

The main symptom is paroxysms of high fever that occurs every 48-72 hours. People first have a low fever, tiredness, headache, muscle aches, and chilly feeling. Then the cycles of high fever and chills begin.

Liver

PARASITIC INFECTIONS: CEREBRAL MALARIA AND AFRICAN TRYPANOSOMIASIS

CEREBRAL MALARIA

Humans bitten by *Anopheles* mosquitoes infected with *Plasmodium falciparum, P. vivax, P. ovale,* or *P. malariae* are at risk of developing malaria, a disorder that occurs mainly in Africa, Asia, and Central and South America, causing up to 1 million deaths annually. Cerebral malaria—typically caused by *P. falciparum*—is the most deadly form of the disease. Fever and nonspecific symptoms give way to seizures and disorders of consciousness, ranging from irritability to obtundation and coma. Progression may be acute or more gradual. Accompanying hypoglycemia, acidosis, and anemia may exacerbate the neurologic symptoms.

Diagnosis is confirmed by examination of peripheral blood smears every 8 to 24 hours. The CSF is examined to exclude other possible causes of symptoms in patients with suspected cerebral malaria. Antimalarial chemotherapy, consisting of intravenous quinine or quinidine (in an intensive care unit [ICU] setting) or artesunate, plus doxycycline, tetracycline, or clindamycin, is started without awaiting laboratory confirmation of the clinical diagnosis. Untreated cerebral malaria is generally fatal. Neurologic sequelae are common in survivors and may include motor, sensory, cognitive, or language deficits and seizures.

AFRICAN TRYPANOSOMIASIS

African trypanosomiasis in humans ("sleeping sickness") is transmitted by infected tsetse flies and takes two forms; in each, meningoencephalitis may develop. An initial inflammatory skin lesion or chancre may occur a few days after a bite by the infected fly. Infection by *T. brucei gambiense* (in West and Central Africa) may otherwise be asymptomatic for months or years. Presentation with fever, headache, arthralgia, lymphadenopathy,

African Trypanosomiasis

Infected Tsetse fly transmits trypanosome to human

Trypanosomes further divide and develop in gut of the fly, migrate to salivary glands, and undergo further development into infective stage

Trypanosomes enter lymphatics, transform into mature trypomastigote stage and begin to multiply

Trypanosomes ingested by Tsetse fly feeding on infected blood

Lethargy

"Winterbottom sign" (enlargement of posterior cervical lymph nodes)

Encephalitis

Trypomastigotes enter bloodstream and multiply

Trypomastigotes enter brain via CSF or bloodstream

and hepatosplenomegaly is followed in late stages by neurologic involvement, with lethargy, headache, personality changes, poor concentration, tremor, unsteadiness, and daytime somnolence. With further progression, the patient becomes obtunded; worsening coma leads to death. Infection by *T. brucei rhodesiense* (in East Africa) leads to a similar but more acute disorder.

Diagnosis requires identification of the trypanosome, typically in a blood smear. The CSF must be examined to confirm the diagnosis and stage the disease. Pleocytosis or increased protein concentration, or both, indicate neurologic involvement; IgM levels may be increased, and trypanosomes may be present. Serologic tests for the West but not East African disease are available; PCR is investigational. Treatment regimens with antiprotozoal agents depend on the offending organism and whether neurologic involvement has occurred.

Plate 11.20

Infections of the Nervous System

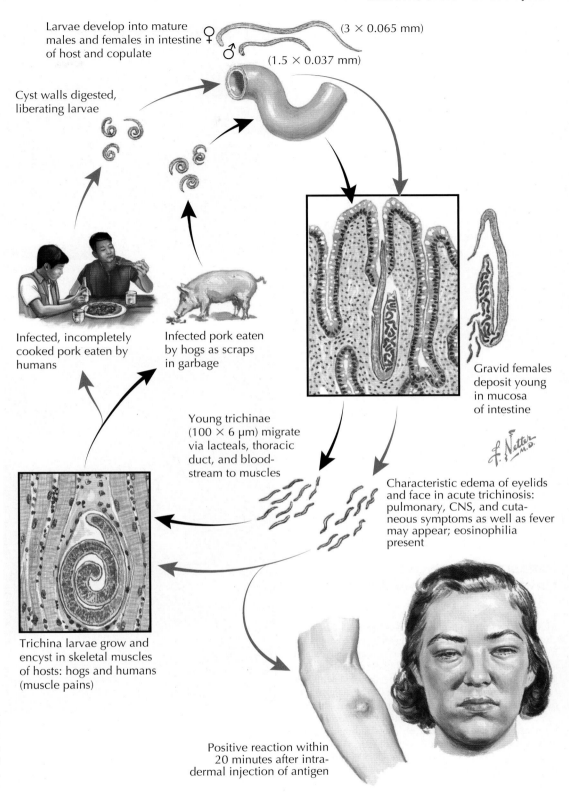

Larvae develop into mature males and females in intestine of host and copulate

(3 × 0.065 mm)

(1.5 × 0.037 mm)

Cyst walls digested, liberating larvae

Infected, incompletely cooked pork eaten by humans

Infected pork eaten by hogs as scraps in garbage

Gravid females deposit young in mucosa of intestine

Young trichinae (100 × 6 μm) migrate via lacteals, thoracic duct, and bloodstream to muscles

Characteristic edema of eyelids and face in acute trichinosis: pulmonary, CNS, and cutaneous symptoms as well as fever may appear; eosinophilia present

Trichina larvae grow and encyst in skeletal muscles of hosts: hogs and humans (muscle pains)

Positive reaction within 20 minutes after intradermal injection of antigen

PARASITIC INFECTIONS: TRICHINOSIS (TRICHINELLOSIS)

Human infection with *Trichinella spiralis* or certain other species of *Trichinella,* a nematode (roundworm), occurs most commonly by ingestion of contaminated raw or undercooked meat, especially from domestic pigs. In pigs, the larvae of *T. spiralis* are liberated from cysts in ingested meat by gastric digestion and then invade the small bowel mucosa. They develop into adult worms in the small intestine; the females are fertilized and release larvae that migrate to striated muscles, where they encyst. Thus adult worms and encysted larvae develop within the same host. Humans eating the infected pork develop trichinosis. The disorder is worldwide.

The incubation period varies with severity of infection. Abdominal pain and gastrointestinal symptoms may develop in the first week. Periorbital edema may occur for a few days. Subsequently, muscle and joint pain, muscle weakness, fever, skin rashes, headache,

and other manifestations develop. Severe infections may cause meningitis or encephalitis. Myocarditis may lead to fatal cardiac arrhythmias. Pulmonary or renal involvement occurs occasionally.

The diagnosis is suggested by the concurrence of periorbital edema, myositis, and eosinophilia and can be confirmed serologically, but serologic tests are usually unhelpful for the first 2 or 3 weeks after infection. If

necessary, skeletal muscle biopsy is performed to detect the presence of larvae. Mild infection requires only symptomatic therapy; the clinical course is self-limited. Definitive treatment is required for severe infections or neurologic involvement and consists of corticosteroids plus mebendazole or albendazole. Preventive approaches involve education about the dangers of consuming undercooked meats and control of farming techniques.

Plate 11.21

Brain: PART I

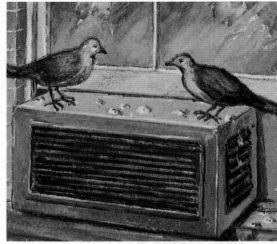

Infection is by respiratory route. Pigeon dung and air conditioners may be factors in dissemination.

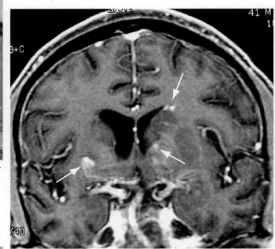

Coronal spoiled gradient T1-weighted MRI after gadolinium enhancement demonstrates multiple small enhancing lesions in both basal ganglia *(arrows)*.

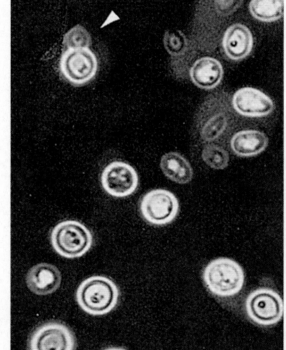

India ink preparation showing budding and capsule

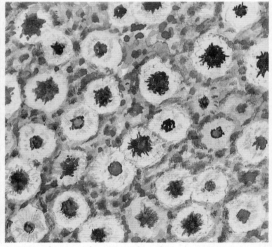

Accumulation of encapsulated cryptococci in subarachnoid space (periodic acid–Schiff or methenamine-silver stain)

PARASITIC INFECTIONS: CRYPTOCOCCAL MENINGITIS

Much of the human population has been infected subclinically by inhalation with *Cryptococcus neoformans*, a yeastlike fungus. The fungus is distributed in soil samples worldwide in areas inhabited especially by pigeons, but pigeons do not become infected with the fungus, transmission from pigeons to humans is not described, and the role of pigeon excreta in human infection is unclear. Focal pneumonitis develops in humans and may be evident on chest radiographs but only occasionally becomes symptomatic. Hematogenous spread from the lungs to the CNS is rare in immunocompetent persons unless there are very high cryptococcal antigen titers in the serum. In the immunocompromised, however, reactivation of latent infection or a new primary infection may cause a meningitic illness that is typically subacute or chronic. Thus cryptococcal meningitis is encountered most commonly in patients with HIV infection and neoplastic disease or who are on long-term immunosuppressant therapy or are transplant recipients.

Patients present with headache, personality changes, irritability, somnolence, and cognitive changes. Intracranial pressure may be increased. There may be cranial nerve deficits. The diagnosis can only be made definitively by lumbar puncture, which typically shows increased opening pressure, mononuclear pleocytosis, elevated protein concentration, and reduced glucose level in the CSF. India ink preparations can define the yeast, but this is now rarely performed; cultural isolation is preferred but may take several days. Measurement of cryptococcal capsular antigen in the CSF is helpful in suggesting cryptococcal infection while the cultures are still pending. The clinical context generally requires that the brain be imaged before lumbar puncture to exclude space-occupying lesions; when present, these are typically the result of other disorders, such as lymphoma.

A fatal outcome is likely in the absence of treatment, which generally involves intravenous amphotericin B and oral flucytosine for at least 2 weeks, followed by high-dose fluconazole therapy for 2 months. Maintenance lower-dose therapy with fluconazole is then continued for at least 1 year, when discontinuation can be considered, depending on the response to antiretroviral therapy in HIV-infected patients.

Plate 11.22

Infections of the Nervous System

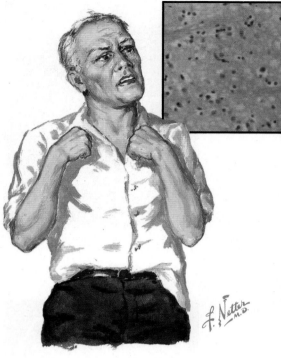

Section from putamen showing extensive loss of neurons and spongiform brain tissue. Spinal cord usually shows similar loss of motor neurons.

Myoclonus being exhibited in demented patient

Electroencephalogram showing characteristic diffuse periodic wave pattern

CREUTZFELDT-JAKOB DISEASE

Creutzfeldt-Jakob disease (CJD) is the most common prion disease. The word *prion* denotes the protein-aceous "infectious" nature of the pathogenic agent. The initial event in the pathogenesis of prion diseases is the conversion of a normal cellular protein (PrP^C) to a pathogenic isoform (PrP^{Sc}). CJD was labeled a transmissible spongiform encephalopathy because of the pathologic evidence of extensive vacuolation (spongiform changes) and amyloid plaques in the brains of afflicted individuals.

There are a number of human prion diseases: sporadic CJD, iatrogenic CJD, variant CJD, kuru, Gerstmann-Straussler-Scheinker disease, and fatal familial insomnia.

SPORADIC CREUTZFELDT-JAKOB DISEASE

The cardinal manifestations of CJD are dementia, myoclonus, and ataxia. Patients typically present with cognitive difficulty and ataxia and subsequently develop myoclonus. Diffusion-weighted and FLAIR MRI show increased signal in the cortical ribbon, putamen, caudate nuclei, and thalamus. Electroencephalography shows bisynchronous periodic sharp-wave discharges that may be time locked to myoclonus. The presence of CSF pleocytosis should initiate a search for another

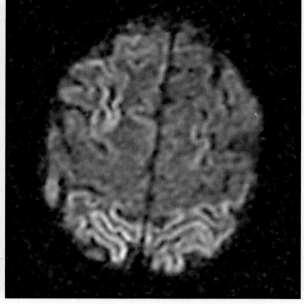

Axial diffusion-weighted MRIs showing marked abnormal hyperintense gyral cortical ribboning within both frontal and both (right > left) parietal lobes

disease because an inflammatory response is characteristically absent. The CSF 14-3-3 protein has a low specificity and can be increased in a number of CNS disorders. CSF 14-3-3 protein is elevated in 95% of patients with sporadic CJD.

Iatrogenic CJD is due to prion exposure from contaminated surgical equipment, electrode implantation, dural mater grafts, cadaveric-derived human growth hormone, and corneal or organ transplantation.

The clinical presentation of iatrogenic CJD depends somewhat on the route of intracerebral inoculation, with some cases resembling that described for sporadic CJD and others resembling a cerebellar syndrome.

Variant CJD is acquired from ingestion of contaminated meat and typically consists of behavioral and psychiatric symptoms, peripheral sensory disturbances, and cerebellar ataxia.

Plate 11.23

Brain: PART I

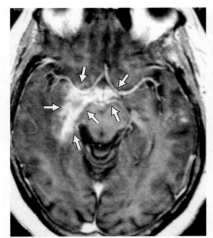
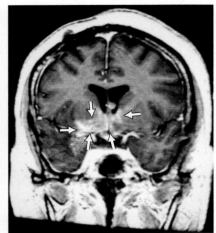

Axial and coronal T1-weighted fast spin echo MRIs after gadolinium demonstrating intense enhancement of hypothalamic region, adjacent basal ganglia, right temporal lobe, and dura *(arrows).*

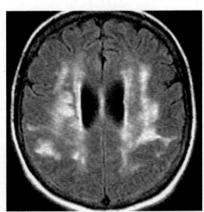
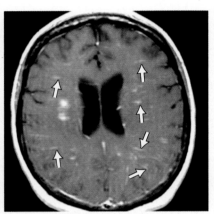

Axial FLAIR MRI demonstrating a patchy confluent pattern of involvement of paraventricular and central white matter, with extension into subcortical hemispheric white matter

Axial T1-weighted fast spin echo MRI after gadolinium showing some globular enhancement and a linear pattern consistent with infiltration of Virchow-Robin spaces *(arrows)*

NEUROSARCOIDOSIS

Although this systemic noncaseating granulomatous disorder has not been associated with a specific infecting microorganism, it has many similarities to a chronic infective or inflammatory disease and is thus being considered in this section. Sarcoidosis is more common in Black people than in White people. It is often asymptomatic, being discovered by the presence of hilar adenopathy on a chest radiograph. Neurologic involvement is less common and may present acutely, subacutely, or more insidiously. The disease is usually monophasic but can follow a relapsing-remitting or progressive course.

Presentation may be with cranial nerve deficits from a basal meningitis, the most common being neuropathies that affect CNs VII, V, VIII, and II. Facial nerve (CN VII) involvement may be unilateral or bilateral; when bilateral, it may occur simultaneously or sequentially on the two sides. Endocrine disturbances from hypothalamic-pituitary involvement may manifest as hypothyroidism, hypogonadism, hypoadrenalism, or hypopituitarism; diabetes insipidus sometimes occurs. An intraparenchymal lesion may lead to seizures; masquerade as a cerebral tumor, producing focal deficits and increased intracranial pressure; lead to a nonspecific encephalopathy; cause obstructive hydrocephalus; or result in myelopathy or myeloradiculopathy if the spinal cord is affected. Neurosarcoid may affect the peripheral nervous system, causing multiple mononeuropathy or polyneuropathy. Myopathy has also been described.

The diagnosis is established with certainty only by histopathologic examination of a biopsy specimen. All patients with suspected neurosarcoidosis require evaluation for extraneural involvement that may serve as a site for biopsy. An elevated serum angiotensin-converting enzyme (ACE) level may be helpful for diagnosis but is not specific, and normal findings do not exclude the diagnosis. CSF is often abnormal and may simulate an infective process, with an increased cell count (usually a mononuclear pleocytosis) and elevated protein concentration; glucose level is normal or reduced. The IgG index may be increased, and oligoclonal bands may be present. The CSF ACE level is sometimes elevated, a suggestive but nonspecific finding. Chest radiographs or CT scans often reveal hilar adenopathy and allow for mediastinal lymph node biopsy. Cranial CT or MRI may document the site and extent of neurologic involvement and also identify a site for biopsy if diagnostic uncertainty persists or the response to therapy is poor.

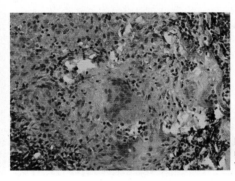

Hilar node biopsy. Noncaseating granuloma with lymphocytes, macrophages, and epithelioid, mast, and plasma cells compatible with sarcoidosis.

Controlled treatment trials are not available to guide therapy, but treatment with corticosteroids is the generally accepted approach. The duration of treatment is determined individually depending on disease location, severity, and response to therapy. Other immunomodulatory approaches have also been used in patients who do not respond to or are unable to tolerate corticosteroids. In only rare instances is resection of a mass lesion necessary, although placement of a ventricular drain may be needed in patients with hydrocephalus. Endocrinologic abnormalities require correction.

Plate 11.24

Infections of the Nervous System

NEUROLOGIC COMPLICATIONS OF COVID-19

The first case of SARS-CoV-2 infection was discovered in Wuhan, China, in December 2019, and the clinical syndrome caused by this virus has been named coronavirus disease 19 (COVID-19). The virus caused a global pandemic claiming millions of lives. Despite the advancements in medicine since the 1918–1919 pandemic, most notably the ability to care for patients in ICUs, the healthcare system was strained beyond its capacity to care for the ever-increasing numbers of patients with COVID-19, leading to lockdowns, quarantines, social distancing, and mask mandates. Families could not visit their dying loved ones, and visiting the elderly in senior living facilities was prohibited. Despite these aggressive measures, it was impossible to prevent the worldwide spread of the virus or to prevent the development of variants that were more transmissible.

The most common initial symptoms of COVID-19 are cough, fever, fatigue, headache, myalgias, and diarrhea. SARS-CoV-2 enters cells of the respiratory tract through an interaction between the spike protein of the virus and the angiotensin-converting receptor-2 (ACE2) in lung epithelium. ACE2 receptors are abundant in the respiratory tract.

The early neurologic symptoms of COVID-19 are anosmia (loss of smell) and ageusia (loss of taste). The symptoms of cough, fever, fatigue, and headache are nonspecific, but the loss of smell is specific and the first symptom that led to testing and diagnosis. Anosmia is attributed to viral entry, infection, and death of olfactory sustentacular epithelial cells and not infection of the olfactory nerve. The loss of taste is due to the loss of smell.

Severe illness usually begins approximately 1 week after the onset of symptoms. Dyspnea is the most common symptom of severe disease and is often accompanied by hypoxemia. Severe illness is associated with high levels of proinflammatory cytokines referred to as *cytokine storm*. The proinflammatory cytokines are interleukins (IL-1, IL-2, and IL-6), tumor necrosis factor, granulocyte-colony stimulating factor, and macrophage inflammatory protein-1.

The neurologic complications of COVID-19, which develop in patients with more severe disease, are encephalopathy, acute necrotizing hemorrhagic encephalopathy, hemorrhagic and ischemic stroke, cerebral venous thrombosis, seizures, and Guillain-Barré syndrome (GBS).

Encephalopathy is the most common complication and is due to hypoxia, metabolic abnormalities as multiorgan failure develops, and the immune-mediated systemic inflammatory response. Hypoxia is often an indication of impending respiratory failure. The neurologic complications of COVID-19 are not the result of viral infection of the nervous system because SARS-CoV-2 has rarely been detected in CSF by PCR assays. The high level of proinflammatory cytokines and chemokines that causes the neurologic complications of bacterial meningitis is the same inflammatory response that contributes to the neurologic complications of COVID-19. The severe inflammatory response causes multiorgan failure, disseminated intravascular coagulation, and coagulopathy and stroke. Common laboratory abnormalities in patients with stroke are elevated D-dimer and ferritin levels. Patients with severe disease are treated with subcutaneous

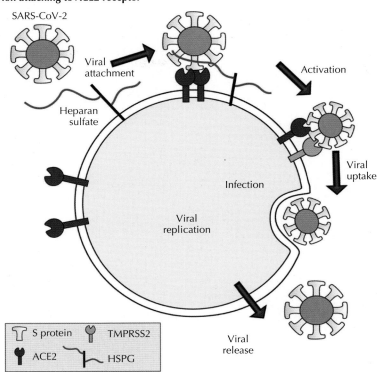

SARS-CoV-2 virion attaching to ACE2 receptor

Transmembrane serine protease 2 (TMPRSS2) is needed for viral entry to epithelial cells. *From Clausen TM, Sandoval DR, Spliid CB, et al. SARS-CoV-2 infection depends on cellular heparan sulfate and ACE2. Cell. 2020;183(4):1043-1057.e15.*

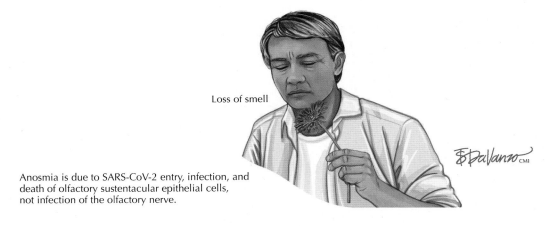

Loss of smell

Anosmia is due to SARS-CoV-2 entry, infection, and death of olfactory sustentacular epithelial cells, not infection of the olfactory nerve.

low-molecular-weight heparin for thromboprophylaxis. This approach has decreased the incidence of stroke.

GBS is a postinfectious neurologic complication of COVID-19. As is so often the case, the etiology is believed to be a molecular mimicry mechanism. SARS-CoV-2 epitopes are similar to components of peripheral nerves. Antibodies produced by the immune system to attack the virus bind to components of the peripheral nervous system, causing GBS. The clinical syndrome resembles classic GBS, and examination of the CSF demonstrates an albuminocytologic dissociation. The virus has not been detected by PCR in CSF in patients with COVID-19–associated GBS.

Children, in general, had significantly less morbidity and mortality from SARS-CoV-2. It is not known whether this is due to their ability to produce antibodies from other milder coronavirus respiratory infections that children have had or due to a lack of ACE2 receptors for binding of the spike protein of SARS-CoV-2. Some children developed multisystem inflammatory syndrome, which can also follow other infectious diseases in children.

Between the availability of vaccines and the development of herd immunity from both infection and vaccines, 2 years after the beginning of the pandemic, the number of cases and hospitalizations began to decrease.

Therapeutics were as challenging as the inability to contain the spread of the virus. Dexamethasone was used to treat the severe inflammatory process. As is true of every infectious disease, the earlier treatment is begun before more severe disease develops, the higher the likelihood of preventing severe disease. Intravenous monoclonal antibody therapy helped decrease hospitalizations but was most efficacious in patients whose immune system had not yet been activated. In a double-blind, randomized, placebo-controlled trial, remdesivir showed faster time to recovery in hospitalized patients but did not decrease mortality. But even in the era of "modern medicine," the development of antiviral therapy was painstakingly slow. The FDA approved Paxlovid in May 2023 for mild to moderately symptomatic patients.

Some symptoms may persist on a long-term basis but are of uncertain etiology.

NEURO-ONCOLOGY

Plate 12.1

Brain: PART I

SOME COMMON MANIFESTATIONS OF BRAIN TUMORS

CLINICAL PRESENTATIONS OF BRAIN TUMORS

Brain tumors commonly present with symptoms of elevated intracranial pressure or focal neurologic dysfunction. Elevated intracranial pressure can directly result from an enlarging mass or can be secondary to the development of hydrocephalus stemming from obstruction of the ventricular system and cerebrospinal fluid (CSF) flow by the tumor. The specific neurologic dysfunction results from the local mass effect of the tumor. Occasionally, clinically silent tumors are found incidentally on imaging studies done for other reasons, such as head trauma.

Clinical Manifestations. Traditionally, headaches, nausea and vomiting, and papilledema constitute the clinical triad of increased intracranial pressure. Although headaches themselves are nonspecific, headaches resulting from elevated intracranial pressure are generalized in location and usually are worst upon awakening, occasionally even waking a patient from sleep. The vomiting is ascribed to pressure in the region of the fourth ventricle, though the "classic" projectile vomiting is rarely seen. Papilledema, or blurring of the optic disc margin due to swelling of the optic nerve (cranial nerve II) from the increased intracranial pressure, can be detected by ophthalmoscopic examination.

Local mass effect can result in a variety of neurologic symptoms, depending on what structures are affected. Symptoms may stem from local neural tissue invasion or compression of adjacent structures. Often these focal signs and symptoms will manifest before the tumor is large enough to cause significant increased intracranial pressure. Clinical presentations depend on the function of the affected tissue. For instance, *headaches* may also result from local mass effect. Typically, these headaches localize to the side of the tumor. They are usually dull and constant in character. Occasionally they may be severe. The combination of headaches associated with new neurologic abnormalities, or changes in headache characteristic suggestive of increased intracranial pressure, should warrant consideration of an underlying neoplasm.

Seizures are another common sign that occur in association with an underlying malignancy. They can be either generalized or focal, with focal seizures representative of the underlying location of the tumor. For example, distinct *motor or sensory symptoms*, such as focal shaking or episodic numbness or paresthesia, relate to the functions of the cortical areas affected by the tumor. *Cognitive changes* may herald an underlying intracranial neoplasm, especially if they are frontal in location. Often these changes are subtle, with patients experiencing fatigue, memory difficulties, personality changes, or apathy. *Difficulties with balance* or *disequilibrium* often localize to the posterior fossa. *Visual field defects* such as homonymous hemianopsia may result from damage to the optic tracts, and bitemporal hemianopsia is often seen with compression of the optic chiasm by pituitary tumors. Occasionally, patients will be asymptomatic but the physical examination may reveal subtle neurologic abnormalities such as a drift of an upper extremity, asymmetric reflexes, or a positive Babinski sign.

Diagnostic Studies. Once suspicion is raised of an intracranial malignancy, neuroimaging is warranted. Contrast-enhanced magnetic resonance imaging (MRI)

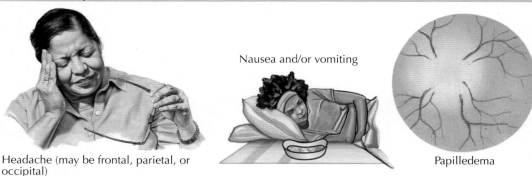

Intracranial pressure triad

Headache (may be frontal, parietal, or occipital)

Nausea and/or vomiting

Papilledema

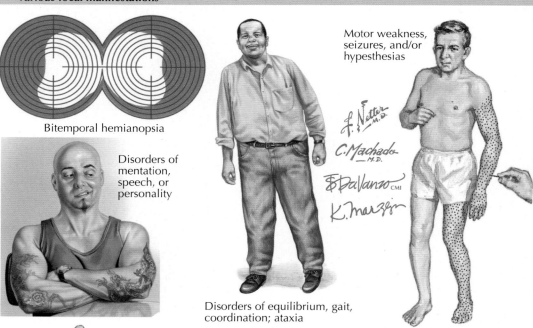

Various focal manifestations

Bitemporal hemianopsia

Disorders of mentation, speech, or personality

Motor weakness, seizures, and/or hypesthesias

Disorders of equilibrium, gait, coordination; ataxia

Reflex abnormalities (Babinski sign)

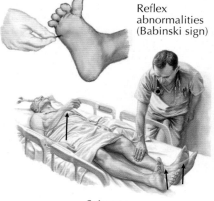

Seizures

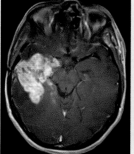

MRI of right temporal glioblastoma causing left homonymous hemianopsia

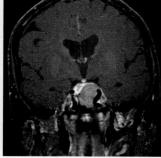

MRI of pituitary macroadenoma causing bitemporal hemianopsia

is the diagnostic modality of choice as it allows for visualization of the tumor in relation to the surrounding brain parenchyma, especially in the posterior fossa. Computed tomography (CT) is still used in patients for whom MRI is contraindicated or in emergent situations where time is of the essence. In addition, it is superior to MRI in the detection of bony involvement, particularly in the region of the skull base. Other imaging modalities include magnetic resonance spectroscopy (MRS), which analyzes the chemical composition of the area of interest in an effort to differentiate tumors from other abnormalities, and positron emission tomography (PET) with fluorodeoxyglucose or amino acid tracers, which detects metabolically active tumors. Finally, perfusion MRI has emerged as a potentially useful technique as it identifies areas of increased vascularity, which can be useful for planning surgical removal.

Plate 12.2

Neuro-Oncology

Change Between 2016 and 2021 WHO Classification of CNS Tumors

2016 Classification	2021 Classification
Grading via Roman numerals (WHO I–IV)	Grading via Arabic numerals (WHO 1–4)
Graded across different tumor types	Graded within tumor types - Loss of modifiers such as anaplastic; using grades of 2–4 instead - Revised terminology of 13 tumors
Diffuse gliomas include tumors seen in both adult and pediatric population	Separated diffuse gliomas into adult-type and pediatric-type diffuse glioma - Pediatric tumors divided into four types of low-grade diffuse gliomas and four types of high-grade diffuse gliomas, all defined by specific molecular features
Glioblastoma subclassified as primary (*IDH* wildtype) vs. secondary (*IDH* mutant)	Glioblastoma now defined only as *IDH* wildtype astrocytoma (*CDKN2A/B* homozygous loss, *TERT* promoter mutation, *EGFR* mutation, gain of chromosome 7 or loss of chromosome 10)
Grading still defined by histopathologic features	Certain molecular parameters automatically upgrade to grade 4: molecular GBM, *IDH* wildtype; *IDH* mutant astrocytoma with *CDKN2A* deletion; DMG with H3K27 alteration; DHG with H3G34 mutation; pediatric high-grade glioma, *IDH* wildtype and H3 wildtype

CDKN2A/B, Cyclin-dependent kinase inhibitor; *DMG*, diffuse midline glioma; *DHG*, diffuse hemispheric glioma; *EGFR*, epidermal growth factor receptor; *GBM*, glioblastoma; *IDH*, isocitrate dehydrogenase; *TERT*, telomerase reverse transcriptase.

Modified from Louis DN, Perry A, Wesseling P, et al. The 2021 WHO Classification of Tumors of the Central Nervous System: a summary. *Neuro Oncol.* 2021;23(8):1231–1251.

2021 WHO Changes to Classification of Central Nervous System Tumors

In 2016 the World Health Organization (WHO) Classification of Tumors of the Central Nervous System (CNS) updated its classification schema of brain tumors, incorporating molecular data for the first time. The premise is that the inclusion of molecular markers will provide greater objectivity to the diagnosis of these tumors and improve the grouping of tumors based on underlying biology. For instance, isocitrate dehydrogenase (*IDH*) 1 and 2 genes emerged as a key marker for gliomas. This in conjunction with co-occurrence of codeletion of the p arm of chromosome 1 and the q arm of chromosome 19 (1p/19q codeletion) or mutation of the alpha thalassemia mental retardation X-linked (*ATRX*) gene have resulted in more narrowly defined subcategories of oligodendrogliomas and astrocytomas, respectively. The combination of molecular parameters with traditional histology restructured the classification of many tumors, including gliomas, medulloblastomas, and ependymomas, as well as highlighted new distinct entities. The fifth edition of the WHO classification was published in 2021 and continues to advance the role of molecular diagnostics in the classification of CNS tumors while adhering to traditional histologic characterization. This has resulted in simplification of nomenclature with grading based on histologic and molecular parameters.

Significant changes have been made with the most recent updated 2021 WHO classification. For instance, the numerical grade of tumors has converted from Roman numerals to Arabic numerals in keeping with the classification of other solid tumors. Most importantly, approaches to tumor nomenclature and grading have been made, resulting in changes in categorization of tumors and the emergence of new tumor types. This has especially affected gliomas, including ependymomas, glioneuronal tumors, and neuronal tumors. Now there are six families: adult-type diffuse gliomas, pediatric-type diffuse low-grade gliomas (LGGs), pediatric-type diffuse high-grade gliomas (HGGs), circumscribed astrocytic gliomas, glioneuronal and neuronal tumors, and ependymomas. What is especially striking with this approach is the division of diffuse gliomas into adult type and pediatric type based on the clinical and molecular distinctions of these tumors that occur in each population.

Classification of adult-type diffuse gliomas has also been simplified. Oligodendrogliomas are now defined by the presence of both *IDH* mutation and 1p/19q codeletion, whereas the rest of the *IDH* mutated gliomas are considered *IDH* mutant diffuse astrocytomas, further graded 2 to 4. The term "anaplastic" has been replaced by the numerical grade of the tumor. Thus what were previously called anaplastic astrocytomas, anaplastic oligodendrogliomas, and anaplastic pleomorphic xanthoastrocytomas are now designated, respectively, as WHO 3 astrocytoma, *IDH* mutant; WHO 3 oligodendroglioma, *IDH* mutant and 1p/19q codeleted; and WHO 3 pleomorphic xanthoastrocytoma. The incorporation of molecular findings, such as cyclin-dependent kinase inhibitor (*CDKN*) 2A and 2B homozygous deletion in *IDH* mutant gliomas, automatically delineates these tumors as *IDH* mutant astrocytoma, grade 4, bypassing the need for traditional histologic features required of a grade 4 designation. *IDH* wildtype diffuse astrocytomas are now categorized as a glioblastoma (GBM) rather than an astrocytoma, grade 4, if traditional histologic features such as microvascular proliferation and necrosis are seen or if molecular parameters (defined later) are met, regardless of histology. *IDH* mutant GBMs have now been classified as astrocytoma, *IDH* mutant, grade 4.

The emergence of the pediatric low-grade and high-grade diffuse gliomas highlights the importance of separating pediatric gliomas from other diffuse gliomas. Pediatric low-grade diffuse gliomas have been subdivided into four entities categorized by molecular features such as alterations in the mitogen-activated protein kinase pathways. The pediatric high-grade diffuse gliomas are also subclassified into four types, with each relying on molecular features, whether epigenetic changes or fusion proteins, for their classification. Recognition of epigenetic changes to histones such as histone 3 (H3), as well as the more recently discovered enhancer of zeste homolog inhibitory protein (EZHIP), allows for more accurate diagnosis of these aggressive tumors.

Plate 12.3

Brain: PART I

GLIOMAS

Gliomas represent tumors arising from glial cells that comprise the supporting tissue in the brain. Gliomas can be classified as low grade or high grade depending on the degree of aggressive features seen on histology. One caveat to this classification scheme is that it may not reflect the underlying biology. Traditionally, LGGs are slower growing tumors, whereas HGGs are more aggressive with a faster rate of recurrence. They are further subdivided based on their histopathologic appearance. For example, astrocytomas represent tumors arising from astrocytes, whereas oligodendrogliomas have features consistent with oligodendrocytes. Other tumors falling under the category of gliomas include ependymomas, GBMs, and rarer tumors such as gangliogliomas. As noted earlier, the updated classification schema from 2021 has reduced gliomas to only three subtypes: GBM, *IDH* wildtype; astrocytoma, *IDH* mutant; and oligodendroglioma, *IDH* mutant, 1p/19q-codeleted.

LGGs are less common than HGGs and tend to affect younger patients. Many of the LGGs are considered pediatric tumors. Historically, LGGs include tumors designated as WHO grade 1 or 2. The most common LGGs are diffuse astrocytomas, oligodendrogliomas, and pilocytic astrocytomas. Rarer tumors include ganglioglioma and pleomorphic xanthoastrocytoma (PXA). Gangliogliomas and PXA, considered a WHO 1 tumor, may occasionally harbor *BRAF* mutations, which may be an appropriate therapeutic target. Subependymal giant cell astrocytomas (SEGAs) are benign tumors consisting of large ganglionic astrocytes arising from the wall of the lateral ventricles. They are most often found in patients with tuberous sclerosis. Though ependymomas are considered gliomas, they are traditionally considered separate from the other LGGs. Molecularly, the low-grade diffuse astrocytomas and oligodendrogliomas harbor *IDH* mutations. HGGs include those tumors of WHO grade 3 or higher. Interestingly, the WHO 3 astrocytomas and oligodendrogliomas in the 2021 WHO classification all harbor *IDH* mutations and behave biologically more akin to their grade 2 counterparts.

Clinical Manifestations. The neurologic presentation depends on the location and size of the tumor and its rate of growth. Very slow growing tumors can become impressively large without causing significant symptoms. More rapidly growing small tumors located near sensitive areas such as the cerebral cortex may cause seizures or difficulties with language or vision. Tumors located deep within the frontal lobe may reach significantly larger size before producing focal neurologic symptoms, even if they grow rapidly. Headache and cognitive dysfunction with memory loss and apathy may develop as early symptoms of these deep tumors, especially if the corpus callosum is involved. Tumors within the brainstem produce symptoms such as double vision, facial weakness, or difficulty swallowing related to local involvement of the brainstem nuclei. Gangliogliomas, which commonly arise in the temporal lobe, are notable for causing seizures.

Diagnostic Studies. On MRI, LGGs often present as an infiltrative nonenhancing lesion. Pilocytic astrocytomas have a large cystic component with an enhancing mural nodule (see Pediatric Brain Tumors) and classically are found in the posterior fossa. Calcifications are most commonly seen with oligodendrogliomas of all grades. Grade 3 gliomas may resemble GBMs on MRI, highlighting the necessity of obtaining tissue for a definitive neuropathologic diagnosis. Ependymomas

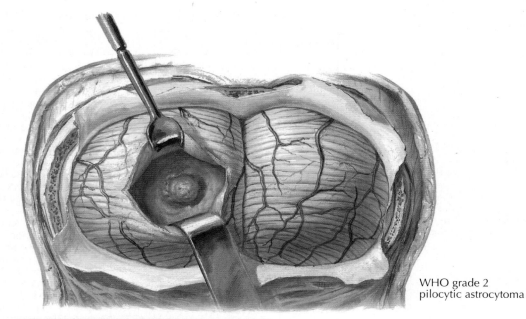

WHO grade 2 pilocytic astrocytoma

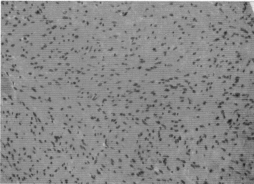

Astrocytoma, *IDH* mutant, grade 2

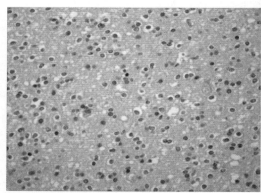

Oligodendroglioma, *IDH* mutant, 1p/19q codeleted, grade 2

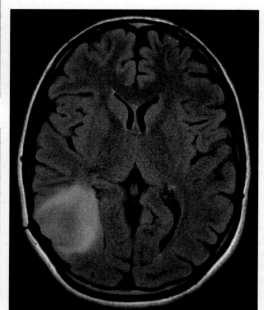

MRI of WHO grade 2 astrocytoma

usually strongly enhance with cystic and calcification components commonly seen. Often, the presence of calcifications in a fourth ventricle tumor is suggestive, although nondiagnostic, of an ependymoma. Because 10% of ependymomas have disseminated upon presentation, it is necessary to image the entire brain and spine by MRI and examine the CSF for the presence of malignant cells.

Treatment. The treatment of gliomas is highly variable and depends on the histopathologic subtype. For pilocytic astrocytomas and gangliogliomas, complete surgical resection is potentially curative. Tumors harboring a *BRAF* mutation, such as pleomorphic xanthoastrocytomas and gangliogliomas, may respond to targeted therapy. Currently, there are trials examining the efficacy of *IDH* inhibitors for *IDH* mutant LGGs (https://clinicaltrials.gov, NCT04164901). For LGGs with significant residual disease after resection, the standard treatment consists of radiation therapy followed by adjuvant chemotherapy. The standard of care for grade 3 gliomas is radiation therapy and chemotherapy. Adjuvant temozolomide has been found to improve survival for non-codeleted 1p/19q grade 3 tumors, and PCV (procarbazine, CCNU, and vincristine) chemotherapy has shown survival benefit for 1p/19q codeleted grade 3 tumors.

Plate 12.4

Neuro-Oncology

GLIOBLASTOMAS

GBMs are the most frequently occurring subtype of glioma and the most aggressive. They are now officially classified as a WHO 4 GBM, *IDH* wildtype tumors. Histopathologic features include nuclear atypia, hyper-cellularity, mitoses, microvascular proliferation, and necrosis. The updated 2021 WHO classification has in-cluded additional molecular markers such as homozy-gous deletion of *CDKN2A/B* gene, promoter mutation in telomerase reverse transcriptase *(TERT)* gene, and amplification of the epidermal growth factor receptor *(EGFR)* gene as sufficient to render a diagnosis of GBM in IDH wildtype astrocytoma, regardless of histologic grade. The median age of diagnosis is 65 years. GBMs are preferentially localized to the cerebral hemispheres; very rarely they occur in the brainstem, meninges, or spinal cord. For primary or de novo GBMs (*IDH* wild-type) that arise with no preexisting lesion, the natural history is usually short, with a median survival of 15 to 18 months. The previously coined "WHO IV GBM, *IDH* mutant" tumor is now reclassified as a WHO 4 astrocytoma, *IDH* mutant and is thought to develop through progression from lower-grade gliomas. These are much less frequent (5%–10%), typically occur in younger patients, and are associated with longer sur-vival than primary GBM. Comparisons of the molecu-lar profiles of primary and secondary GBMs indicate that they represent distinct entities with evolution through different genetic abnormalities and through activation of different molecular signaling pathways.

GBMs are characterized by molecular heterogeneity. Through molecular profiling, three subgroups have been identified based on commonly mutated genes and pathways, though the clinical application remains unclear. Moreover, the discovery of key genes and path-ways affected in GBM development have led to the proposal for the diagnostic entity of "molecular GBM," even when traditional histologic criteria are not met.

Clinical Manifestations. As discussed earlier, signs and symptoms of underlying GBMs reflect the location of the tumor and its rate of growth. Because of the rapid rate of growth, symptoms tend to be of shorter duration before diagnosis. The most frequent present-ing symptoms are headaches, focal neurologic deficits, and seizures.

Diagnostic Studies. On MRI, GBMs commonly present with heterogeneous or ring-like enhancement admixed with central areas of necrosis. Fluid attenu-ated inversion recovery (FLAIR) and T2-weighted MRI images illustrate infiltrative tumor and surrounding edema, which is often significant. If MRI is contraindi-cated, CT with and without contrast is acceptable, though the anatomy is less defined.

Treatment. Treatment of GBMs is multimodal, in-volving surgery, radiation, and chemotherapy. Initial neurosurgical resection allows for definitive diagnosis, alleviation of neurologic symptoms, and debulking, which can improve outcome. After surgery, patients undergo radiation in combination with chemotherapy. External-beam radiation has been shown to be the sin-gle most effective treatment for GBMs. The addition of temozolomide, an alkylating agent, has shown to sig-nificantly extend survival. Despite combined therapy, the tumors almost inevitably recur and progress. Prog-nostic factors associated with increased survival include younger age, higher performance status, greater extent of resection, and some genetic factors, such as the pres-ence of the methylation of the DNA repair enzyme O6-methylguanine DNA-methyltransferase (MGMT) or *IDH* mutation. Experimental therapies targeting

Large, hemispheric glioblastoma multiforme. With central areas of necrosis; brain distorted to opposite side.

MRI of left frontal glioblastoma

Coronal section and corpus callosum glioma

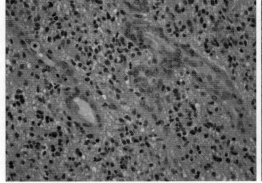

Histopathology of glioblastoma showing microvascular proliferation

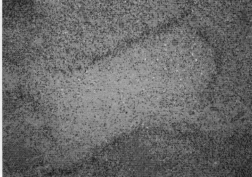

Histopathology of glioblastoma showing pseudopalisading necrosis

angiogenesis (the formation of new blood vessels from preexisting adjacent vessels) have emerged as novel an-ticancer agents. For example, bevacizumab, a human-ized monoclonal antibody to vascular endothelial growth factor (VEGF), was granted approval by the US Food and Drug Administration (FDA) for recurrent GBM; however, although progression-free survival is improved, there is no benefit to overall survival. Tumor-treating fields, which inhibit mitosis by changing the intracellular electric fields, were approved by the FDA for recurrent and newly diagnosed GBM in 2011 and 2015, respectively. Current research has focused on the development and use of small-molecule inhibitors to

target molecular signaling pathways implicated in tu-morigenesis, as well as immunotherapy.

In addition to treatment of tumor growth, symptom-atic treatment is equally as important. Corticosteroids are often used to relieve the surrounding edema. Anti-epileptic agents are only necessary when patients expe-rience seizures. As a rule, non–enzyme-inducing agents are preferred to minimize interactions with chemo-therapy or other therapeutic agents. Stimulants may be considered to help address fatigue, though the evidence supporting this is modest at best. Mood disorders are quite common in patients with primary brain tumors and may be managed with antidepressants.

Plate 12.5

Brain: PART I

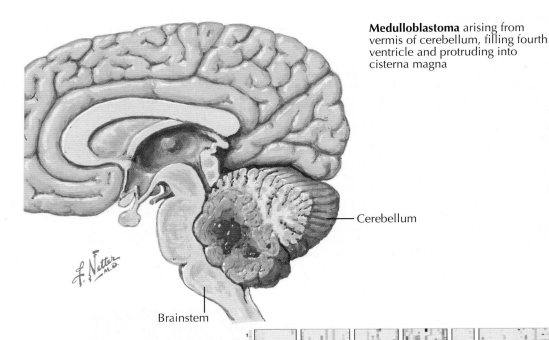

Medulloblastoma arising from vermis of cerebellum, filling fourth ventricle and protruding into cisterna magna

Cerebellum

Brainstem

PEDIATRIC BRAIN TUMORS

Brain tumors are the second most common type of cancer in children and the most common type of solid tumor. These tumors often occur in the posterior fossa; the most common types include pilocytic astrocytomas, malignant gliomas, and medulloblastomas. Plates 12.5 and 12.6 focus on brainstem gliomas and medulloblastomas.

Brainstem gliomas encompass a number of tumor subtypes, each with its own pathologic and clinical characteristics. Though they can be seen in adult patients, they are far more common in children. There are four types: dorsal exophytic gliomas, tectal gliomas, cervicomedullary gliomas, and diffuse midline gliomas, under which fall the diffuse infiltrating pontine gliomas (DIPGs). Dorsal exophytic gliomas are slow-growing astrocytomas arising from the floor of the fourth ventricle. Intrinsic midbrain tectal gliomas tend to be low-grade astrocytomas, occurring next to the third ventricle and aqueduct of Sylvius. Cervicomedullary tumors typically are low-grade astrocytomas of the upper spinal cord and lower brainstem, though other tumor types can be seen.

Diffuse midline gliomas are the most aggressive types of tumors. The median age of diagnosis is 5 to 9 years with a very slight female sex predominance. These tumors have the worst prognosis and account for most childhood brain tumor–related deaths. They occur in the midline structures such as the pons, thalamus, and spinal cord. Diffuse midline gliomas typically harbor mutations in genes encoding histone H3 (H3K27M). DIPGs harbor H3K27M mutations in 80% of cases. In 2016 the H3K27M mutant diffuse midline glioma was recognized in the updated WHO classification of CNS tumors as a new entity. Unlike adult gliomas, *IDH* mutations are notably absent in DIPG. Patients often present with cranial nerve palsies (especially cranial nerve VI), long trace signs, and cerebellar dysfunction. Diagnosis is typically made radiographically, especially in

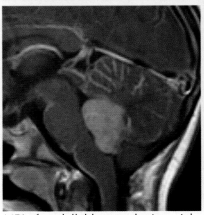

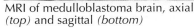
MRI of medulloblastoma brain, axial *(top)* and sagittal *(bottom)*

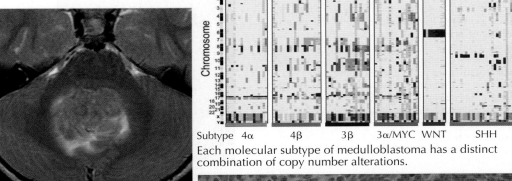

| Subtype | 4α | 4β | 3β | 3α/MYC | WNT | SHH |

Each molecular subtype of medulloblastoma has a distinct combination of copy number alterations.

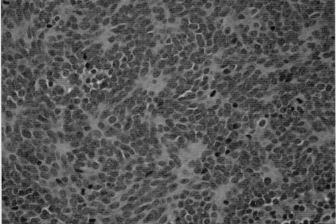
Medulloblastoma histopathology

the appropriate demographic setting. Radiation is the main treatment of DIPG; unfortunately, responses are transient with a median survival of 10 months.

Medulloblastomas are WHO grade 4 embryonal brain tumors that arise in the cerebellum and tend to disseminate through CSF pathways throughout the brain and spine. They are highly cellular tumors with a highly variable prognosis that is not predicted by histologic features, which typically consist of tightly packed

small round blue cells. Analysis of their molecular profiles has revealed that this heterogeneity arises because they consist of four main subclasses associated with distinct demographics, genetics, clinical presentation, and outcome. This may actually influence treatment recommendations to balance survival and morbidity of treatment. For instance, WNT (wingless/INT) medulloblastomas typically have a good prognosis with 5-year survival of greater than 90%. Thus there is interest in

Plate 12.6

Neuro-Oncology

BRAINSTEM GLIOMA

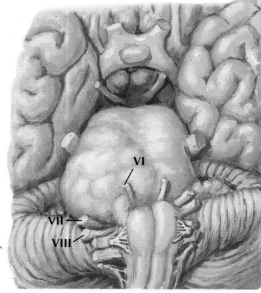

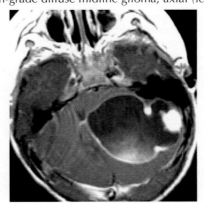

Child with cranial nerve (VI, VIII) palsy on same side as tumor, with contralateral limb weakness

Glioma distorts brainstem and cranial nerves VI, VII, VIII

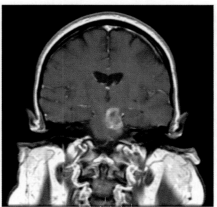

MRIs of pediatric high-grade diffuse midline glioma, axial *(left)* and coronal *(right)*

MRI of juvenile pilocytic astrocytoma

PEDIATRIC BRAIN TUMORS (Continued)

potentially reducing the dose of radiation in patients with no high-risk features. Targeted agents including sonic hedgehog (SHH) inhibitors are being tested for the SHH class of medulloblastoma.

Clinical Manifestations. In general, brainstem gliomas produce symptoms reflecting the exact location of the tumor in the brainstem, rate of growth, and presence of CSF flow obstruction. Patients with tectal gliomas often display signs and symptoms of isolated hydrocephalus. Dorsal exophytic brainstem tumors may manifest with headaches due to hydrocephalus combined with ataxia from cerebellar dysfunction. Diffuse pontine gliomas often present with double vision and facial weakness due to cranial nerve VI and VII palsies, accompanied by motor and cerebellar dysfunction of the contralateral limbs. Medulloblastomas can present with ataxia from cerebellar dysfunction, cranial nerve deficits, headache and vomiting from hydrocephalus, or occasionally signs and symptoms attributable to spinal cord or nerve root compression from extensive tumor dissemination.

Diagnostic Studies. With the advent of MRI, the ability to diagnose brainstem tumors has improved tremendously. Tectal gliomas and diffuse intrinsic pontine gliomas frequently are diagnosed based on MRI appearance alone without biopsy. This is especially important given the high risk of neurologic injury from the biopsy procedure. Dorsal exophytic brainstem tumors tend to have sharp borders and are relatively homogeneous.

Medulloblastomas are generally well-defined midline cerebellar lesions with regions of mineralization, intratumoral cysts and blood vessels, and heterogeneous enhancement. Because of the propensity for medulloblastomas to disseminate, the entire neuroaxis must be imaged. In addition, the CSF should be analyzed, as the tumor tends to spread along the CSF pathways.

Treatment. Dorsal exophytic brainstem tumors and cervicomedullary tumors are amenable to surgical resection, followed by chemotherapy or radiation for progressive or symptomatic tumors that cannot be completely removed. Tectal gliomas are generally managed by treating the hydrocephalus, although larger or progressive tumors may need radiation or chemotherapy. Diffuse infiltrating pontine lesions are treated with fractionated radiotherapy.

Initial treatment of medulloblastomas consists of maximal surgical resection, with the extent of surgical resection a significant prognostic factor. Subsequent treatment depends on whether patients fall into "average risk" (older than 3 years with near or total resection of the tumor and no evidence of disseminated disease) or "high risk" (younger than 3 years, less than neartotal resection, and evidence of disseminated disease) categories. Average-risk patients are treated with lower doses of radiation and less chemotherapy. However, all patients undergo craniospinal irradiation with a boost to the posterior fossa.

Plate 12.7

Brain: PART I

EPENDYMOMAS

Although technically considered a type of glioma, ependymomas are usually considered separately. Glial tumors of this type arise within or adjacent to the ependymal lining of the ventricles. They may arise anywhere along the CNS axis and comprise a heterogeneous group of tumors. Similar to other primary brain tumors, there is a shift toward incorporating molecular markers to better classify ependymomas in groups that will reflect underlying biologic behavior. Multiple subtypes have been added in the updated WHO 2021 classification.

Intracranial ependymomas may occur in the supratentorial (less common) or infratentorial (more common) compartments. Peak incidence occurs in early childhood, but these tumors can occur at any age. They are quite infrequent in adults and tend to occur before the age of 40 years. Conversely, spinal ependymomas are more common in adults, with a median age of 30 to 40 years at diagnosis. Subependymomas are typically incidental findings and tend to occur in middle-aged and older adults.

Histologically, ependymomas are graded from WHO 1 to 3. The tumors are usually well demarcated with areas of calcification, hemorrhage, and cysts. Tumor ependymal rosettes can be seen but are not always present, as shown in Plate 12.7. Myxopapillary ependymomas arise almost exclusively in the conus medullaris and filum terminale, though they can disseminate and be found intracranially as well. Historically, myxopapillary ependymomas and subependymomas were considered WHO grade 1 tumors; the classic ependymoma was categorized as WHO grade 2, and the anaplastic ependymoma was given a designation of WHO grade 3. However, the grade of the tumor does not always reflect the underlying biology, nor does it always correlate with clinical outcome. The updated WHO 2021 classification scheme proposed nine different subgroups of ependymomas across three key anatomic compartments of the CNS, including the supratentorial, posterior fossa, and spinal cord. Although the myxopapillary ependymoma and subependymoma were retained as histopathologically distinct types, this new classification schema dropped the distinction between classic and anaplastic ependymoma. Moreover, it proposed that myxopapillary ependymomas be upgraded to WHO grade 2 based on clinical behavior.

Clinical Manifestations. Intracranial tumors may present with focal neurologic deficits depending on their location. Tumors occurring in the posterior fossa may cause obstructive hydrocephalus resulting in headache, nausea, and vomiting. Spinal tumors may cause myelopathic or radicular signs.

Diagnostic Studies. On MRI, ependymomas typically are hypointense on T1 and hyperintense on T2. They typically enhance with contrast administration. On CT,

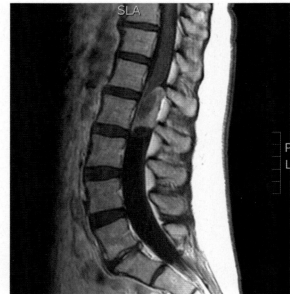

Grade 2 ependymoma; post T1 image

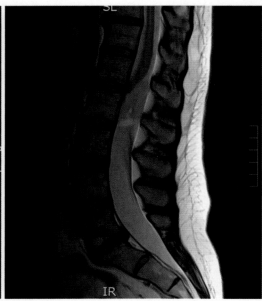

Grade 2 ependymoma; T2 image

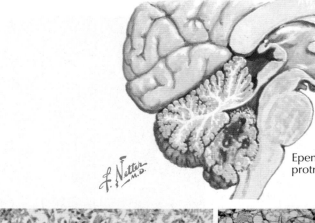

Ependymoma of fourth ventricle protruding into cisterna magna

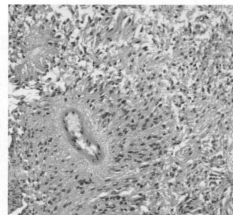

Ependymal true rosettes

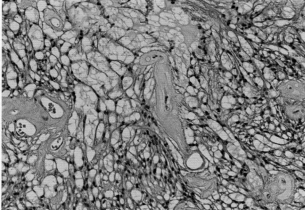

Myxopapillary ependymoma

calcifications and cysts may be seen. Calcifications in a fourth ventricular tumor are typically considered highly suggestive of an ependymoma. In contrast, subependymomas are nonenhancing, nodular, well-demarcated tumors.

Treatment. Surgical resection is the primary modality of treatment. Typically, patients who have had a gross total resection have a lower rate of recurrence and overall better prognosis. After surgery, intracranial tumors are typically treated with radiation and adjuvant chemotherapy in children older than 1 year. Occasionally, grade 2 supratentorial ependymomas are just observed after gross total resection, as these tumors are thought to be bear a favorable prognosis. Because of concerns about the effects of radiation on neurologic development, adjuvant chemotherapy alone is recommended for children younger than 1 year. For adults with intracranial ependymomas, maximal resection is the goal, and adjuvant radiation is typically suggested for those with WHO 3 ependymomas.

Plate 12.8

Neuro-Oncology

METASTATIC TUMORS TO BRAIN

Metastasis to the brain constitutes the most common type of intracranial neoplasm in adults. The incidence appears to be increasing secondary to better control of systemic disease and to improved imaging techniques. In adults, the most common primary tumors to spread to the brain include carcinomas of the lung and breast and melanoma. Renal carcinoma and pelvic/abdominal tumors also frequently disseminate to the brain. Metastasis to the brain occurs only rarely in children, with sarcomas and neuroblastomas the most common primary source. Typically, patients have a known diagnosis of cancer before the development of neurologic symptoms, though occasionally metastasis to the brain may be the first manifestation of the malignancy.

Three mechanisms have been described for the development of metastases. For parenchymal lesions, the most common is hematogenous spread. Metastatic lesions are usually found at the junction between gray and white matter where the vessel diameter is significantly reduced, effectively "trapping" tumor cells. Metastasis can also occur via local extension from the primary tumor, such as in head and neck cancer, and via bodily fluids such as the CSF.

Clinical Manifestations. Patients with brain metastases can present with a variety of clinical features. Thus any patient with a history of cancer who develops new neurologic symptoms warrants careful examination. About half of the patients will present with headaches with increasing frequency when multiple lesions or posterior fossa lesions are present. Other common symptoms include focal weakness and mental status changes. Up to one-fifth of patients will present with seizures. Strokes can also occur in the setting of metastasis. This may be due to general hypercoagulability, disturbance of arterial flow, tumor embolization, or hemorrhage into a lesion. Melanoma, renal cell carcinoma, thyroid cancer, and choriocarcinoma have a propensity to bleed.

Diagnostic Studies. Contrast MRI is preferred for the diagnosis of brain metastasis, as it is more sensitive in detecting lesions and differentiating metastatic lesions from other CNS abnormalities. Parenchymal brain metastasis tends to be circumscribed, with large amounts of surrounding vasogenic edema relative to the size of the lesion. The presence of multiple lesions and location at the gray and white matter junction further supports a diagnosis of metastasis. Because metastatic lesions can also spread via CSF fluid, examination of CSF fluid may be necessary in some patients to evaluate for the presence of leptomeningeal involvement. Finally, if the diagnosis of metastasis is still in doubt, a biopsy should be performed for confirmation.

Treatment. The treatment plan for patients with brain metastases depends on their prognosis, which is based on their performance status, extent of extracranial disease, age, and primary diagnosis. In patients with a favorable prognosis, treatment is aimed toward eradication or control of brain metastasis. This may involve surgical resection (depending on the number of lesions) combined with radiotherapy to eliminate residual cancer cells. Randomized trials have shown that the addition of whole brain radiation (WBRT) to surgery reduces recurrence rate but does not improve overall survival. Because of ongoing concerns about the neurotoxicity of WBRT, adoption of stereotactic radiosurgery (SRS) has become more prevalent. SRS is favored for patients with a limited number of brain lesions. A recent phase III study showed that, although there was no survival difference between SRS and WBRT compared with SRS alone, there was a significant increase in cognitive failure in the combination group. In patients considered to have poor prognosis, treatment is focused on symptom management and maintenance of neurologic function. In these cases, WBRT is preferred to improve neurologic deficits and prevent further deterioration. Addition of memantine to WBRT may provide neuroprotection, and hippocampal avoidance during WBRT may also help preserve cognitive function. Corticosteroids are often used to control symptoms from mass effect and edema.

Chemotherapy traditionally is not used in the treatment of brain metastases, often because of the inability of chemotherapeutic agents and targeted drugs to penetrate the blood-brain barrier. However, newer-generation agents have better penetration to overcome the blood-brain barrier and thus have generative objective radiographic responses. The introduction of immunotherapy in the form of checkpoint inhibitors has generated radiographic responses in lung cancer and melanoma.

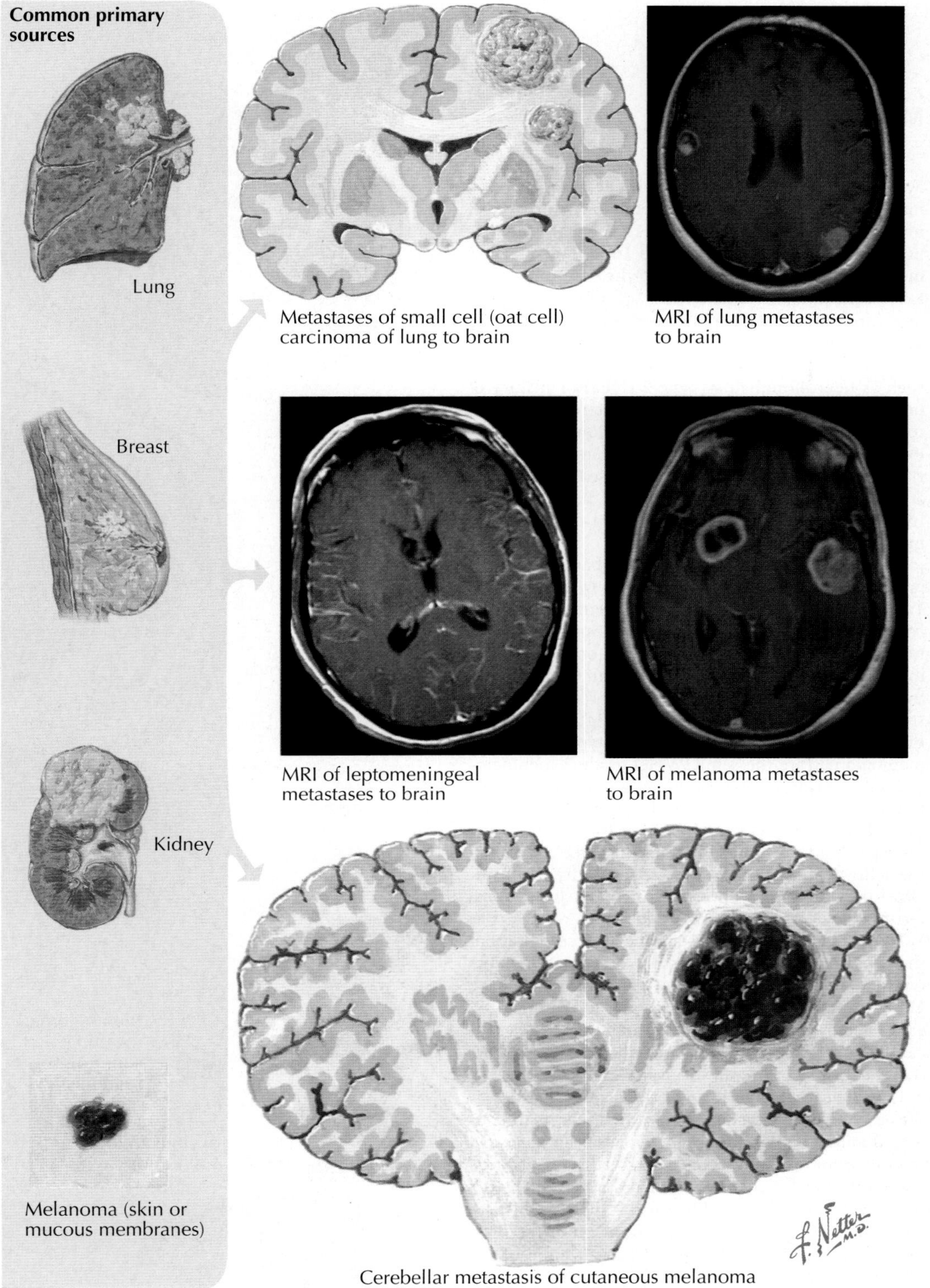

Common primary sources

Lung

Breast

Kidney

Melanoma (skin or mucous membranes)

Metastases of small cell (oat cell) carcinoma of lung to brain

MRI of lung metastases to brain

MRI of leptomeningeal metastases to brain

MRI of melanoma metastases to brain

Cerebellar metastasis of cutaneous melanoma

Plate 12.9

Brain: PART I

MENINGIOMAS

Meningiomas are the most common primary intracranial neoplasm and constitute about one-third of all intracranial tumors. These tumors arise from the meningothelial cells and are graded from 1 to 3. Their incidence increases with age, and they are more than twice as common in females. This sex difference is even more pronounced with spinal meningiomas, which are quite rare in males. Meningiomas are infrequently seen in children, except in those with genetic syndromes such as neurofibromatosis type 2 (NF2) or history of prior radiation exposure. Much interest has surrounded the epidemiology of meningiomas. Thus far, ionizing radiation and hormonal use have emerged as risk factors for the development of these tumors. Radiation-induced meningiomas tend to have a higher frequency of multiplicity and of atypia than sporadic meningiomas.

The WHO classification schema is based on histopathologic morphology and correlates with prognosis. WHO grade 1 lesions are considered benign and by far constitute the majority of meningiomas. These are further subdivided based on their morphology into meningotheliomatous (which includes the psammomatous tumors with the characteristic whorl pattern of the stroma), fibromatous, and angioblastic types. Treatment approaches for all of these subtypes of benign meningiomas are the same. WHO grade 2 meningiomas are considered atypical meningiomas and constitute about 10% to 20% of cases. These are characterized by higher mitotic activity, defined as four or more mitoses per high-power field and having three or more of the following features: increased cellularity, high nuclear-to-cytoplasmic ratio, prominent nucleoli, uninterrupted sheet-like growth, and areas of necrosis. WHO grade 3 meningiomas are the least common but the most ominous. These tumors exhibit loss of the typical meningioma growth patterns, infiltrative growth, abundant mitosis with atypia, and multiple areas of necrosis. Grade 2 and 3 meningiomas are significantly more likely to have invasive disease, local recurrence, and shorter overall survival.

It is unclear whether histopathologic classification is the best methodology for risk assessment for meningiomas. Similar to other tumor types, it has been suggested that incorporation of molecular markers may improve the ability to identify meningiomas at risk for recurrence. Various mutations identified indicate that there are distinct pathways for the development of these tumors. This, in turn, may affect the localization of the tumors (convexity of brain vs. skull base vs. spinal cord) and the histologic subtype.

Clinical Manifestations. Presenting signs and symptoms depend on the location and growth rate of the tumor. Because most meningiomas are slow growing, patients are frequently asymptomatic, with the discovery of the tumor an incidental finding. Any signs or symptoms that do develop are usually secondary to compression of underlying structures.

Seizures are often presenting signs of meningiomas, especially those located near the cerebral cortex. Focal weakness is another frequent complaint, with the pattern of weakness a potential clue as to the location of the tumor. For example, bilateral lower extremity weakness in the absence of a spinal cord lesion can often be

Meningioma with attached matter removed from brain

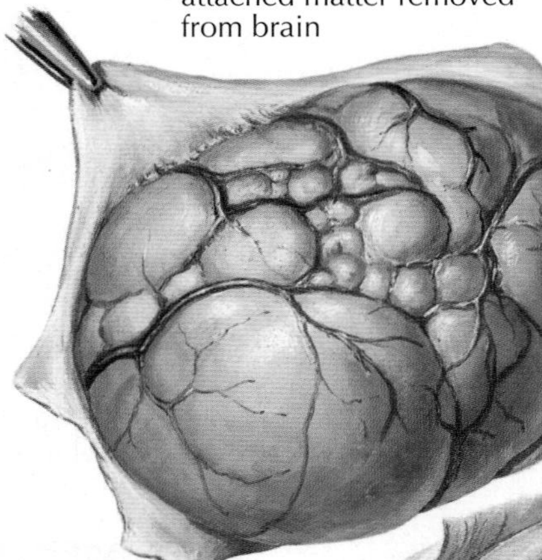

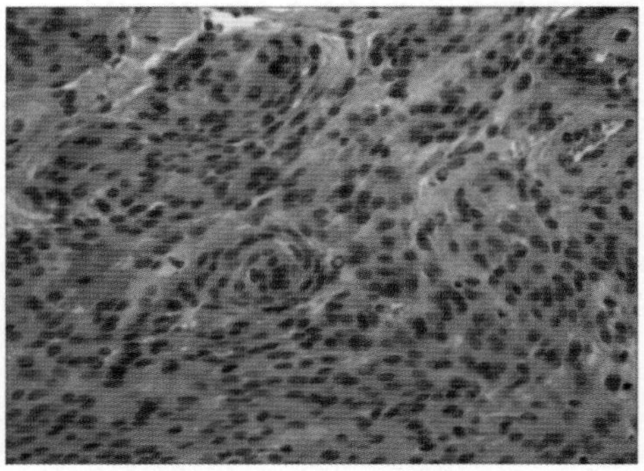

Meningioma histopathology

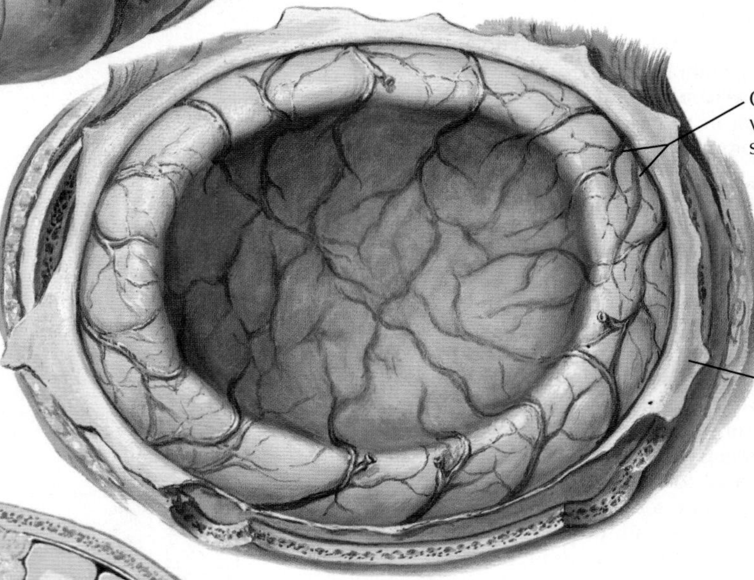

Superior view of brain showing depressed bed left behind after removal of meningioma

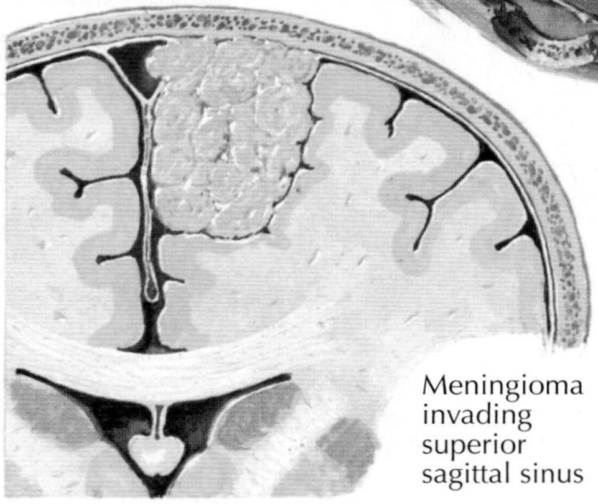

Cerebral vessels on surface

Dura mater

Meningioma invading superior sagittal sinus

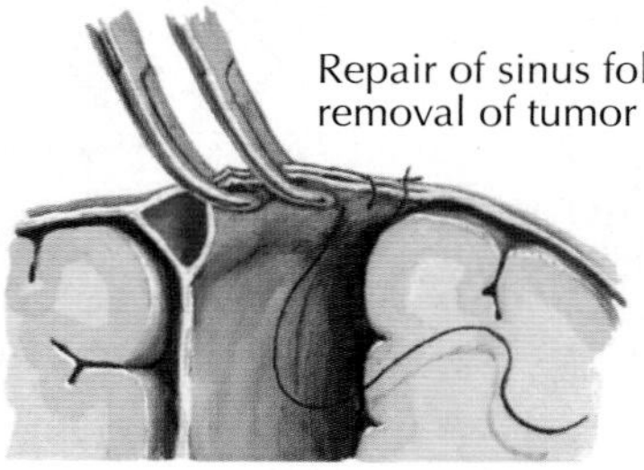

Repair of sinus following removal of tumor

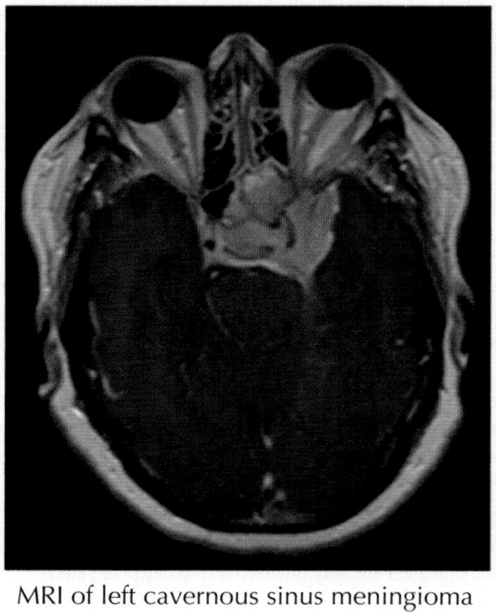

MRI of left cavernous sinus meningioma

seen with parasagittal lesions arising from the falx and compressing the adjacent motor strips of both hemispheres. A potential concern with these lesions is involvement of the sagittal sinus, which can lead to venous infarction. Spinal meningiomas can also cause bilateral leg weakness, but this is often accompanied by numbness. Foramen magnum meningiomas can present with insidious weakness of the arm and leg, which progresses to involve the contralateral limbs. This is accompanied by neck pain, worsened with neck flexion or Valsalva maneuvers. Because of the subtly progressive symptoms, meningiomas can be hard to diagnose and can be confused with multiple sclerosis (MS).

Visual changes can be subtle but are commonly seen with meningiomas. Deficits may include visual loss, field deficits, and diplopia. Olfactory groove, medial sphenoid wing, and other parasellar tumors can compress the optic nerve (CN II), resulting in blindness

Plate 12.10 Neuro-Oncology

MENINGIOMAS
(Continued)

with optic atrophy in one eye and papilledema in the other. This is also known as Foster Kennedy syndrome. Parasellar lesions can also cause visual field deficits. When tumors involve the cavernous sinus, ocular palsies can be seen, frequently accompanied by facial numbness. Finally, meningiomas can arise from the optic sheath, resulting in slowly progressive loss of vision.

Other signs and symptoms include ataxia and hemiparesis secondary to lesions in the posterior fossa causing brainstem compression. Meningiomas arising at the cerebellopontine angle (CPA) can produce sensorineural hearing loss. Occasionally, they can be quite adherent to adjacent cranial nerves and vasculature, rendering them difficult to remove. Large tumors in the posterior fossa can cause obstructive hydrocephalus.

Because the majority of meningiomas are very slow growing, the brain has time to adapt to the enlarging mass. Thus tumors in the frontal or occipital lobe can become quite large before the tenuous pressure relationships decompensate, resulting in symptomatic presentation. Tumors arising in the frontal lobe may present with cognitive or personality changes or other mental status changes.

Diagnostic Studies. Both MRI and CT can be used to diagnose meningiomas, although MRI is the preferred imaging modality. Typically, meningiomas are iso- to hypointense on T1 and iso- to hyperintense on T2 with strong homogeneous enhancement. Often, there is a characteristic dural tail, the marginal dural thickening that tapers at the periphery. On CT, the meningioma appears as a well-circumscribed extraaxial mass that is sometimes calcified. Similar to the MRI, homogenous enhancement is seen when intravenous contrast is administered. Occasionally, areas of necrosis, cyst formation, or hemorrhage is seen. CT is also helpful to evaluate for bony involvement. Though bony involvement from cerebral convexity tumors is rare, almost 50% of skull base tumors will have secondary involvement of the bone.

Treatment. With the availability of imaging modalities such as MRI, meningiomas are often asymptomatic incidental findings. Frequently, these tumors are unchanging or slow growing. It is reasonable to follow these patients conservatively with active surveillance, withholding treatment until the tumor becomes symptomatic or increases in size significantly. This is especially true for elderly patients (>70 years) or those with multiple surgical comorbidities.

The threshold for surgical intervention in younger patients is lower because morbidity is less than in older patients and because it is assumed that these lesions will eventually progress. Thus surgical intervention may be recommended for lesions in surgically accessible locations even if they are asymptomatic. In patients with symptomatic lesions or asymptomatic tumors that appear to be infiltrative or associated with vasogenic edema, surgical resection is recommended. Complete surgical resection is potentially curative, and the extent of resection correlates with prognosis. Advances in neurosurgery such as microsurgery, intraoperative imaging, and the widespread use of MRI have improved a surgeon's ability to successfully resect these

lesions while minimizing injury to surrounding normal tissue.

In some cases, only a subtotal resection can be achieved. In these cases, adjuvant radiotherapy should be considered, as retrospective studies have reported improved progression-free survival, though not overall survival. Radiotherapy alone can be effective for lesions that are surgically inaccessible, with local control rates of greater than 90% in 5 years. For WHO

grade 2 tumors, the frequency of recurrence is increased. Despite the lack of large prospective trials, adjuvant radiotherapy is recommended for incompletely resected tumors and possibly even for newly diagnosed gross totally resected tumors. Grade 3 tumors invariably require irradiation. There is very little role for systemic therapy for meningiomas. Bevacizumab has been used on occasion for treatment-refractory tumors.

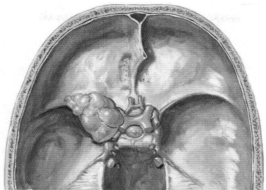

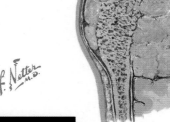
Convexity meningioma eroding through skull and producing distinct prominence

Meningioma of left medial sphenoid wing compressing optic (II) nerve and internal carotid artery

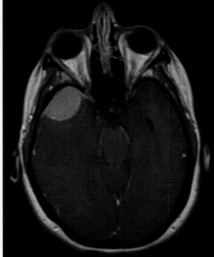
MRI of sphenoid wing meningioma

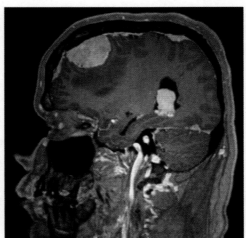
MRI of right frontal meningioma (sagittal)

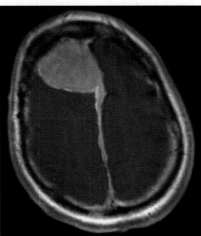
MRI of right frontal meningioma (axial)

Plate 12.11

Brain: PART I

PITUITARY TUMORS

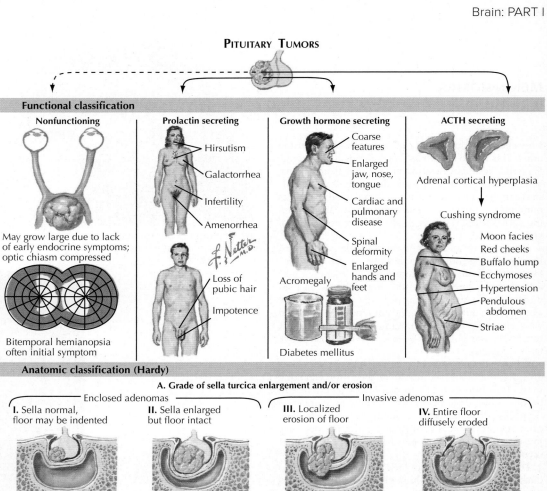

Functional classification

| Nonfunctioning | Prolactin secreting | Growth hormone secreting | ACTH secreting |

Nonfunctioning

May grow large due to lack of early endocrine symptoms; optic chiasm compressed

Bitemporal hemianopsia often initial symptom

Prolactin secreting

Hirsutism
Galactorrhea
Infertility
Amenorrhea
Loss of pubic hair
Impotence

Growth hormone secreting

Coarse features
Enlarged jaw, nose, tongue
Cardiac and pulmonary disease
Spinal deformity
Enlarged hands and feet

Acromegaly

Diabetes mellitus

ACTH secreting

Adrenal cortical hyperplasia

Cushing syndrome

Moon facies
Red cheeks
Buffalo hump
Ecchymoses
Hypertension
Pendulous abdomen
Striae

PITUITARY TUMORS AND CRANIOPHARYNGIOMAS

Pituitary tumors account for the third most common primary intracranial tumor, with males and females equally affected. Patients often present with a variety of neurologic and endocrinologic abnormalities depending on the tumor type and growth characteristics. Although the pituitary adenoma is the most common sellar tumor, other tumor types exist, including pituitary carcinomas, craniopharyngiomas, and Rathke cleft cysts.

The pituitary gland is located in the sella turcica in the body of the sphenoid bone. The tuberculum sellae forms the anterior border of the sella turcica, and the dorsum sella demarcates the posterior border. The cavernous sinus is found in the lateral sellar compartment and borders each side of the pituitary. The optic apparatus lies above the sella.

The pituitary gland is formed by two distinct lobes: anterior (adenohypophysis) and posterior (neurohypophysis). The anterior lobe contains glandular epithelial cells that secrete endocrine hormones such as adreno-corticotropic hormone (ACTH), thyroid-stimulating hormone (TSH), prolactin, growth hormone (GH), luteinizing hormone (LH), and follicle-stimulating hormone (FSH). The posterior lobe represents the termination of the hypothalamohypophysial tract and stores oxytocin and vasopressin. In general, pituitary adenomas represent benign neoplasms of the anterior lobe.

Pituitary tumors are classified according to size, with microadenomas referring to adenomas 10 mm or smaller and macroadenomas to adenomas larger than 10 mm. The tumors can also be categorized according to function, with nonfunctioning adenomas including gonadotroph adenomas, null cell adenomas, and oncocytomas. Hyperfunctioning tumors secrete GH, prolactin, ACTH, and TSH.

Craniopharyngiomas are solid or mixed solid-cystic tumors that arise from the remnants of Rathke's pouch. They are relatively rare and have a bimodal age distribution, with the first peak occurring in children between 5 and 14 years of age and the second peak developing in adults between 50 and 75 years of age. Males and females appear to be equally affected. Although these tumors are considered benign by histology, they frequently shorten life. Malignant transformation is a rare occurrence.

Clinical Manifestations. In general, nonfunctioning adenomas cause clinical symptoms by exerting mass effects on neighboring structures. The most common symptom is progressive visual impairment secondary

Anatomic classification (Hardy)

A. Grade of sella turcica enlargement and/or erosion

Enclosed adenomas

I. Sella normal, floor may be indented

II. Sella enlarged but floor intact

Invasive adenomas

III. Localized erosion of floor

IV. Entire floor diffusely eroded

B. Type of suprasellar extension

A. No suprasellar extension of tumor

B. Suprasellar bulge does not reach floor of third ventricle

C. Tumor reaches third ventricle, distorting its chiasmatic recess

D. Tumor fills third ventricle almost to interventricular foramen (of Monro)

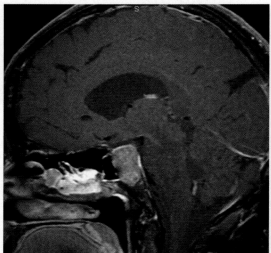
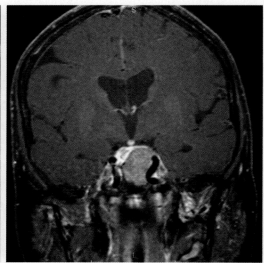
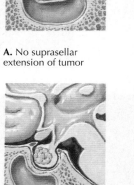
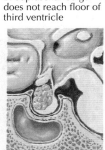
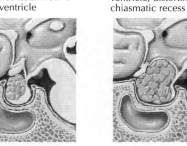
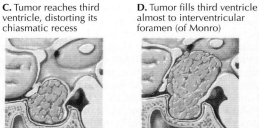

MRI of pituitary macroadenoma with suprasellar extension causing compression of the optic nerve

Plate 12.12

Neuro-Oncology

PITUITARY TUMORS AND CRANIOPHARYNGIOMAS (Continued)

to compression of the optic chiasm from suprasellar growth of the adenoma. Patients may report diminished vision in the temporal fields (bitemporal hemianopsia) or decreased visual acuity. Other symptoms caused by a sellar lesion include headaches and diplopia from oculomotor compression. Patients may also present with hyposecretion of hormones resulting from compression of different pituitary cell types by the adenoma. Impaired secretion of LH is the most common deficiency, with females reporting amenorrhea and males reporting decreased libido.

Hyperfunctioning tumors result in oversecretion of a particular hormone. The most common are corticotroph adenomas, lactotroph adenomas, and somatotroph adenomas. Corticotroph adenomas produce an excess of ACTH, resulting in Cushing disease. This is the most serious condition produced by any pituitary tumor and leads to body deformities, hyperglycemia, skin hyperpigmentation, hypertension, infertility, and electrolyte imbalances. Lactotroph adenomas cause hypersecretion of prolactin, resulting in hypogonadism in males and females. Females experience amenorrhea, infertility, and galactorrhea, and males report impotence. Somatotroph adenomas secrete excess GH. Gigantism develops in children, whereas adults manifest with acromegaly, causing tissue overgrowth, metabolic disturbances, cardiovascular problems, sleep apnea, and neuropathy.

Craniopharyngiomas are typically slow growing with slow onset of symptoms. Visual deficits are common because of direct pressure of the tumor on the optic chiasm. Hormonal abnormalities can occur with compression of normal pituitary structures. In children, growth failure from hypothyroidism or GH deficiency is the most common presentation, whereas sexual dysfunction is the most common presenting symptom in adults. Other symptoms include headache, depression, and lethargy.

Diagnostic Studies. MRI has supplanted CT as the imaging procedure of choice for most sellar masses. On noncontrast images, the normal pituitary gland and pituitary adenomas are isointense to the rest of the brain parenchyma. With dynamic administration of gadolinium contrast, the majority of pituitary adenomas exhibit early enhancement before the normal gland; when this washes out, the normal pituitary gland will enhance more intensely than the adenoma. Because of the increased risk of associated hormonal dysfunction, a thorough evaluation of the hypothalamic-pituitary axis must

be conducted to assess for hormonal excess or deficiency. Ophthalmologic and endocrine screening should be performed in patients with an incidentally discovered pituitary lesion.

On imaging, craniopharyngiomas typically present as a parasellar mass with calcification and cystic components. In these cases CT may be the superior diagnostic modality, as it highlights calcifications and cystic lesions better than MRI. Occasionally, calcifications are

not readily identified on imaging; thus a histologic diagnosis is warranted. Many patients with craniopharyngiomas have symptoms of hypopituitarism; thus a thorough endocrine evaluation is recommended.

Treatment. The primary treatment for nonfunctioning macroadenomas and most hypersecreting adenomas is transsphenoidal surgery. Traditionally, most surgeons enter the sphenoid sinus through a variant of the transseptal approach, which exposes the anterior

CLINICALLY NONFUNCTIONING PITUITARY TUMOR

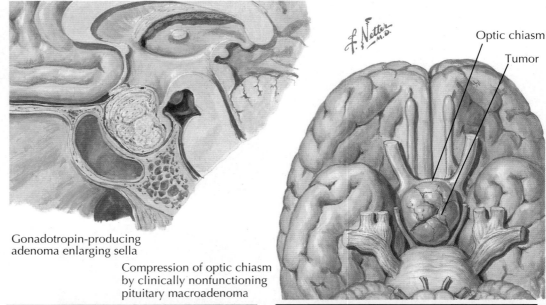

Optic chiasm

Tumor

Gonadotropin-producing adenoma enlarging sella

Compression of optic chiasm by clinically nonfunctioning pituitary macroadenoma

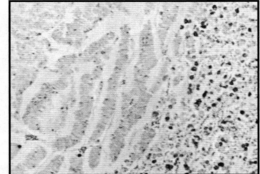

Null cell adenoma (Mann stain, x100)

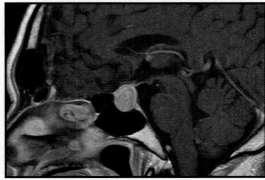

MRI (sagittal view) showing suprasellar extension of a clinically nonfunctioning pituitary macroadenoma

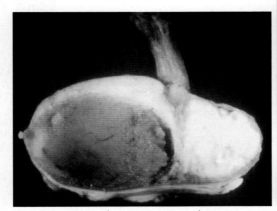

Gross specimen of pituitary microadenoma

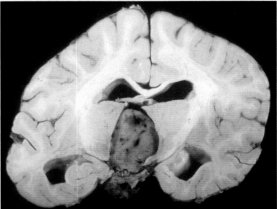

Gross specimen of pituitary microadenoma

Plate 12.13

Brain: PART I

CRANIOPHARYNGIOMA

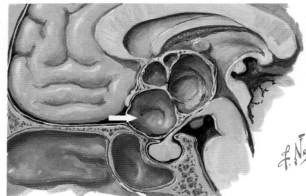

Large cystic suprasellar craniopharyngioma compressing optic chiasm and hypothalamus, filling third ventricle up to interventricular foramen (of Monro), thus causing visual impairment, diabetes insipidus, and hydrocephalus

PITUITARY TUMORS AND CRANIOPHARYNGIOMAS (Continued)

wall of the sphenoid bone. After the removal of the anterior wall, the bony floor of the sella turcica is removed, and the sella dura is then opened to allow for tumor removal. The most important aspect of the surgery is the preservation of the arachnoid membrane. Low postoperative morbidity depends on preventing blood from entering the CSF during the operation and leakage of CSF postoperatively. Afterward the muscle is placed in the tumor cavity, occasionally with a piece of nasal cartilage. The mucosal flaps are reapproximated and the nose is packed.

In the 1990s, the use of endoscopy to remove pituitary tumors became revitalized. Advantages with this approach include less postoperative swelling, the avoidance of nasal packing, decreased discomfort to the patient, and improvement of intra- and suprasellar visualization. In general, the endoscope is advanced into the choana and the sphenoid ostium is identified. With the bilateral approach, the nasal septum is removed, revealing the sphenoid sinus. This allows for visualization of the floor of the sella, which is then opened. After the dural covering is opened, the pituitary tumor is exposed, allowing for removal. Before closure, careful examination for CSF leak is performed. If there is no evidence of a leak, the floor of the sella is reconstructed. Occasionally, the transsphenoidal approach is not ideal, such as when there is significant tumor extension into the cranial fossa or with extreme suprasellar extension. In those cases, a transcranial approach is used via craniotomy. The tumor is then carefully removed via microdissection.

With surgery, about 87% of patients report improvement in preoperative visual deficits, and many patients report improvement in preoperative endocrine deficits. Recurrence can occur but is rare in those who have undergone a complete resection. In patients with residual disease, adjuvant radiotherapy or medical therapy can be considered, including dopamine, gonadotropin-releasing hormone, and somatostatin agonists. Radiation treatment runs the risk of affecting critical neighboring structures and does not have the advantage of significant cytoreduction. SRS and stereotactic radiotherapy have improved the safety and effectiveness of irradiation.

Prolactinomas, on the other hand, respond well to medical therapy. Dopamine agonists can effectively normalize prolactin levels, normalize vision, and decrease tumor size in the majority of patients. Occasionally the tumors are resistant to medical therapy or patients are unable to tolerate them; in those cases transsphenoidal

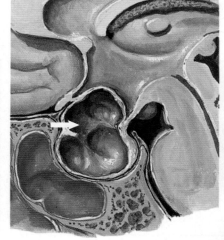

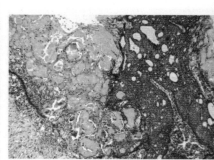

Intrasellar cystic craniopharyngioma compressing pituitary gland to cause hypopituitarism

Histology of craniopharyngioma

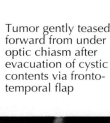

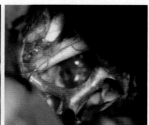

Tumor gently teased forward from under optic chiasm after evacuation of cystic contents via fronto-temporal flap

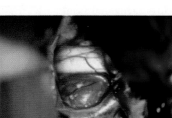

Intraoperative craniopharyngioma dissection before (left) and after (right)

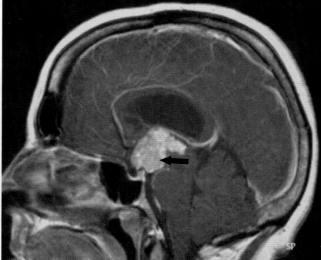

MRI (sagittal) of craniopharyngioma

surgery is advocated. Much interest has surrounded the role of medical therapy with GH-secreting adenomas; however, no drug has been found to consistently reduce tumor volume by a significant amount.

Pituitary adenomas found incidentally are increasingly common. Conservative management is reasonable if the lesion is less than 10 mm and there is no evidence of neurologic or endocrinologic abnormalities.

Craniopharyngiomas can be treated either with aggressive surgery or a combination of surgery followed by radiotherapy. Surgery allows for a diagnosis, debulking of the tumor, and a chance of surgical cure. Radiation, either stereotactic radiotherapy or radiosurgery, is used to treat incompletely resected tumors or those that have recurred after prior surgery. With modern advances in both the surgical and radiation fields, the risk of treatment-related side effects has decreased significantly. Papillary craniopharyngiomas frequently have *BRAFv600E* mutations and respond to Raf inhibitors.

Plate 12.14

Neuro-Oncology

TUMORS OF PINEAL REGION

Pineal tumors can be generally divided into primary intracranial germ cell tumors (GCTs) and non-GCTs. GCTs typically arise in midline structures such as the pineal and suprasellar regions. They commonly spread via the ventricular and subarachnoid space to the third ventricles and spinal cord, although extraneural spread outside the CNS is quite rare. GCTs are further subdivided into germinomas and nongerminomas. Germinomas are distinguished by their undifferentiated histopathology but are cured more readily by radiation. They tend to occur in adolescence and young adulthood. Nongerminomas are composed of several subtypes but are distinguished by their relative radioresistance and poorer prognosis. They predominate in younger children. Mature teratomas should be considered separately, as they behave very differently and generally have a good prognosis after total surgical resection.

Non-GCTs include pineal parenchymal tumors, glial tumors, and metastasis from systemic tumors. Pineal parenchymal tumors are traditionally classified as the lower-grade pineocytoma; the pineal parenchymal tumor of intermediate differentiation (PPID), which can have a relatively good prognosis; and the malignant pineoblastoma. Pineocytomas occur in middle-aged adults and are thought to be locally invasive. They are frequently managed with aggressive surgical resection and local radiotherapy for any residual tumor. Pineoblastomas resemble medulloblastomas and predominate in the pediatric population. They are treated with multimodal therapy consisting of maximal surgical resection followed by craniospinal irradiation and adjuvant chemotherapy. The treatment of PPID is controversial, and it is unclear whether radiotherapy and chemotherapy are needed after gross total resection. Glial tumors may be low grade or high grade and are identical to glial neoplasms that occur elsewhere in the CNS. Because of their location, which is less accessible by surgery, they tend to have a poorer prognosis. Finally, cysts and meningiomas can also be found in the pineal region.

Clinical Manifestations. Clinical presentation of pineal region tumors includes increased intracranial pressure from hydrocephalus, tectal dysfunction, and endocrinopathies. Obstruction of the third ventricle and cerebral aqueduct results in increased intracranial pressure, which manifests as headache, nausea and vomiting, lethargy, and papilledema. Because the lesions are located in the posterior aspect of the third ventricle, compression of the tectum often ensues. This can lead to Parinaud syndrome, which consists of vertical upward gaze paralysis, decreased or absent pupillary response to light, and convergence retraction nystagmus. Occasionally, cerebellar signs, such as ataxia and tremor, are seen with more extensive growth.

Diagnostic Studies. Neuroimaging is the first step in identifying a pineal region lesion. MRI with and without contrast is preferred, as it outlines the tumor anatomy better than CT. Germinomas and pineal parenchymal tumors tend to have mixed T1 signal and increased T2 signal. Calcifications occur less frequently than in teratomas. Benign teratomas are well circumscribed and have mixed densities secondary to large cysts, areas of calcifications, and the occasional presence of teeth and hair. Though characteristic radiographic findings may be seen, they cannot substitute for histologic diagnosis.

Other studies include examination of tumor markers in the CSF. Elevated alpha-fetoprotein levels confirm the

Tumor compressing mesencephalic tectum and corpora quadrigemina, occluding cerebral aqueduct (of Sylvius) and invading third ventricle

Parinaud syndrome: paresis of upward gaze, unequal pupils, loss of convergence

Diabetes insipidus in some patients

Possible sexual precocity in boys

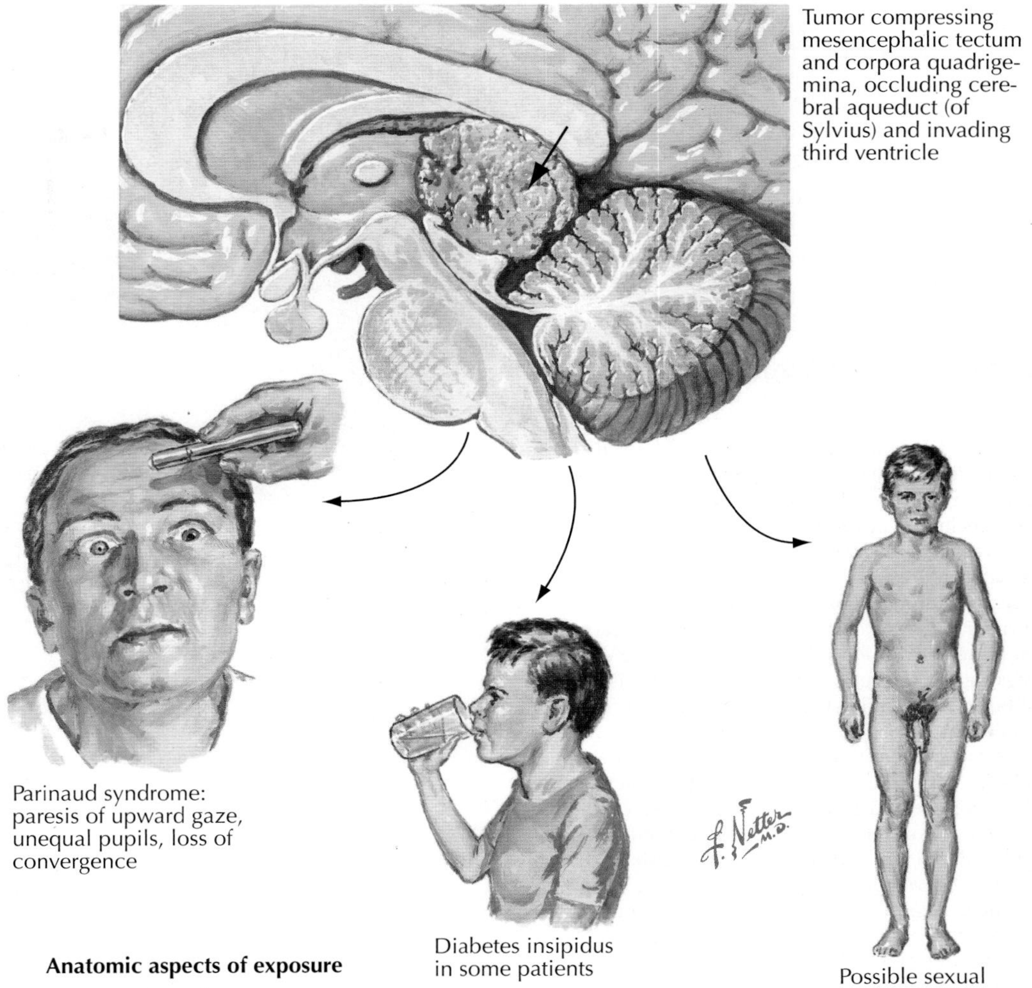

Anatomic aspects of exposure

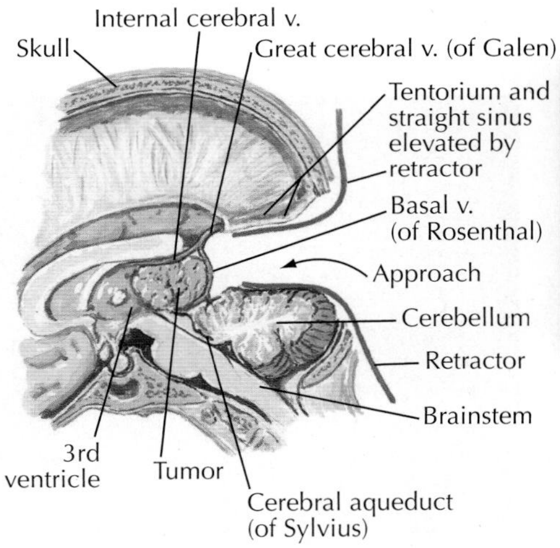

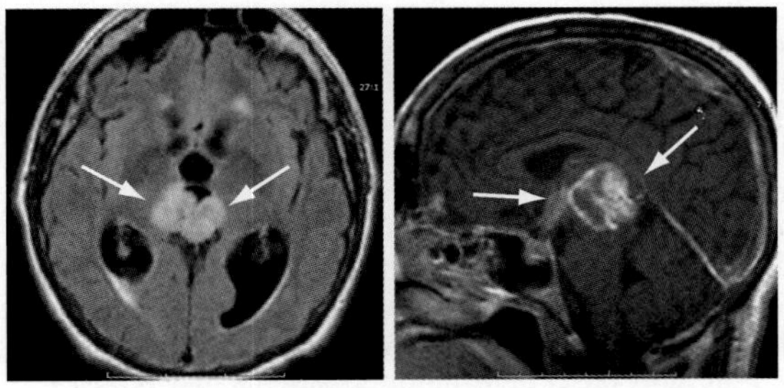

Skull

Internal cerebral v.

Great cerebral v. (of Galen)

Tentorium and straight sinus elevated by retractor

Basal v. (of Rosenthal)

Approach

Cerebellum

Retractor

Brainstem

3rd ventricle

Tumor

Cerebral aqueduct (of Sylvius)

Pineoblastoma. Axial FLAIR and sagittal T1-weighted gadolinium-enhanced MRI showing a large mass in the pineal region, bright on FLAIR imaging and heterogeneous after gadolinium enhancement, compressing the aqueduct with enlargement of the third and lateral ventricles.

presence of nongerminoma elements, and high human chorionic gonadotropin levels indicate a diagnosis of choriocarcinoma. The CSF should also be examined for the presence of malignant cells as a means to confirm the extent of disease, which can influence treatment planning.

Treatment. In general, surgery is almost always indicated for several reasons: establishment of a tissue diagnosis, symptomatic relief of hydrocephalus, and therapeutic resection in anticipation of adjuvant treatment. For germinomas, extensive resection is not indicated; however, there is debate whether patients with nongerminomas benefit from radical surgery

because of their decreased responsiveness to radiotherapy.

Radiation treatment is the standard treatment for pure germinomas. With radiation, long-term survival rates approximate 80% to 90%. However, this leads to genuine concerns for the potential delayed effects of therapy, such as neuroendocrine deficits and neurocognitive slowing. Currently, there is much interest surrounding the use of chemotherapy in an effort to reduce the dose of irradiation used. Because nongerminomas are less responsive to radiation, radiotherapy is often combined with chemotherapy, although survival rates seem to vary among patients with this regime.

Plate 12.15

Brain: PART I

VESTIBULAR SCHWANNOMAS

Vestibular schwannomas are tumors derived from Schwann cells surrounding the vestibular portion of the eighth cranial nerve. They are known by many different names, including acoustic neuromas, acoustic schwannomas, acoustic neurinomas, and vestibular neurilemmomas. They are more common in adults and constitute the overwhelming majority of tumors found at the CPA. The median age of diagnosis is around 50 years, and most tumors are unilateral. Bilateral vestibular schwannomas usually indicate an underlying diagnosis of NF2. Vestibular schwannomas are quite rare in children except in cases of NF2.

Histologically, vestibular schwannomas appear quite similar to peripheral schwannomas. On a microscopic level, there are zones of dense and sparse cellularity, identified as Antoni A and B areas, respectively. They are typically benign, with malignant transformation a very rare occurrence.

Clinical Manifestations. Clinical signs and symptoms result from cranial nerve involvement or mass effect on the cerebellum and other posterior fossa structures. Symptom onset is usually insidious given the slow rate of growth of these tumors. Almost all patients present with hearing loss and tinnitus secondary to cochlear nerve involvement, although patients may not necessarily be aware of their deficits. In a study of 1000 patients, 95% were found to have hearing loss, but only two-thirds of patients recognized their limitations. Rarely, patients have the acute onset of hearing loss secondary to compression of the vascular supply to the auditory nerve. More than half of patients also have involvement of the vestibular nerve with complaints of gait unsteadiness. Although true vertigo is uncommon given the slow onset of symptoms, patients may report nonspecific dizziness. A minority of patients have trigeminal involvement, which can range from facial numbness to trigeminal neuralgia. Involvement of the seventh cranial nerve is rare but can occur with the onset of facial paresis, hemifacial spasm, or taste disturbance. Finally, mass effect of the tumor can cause various types of neurologic dysfunction. Compression of the cerebellum can result in ataxia, and disruption of the lower cranial nerves can cause dysarthria, dysphagia, and aspiration. Involvement of the brainstem can lead to hydrocephalus, coma, and even death.

Diagnostic Studies. When suspicion for a vestibular schwannoma is raised, pure tone and speech audiometry should be performed as an initial screening test. Typically, results will reveal asymmetric hearing loss, especially with high frequencies. Speech discrimination is reduced in the affected ear and is usually out of proportion to the measured hearing loss. Another screening measure used is brainstem-evoked response, which detects a delay on the affected side. However, it has a relatively low sensitivity and specificity compared with

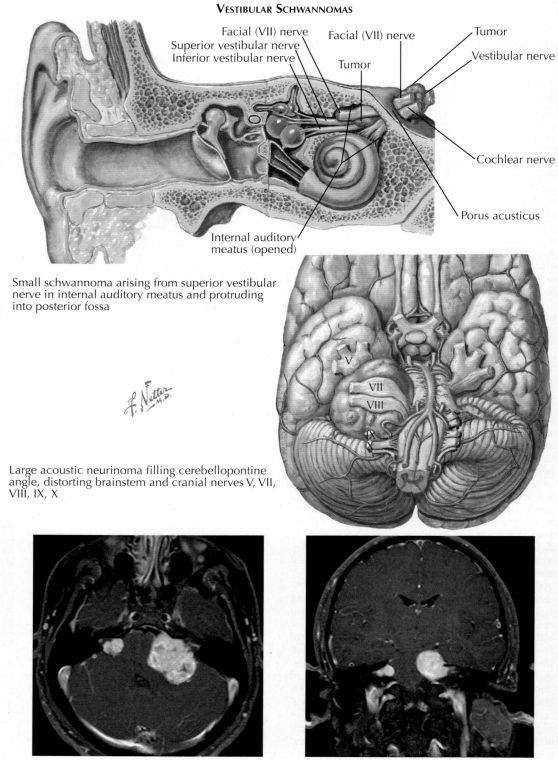

VESTIBULAR SCHWANNOMAS

Small schwannoma arising from superior vestibular nerve in internal auditory meatus and protruding into posterior fossa

Large acoustic neurinoma filling cerebellopontine angle, distorting brainstem and cranial nerves V, VII, VIII, IX, X

MRI of vestibular schwannoma, axial (*left*) and coronal (*right*)

MRI, especially with smaller lesions. Thus MRI has become the diagnostic modality of choice when suspicion for a vestibular schwannoma is raised. Specifying fine cuts (≤3-mm slices) through the internal auditory canal (IAC) may increase the sensitivity and specificity even further. CT scans with bone windows are also useful, as the extent of tumor growth in the IAC has prognostic significance. It should be noted that the diagnosis of a vestibular schwannoma is based on the clinical history (asymmetric hearing loss) in conjunction

with audiometry and imaging, as they constitute the majority of posterior fossa lesions that behave in this manner. Rarely are these lesions biopsied. Nonetheless, other considerations include meningiomas, schwannomas of other cranial nerves, hemangiomas, gliomas, metastatic tumors, aneurysms, and arachnoid cysts.

Treatment. The natural history of vestibular schwannomas is highly variable, with some tumors experiencing little to no growth and others enlarging quite rapidly. The main treatment is surgery, which is potentially

Plate 12.16

Neuro-Oncology

REMOVAL OF VESTIBULAR SCHWANNOMA: TRANSLABYRINTHINE APPROACH

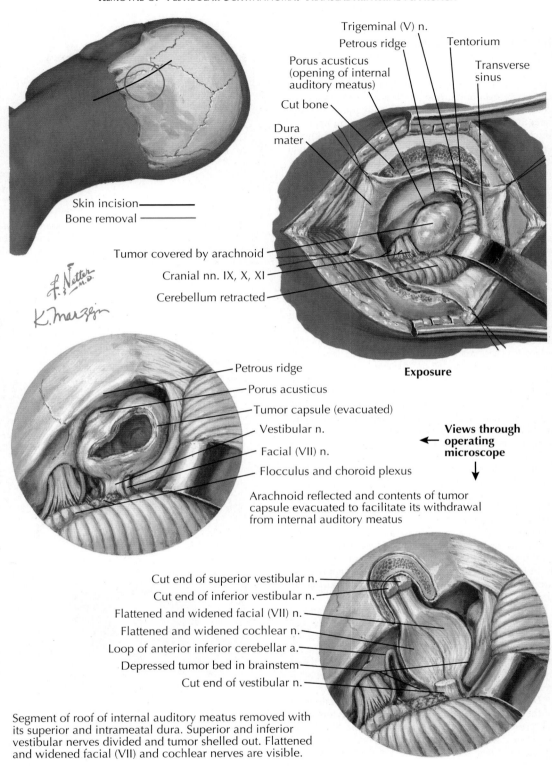

Trigeminal (V) n.

Petrous ridge

Tentorium

Porus acusticus
(opening of internal
auditory meatus)

Transverse
sinus

Cut bone

Dura
mater

Skin incision

Bone removal

Tumor covered by arachnoid

Cranial nn. IX, X, XI

Cerebellum retracted

Exposure

Petrous ridge

Porus acusticus

Tumor capsule (evacuated)

Vestibular n.

Facial (VII) n.

Flocculus and choroid plexus

**Views through
operating
microscope**

Arachnoid reflected and contents of tumor
capsule evacuated to facilitate its withdrawal
from internal auditory meatus

Cut end of superior vestibular n.

Cut end of inferior vestibular n.

Flattened and widened facial (VII) n.

Flattened and widened cochlear n.

Loop of anterior inferior cerebellar a.

Depressed tumor bed in brainstem

Cut end of vestibular n.

Segment of roof of internal auditory meatus removed with
its superior and intrameatal dura. Superior and inferior
vestibular nerves divided and tumor shelled out. Flattened
and widened facial (VII) and cochlear nerves are visible.

VESTIBULAR SCHWANNOMAS (Continued)

curative after gross total resection. Three standard approaches are used: retromastoid suboccipital (retrosigmoid), translabyrinthine, and middle fossa. The choice of a particular approach depends on size of the tumor and whether hearing preservation is attempted. The translabyrinthine approach is reserved for tumors 3 mm or smaller when hearing preservation is not an issue, and the middle fossa approach attempts to preserve hearing while resecting tumors 1.5 mm or smaller. Surgical morbidity includes hearing loss, facial weakness, vestibular dysfunction, CSF leakage, and persistent headaches.

The retromastoid suboccipital approach (see Plate 12.16) can be used for any size tumor with or without attempts to preserve hearing. This technique allows the tumor and the important structures medial and lateral to it to be in full view in the surgical field. In general, an incision is made to the tip of the mastoid eminence. After separation of the underlying muscles, a bony opening is made, extending laterally to the sigmoid sinus. The surgeon carefully tries to preserve the planes of the arachnoid over the tumor to protect the delicate cranial nerves and brainstem. To the right, the fifth cranial nerve and petrosal vein are seen; toward the lower portion of the field, the glossopharyngeal (IX), vagus (X), and accessory (XI) nerves are visible.

When the tumor grows in the posterior portion of the canal, the facial nerve tends to be pushed forward. Knowing this relationship is important in preserving the facial nerve, which is markedly flattened and often quite adherent just medial to the internal auditory meatus. The vestibular nerves, from which the tumor is arising, must be sectioned. If hearing has not already been irreversibly damaged, preservation of hearing may be attempted by minimizing manipulation of the cochlear nerve and protecting the labyrinthine artery, which may be a source of blood supply to the tumor. The anterior inferior cerebellar artery, which supplies the lateral portion of the brainstem and cerebellar peduncles, is another important structure of which the surgeon must be mindful.

With a larger tumor, the capsule is gutted at an early stage to facilitate atraumatic manipulation. Plate 12.16 shows the ninth, tenth, and eleventh cranial nerve complex passing through the jugular foramen with the accompanying sigmoid sinus, as well as a view after the tumor has been excised. The labyrinthine artery has been preserved, and the relationship of the four main nerves in the canal is seen. Because a CSF leak through the lateral portion of the canal can develop, the lateral canal is plugged with fat and bone wax.

For patients who are not surgical candidates, SRS and stereotactic fractionated radiotherapy have been used. SRS focuses the beams in a single dose to a discrete tumor volume in an effort to decrease the risk of damage to neighboring structures. One large series documented a 97% tumor control rate at 10 years with SRS. Fractionated stereotactic radiation focuses the radiotherapy over a series of treatments to minimize the risk of damage to critical structures. One prospective study comparing SRS with stereotactic radiotherapy documented a 97% tumor control rate for both treatments with a higher rate of hearing preservation with the fractionated stereotactic radiotherapy. Potential concerns for radiotherapy are the risk of cranial nerve injury, secondary tumor formation, and scarring rendering future surgeries more precarious. There is very little role for systemic therapy with the exception of tumors that arise in patients with NF2.

Finally, conservative management is used in select patients, especially those with small symptomatic tumors or who are deemed poor candidates for immediate intervention. In these cases, close monitoring with surveillance MRI is warranted.

Plate 12.17

Brain: PART I

INTRAVENTRICULAR TUMORS

Intraventricular tumors are composed of a histologically heterogenous group of tumors, with the most common being ependymomas. Ependymomas are frequently found within the fourth ventricle and are thought to derive from the primitive neuroepithelial cells lining the ventricles and central canal of the spinal cord. They are generally well demarcated with a low incidence of CSF dissemination. In adults, the most common intracranial location affected is the fourth ventricle. Other intraventricular tumors include gliomas, subependymomas, neurocytomas, GCTs, choroid plexus tumors, meningiomas, and pineal region tumors. Most of the other histologic subtypes tend to occur in the lateral ventricles, with the exception of GCTs, which can be seen in the third ventricle.

Lateral ventricle tumors, although varying in pathology, all arise from cells located within or around the ventricular walls. About half of lateral ventricular tumors consist of LGGs, with choroid plexus papillomas and meningiomas accounting for about 35%. SEGA is a variant of astrocytoma and is found in patients with tuberous sclerosis. These are generally asymptomatic lesions but can obstruct CSF flow. Choroid plexus tumors are most commonly seen in children, though they can occur in adults. Histology is the most important prognostic factor, with choroid plexus papillomas having a much better prognosis than choroid plexus carcinomas. The remainder include neurocytomas, congenital tumors, ependymomas, and metastasis. Neurocytomas are rare tumors, commonly found near the septum pellucidum near the foramen of Monro. They are very slow growing and histologically low grade.

Not all intraventricular lesions represent neoplasm. The colloid cyst is a benign remnant of the embryonic paraphysis and often seen in the intraventricular foramen of Monro, producing obstructive hydrocephalus. Some neurosurgeons approach the cyst through a cortical incision into the hydrocephalic right lateral ventricle or through the corpus callosum. Both approaches are satisfactory, although there is risk of neurologic damage.

Clinical Manifestations. The most common sign and symptom with intraventricular tumors is hydrocephalus. The onset is usually insidious as the majority of the tumors are slow growing. Lesions occurring in the pineal region and third ventricle can cause Parinaud syndrome secondary to compression of the quadrigeminal plate.

Diagnostic Studies. MRI allows for easy visualization of the tumor. Subependymomas and neurocytomas often present as a heterogenous cystic lesion. SEGAs are found near the foramen of Monro and are characterized by calcifications and intense enhancement in the context of other signs associated with tuberous sclerosis. The choroid plexus tumor is heavily lobulated and appears as a vascular tumor centered on the choroid. As stated earlier, a complete diagnostic evaluation for ependymoma includes imaging of the entire neuroaxis and examination of the CSF.

Treatment. Treatment varies depending on the histology. Surgery is the mainstay of treatment for ependymomas with a total or near-total resection a favorable prognostic factor. Resection of an infratentorial ependymoma is technically more challenging than that of its supratentorial counterpart and is associated with higher

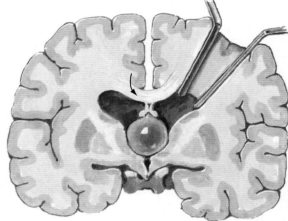

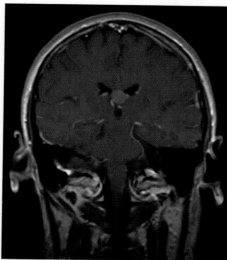

Colloid cyst of third ventricle and surgical approach via right prefrontal (silent) cerebral cortex. May also be approached through corpus callosum (arrow). Note enlarged lateral ventricles (posterior view).

MRI colloid cyst

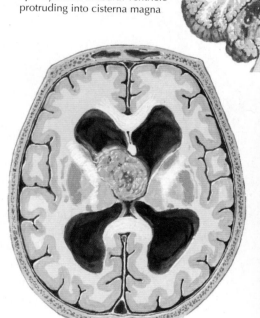

Ependymoma of fourth ventricle protruding into cisterna magna

Subependymoma of anterior horn of left lateral ventricle obstructing interventricular foramen (of Monro), thus producing marked hydrocephalus

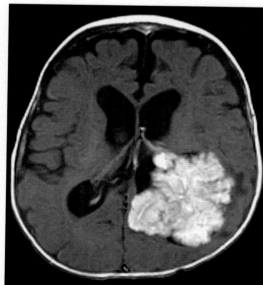

MRI of choroid plexus papilloma

surgical morbidity. Nonetheless, attempt at gross total resection is crucial for management of ependymomas. Historically, adjuvant radiation treatment has been used based on results from retrospective studies showing that patients who received postoperative radiation had a better prognosis than patients who only had surgery. The role of chemotherapy remains unclear, although it has been used in young children in an attempt to defer radiation. Subependymomas and neurocytomas have

excellent prognosis with surgical resection without a need for adjunct therapy. Choroid plexus tumors that can be completely excised have improved prognosis compared with those treated with subtotal resection. Radiotherapy has been associated with significantly better survival in choroid plexus carcinomas. Unfortunately, the rarity of these tumors results in limited information regarding their natural history and the optimal treatment.

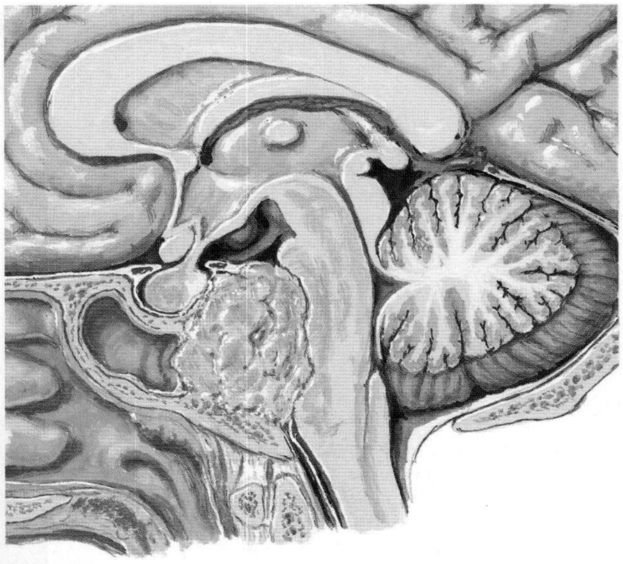

Plate 12.18

Neuro-Oncology

CHORDOMAS

Chordomas are slow-growing, locally aggressive neo-plasms that arise from the unabsorbed remnants of the embryonic notochord, a mesodermal structure running through the center of the vertebrae and into the clivus. These tumors may occur anywhere along the axial skeleton but are most common in the spheno-occipital region of the skull base and sacral regions of the spine. In adults, 35% arise in the skull base, 50% involve the sacrococcygeal region, and the rest occur elsewhere along the vertebral column. In general, skull base chordomas affect younger adults, whereas older patients tend to develop the tumors in the sacrococcygeal region. There appears to be a male predominance.

Chordomas can be classified into three subgroups. The most common are the conventional chordomas, which are distinguished by the absence of mesenchy-mal elements such as cartilage. On histologic examina-tion, lobules of epithelioid cells are arranged in cords separated by a mucinous matrix. Tumor cells have a vacuolated, bubbly cytoplasm, earning the name *phys-aliphorous cells*. Nuclear pleomorphism and mitoses are rare. Chondroid chordomas contain chordomatous and chondromatous features and often occur in the spheno-occipital region. Both conventional chordo-mas and chondroid chordomas have similar a progno-sis. The third type includes chordomas that undergo sarcomatous transformation; these have a worse prog-nosis as they behave more aggressively. Histologically, the sarcomatous component is interspersed between areas of conventional chordoma. Although chordomas are slow growing, they tend to recur and occasionally metastasize.

Clinical Manifestations. Signs and symptoms de-pend on location of the tumor and its effect on neigh-boring structures. Local pain is a common complaint. With skull base involvement, patients often report headache and diplopia secondary to invasion of the cavernous sinus. Involvement of the lower clivus may affect the lower cranial nerves, resulting in dysphagia or hoarseness followed by brainstem compression. Be-cause the onset of symptoms is quite insidious and vague, diagnosis is often delayed. Tumors of the spinal column and sacrum can cause back pain. Direct com-pression from spinal column tumors can lead to cord compression. Occasionally, the tumors of the sacrococ-cygeal region may reach enormous proportions and result in bladder and bowel dysfunction due to direct pressure on the rectum and involvement of sacral nerves.

Diagnostic Studies. Both MRI and CT are used for diagnostic purposes. MRI provides detailed anatomy, offering the ability to assess the extent of soft tissue and dural involvement. CT is more effective for delineating bony lesions. There are no pathognomonic imaging findings; thus histopathologic examination from a tis-sue specimen is required for a definite diagnosis.

Treatment. Because of the rarity of the tumor, there are no set guidelines for treatment of chordomas. Based

Chordomas of clivus compressing pons and encroaching on sella turcica and sphenoid sinus

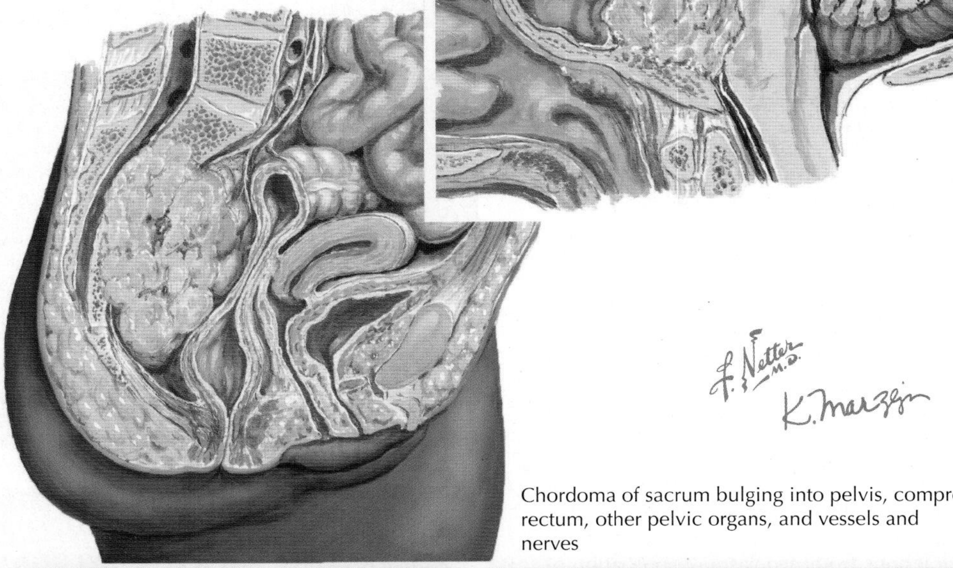

Chordoma of sacrum bulging into pelvis, compressing rectum, other pelvic organs, and vessels and nerves

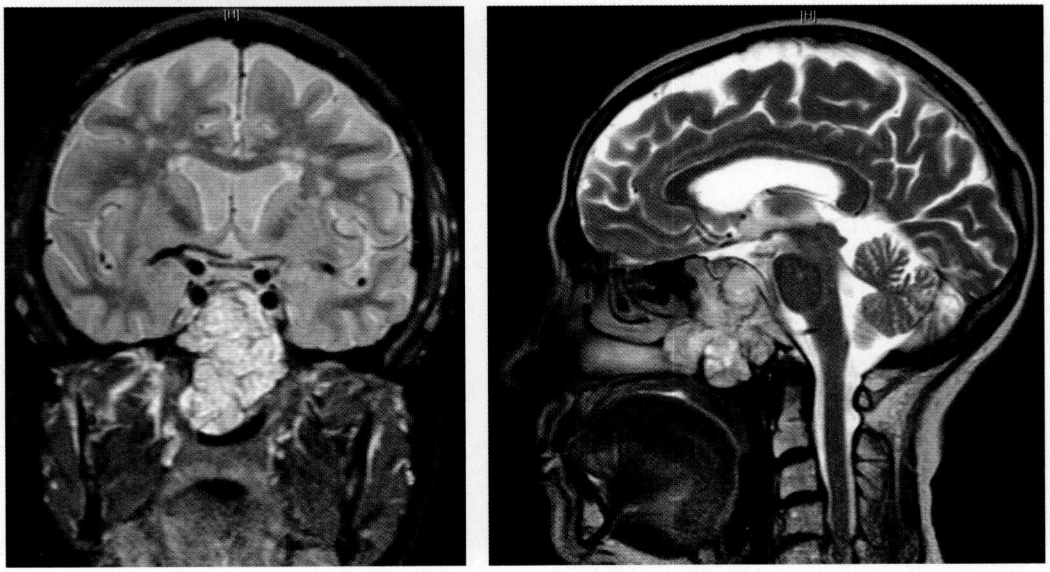

Coronal *(left)* and sagittal *(right)* MRIs of chordoma

on small retrospective studies, a multimodal approach combining surgery with radiotherapy is recommended. Surgery is used for both diagnostic and therapeutic purposes; it allows for a tissue diagnosis and reduces tumor burden. Complete resection is the goal but is often not feasible because of the anatomic constraints of the tumor. Their invasive nature results in a high incidence of local recurrence, and about 2% to 8% of chordomas will undergo sarcomatous transformation. Salvage therapy may include repeat surgery or radiation treatment.

Adjuvant radiotherapy has been used with increasing frequency, especially with current advances in radiation equipment and technique. Historically, conventional radiation with photons was difficult to administer be-cause the required doses were often associated with in-creased risk of damage to important structures such as the brainstem or cranial nerves. With newer techniques using proton therapy, SRS, or intensity-modulated ra-diation therapy (IMRT), outcomes have significantly improved by allowing higher doses of radiation while minimizing injury to neighboring structures.

Plate 12.19

Brain: PART I

DIFFERENTIAL DIAGNOSIS OF CENTRAL NERVOUS SYSTEM TUMORS

Although advances in imaging have increased the incidence of CNS tumor diagnosis, other brain lesions can appear similar to neoplasms. Mimics include inflammatory lesions, demyelination, autoimmune disease, radiation necrosis, and infection. These lesions are often expansile masses, resulting in similar clinical manifestations, highlighting the importance of histopathologic examination.

MULTIPLE SCLEROSIS

MS is the most common demyelinating disease of the CNS. Imaging typically reveals multiple lesions in a characteristic pattern, such as "Dawson fingers" (periventricular lesions oriented perpendicular to the long axis of the lateral ventricle on FLAIR sequences). These plaques have very little mass effect. Active lesions are usually enhancing, representing the breakdown of the blood-brain barrier. Tumefactive MS is a special subtype that affects patients in the second or third decades of life. Imaging reveals large (>2 cm) tumor-like masses that demonstrate incomplete ring enhancement with the incomplete area abutting the cortical gray matter or basal ganglia. These lesions can be associated with mass effect and vasogenic edema. Unlike hypercellular brain tumors, these lesions tend to have a relatively low cerebral blood volume on perfusion imaging and an increased apparent diffusion coefficient on diffusion sequences. Furthermore, MRS may help distinguish demyelinating lesions from neoplasm. Appreciation of the clinical history in conjunction with ancillary testing, such as CSF studies or evoked potentials, may aid in the differentiation of demyelinating disease from CNS tumors.

SARCOIDOSIS

Sarcoidosis is a multisystem granulomatous disease that can affect the CNS. About 5% of patients with known sarcoidosis manifest with neurosarcoidosis, although de novo presentation is also possible. It initially develops in the leptomeninges, allowing entry of the inflammatory process into the brain parenchyma, where granulomatous masses can develop. It has a predilection for cranial nerves, hypothalamus, and the pituitary gland, but any part of the CNS can be affected. On imaging, neurosarcoidosis can present with meningeal or pachymeningeal enhancement in association with nonenhancing periventricular white matter lesions. With cranial nerve involvement, enhancement along the nerves can be seen, although the extracranial portion is affected more often. Less common are enhancing granulomatous nodules in the parenchyma and dural mass lesions. With the relatively high frequency of leptomeningeal involvement, neurosarcoidosis can be mistaken for carcinomatous meningitis. Again, clinical history, systemic imaging, and CSF studies must be considered in distinguishing between the two.

RADIATION EFFECTS

Since the establishment of chemoradiation as the standard of care for GBM, there has been an increasing awareness of a phenomenon termed *pseudoprogression,* in which posttreatment imaging reveals the presence of enhancing lesions secondary to radiation injury, resulting in

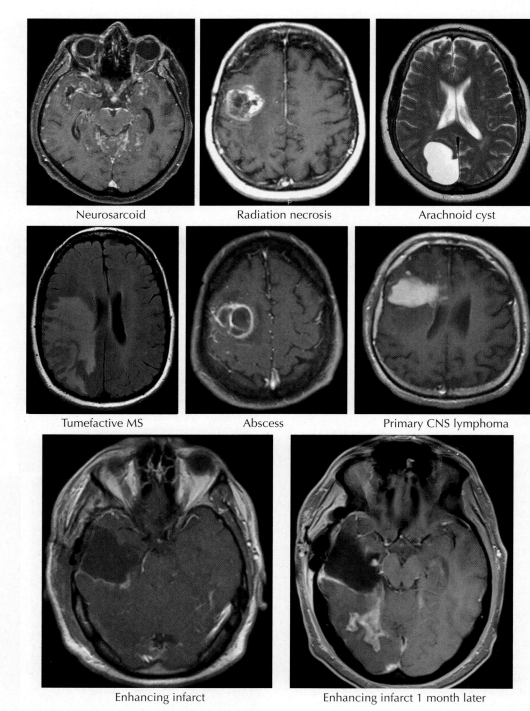

Neurosarcoid

Radiation necrosis

Arachnoid cyst

Tumefactive MS

Abscess

Primary CNS lymphoma

Enhancing infarct

Enhancing infarct 1 month later

increased capillary permeability and breakdown of the blood-brain barrier. Eventually, these lesions decrease in size or stabilize without the need for further treatment. Evidence suggests that these treatment-related effects occur more frequently with the use of temozolomide and significantly correlate with MGMT promoter methylation status. Clinically and radiographically, pseudoprogression can appear and behave identically to true tumor progression. Adjunct studies such as dynamic susceptibility-weighted contrast-enhanced MRI and PET scans may be useful. Pseudoprogression typically exhibits low cerebral blood volume and is "cold" on PET imaging, whereas tumor progression will have elevated cerebral blood volume and be metabolically active. Occasionally, biopsy of the lesion may be necessary to establish the correct diagnosis and appropriate management.

CEREBRAL ABSCESS

Intracranial abscesses can appear very similar to cystic or necrotic brain tumors. Both appear as ring-enhancing lesions with associated mass effect, causing associated neurologic deficits. Fever is not always present and is found in fewer than half of patients. Other parameters diagnostic for infection, such as leukocytosis, elevated erythrocyte sedimentation rate, and positive blood cultures, are not reliably present in patients affected by cerebral abscess. Studies such as lumbar puncture are less useful because findings are often nonspecific and cultures are rarely positive. Proton MRS and diffusion-weighted imaging have been reported to be helpful in distinguishing abscesses from nonpyogenic lesions, with abscesses displaying a specific metabolite profile on MRS and hyperintense signal on diffusion imaging.

Plate 12.20

Neuro-Oncology

CLASSIFICATION OF SPINAL TUMORS

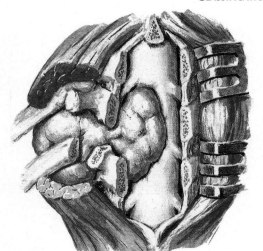

Extradural tumors.
Lymphoma invading spinal canal via intervertebral foramen, compressing dura mater and spinal cord.

Intradural extramedullary tumors.
Meningioma compressing spinal cord and distorting nerve roots.

Intramedullary tumors.
Astrocytoma exposed by longitudinal incision in bulging spinal cord.

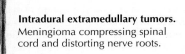

SPINAL TUMORS

Tumors involving the spine are classified according to their anatomic location. They can occur extradurally or intradurally. Intradural lesions are further subdivided into extramedullary or intramedullary lesions. Extramedullary lesions refer to tumors arising within the dura but outside the actual spinal cord, whereas intramedullary lesions are tumors arising from the spinal cord itself. Similar to brain lesions, spinal cord tumors can be either primary or metastatic. Primary spinal cord neoplasms constitute about 2% to 4% of all intrinsic CNS tumors. About one-third of these tumors are found in the intramedullary compartment. Metastatic tumors typically occur as extradural lesions and account for the majority of spinal cord compression cases.

The majority of extradural tumors consist of metastatic lesions to the bony vertebrae with subsequent invasion of the epidural space. Although any neoplasm could potentially spread to the spine, the most common primary tumors include the lung, breast, and prostate. Mechanisms of metastasis to the spine include hematologic spread either through the arterial circulation or Batson's venous plexus and direct extension of the tumor. Primary bone tumors, such as chordomas or sarcomas, can also arise in the vertebrae, producing symptoms of epidural compression. Benign lesions, such as osteomas, hemangiomas, giant cell tumors, and aneurysmal bone cysts, can be found in the spine and must be distinguished from malignant neoplasms. Other rare primary tumors that can occur in the epidural space include lymphoma, multiple myeloma, and plasmacytoma.

Intradural extramedullary tumors include meningiomas and nerve sheath tumors such as neurofibromas and schwannomas. Spinal meningiomas most often occur in the thoracic spine. They are usually slow-growing lesions that are adherent to the dura. Local invasion may cause remodeling or erosion of the bone. Spinal nerve sheath tumors may occur sporadically or as a manifestation of neurofibromatosis. On MRI, they often appear as dumbbell-shaped lesions. Schwannomas derive from proliferating Schwann cells, whereas neurofibromas are composed of a mix of cellular elements including Schwann cells, perineural elements, and fibroblasts. They are benign lesions but, rarely, de-differentiation into malignant nerve sheath tumors may occur.

Intramedullary tumors are the most difficult tumors to diagnose and treat. They may involve only a short segment of the cord or extend almost the whole length of the cord. The most common intradural intramedullary tumors are gliomas, specifically ependymomas and astrocytomas. Ependymomas are the most common intramedullary tumor in adults, with peak incidence in the fourth and fifth decades. About 50% occur in the lumbosacral spinal cord or filum terminale; the rest occur in the cervical and thoracic cord. It has been recently proposed that there are three subtypes to the

spinal ependymomas: myxopapillary tumors, classic ependymomas, and spinal subependymomas. Although myxopapillary ependymomas are typically benign and located in the conus and filum terminale, there are data that indicate that they have similar outcomes to classic ependymomas, thereby suggesting that they are more of a grade 2 tumor. Astrocytomas can occur anywhere in the cord. About one-half are pilocytic astrocytomas, and the other half are infiltrative. Similar to astrocytomas in the brain, prognosis depends on the grade of the tumor. Other prognostic

Plate 12.21

Brain: PART I

SYMPTOMS OF ACUTE SPINAL CORD SYNDROME EVOLUTION

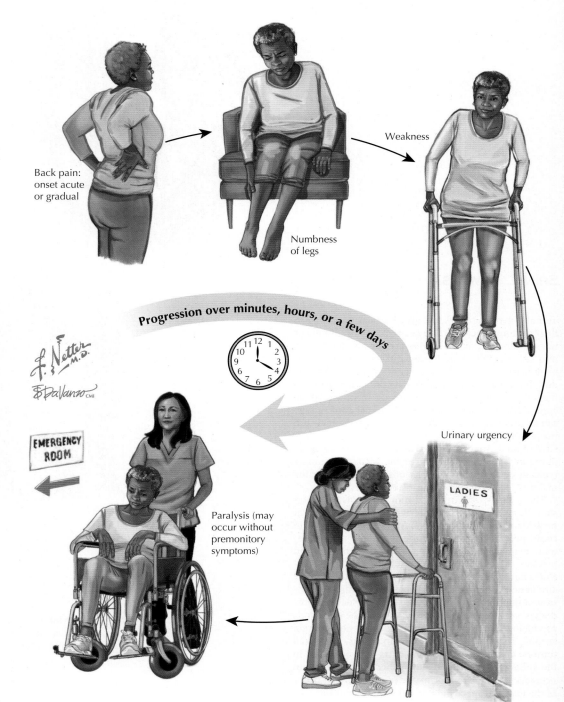

Back pain: onset acute or gradual

Numbness of legs

Weakness

Progression over minutes, hours, or a few days

EMERGENCY ROOM

Paralysis (may occur without premonitory symptoms)

Urinary urgency

LADIES

SPINAL TUMORS
(Continued)

factors include location of the tumor (with the exception of the cervical cord), extent of tumor involvement along the spinal cord, and duration of symptoms.

Clinical Manifestations. Symptoms of spinal cord tumors result from the compressive effect on neighboring structures disrupting both parenchymal elements and pathways. This can cause local and distal effects. In general, pain is a common complaint. Epidural tumors present with unremitting back pain, whereas intradural intramedullary lesions cause local and radicular pain. Onset of symptoms is gradual with the one exception of spinal cord infarction from compression of the tumor on the vasculature. Neurologic symptoms often consist of dysesthesia and muscular weakness followed by increased difficulty with ambulation. Other possible manifestations include cauda equina syndrome, conus medullaris syndrome, or Brown-Séquard syndrome when half the cord is affected. The clinical presentation may begin unilaterally with progression to bilateral involvement once both sides of the cord are involved. Spinal cord compression is one of the few neurologic emergencies and warrants immediate evaluation.

Diagnostic Studies. MRI with and without contrast is the diagnostic modality of choice because of its superiority in highlighting the cord anatomy in relation to the tumor. Almost all intrinsic tumors and metastases enhance upon administration of gadolinium. CT of the spine may be used in conjunction with MRI to delineate any bony involvement by the tumor. Occasionally, analysis of the CSF is performed when a diagnosis of ependymoma is established, as 10% will disseminate tumor cells in the spinal fluid.

Treatment. Complaint of back pain in any patient with an oncologic history should prompt an expedited evaluation for spinal metastasis to prevent irreversible neurologic damage. For epidural metastases, one of the most important prognostic factors for regaining the ability to ambulate is pretreatment neurologic function. Thus timely evaluation is required to preserve neurologic function and to prevent further neurologic deterioration. Treatment consists of pain management, usually with a combination of high-dose steroids and opiates, and treatment directed at the tumor. In patients with epidural spinal cord compression who are appropriate surgical candidates,

radical resection followed by radiotherapy seems to have improved outcome compared with those patients undergoing radiotherapy alone. For patients who are not candidates for aggressive surgery, external-beam radiotherapy is effective for palliative symptom management and local tumor control.

Intradural extramedullary tumors are treated with surgical resection, which is potentially curative if gross total resection is achieved. Radiotherapy is generally reserved for patients with incomplete resection or as salvage therapy. The role of chemotherapy has yet to be established. Ependymomas are treated with

surgical excision; often a total or near-total resection can be achieved with little to no neurologic deficits. Though rare, CSF dissemination is possible. It is unclear whether adjuvant radiotherapy is beneficial, although some studies have shown it to improve local control in subtotally resected ependymomas. There are no randomized trials offering guidelines for the treatment of spinal cord astrocytomas. For pilocytic astrocytomas, total surgical excision is recommended, similar to its intracranial counterpart. Higher-grade gliomas may benefit from adjuvant radiotherapy after surgery.

Plate 12.22

Neuro-Oncology

Treatment Modalities

The treatment of brain tumors requires a multidisciplinary approach that consists of neurosurgery, radiotherapy, and/or chemotherapy. In all three fields, technological advances have improved the efficacy of each individual treatment modality. For instance, radiographic innovations have expanded neurosurgical capabilities. Functional MRI, a noninvasive imaging modality that uses cortical blood flow changes as a marker for increased or decreased neuronal activity, has improved presurgical planning by delineating tumor margins from eloquent cortex. Intraoperative MRI brings the ability to update images as necessary as intraoperative deformation from secondary fluid shifts, changes in intracranial pressure, and/or the use of retractors may render preoperative images inaccurate. Fluorescence-guided surgery with 5-aminolevulinic acid allows more extensive resections of GBM with the hope of improved overall survival. The advent of endoscopy has transformed previously complex craniotomies to elegant outpatient procedures. Finally, the development of short-acting analgesic and anesthetic agents has paved the way for intraoperative mapping, allowing for maximum excision of tumors in regions of eloquent cortex while minimizing neurologic damage.

Radiation therapy is frequently used as adjunctive therapy or primary therapy. Primary therapy may be for curative intent, palliation, or stabilization. Ionizing radiation is the mainstay of treatment in neuro-oncology, with the most common types of radiation being photons and protons. Radiation can be delivered either in multiple treatments as "fractions" or in a single treatment dose. Advances in radiation oncology have improved its effectiveness and decreased its complications by honing its precision in an effort to minimize surrounding neurotoxicity. This has been achieved with the advent of stereotactic treatment, which is a specialized method of targeting, and the use of three-dimensional (3D) conformal treatment in which the volumetric distribution of the desired dose mimics the shape of the target. Stereotactic IMRT is a type of 3D conformal therapy that delivers radiation (usually photons) in a controlled and precise fashion, limiting the toxicity to the rest of the brain. Advantages include reducing the radiation dose to at-risk dose-limiting organs, such as the optic apparatus, brainstem, and inner ear, and improving dose delivery to target organs. More recently, proton beams have garnered much attention because of their ability to limit the amount of scatter to normal tissue. This has allowed radiotherapists to deliver sufficient radiation to specific areas. SRS, using either the linear accelerator, gamma knife, or cyber knife, delivers a large single dose of radiation in a highly focused manner, achieving a similar biologic effect as several weeks of fractionated radiation therapy. Gamma knife uses gamma radiation derived from 201 cobalt-60 sources arranged in a circular array directed at the center of the unit, where the head is rigidly fixed. A linear accelerator targets its radiation beams by simultaneously rotating the patient and treatment unit gantry. Cyber knife uses an image guidance system in conjunction with a linear accelerator mounted on a robotic arm. To date, a clinically meaningful advantage has not been demonstrated among these apparatuses.

The realm of chemotherapy has also seen some advances that have improved overall survival and progression-free survival. Temozolomide, an oral alkylating agent, received FDA approval in 1999 for recurrent anaplastic astrocytoma and approval in 2005 for use in newly diagnosed GBM. Compared with previous alkylating agents, the adverse effects associated with temozolomide are generally mild to moderate and predictable. Moreover, the EORTC-NCIC Phase III trial demonstrated a significant improvement in survival with the addition of temozolomide to radiation compared with radiation alone. In 2009 the FDA granted accelerated approval to bevacizumab (Avastin), a monoclonal antibody against human VEGF as monotherapy for recurrent GBM. Although its effect on overall survival remains modest, phase II trials have reported increased response rates and improved 6-month progression-free survival with this drug, although there is no benefit to overall survival. Tumor-treating fields are a novel antitumor treatment that has influenced overall survival. This technique uses alternating electric fields at intermediate frequencies to inhibit cancer cell proliferation. Currently, small-molecule inhibitors are subject to much investigation as potential therapeutics for malignant glioma. Immunotherapy is also being explored, whether in the form of checkpoint blockade, oncolytic viruses, or vaccines, especially as GBM is a uniquely immunosuppressive tumor.

Surgical Approaches

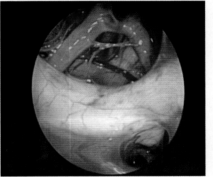

Sublabial transseptal transsphenoidal surgical approach

Endoscopic transnasal transsphenoidal surgical approach

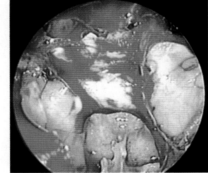

Endoscopic view

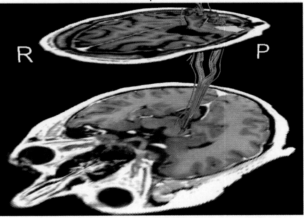

Functional MRI

HEADACHE

Plate 13.1

Brain: PART I

OVERVIEW OF HEADACHES

Headache is one of the most common reasons for consulting a physician and is considered the most prevalent neurologic disorder worldwide. Rather than a disease, headache is a symptom, frequently providing a valuable warning of hidden pathology.

Physicians treating patients for headache must decide whether the headache represents a primary or secondary headache syndrome. *Primary headaches* are more common and include disorders such as migraine, tension-type headache (TTH), and trigeminal autonomic cephalalgias (TACs). The patient with primary headaches may have severe and incapacitating pain, but there is no identifiable cause leading to activation of nociception. In contrast, *secondary headaches* are symptomatic of a cranial or extracranial pathology, such as a brain tumor, ruptured aneurysm, meningitis, or hematoma. Headache diagnosis depends on a thorough history and neurologic and medical examinations. The history should seek information on premonitory symptoms, timing of onset (gradual vs. sudden) and duration, pain quality and severity, location of pain, provoking factors, any associated symptoms, clinical circumstances, and details of previous investigations and treatments. A past medical history, family history, trauma history, social history, current medications, drug allergies, and review of systems are also indispensable. If a new headache is unlike any headache the patient has had in the past, it requires very expeditious evaluation, which may include ancillary laboratory and neuroradiologic imaging.

Secondary headaches, and possibly primary headaches, are thought to occur when primary afferent nociceptive neurons arising from either the trigeminal ganglion or upper cervical spinal ganglia (C1–C3) are depolarized. These neurons innervate both extracranial and intracranial pain-sensitive structures. The first and second trigeminal nerve divisions provide sensory innervation for the anterior head and upper face. The trigeminal nerve innervates pain-sensitive dural structures, including the dural sinuses and tentorium cerebelli, as well as many arteries, including the middle meningeal, temporal, and proximal portions of the anterior and posterior cerebrals, and the internal/external carotid. The cervical spinal nerves (C1–C3) provide innervation to the dural structures of the posterior fossa, the basilar and vertebral arteries, and muscular structures in the upper neck and posterior portion of the head.

The cause of prolonged head pain is usually apparent when a secondary headache develops related to a tumor or other intracranial lesion producing ongoing traction upon a dural or vascular structure. However, patients with a primary headache disorder do not have a clearly discernible source for ongoing activation of nociceptive neurons. Therefore pathophysiologic mechanisms leading to a persistent primary headache are less clear. It is likely that the neurons within the trigeminal-cervical pain system are more than passive conduits for depolarization because they also seem to play a role in pain sensitization. Sensitization is a process by which, after repeated activation, neurons become increasingly responsive to painful and nonpainful stimulation. *Peripheral sensitization* (in the primary afferent neurons) and *central sensitization* (within second-order neurons in the trigeminal nucleus caudalis and higher-order neurons within the central nervous system [CNS]) may play a role in prolonging headaches and may contribute to the transformation of episodic migraine into the chronic form of migraine.

The evidence of peripheral sensitization of the primary afferents comes from both animal and human studies. In animal models, stimulation of the trigeminal system leads to increased concentrations of vasoactive peptides, including substance P, neurokinin A, and calcitonin gene–related protein (CGRP) in sagittal sinus blood. Similarly, in humans, internal jugular CGRP levels reportedly rise during migraine attacks. Release of these neuropeptides is a marker for neuronal activation in primary afferents. Primary afferent neurons exposed to activating stimuli show increased spontaneous firing and lowered activation thresholds.

There is also evidence that initial activation of the primary afferent neurons leads to sensitization of second- and possibly higher-order neurons. Chemical irritation of the meninges in animal models (peripheral nociceptors) causes sensitization of both trigeminovascular fibers innervating dura and central trigeminal neurons receiving convergent input from dura mater and skin. After sensitizing activation of the meninges, central trigeminal neurons respond to low-intensity mechanical and thermal stimuli from skin that previously induced minimal or no response. This change in activation threshold for central neurons receiving input from skin (which was not directly irritated) strongly implicates sensitization of second-order neurons within the CNS.

PAIN-SENSITIVE STRUCTURES AND PAIN REFERRAL

Pain sensation
Dural sinus
Middle meningeal artery
Temporal artery
Proximal cerebral arteries
Tentorium cerebelli
Internal and external carotid arteries
Ophthalmic (V₁) nerve
Central pain pathway
Spinal nucleus of trigeminal (V) nerve
Spinal ganglia C1–3
Dura of posterior fossa
Vertebrobasilar arteries

JOHN A. CRAIG—MD
C. Machado—M.D.

Anterior head
Afferent nerves from intracranial and extracranial structures of anterior two-thirds of head and somatic pain afferent nerves from forehead and scalp are carried by ophthalmic nerve. These neurons refer pain from intracranial structures to forehead, scalp, or retrobulbar sites.

Posterior head
Afferent nerves from occipital region, ear, and neck and from dura of posterior fossa and vertebrobasilar arteries are carried by dorsal roots of C1–3 spinal ganglia, accounting for pain referral to these sites.

Plate 13.2

Headache

MIGRAINE PATHOPHYSIOLOGY

Migraine pathophysiology is not well understood. At present, migraine is viewed as a complex, often genetically based disorder that confers a susceptibility to the initiation of a cascade of events within the CNS, resulting in a clinical migraine attack.

Until the 1980s, the accepted explanation for migraine attacks was the *vascular theory of migraine,* which suggested that migraine headache was caused by the dilation of cranial blood vessels, whereas the aura of migraine resulted from vasoconstriction. The vascular theory was based on four observations: (1) the only effective treatment of acute migraine at the time, ergotamine, was a potent vasoconstrictor; (2) nitroglycerin, a vasodilating agent, caused headaches; (3) the branches of the external carotid arteries often became distended and pulsated during a migraine attack; and (4) stimulation of intracranial vascular structures (but not the brain) in awake patients undergoing surgical procedures caused headache. However, this vascular theory did not appear to account for all the elements of migraine pathophysiology.

A *neurogenic theory* evolved next, suggesting that the migraine aura was caused by a cortical wave of neuronal and glial depolarization, referred to as *cortical spreading depression* (CSD). From its cerebral cortical origin, this CSD wave spreads across the cortex at a rate of 3 to 5 mm/min, a rate similar to the estimated speed of visual aura of migraine as it progresses across the primary visual cortex. In experimental CSD, there are characteristic cerebral blood flow changes, with an initial increase in blood flow (hyperemia) followed by a decrease in blood flow (oligemia) and relative tissue hypoxia. Imaging studies using functional magnetic resonance imaging (MRI) seem to corroborate these hemodynamic changes in migraineurs during visual aura. In addition to contributing to aura, CSD may also act as a trigger for the headache pain. Experimental evidence demonstrates that CSDs may result both in activation of nociceptive second-order neurons within the medullary *trigeminal nucleus caudalis* and in changes within the vessel caliber of dural vessels innervated with pain-sensitive neurons. This mechanism might certainly account for activation of the headache in patients who experience the migraine aura but would not explain headache in patients with migraine without aura. It has been suggested that migraine without aura occurs when CSD takes place in noneloquent brain areas (such as the cerebellum), where depolarization is not consciously perceived; however, there is insufficient evidence to support this possibility currently.

The headache of migraine likely arises upon activation of nociceptive neurons in the *trigeminovascular system* (TVS). The TVS consists of small caliber pseudounipolar sensory neurons arising from the trigeminal ganglion and upper cervical dorsal roots and project to innervate pial vessels, dura mater, large cerebral vessels, and venous sinuses. Once activated, the neurons transmit the nociceptive information to the *trigeminal nucleus caudalis* of the medulla, where they synapse on second-order neurons.

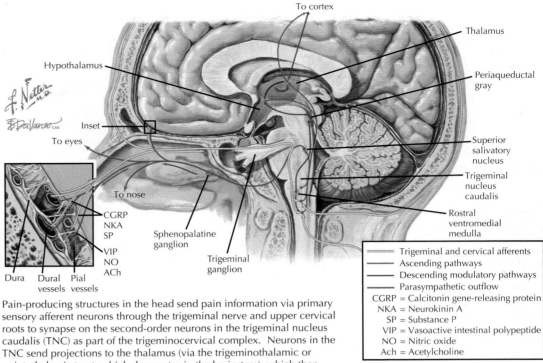

Pain-producing structures in the head send pain information via primary sensory afferent neurons through the trigeminal nerve and upper cervical roots to synapse on the second-order neurons in the trigeminal nucleus caudalis (TNC) as part of the trigeminocervical complex. Neurons in the TNC send projections to the thalamus (via the trigeminothalamic or quintothalamic tract, which decussates in the brainstem), which then projects to the cortex. The TNC is thought to project to other structures as well, including the periaqueductal gray (PAG), which also send signals to the thalamus and hypothalamus, with projections to the cortex. There are descending projections from the cortex back to the thalamus and hypothalamus. Descending modulation of the TNC takes place via nuclei in the hypothalamus, as well as direct projections from the PAG through the rostral ventromedial medulla (RVM).

Cranial parasympathetic outflow stems from a reflex connection from the TNC to the superior salivatory nucleus (SSN) in the pons. Efferents from the SSN (via the facial nerve) connect with neurons in the sphenopalatine ganglion (SPG; pterygopalatine). The SPG then projects to innervate intracranial vessels (vasodilation), as well as the nasal and lacrimal glands.

Pathophysiology of aura

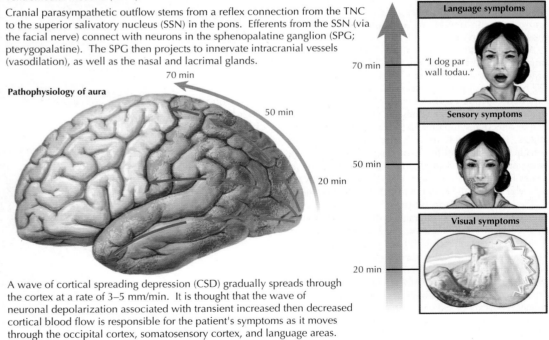

A wave of cortical spreading depression (CSD) gradually spreads through the cortex at a rate of 3–5 mm/min. It is thought that the wave of neuronal depolarization associated with transient increased then decreased cortical blood flow is responsible for the patient's symptoms as it moves through the occipital cortex, somatosensory cortex, and language areas.

From the trigeminal nucleus caudalis, neurons that are involved in localization of pain project to the *thalamus* and then to the *sensory cortex,* where pain reaches consciousness. Central signals can be modulated by projections from several sources, including the *periaqueductal gray,* the *nucleus raphe magnus* in the *rostral ventromedial medulla,* and by *descending cortical inhibitory systems.* Other activated second-order neurons within the trigeminal nucleus caudalis project to numerous *subcortical nuclei* and to *limbic areas* of the brain involved in the emotional and vegetative responses to pain.

There is ongoing debate as to whether initial activation of primary afferent neurons is necessary for the occurrence of migraine headaches. Increases in measured levels of CGRP (a neuropeptide known to be released by activated first-order neurons) are observed in external jugular venous blood during migraine in humans, implicating activation of primary afferent neurons. In some individuals, however, it would seem the abnormal activation or lack of regulating inhibitory tone could result in the propensity of a migraine attack.

Plate 13.3

Brain: PART I

TRIGGERS OF MIGRAINE

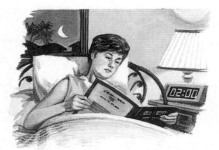

Lack of sleep

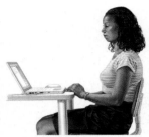

Flickering, glaring, or fluorescent lights

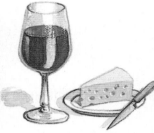

Alcohol, certain foods, or missing a meal

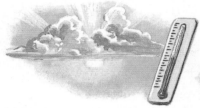

Changes in weather or barometric pressure

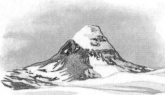

High altitude

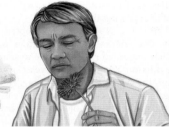

Strong odors

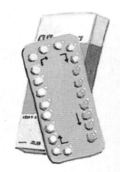

Oral contraceptives, other hormonal changes

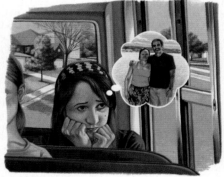

Stress, anxiety

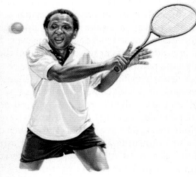

Exertion, fatigue

Common symptoms and signs

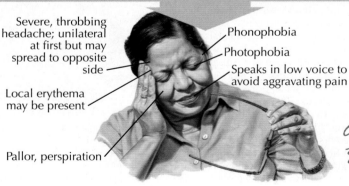

Severe, throbbing headache; unilateral at first but may spread to opposite side

Phonophobia

Photophobia

Speaks in low voice to avoid aggravating pain

Local erythema may be present

Pallor, perspiration

JOHN A. CRAIG—MD
C. Machado—M.D.
DaVanzo CMI

MIGRAINE PRESENTATION

Migraine is a very common disorder, with a 3-month prevalence of 21% in females and 10% in males, based on data reported in the US population. It is most common in the third and fourth decades, although it may occur at any time of life from early childhood onward. Migraine is divided into two types based on the presence or absence of transient neurologic symptoms referred to as aura. *Migraine without aura* (formerly *common migraine*) is more common than *migraine with aura* (formerly *classic migraine*) and accounts for about three-quarters of patients with migraine. Both migraine with aura and migraine without aura occur in either an episodic form (<15 headache days/month) or a chronic form (≥15 headache days/month). Over the course of a lifetime, a migraine sufferer may move back and forth between the chronic and episodic forms. The factors determining susceptibility to the development of the chronic form of migraine are poorly understood. Motion sickness and *cold stimulus headache* (also known as brain freeze) are common comorbidities in those with migraine.

Although head pain is the most debilitating aspect of migraine, a migraine attack may unfold through a series of four phases: (1) prodrome, (2) aura (when present), (3) headache, and (4) postdrome. Not all individuals experience all phases. The *prodrome* occurs in up to 60% of patients with migraine and consists of vague vegetative or affective symptoms that herald the onset of the attack. These symptoms may include food cravings, constipation, neck stiffness, increased yawning, irritability, euphoria, or depression. With resolution of the prodrome, the *aura* (when present) occurs generally just before or during the opening minutes of the headache.

The *migraine headache* is usually (but not always) unilateral. In fact, the term migraine is derived from the ancient Greek word, *hemikranos*, which means "half head." A migraine headache tends to have a throbbing or pulsatile quality that at times is superimposed on a constant pressure-like sensation. As the attack severity increases over the course of one to several hours, patients may experience nausea and sometimes vomiting. Most individuals report abnormal sensitivity to light (*photophobia*), sound (*phonophobia*), and/or smell (*osmophobia*) during attacks. Individuals may also report *cutaneous allodynia* over the face or scalp on the same side as the headache. Allodynia is a tenderness or hypersensitivity in the context of which even a light touch may be perceived as painful. In adults, an untreated migraine headache will attain at least a moderate level of pain intensity that can persist from 4 hours to 3 days. Many attacks resolve with sleep that can occur as a part of the natural course of the migraine attack or as the result of treatment of the headache with sedating medications.

As the headache is resolving, many patients experience a *postdromal* phase during which they feel drained or exhausted, although some report a feeling of mild elation or euphoria. During the postdromal phase, sudden head movement may cause transient pain in the location of the recently resolved headache.

Frequently cited precipitating factors (triggers) of migraine headache include stress, fasting, sleep disturbances, weather changes, bright light or glare, ingestion of alcohol, strong odors, smoke, nitroglycerin or other vasodilating drugs, nasal congestion, withdrawal from caffeine or ergotamine-containing medicines, exercise, sexual intercourse, and certain food substances, such as chocolates, aged cheeses, processed meats, and hot dogs. However, for most patients migraine attacks occur unpredictably.

One of the most potent and frequent triggers of migraine in females is the monthly fluctuation of gonadal hormones that underlies the menstrual cycle. Typically, the headaches appear 1 to 2 days before or the first day of menstrual flow, although they may appear at midcycle with ovulation. The headaches can be quite severe and are usually without aura, although females can also have headaches preceded by aura at other times of the month.

Plate 13.4

Headache

Migraine Aura

Migraine aura consists of transient focal neurologic symptoms that tend to last for 5 minutes to 1 hour and may occur before or during the headache phase. There are four types of migraine aura: visual, sensory, language, and motor. Patients may have one or more types, and auras may occur even in the absence of headache. The most common aura type is *visual,* consisting of positive (shimmering, sparkling, flashes of light) or negative (blurred vision or loss of vision) symptoms in both eyes. The classic visual aura is a *scintillating scotoma* that starts as a small shimmering or blurred spot just lateral to the point of visual fixation. This spot expands over 5 minutes to 1 hour to involve a quadrant or half of the visual field. It often assumes a curved or sickle shape with a zigzagging or serrated border, sometimes multicolored or sparkling in appearance. This jagged edge has also been referred to as *fortification spectra* based on its resemblance to the top of a medieval fortress. Over time, the positive visual phenomena tend to move toward the periphery, leaving a blind spot (scotoma) in their wake.

When a *sensory aura* accompanies a visual aura, it tends to follow the visual symptoms within minutes and typically begins as unilateral paresthesias in a limb or one side of the face. From their origin, the paresthesias may gradually march up or down the limb or face, often with a subsequent feeling of numbness that may last up to an hour. The sensory aura may also expand to involve the inside of the mouth, affecting the inside of one cheek and half the tongue. The slow spread of positive symptoms (the scintillations or the tingling) followed by negative symptoms (scotoma or numbness) is very suggestive of migraine aura and contrasts significantly with an ischemic event, such as a transient ischemic attack during which all symptoms begin concomitantly.

A *language aura* occurs much less commonly than the visual and sensory type auras. This consists of transient language problems that may range from mild word-finding difficulties to frank dysphasia with paraphasic errors.

The *motor aura* is least common, presenting as unilateral weakness in the limbs and possibly the face. Most patients with motor aura also report sensory symptoms and may have other attacks, including visual, sensory, or language aura. The weakness of a motor aura must be distinguished from clumsiness based on proprioceptive loss from a sensory aura. To date, research studies have linked motor aura to at least three separate genetic mutations. As a result, a motor aura is classified separately from the other forms of migraine aura and is referred to as *hemiplegic migraine.* Hemiplegic migraine can be further classified as either familial or sporadic. Patients with *familial hemiplegic migraine* have at least one first- or second-degree relative with the same disorder. *Sporadic hemiplegic migraine* (SHM) is thought to be the result of a new mutation, and a patient with SHM may or may not carry one of the three gene variants already linked to the familial form.

Migraine with brainstem aura (previously known as basilar-type migraine) is a variant of migraine with aura during which the symptoms mimic occlusive disease in the posterior cerebral circulation. These include reversible vertigo, ataxia, diplopia, dysarthria, and decreased consciousness. By definition, migraine with

Visual Auras

Scintillating scotoma and fortification phenomena

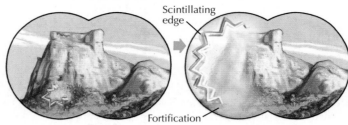

Scintillating edge

Early phase; isolated paracentral scintillating scotoma

Fortification spectra

Spread of scotoma to involve entire unilateral visual field

Wavy lines (heat shimmers)

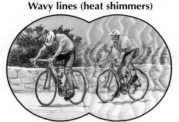

Wavy line distortions in part of visual field similar to shimmers above hot pavement

Metamorphopsia

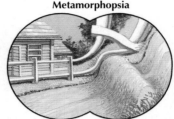

Distortions of form, size, or position of objects or environment in part of visual field

Hemianopsia

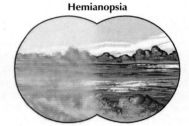

Sensory aura
Unilateral spreading paresthesias followed by numbness; often involve an arm and lower face and oral region (cheiro-oral paresthesias)

Hemiplegic migraine
Transient unilateral weakness can accompany migraine as motor aura

JOHN A. CRAIG—AD
C. Machado—M.D.
B. DaVanzo CMI

"Can't think of right weird."

Language aura
May have transient difficulty with language comprehension or production of speech

brainstem aura should not have associated hemiplegia. If motor aura symptoms are present, the diagnosis remains hemiplegic migraine.

PROLONGED OR FREQUENT MIGRAINE AURA

An aura lasting substantially longer than the typical 5 to 60 minutes requires consideration for an alternative cause. Prolonged or persistent neurologic symptoms should be evaluated for cerebral infarction (stroke) or inflammatory disorder with an MRI with contrast enhancement and diffusion-weighted sequences. Very rarely, patients have been described as having prolonged aura lasting longer than 1 week, referred to as *persistent aura without infarction.*

A new-onset marked increase in the frequency of aura is also concerning. *Migraine aura status,* defined as more than three auras in 3 days, is a red flag requiring further evaluation. Possible causes include reversible cerebral vasoconstriction syndrome, posterior reversible encephalopathy syndrome (PRES), arterial dissection, and embolic stroke, among others.

Plate 13.5

Brain: PART I

Migraine Management

The medical management of migraine involves two types of therapy: acute or abortive therapy at the time of an attack to truncate it, and prophylactic treatment taken daily to decrease the intensity and frequency of the migraine headaches.

When migraine attacks occur infrequently (3 days or fewer per month) and are not associated with prolonged neurologic symptoms, abortive management is usually sufficient. However, daily prophylactic treatment should be considered if (1) headaches are usually disabling to the patient for 4 or more days per month; (2) the severity of the attacks, or even the dread of an attack, negatively affects the patient's ability to carry out normal activities of daily living between attacks; (3) headaches are associated with neurologic deficits that persist beyond the duration of the headache phase of the attack; (4) there is a history of migraine-associated cerebral infarction; or (5) the patient obtains only incomplete relief from all tolerated abortive treatments.

The initial management of acute migraine treatment is with nonsteroidal antiinflammatory drugs (NSAIDs), such as naproxen sodium or ketoprofen, or with serotonin agonists such as dihydroergotamine and 5-hydroxytryptamine (5-HT) 1B/1D/1F serotonin agonists (triptans such as sumatriptan, zolmitriptan, naratriptan, rizatriptan, almotriptan, eletriptan, and frovatriptan).

Two new medication classes have been developed for acute migraine treatment, including *ditans,* which act as selective 5-HT 1F agonists (e.g., lasmiditan), and *gepants,* which act as CGRP receptor antagonists (e.g., rimegepant and ubrogepant). Unlike the ergotamine derivatives and triptans, these newer classes are not thought to contribute to vasoconstriction and therefore may be safer in patients with a history of vascular disease. Ditans are specifically thought to be a safe option if there is a history of cardiovascular or cerebral ischemia.

For difficult-to-treat headaches, the combination of an NSAID with a triptan or newer abortive may provide better relief than either medicine alone. The addition of an antiemetic, such as prochlorperazine or promethazine, may further increase the effectiveness of acute treatment. Importantly, the use of acute headache medications more than 2 days per week may contribute to an increasing frequency and severity of headaches over time. This includes over-the-counter analgesics, triptans, and ergotamine derivatives. Gepants may be an exception to this limitation, with some evidence suggesting that the regular use of gepants may help with migraine prevention.

When *prophylactic or preventive treatment* is necessary, several general principles should be remembered. To minimize side effects, prophylactic medications need to be started at a low dose and gradually increased over a period of a few weeks toward a therapeutic target dose. Once the therapeutic dose is attained, maintaining treatment for at least 8 to 12 additional weeks is needed to reliably assess effectiveness. Early discontinuation may deprive the patient of a potentially effective therapy. If drugs are not completely effective but are well tolerated as monotherapies, a combination of two agents may be tried, each from a different class, despite the greater risk of side effects. The additional benefit to be gained from the use of combination therapy has not been fully assessed in a prospective evidence-based

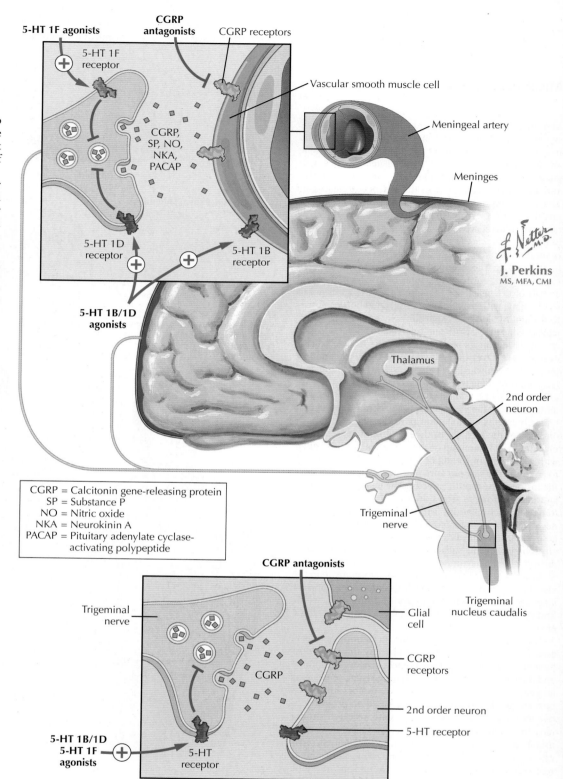

CGRP = Calcitonin gene-releasing protein
SP = Substance P
NO = Nitric oxide
NKA = Neurokinin A
PACAP = Pituitary adenylate cyclase-activating polypeptide

fashion. To be considered successful, the prophylactic treatment should reduce the number of headache days per month by at least 50%.

Migraine preventive treatments come from multiple classes of medications, including *beta-adrenergic blockers* (atenolol, metoprolol, nadolol, propranolol, and timolol), *tricyclic antidepressants* (amitriptyline and nortriptyline), *calcium channel blockers* (verapamil), *anticonvulsants* (divalproex sodium, topiramate, and gabapentin), *serotonin and norepinephrine reuptake inhibitors* (venlafaxine), botulinum toxin A injections (chronic migraine only), *CGRP monoclonal antibodies* (erenumab, fremanezumab, galcanezumab, and eptinezumab), *CGRP receptor antagonists* (rimegepant, atogepant), and *nutritional supplements* (riboflavin, feverfew, magnesium, and butterbur). Individual patients may find that one preventive agent is more effective than another. Unfortunately, at present there is no method for drug selection other than trial and error. For some individuals nonpharmacologic treatments such as cognitive-behavioral therapy, biofeedback, and noninvasive neurostimulation devices can play a role in migraine management.

Plate 13.6

Headache

TRIGEMINAL AUTONOMIC CEPHALALGIAS

Trigeminal autonomic cephalalgias (TACs) are a category of primary headache disorders distinguished by *one-sided pain* in the trigeminal distribution that is present in combination with *ipsilateral cranial autonomic* signs and symptoms, including:

- Ipsilateral conjunctival injection and/or lacrimation
- Ipsilateral nasal congestion and/or rhinorrhea
- Ipsilateral forehead and facial sweating or flushing
- Ipsilateral eyelid edema
- Ptosis and/or miosis (less common)

The TAC disorders include (1) cluster headache (CH), (2) paroxysmal hemicrania (PH), (3) short-lasting unilateral neuralgiform headache attacks with conjunctival injection and tearing (SUNCT), (4) short-lasting unilateral neuralgiform headache attacks with cranial autonomic symptoms (SUNA), and (5) hemicrania continua (HC). Although sharing several features, the TACs differ in attack duration and frequency as well as in their therapeutic response (see Plate 13.7). CH has a long attack length and a relatively low attack frequency. PH has an intermediate attack length and an intermediate attack frequency. SUNCT/SUNA headache attacks have the shortest attack length and the highest attack frequency. HC is a continuous headache with superimposed attacks that are moderate to severe in intensity. Most importantly, underlying structural brain lesions can mimic these disorders. Therefore brain MRI and MR angiography (MRA) are indicated when a TAC diagnosis is considered.

CLUSTER HEADACHE

Although rare, CH is nevertheless the most common of the TAC disorders with a prevalence of less than 1% and a male-to-female ratio of around 2:1 to 5:1. In addition to the cranial autonomic symptoms, several clinical features help characterize CH. The pain is usually piercing, boring, or stabbing; it usually begins precipitously without premonitory symptoms, rapidly reaching crescendo and becoming excruciatingly severe. The pain may begin in the temporal, lower facial, or occipital region; remains unilateral; and is typically maximal behind and around the eye. The headache usually lasts 60 to 90 minutes, with a range of 15 to 180 minutes, and occurs from every other day to eight times per day, often at the same time each day or night. Photophobia and phonophobia occur in 50% to 90% of CH individuals, typically ipsilateral to the pain. In contrast to migraine, where activity typically aggravates the pain, most patients with CH report restlessness and agitation and avoid remaining recumbent.

The term "cluster" headache was coined because, in its prototypical form, it is episodic and usually occurs at least once every 24 hours for weeks to months at a time—that is, in clusters. During an active cluster period, attacks can usually be precipitated by ingestion of alcohol. A frequent pattern is for cluster periods to occur seasonally, often in the spring or fall. This periodicity may decrease after a few years as periods of cluster activity become less predictable, occurring any time of the year. Approximately 10% of sufferers develop chronic CH characterized by the absence of prolonged remissions.

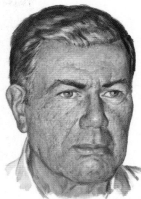

Face may have peau d'orange skin, telangiectasis

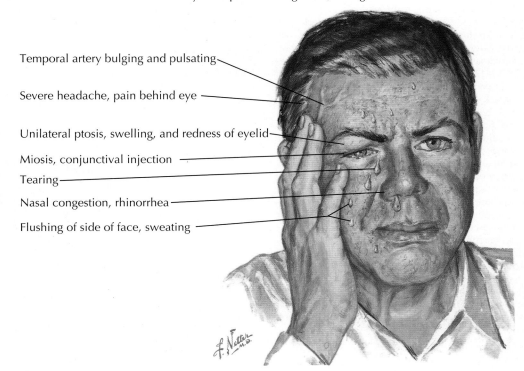

Temporal artery bulging and pulsating

Severe headache, pain behind eye

Unilateral ptosis, swelling, and redness of eyelid

Miosis, conjunctival injection

Tearing

Nasal congestion, rhinorrhea

Flushing of side of face, sweating

Mechanisms of Cluster Headache

Pathophysiology of CH is not well understood. The recurrence of attacks at similar times of day during cluster bouts is one of this syndrome's most striking characteristics and suggests possible hypothalamic involvement. Positron emission tomography (PET) studies support this, demonstrating activation in the posterior hypothalamus during CHs. The hypothalamus is functionally connected to the ipsilateral trigeminal system and other areas of the pain matrix. Once the hypothalamus is activated, it may activate the trigeminal-autonomic reflex, leading to unilateral pain mainly within the ophthalmic division of the trigeminal nerve, as well as ipsilateral autonomic features including tearing, rhinorrhea, partial Horner syndrome, and orbital vasodilation. Activation of the trigeminovascular pathway during CH is supported by evidence of elevated CGRP during both spontaneous and nitroglycerin-triggered cluster attacks.

Cluster Headache Management

Management is divided into treatment of acute cluster attacks as well as therapeutic options to transition out of a cluster period or prophylactic therapy to prevent future attacks. Options for the acute treatment of CH

include inhalation of 100% oxygen, subcutaneous or nasal sumatriptan, oral or nasal zolmitriptan, octreotide, nasal lidocaine, and subcutaneous dihydroergotamine. Noninvasive vagus nerve stimulation may also be helpful as an acute treatment for CH.

Transitional prophylaxis may be used for a few weeks to quickly end or markedly reduce the frequency of attacks. A 2- to 3-week course of corticosteroids often leads to a substantial reduction of attacks. Greater occipital nerve blockade with a local anesthetic and a corticosteroid may significantly reduce attacks and sometimes leads to a remission. Galcanezumab, one of the CGRP antibodies, has also been shown to reduce the frequency of attacks in episodic CH. For longer-term prophylaxis, verapamil is usually the drug of choice because of its efficacy and side effect profile. Lithium carbonate can also be efficacious but is usually reserved for chronic, intractable CH. The use of other agents, such as topiramate, divalproex sodium, and pizotifen, may occasionally be useful. For medically intractable chronic CH, wherein the patient's activities of daily living are totally incapacitated by the pain, occipital nerve stimulation, sphenopalatine ganglion

Plate 13.7

Brain: PART I

Trigeminal autonomic cephalalgias				
	Cluster headache	Paroxysmal hemicrania	SUNCT/SUNA	Hemicrania continua
Sex (M:F)	2–5:1	M≈F	1.5:1	1:2
Pain severity	++++	++++	+++/++++	++/+++
Attack duration	15–180 minutes	2–30 minutes	1–600 seconds	Months to years
Typical attack frequency/day	1–8	>5	3–200	Continuous with exacerbations
Alcohol as trigger	++++	+	–	+
Cutaneous triggers	–	–	++	–
Agitation/restlessness in attack	++++	+++	++	++/+++
Autonomic features	++++	++++	++++	+++
Migrainous symptoms (photo/phonophobia, nausea)	+++	+++	+	+++
Indomethacin responsiveness	–	Required for diagnosis	–	Required for diagnosis

TRIGEMINAL AUTONOMIC CEPHALALGIAS (Continued)

stimulation, and deep brain stimulation appear useful as rescue options.

SUNCT AND SUNA

SUNCT and SUNA are very rare TACs characterized by extremely brief episodic, unilateral severe head pain in in orbital, periorbital, or temporal regions accompanied by cranial autonomic features.

There are three distinct patterns of pain: (1) *single stabs* with a mean duration of about 1 minute (range, 1–600 seconds); (2) *a series of stabs* with a mean attack duration of approximately 400 seconds, that is, 6 to 7 minutes (range, 10–1200 seconds); and (3) *Saw-tooth* attacks of persistent pain with multiple superimposed stabs and a mean attack duration of 1200 seconds, that is, 20 minutes (range, 5–12,000 seconds).

SUNCT and SUNA attacks can be episodic with spontaneous remissions lasting 3 months or longer, or chronic with long symptomatic periods without spontaneous remission. Although attacks are often spontaneous, a wide array of attack triggers occur, including touching the face or scalp, coughing, blowing the nose, exercise, and exposure to light. Given the overlap of symptoms with trigeminal neuralgia, evaluation with MRI for trigeminovascular compression is recommended.

Prophylactic medication is the mainstay of treatment. Lamotrigine, topiramate, and gabapentin are probably the most helpful, although a variety of other agents are useful in a few patients. Rapid treatment with lidocaine may be helpful with severe acute episodes of pain. Occipital nerve blockade with a local anesthetic and a corticosteroid are helpful in some individuals.

PAROXYSMAL HEMICRANIA

PH is a rare TAC distinguished by unilateral, short-lived attacks of intense pain associated with cranial autonomic features that repeat many times daily, with an average of approximately 10 to 12 per day. Pain is typically localized to the trigeminal nerve's first division and usually lasts 15 to 20 minutes. Usually the pain is described as "torturous" and is often characterized as boring, burning, sharp, stabbing, throbbing, or shooting. Approximately 20% of patients have episodic PH, diagnosed when remissions last 3 months or longer; the remaining patients have chronic PH, in which a remission does not occur within 1 year.

Although the majority of PH attacks occur spontaneously, approximately 10% may be triggered mechanically, typically by flexing or by rotating the head. Attacks are sometimes elicited by external pressure over the greater occipital nerve, C2 root, or the transverse processes of C4–C5. Alcohol ingestion provokes attacks in approximately 20% of patients.

An absolute unequivocal response to a therapeutic dose of indomethacin is the primary diagnostic criterion for PH. This remains the gold standard for PH treatment. Both cyclooxygenase-2 (COX-2) selective inhibitors (e.g., celecoxib) and topiramate are effective in some patients. Greater occipital nerve block with

Paroxysmal hemicrania

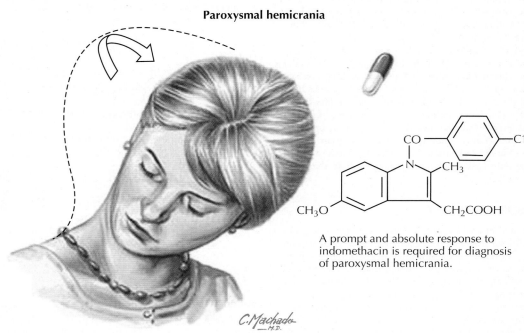

A prompt and absolute response to indomethacin is required for diagnosis of paroxysmal hemicrania.

The typical patient has symptoms that resemble cluster headache, including unilateral headache with cranial autonomic symptoms such as lacrimation, nasal stuffiness, and rhinorrhea. The attacks are shorter in duration and more frequent.

Flexion and rotation of the neck is a trigger for a headache in about 20%.

local anesthetic and a corticosteroid are beneficial in some patients. Finally, in some patients there may be a role for neuromodulation, such as occipital nerve stimulation.

HEMICRANIA CONTINUA

HC is a relatively uncommon yet likely underdiagnosed form of chronic daily headache. It is typified by a continuous, one-sided headache that changes in severity, waxing and waning, yet not resolving entirely. Episodes of worsening are typically associated with ipsilateral cranial autonomic symptoms (conjunctival injection, lacrimation, nasal rhinorrhea) that are milder in severity

than those seen with the other TACs. The exacerbations may also be accompanied by migrainous symptoms, such as nausea, photophobia, and phonophobia. Because of the overlapping features, HC should be considered when evaluating a patient for chronic CH or chronic migraine (especially if the headache is always on the same side).

A diagnosis of this disorder also requires an absolute and marked response to indomethacin. HC sometimes responds well to other NSAIDs, including COX-2 inhibitors. Some patients are reported to have a favorable result with topiramate and occipital nerve blocks. There may also be a role for neuromodulation, such as occipital nerve stimulation in some patients.

Plate 13.8

Headache

TENSION-TYPE HEADACHE AND OTHER BENIGN EPISODIC AND CHRONIC HEADACHES

Tension-type headache (TTH), previously called tension headache, muscle contraction headache, and stress headache, is the most prevalent primary headache disorder and frequently occurs in migraine individuals. Typically TTH is a bilateral, mild-to-moderate severity, nonpulsatile headache not accompanied by nausea, vomiting, or photophobia. Individuals usually describe TTH pain as "pressure," "dull," "band-like," or "like a tight cap," and it is sometimes associated with muscle tenderness of the head, neck, or shoulders. These headaches may be triggered or exacerbated by stress and mental tension.

Chronic TTH (≥15 days monthly) is the most prevalent form of chronic daily headache. *Episodic TTH* usually lasts from 30 minutes to 7 days. It is subclassified into *infrequent episodic TTH* (<1 day monthly) and *frequent episodic TTH* (1–14 days monthly).

TTH pathophysiology is poorly delineated, possibly including peripheral and CNS mechanisms. The previous theory of sustained pericranial muscle contracture has not been substantiated.

Treatment involves two strategies: an acute/abortive agent during an attack and a prophylactic daily to decrease headache frequency and severity. Acetaminophen or NSAIDs are first-line acute treatment agents. Combination analgesics containing caffeine are sometimes more effective. Opiates and butalbital should be avoided given their propensity to lead to overuse and side effects, including the development of worsening headaches.

Prophylactic therapy is appropriate for frequent, disabling, long-lasting headaches. Tricyclic antidepressants are the principal agents used for TTH. Medications that act through serotonin and norepinephrine (mirtazapine and venlafaxine) may also be useful. Behavioral modification using cognitive-behavioral therapy, relaxation, or electromyographic (EMG) biofeedback may help some patients.

Hypnic headache ("alarm clock headache") occurs in older adults and is typified by dull pain stereotypically awakening them from sleep, often occurring nightly at a similar time as well as occasionally from daytime naps. These are unrelated to migraine or TACs. Controlled treatment trials are lacking. Anecdotal successful treatments include evening caffeine, lithium carbonate, or indomethacin.

Primary stabbing headache is typified by spontaneous, transient, single or multiple, variably localized stabs of pain lasting a few seconds, occurring from less than once to multiple times per day. These are often in the first division of the trigeminal nerve and are more frequent in individuals with migraine, sometimes superimposed on an acute migraine. Most patients do not need treatment, but individuals with frequent attacks may benefit from prophylactic indomethacin.

Primary cough headache has an abrupt onset triggered by coughing or straining, typically lasting from 1 second to 30 minutes. Although often benign, an intracranial abnormality, particularly a spinal cerebrospinal fluid (CSF) leak, Chiari malformation, or intracranial tumor, must be excluded with MRI. Prophylactic treatment with indomethacin is often effective; acetazolamide, propranolol, and other NSAIDs are effective in some patients.

Primary exertional headache occurs during or after physical exertion, typically building up over minutes. The pain is pulsatile, lasting minutes to more than a day. Intracranial structural abnormalities, including supratentorial and posterior fossa tumors, aneurysms, and vascular malformations may present with exertional

Tension headache

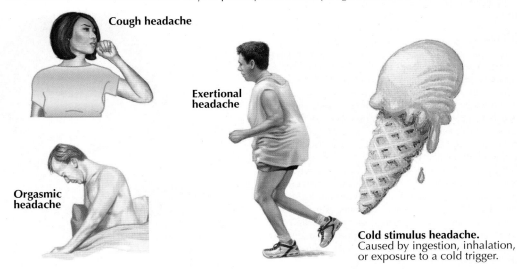

Intermittent, recurrent, or constant head pain, often in forehead, temples, or back of head and neck. Commonly described as "band-like," "tightness," or "vise-like."

Soreness of scalp; pain on combing hair

Occipital tension

Band-like constriction

Temporal tightness or pressure

Pressure on contracted muscle may augment pain

Neck muscle tightness

Hypnic headache or "alarm clock headache" typically wakes the older patient around the same time each night.

All variations of **Valsalva headache** may be primary or secondary (e.g., intracranial mass or CSF leak).

Cough headache

Exertional headache

Orgasmic headache

Cold stimulus headache. Caused by ingestion, inhalation, or exposure to a cold trigger.

headache. Brain MRI and MRA are indicated. Exertional headache may be a manifestation of cardiac ischemia; when suspected, an electrocardiogram and other cardiac testing should be performed. Treatment of recurrent exertional headache includes indomethacin an hour before activity. Other medications that may be helpful include propranolol and naproxen.

Primary headaches associated with sexual activity are of two types. *Preorgasmic headache* begins with mild head and neck aching during sexual activity, builds with sexual excitement, and is often associated with neck and jaw tightness. The average duration is 30 minutes, but it varies between minutes and a few hours. *Orgasmic*

headache is sudden and severe, generalized and explosive or pulsatile, and occurs with or just before orgasm. Primary orgasmic headache must be differentiated from serious causes of thunderclap headache. Recurrent primary orgasmic headaches may be treated with prophylactic indomethacin 1 hour before anticipated sexual activity or daily propranolol. Triptan medications may also be effective for acute treatment of primary orgasmic headache.

Cold-stimulus headache, colloquially called "ice-cream headache" or "brain freeze," is a generalized headache attributed to ingestion or inhalation of a cold stimulus or exposure of the unprotected head to a low environmental temperature.

Plate 13.9

Brain: PART I

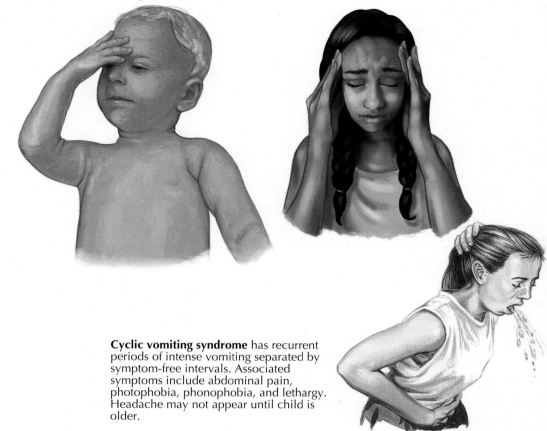

Benign paroxysmal vertigo of childhood

PEDIATRIC HEADACHE

Approximately 2% to 5% of preschool children and 10% of school-aged children will develop significant headaches, including migraine. Compared with adults, headaches in children tend to be shorter in duration and often have a bifrontal or bitemporal location. The typical visual aura of migraine may not be seen until after 9 years of age. Vomiting, abdominal pain, and motion sickness are frequent symptoms in children with migraine. The duration of these episodes may also be shorter in children, sometimes lasting 2 hours or less. The typical avoidance of light (photophobia), sound (phonophobia), and strong odors (osmophobia) is observed.

Commonly, children have episodic syndromes that develop early as precursors to migraine. These periodic syndromes include paroxysmal torticollis of infancy, benign paroxysmal vertigo of childhood, cyclic vomiting syndrome, and abdominal migraine.

Paroxysmal torticollis of infancy is an uncommon disorder characterized by repeated episodes of head tilting associated with nausea, vomiting, and headache. Attacks usually occur in infants and may last from minutes to days. Posterior fossa structural abnormalities must be considered in the differential diagnosis. These symptoms have been linked to mutations in the *CACNA1A* gene in some patients. Optimal treatment is unknown, but antimigraine preventatives are used when necessary.

Benign paroxysmal vertigo of childhood is a condition characterized by brief episodes of vertigo, disequilibrium, and nausea, usually found in children aged 2 to 6 years. The patient may have nystagmus within but not between the attacks, and hearing loss, tinnitus, and loss of consciousness do not occur. Symptoms usually last only a few minutes. A more common form of migraine tends to develop as children mature.

Cyclic vomiting syndrome is manifested by recurrent periods of intense vomiting separated by symptom-free intervals. Many patients with cyclic vomiting have regular or cyclic patterns of illness. Symptoms usually have a rapid onset at night or in the early morning and last 6 to 48 hours. Associated symptoms include abdominal pain, nausea, retching, anorexia, pallor, lethargy, photophobia, phonophobia, and headache. The headache may not appear until later childhood. Cyclic vomiting syndrome usually begins as a toddler and resolves in adolescence or early adulthood; it rarely begins in adulthood. More females than males are affected by cyclic vomiting, and a family history of migraine is often present. These children often experience severe fluid and electrolyte disturbances that require intravenous

Cyclic vomiting syndrome has recurrent periods of intense vomiting separated by symptom-free intervals. Associated symptoms include abdominal pain, photophobia, phonophobia, and lethargy. Headache may not appear until child is older.

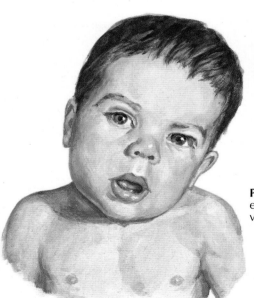

Benign paroxysmal vertigo of childhood occurs in young children and involves brief episodes of vertigo, disequilibrium, and nausea.

Paroxysmal torticollis of infancy involves recurrent episodes of head tilting associated with nausea, vomiting, and headache, lasting minutes to days.

fluid therapy. Some children with cyclic vomiting respond to antimigraine drugs such as amitriptyline or cyproheptadine. Migraine-associated cyclic vomiting syndrome is a diagnosis of exclusion. Other causes of cyclic vomiting include gastrointestinal disorders (malrotation), neoplasms, urinary tract disorders, and metabolic, endocrine, and mitochondrial disorders.

Abdominal migraine manifests as recurrent bouts of generalized abdominal pain with nausea and vomiting but often without headache. Episodes are often relieved by sleep, and later the child awakens feeling better. Abdominal migraine may alternate with typical migraine and can lead to typical migraine as the child matures. Episodes can be treated effectively with migraine prophylactic medication.

The presence of persistent neurologic deficits, papilledema, or seizures should raise concern for a different neurologic condition, requiring neuroimaging.

Plate 13.10

Headache

CRANIAL NEURALGIAS: TRIGEMINAL NEURALGIA

Cranial neuralgias are characterized by brief but intensely severe paroxysms of pain in the distribution of a specific cranial nerve. Any cranial nerve or nerve branch may cause this type of pain, but the trigeminal nerve is the most commonly affected.

Classic trigeminal neuralgia, also known as *tic douloureux,* presents as paroxysmal attacks of severe, sharp, or stabbing pain in the cutaneous distribution of one or more divisions of the trigeminal nerve. This pain usually starts in the second or third divisions, affecting the cheek, jaw lips, gums, or teeth. The first division is affected alone in fewer than 5% of patients. These attacks may last from a fraction of a second to 2 minutes, occur multiple times per day, and tend to be stereotypic in nature.

Attacks of pain are often provoked by sensory stimuli, such as light touch, cold air or cold liquid over the face or gums (especially in small supersensitive areas known as trigger zones), or movements such as talking, chewing, shaving, puckering lips, or brushing teeth. The paroxysm of pain may be followed by a refractory period where stimulation does not trigger pain. The pain is strictly unilateral. In the rare cases of bilateral trigeminal neuralgia, the episodic painful paroxysms are asynchronous and are independently triggered. Between attacks, the patient is usually pain free, although over time some patients notice a dull or burning continuous pain in the same area.

The temporal profile of trigeminal neuralgia may be fluctuating, with exacerbations and spontaneous remissions lasting weeks to months or even years. Patients with classic trigeminal neuralgia have a normal neurologic examination. The presence of a sensory deficit within the distribution of the trigeminal nerve suggests a trigeminal *neuropathy* and may indicate a secondary cause for the pain symptoms.

Although pathogenesis of trigeminal neuralgia is not completely understood, it is thought that the neuralgic pain is related to a chronic focal demyelination secondary to damage to the trigeminal nerve, usually within a few millimeters of where the nerve enters the pons, that is, the *root entry zone.* This damage is most often due to compression of the nerve by an aberrant loop of artery or vein. Rarely, this focal demyelination may also be caused by an aneurysm, arteriovenous malformation, or a neoplasm (i.e., trigeminal neuroma acoustic neuroma, epidermoid, or a meningioma). Demyelination from multiple sclerosis (MS) requires primary consideration in any young adult presenting with trigeminal neuralgia, which is especially suspect in patients presenting with bilateral symptoms. Contrast-enhanced MRI with special sequencing of the trigeminal nerve should be performed to assess the patient for possible demyelination, vascular loop compression, or mass lesion.

There are several therapeutic options for individuals with trigeminal neuralgia. Most patients respond to carbamazepine. Other medications that may be effective include gabapentin, baclofen, or oxcarbazepine.

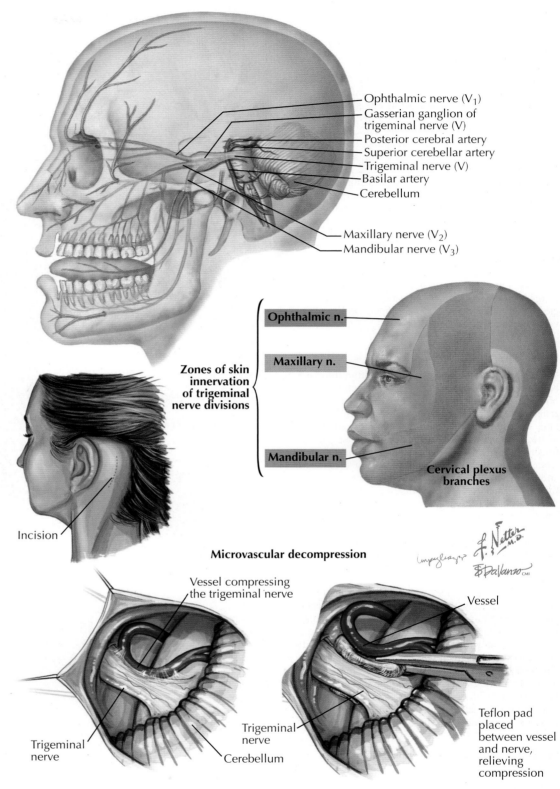

Ophthalmic nerve (V$_1$)
Gasserian ganglion of trigeminal nerve (V)
Posterior cerebral artery
Superior cerebellar artery
Trigeminal nerve (V)
Basilar artery
Cerebellum

Maxillary nerve (V$_2$)
Mandibular nerve (V$_3$)

Zones of skin innervation of trigeminal nerve divisions

Ophthalmic n.
Maxillary n.
Mandibular n.
Cervical plexus branches

Incision

Microvascular decompression

Vessel compressing the trigeminal nerve
Vessel
Trigeminal nerve
Trigeminal nerve
Cerebellum
Teflon pad placed between vessel and nerve, relieving compression

Patients who have not responded or have become intolerant to medical therapy are candidates for a variety of surgical procedures consisting of either *microvascular decompression* or *nerve ablation.* When treating the patient with open surgery, the aberrant vessel is separated from the nerve while a piece of surgical mesh is introduced between the aberrant vessel and the nerve. Surgical risks include damage to the nerve or surrounding structures, including damage to the auditory or facial nerves.

When an ablative procedure is used, the therapeutic goal is to precisely damage the trigeminal nerve so that it no longer transmits the pain signal well. These procedures include radiofrequency thermocoagulation, mechanical balloon compression, chemical (glycerol) injection, or gamma knife radiosurgery. Because the nerve is inherently damaged with these modalities, ablative procedures are accompanied by varying degrees of sensory loss. Unfortunately, trigeminal neuralgia has the potential to recur after any procedure and may require repeat intervention.

Plate 13.11

Brain: PART I

OTHER CRANIAL NEURALGIAS

GLOSSOPHARYNGEAL NEURALGIA

Glossopharyngeal neuralgia is estimated to be 70 times less common than trigeminal neuralgia. This is a severe, paroxysmal, lancinating pain within the glossopharyngeal nerve distribution, usually deep in the throat, at the back of the tongue, and/or in the ear. Characteristic triggers include swallowing, coughing, talking, and yawning. During these painful paroxysms, some patients may experience an associated bradycardia and/or asystole, which may result in syncope. Approximately 10% of patients will have concurrent trigeminal neuralgia.

MRI, with special attention to this nerve, is indicated to rule out secondary causes, including aberrant blood vessels, MS, or various mass lesions. Medical therapies are similar to those for trigeminal neuralgia. Spontaneous remissions also occur. Individuals with medically refractory neuralgia may require microvascular decompression or an ablative procedure, including a rhizotomy. In most cases, a rhizotomy with surgical division of the glossopharyngeal nerve and the upper rootlets of the vagus nerve provides relief.

OCCIPITAL NEURALGIA

This is a paroxysmal, lancinating pain within the distribution of the greater, lesser, and/or third occipital nerve, often starting at the upper neck or base of the skull and radiating to the back, side, or top of the scalp. The stabbing, electric shock–like pain may be provoked by head or neck movement or light touch of the scalp, such as brushing the hair. Neurologic examination may demonstrate local nerve tenderness and percussion (Tinel sign) and may elicit painful paroxysms or paresthesias along the affected nerve's cutaneous distribution.

The occipital nerve is derived from the second cervical (C2) root, and therefore pain from C2 will manifest in a similar distribution. Similarly, skull base and upper cervical joint pathology may refer pain to the upper neck and posterior head. A cranial and/or cervical spine MRI focusing on the craniocervical junction may be helpful in evaluation.

An occipital nerve block with local anesthetic (either alone or combined with steroid) is often the treatment of choice because this can be both therapeutically and diagnostically useful. After a block, the pain should ease temporarily, sometimes for weeks or months. Immediately after the block, pain relief may be accompanied by temporary diminished sensation within the occipital nerve distribution. Relief with an occipital block should be interpreted with caution because other primary headache syndromes, such as migraine and cluster, are also reported to respond to greater occipital nerve blockade.

LESS COMMON CRANIAL NEURALGIAS

Neuralgic-type pain may arise from any nerve or nerve branch within the head or neck. This includes other nerves derived from the cervical plexus, such as the great auricular nerve, as well as terminal branches of the trigeminal nerve such as supraorbital or infraorbital nerves. Neuralgia may develop spontaneously or after nerve trauma. The great auricular nerve, carrying lower ear and jawline sensation, may be damaged during parotidectomy, rhytidectomy (face-lift), or carotid endarterectomy.

It is important to inquire about *neuropathic* in contrast to *neuralgic* symptoms. Persistent pain or sensory dysfunction—that is, paresthesias, hypoesthesia, or allodynia—suggests neuropathy with underlying nerve damage. If an MRI image is normal, evaluation for connective tissue disease and other inflammatory etiologies should be undertaken.

Two other situations deserve special mention. Persistent unilateral facial pain may rarely be the presenting symptom of lung cancer and is speculated to be due to referred pain from compression or invasion of the vagus nerve. Lung malignancy must be suspected in patients with a smoking history who report new unilateral facial pain or when weight loss or persistent cough is present. A chest radiograph or CT scan of the chest may be diagnostic.

Isolated mental or inferior alveolar nerve neuropathies occur in patients with various metastatic cancers, including hematologic malignancies and lung, breast, prostate, and kidney cancers. Patients present with numbness of the chin, lower lip, or the gingiva of the lower teeth, with or without associated pain. This "numb chin syndrome" is usually the consequence of bone metastases or leptomeningeal seeding, but it may manifest without obvious cause.

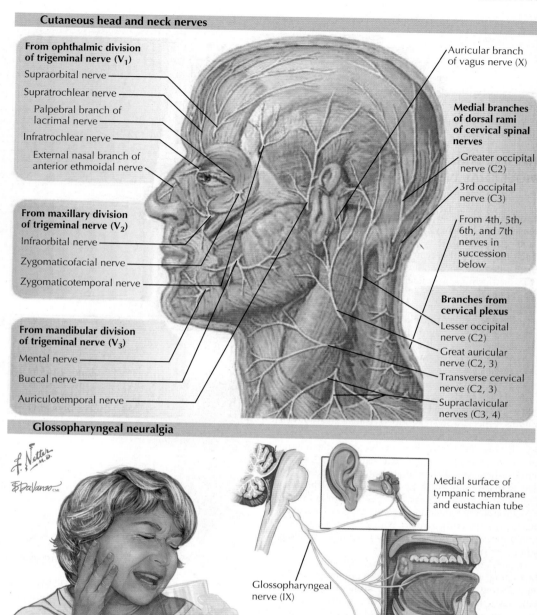

Cutaneous head and neck nerves

From ophthalmic division of trigeminal nerve (V₁)
- Supraorbital nerve
- Supratrochlear nerve
- Palpebral branch of lacrimal nerve
- Infratrochlear nerve
- External nasal branch of anterior ethmoidal nerve

From maxillary division of trigeminal nerve (V₂)
- Infraorbital nerve
- Zygomaticofacial nerve
- Zygomaticotemporal nerve

From mandibular division of trigeminal nerve (V₃)
- Mental nerve
- Buccal nerve
- Auriculotemporal nerve

Auricular branch of vagus nerve (X)

Medial branches of dorsal rami of cervical spinal nerves
- Greater occipital nerve (C2)
- 3rd occipital nerve (C3)
- From 4th, 5th, 6th, and 7th nerves in succession below

Branches from cervical plexus
- Lesser occipital nerve (C2)
- Great auricular nerve (C2, 3)
- Transverse cervical nerve (C2, 3)
- Supraclavicular nerves (C3, 4)

Glossopharyngeal neuralgia

Medial surface of tympanic membrane and eustachian tube

Glossopharyngeal nerve (IX)

Posterior third of tongue, posterior pharynx, tonsils, carotid body, and carotid sinus

Glossopharyngeal neuralgia can cause severe stabbing pain in the throat, back of tongue, tonsils, neck, or deep in the ear on one side. Pain lasts seconds to minutes and may occur spontaneously or be triggered by maneuvers such as swallowing, talking, coughing, or clearing the throat. Some patients may have severe bradycardia or asystole with episodes of pain.

Plate 13.12

Headache

IDIOPATHIC INTRACRANIAL HYPERTENSION

Idiopathic intracranial hypertension (IIH), previously called *pseudotumor cerebri*, is a disorder of elevated intracranial pressure of unknown cause. It most often occurs in obese females of childbearing age, and its incidence has increased in conjunction with rising obesity rates. Patients commonly describe daily severe headaches, often present on awakening, that worsen with cough or strain. Papilledema is a diagnostic hallmark and may be associated with blurred vision, enlarged blind spots, or visual field defects. Additional symptoms include transient visual obscurations (blurring or loss of vision lasting seconds) or photopsia (brief sparkles or flashes of light) in one or both eyes, often provoked by positional changes and Valsalva maneuver. Horizontal diplopia due to unilateral or bilateral sixth nerve palsies may be present. Pulse-synchronous tinnitus, described as a "whooshing sound" like pulsating running water or wind, is common and is thought to represent vascular pulsations transmitted by turbulent CSF in the venous sinuses.

Diagnostic criteria include demonstrating elevated intracranial pressure by lumbar puncture, with an opening pressure greater than 250 mm H_2O. Lumbar puncture should be performed in the lateral decubitus position with legs extended and the patient relaxed. Falsely elevated pressures may occur in a sitting or prone position, with coughing or other Valsalva maneuvers, or with anxiety. CSF composition must be normal. MRI generally shows signs of increased pressure, including dilated optic nerve sheaths, empty sella turcica, enlarged Meckel's caves, or cerebellar tonsillar descent. Diagnosis may require examination by an ophthalmologist because early or mild papilledema can be difficult to detect. Dilated funduscopic exam also helps differentiate true papilledema from pseudopapilledema secondary to optic disc drusen, tilted optic discs, or other mimickers. Images of the optic disc can be used for serial monitoring. Formal visual perimetry should be performed. The most common finding is an enlarged blind spot; arcuate defects, inferonasal visual loss, or generalized visual field constriction may also be seen.

As IIH is idiopathic by definition, secondary causes of intracranial hypertension must be excluded: (1) mass lesions (i.e., intracranial tumor or abscess), (2) decreased CSF absorption via arachnoid granulations (e.g., adhesions after meningitis or subarachnoid hemorrhage [SAH]), (3) increased CSF production (e.g., choroid plexus papilloma), and (4) venous outflow obstruction (e.g., cerebral venous sinus thrombosis). Because venous sinus thrombosis may mimic IIH, imaging of cerebral veins with magnetic resonance venography is indicated along with the routine MRI. Transverse venous sinus stenosis without thrombosis is more common. Of note, intracranial hypertension can also occur with various metabolic, toxic, and hormonal disturbances, including imbalances in growth hormone, thyroid hormone, androgens, or aldosterone. Medications have been implicated, such as tetracycline, vitamin A, lithium, amiodarone, and corticosteroids (especially on withdrawal).

Permanent visual loss is the major morbidity associated with IIH, and management strategies depend on the degree and progression of papilledema. Serial images of the optic disc and serial testing of visual fields help guide treatment. The therapeutic goals are symptomatic relief

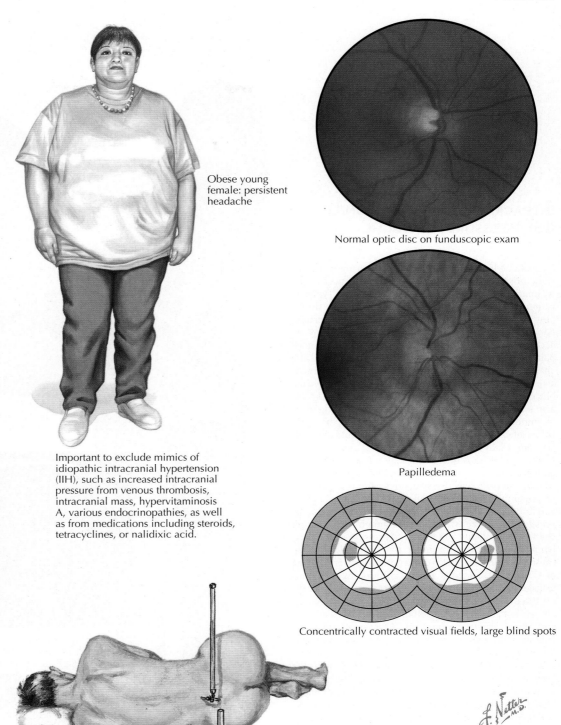

Obese young female: persistent headache

Important to exclude mimics of idiopathic intracranial hypertension (IIH), such as increased intracranial pressure from venous thrombosis, intracranial mass, hypervitaminosis A, various endocrinopathies, as well as from medications including steroids, tetracyclines, or nalidixic acid.

Cerebrospinal fluid pressure elevated

Normal optic disc on funduscopic exam

Papilledema

Concentrically contracted visual fields, large blind spots

by analgesia and reduction of CSF pressure. Weight reduction is very important in the management of overweight patients with IIH. If the patient has no visual loss and mild to moderate headache, weight loss and pain management may be all that is necessary. Medications that exacerbate intracranial hypertension should be discontinued.

Acetazolamide is the most commonly used medical therapy for IIH. It is a carbonic anhydrase inhibitor and is thought to influence intracranial hypertension by inhibiting choroid plexus CSF secretion. It also may

decrease appetite, leading to weight loss. Topiramate has similar effects and may also be used.

Patients with visual loss require urgent treatment with serial lumbar punctures or a short course of corticosteroids to rapidly decrease intracranial pressure. Medically intractable IIH can be treated with surgical procedures, including optic nerve sheath fenestration, venous sinus stenting, CSF shunting, or in select cases, bariatric surgery. Surgery is primarily indicated for visual loss or worsening vision due to papilledema and is not typically performed for isolated headache.

Plate 13.13

Brain: PART I

Headache is orthostatic, worse in an upright position; often aggravated by exertion, bending over, or Valsalva maneuver

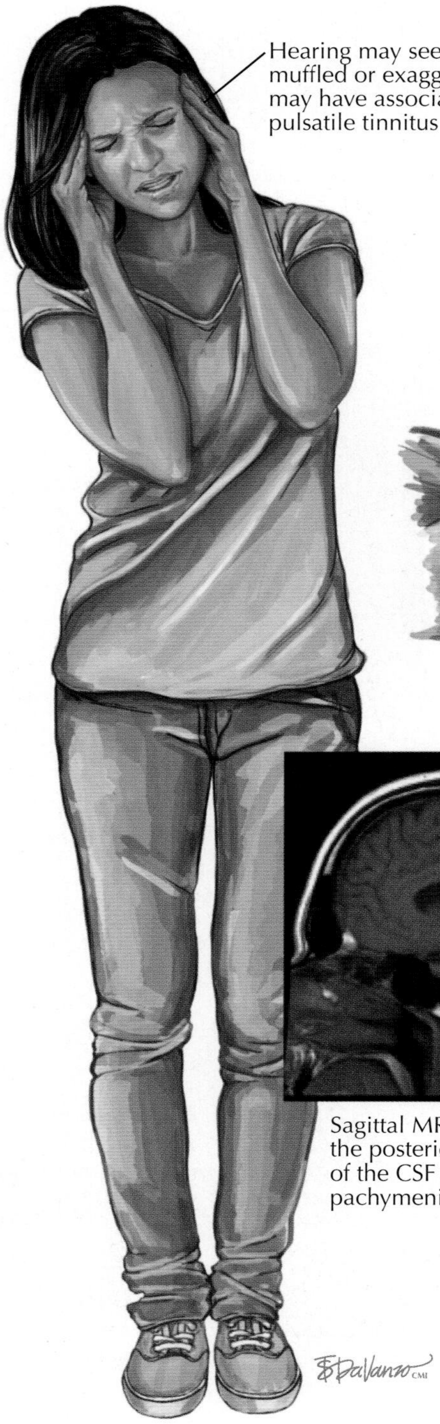

Hearing may seem muffled or exaggerated; may have associated pulsatile tinnitus

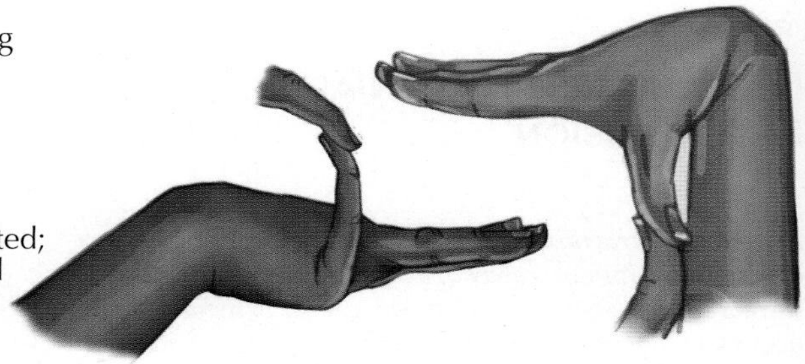

Joint hypermobility may be present

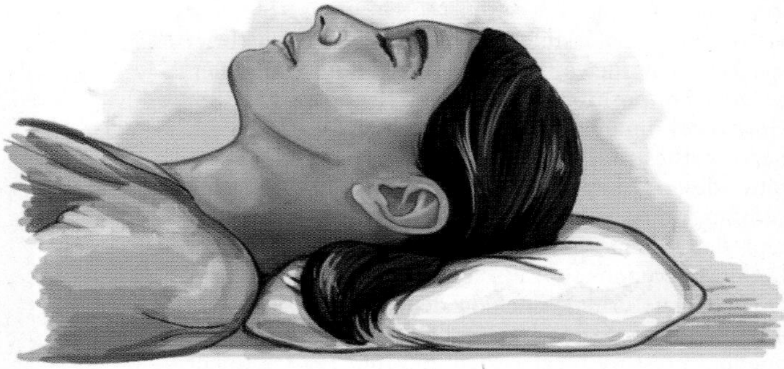

Head pain dramatically improves in a recumbent position (this pattern may be lost over time)

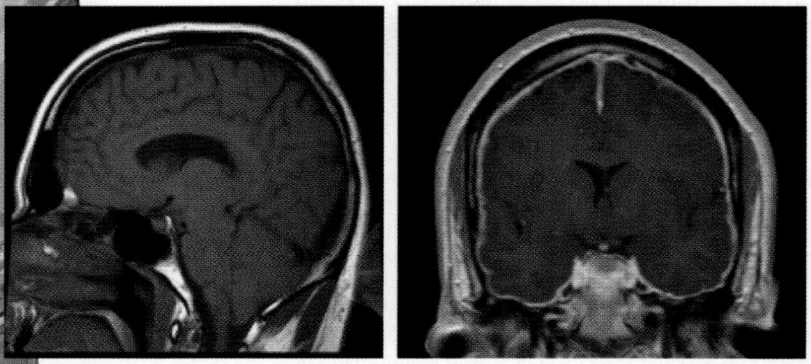

Intracranial Hypotension/Low CSF Pressure Headache

Orthostatic headache, a headache occurring in an upright position and relieved with recumbence, is the hallmark of a low CSF pressure headache. Typically posterior and bilateral, these headaches may be throbbing or constant and are often aggravated by exertion, bending over, or Valsalva maneuvers. They may be accompanied by a variety of symptoms, including neck pain or stiffness, nausea, photophobia, and hearing changes (e.g., "muffled hearing," tinnitus, or hyperacusis). Other reported features include dizziness, visual blurring, diplopia (from sixth nerve palsy), radicular arm symptoms, and, rarely, symptoms mimicking frontotemporal dementia. The headaches may be daily (often late in the day) or intermittent. An acute thunderclap onset may mimic SAH.

The syndrome is due to low CSF volume. When the patient is upright, the loss of brain buoyancy causes traction on pain-sensitive structures, with brain descent or "sagging." Symptoms localizing to the cranial nerves and brainstem are thought to be due to traction or compression of these structures, although the hearing changes may relate to alteration of pressure in the perilymphatic system of the inner ear. CSF leaks may be caused by prior lumbar or dural puncture, overshunting of CSF, or spontaneous spinal CSF leak. Spontaneous leakage can occur because of tears of nerve root sleeve diverticula, dural rents caused by disk osteophyte complexes, and aberrant connections between the thecal sac and spinal epidural veins (i.e., CSF-venous fistulas). Patients with joint hypermobility and connective tissue disorders may be predisposed to CSF leaks. Postural headaches and brain sag result from CSF leakage at the level of the spine. In contrast, intracranial leaks through skull base defects tend to present with clear drainage from the nose (CSF rhinorrhea) or ear (CSF otorrhea).

Patients with an orthostatic headache should be evaluated with a brain MRI with contrast, looking for diffuse pachymeningeal enhancement, descent of the cerebellar tonsils (mimicking a Chiari I malformation), crowding of the posterior fossa, descent of the optic chiasm, pituitary enlargement, engorgement of cerebral venous sinuses, and other signs of brain sag. A normal brain MRI does not rule out low CSF pressure headache and occurs in about 20% of cases. If the clinical history is suggestive, other testing may be useful to identify the presence of a CSF leak. Radioisotope cisternography involves injecting a radionuclide into the CSF and monitoring how fast it ascends and diffuses around the brain. A CSF leak can be demonstrated directly by radiotracer accumulation in the extraarachnoid space, or indirectly by a delay in radiotracer ascent to the cerebral convexities or early appearance in the bladder. Lumbar puncture is not necessary for the diagnosis, as

Sagittal MRI (*left*) shows descent of the cerebellar tonsils, crowding of the posterior fossa, enlargement of the pituitary gland, and obliteration of the CSF spaces. Coronal MRI with gadolinium (*right*) shows diffuse pachymeningeal enhancement.

opening pressure is normal in more than half of cases. When performed, it may show a normal to low (<60 mm H_2O) opening pressure and normal to high CSF protein. Mild pleocytosis (white blood cell count 10–50) may also occur. Superficial siderosis may be associated with a spinal CSF leak, in which case CSF analysis generally shows red blood cells or xanthochromia. The presence of a meningeal diverticulum in the spine does not guarantee that it is the site of CSF leak. Dynamic computed tomography (CT) myelography and digital subtraction

myelography are the most widely used techniques to localize CSF leaks.

Headaches due to low CSF pressure may be self-limited or recalcitrant. Conservative measures such as bed rest, caffeine, and increased fluid intake are advocated as first-line treatments. A persistent headache may require an epidural blood patch. If the site of the leak is known, the blood patch can be targeted toward this site. When more conservative measures fail, surgical intervention or transvenous embolization may be considered.

Plate 13.14

Headache

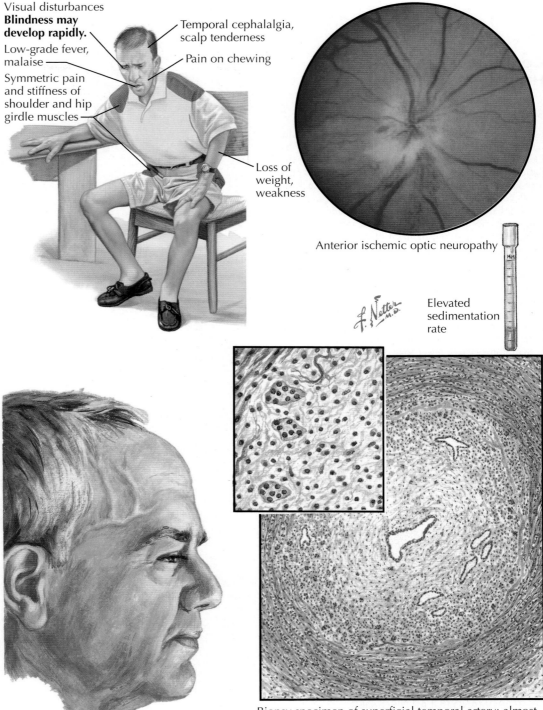

Visual disturbances
Blindness may develop rapidly.

Low-grade fever, malaise

Symmetric pain and stiffness of shoulder and hip girdle muscles

Temporal cephalalgia, scalp tenderness

Pain on chewing

Loss of weight, weakness

Anterior ischemic optic neuropathy

Elevated sedimentation rate

Rigid, tender, nonpulsating temporal arteries may be visible or palpable.

Biopsy specimen of superficial temporal artery: almost total obliteration of the lumen with some recanalization. *High-power inset* shows infiltration with lymphocytes, plasma cells, and giant cells as well as fragmentation of the internal elastic lamina.

GIANT CELL ARTERITIS

Giant cell arteritis (GCA), also known as temporal arteritis, is a generalized vasculitis affecting large- and medium-sized vessels. This arteritis involves the aorta and its extracranial branches, including the external carotid artery with its superior temporal division and, less commonly, the occipital scalp artery. Unlike other forms of vasculitis, GCA rarely involves the skin, kidneys, or lungs.

Signs and symptoms of GCA may begin quite abruptly or gradually develop over several months before becoming clinically recognizable. Its classic symptoms relate to the inflammation of, and reduced blood flow through, the involved arteries. Most patients present with bilateral headache, often complaining of scalp pain with normally nonnoxious stimuli, such as brushing the hair. Transient or permanent vision loss may result from involvement of the posterior ciliary, ophthalmic, or retinal arteries. Painful cramping or claudication often occurs with the use of the jaw while chewing or moving the tongue. Many patients have associated systemic symptoms, such as fever, malaise, sweating, and weight loss. Examination may reveal the temporal and occipital vessels to be firm, tender, and pulseless. Sausage-shaped thickenings or nodularity may be palpable along the vessel walls.

The incidence of GCA increases with advancing age, peaking in the seventh decade, and must be considered in all patients older than 50 years who develop a new headache, have a change in their previous headache characteristics, or have acute-onset transient visual loss. Polymyalgia rheumatica (PMR) is an overlapping disease, and symptoms of PMR are found in up to half of patients with GCA. PMR symptoms include neck pain, morning stiffness, and myalgias in shoulder and hip girdle muscles.

Erythrocyte sedimentation rate (ESR) and C-reactive protein (CRP) are nonspecific markers of inflammation that, when elevated—often to very high levels (60–120 mm/hr for ESR and >40 mg/L for CRP)—are supportive of the diagnosis of GCA. Sedimentation rate is reported to be normal in about 5% of patients with GCA. Normochromic anemia, low albumin, and thrombocytosis are often present.

Diagnosis can only be established with certainty by biopsy of the temporal artery and demonstration of focal inflammation, giant cells, and interruption of the internal elastic lamina. Of importance, none of the testing options has a sensitivity of 100%. Because vessel involvement can be segmental, the biopsy may be falsely negative. If the biopsy is negative but the clinical suspicion remains high, such as in an elderly patient with a new headache and jaw claudication or systemic symptoms, other tests should be performed, looking for signs of vessel inflammation. These would include another site for artery biopsy (such as the contralateral temporal artery or posterior occipital scalp artery), MRA, duplex ultrasonography, or a PET scan.

When unrecognized and untreated, GCA can lead to a variety of complications. The most devastating is sudden permanent unilateral or sequential bilateral vision loss from anterior ischemic optic neuropathy or retinal artery occlusion. Other complications include cerebrovascular ischemia, especially in the vertebrobasilar system, and myocardial infarction. Involvement of the aorta may rarely lead to aortic dissection or aneurysm. Prompt treatment with corticosteroids is required to prevent permanent sequelae, especially visual loss. Headache and systemic symptoms usually improve within 48 hours of starting treatment, but vision loss and other ischemic complications are often irreversible. Biopsy should be obtained as soon as possible but must not delay the initiation of steroids.

Plate 13.15

Brain: PART I

CONTIGUOUS STRUCTURE HEADACHES

SINUS HEADACHE

Most patients presenting with "sinus headache" actually have migraine. Misdiagnosis may arise based on the location of pain and is further complicated if the patient's migraine is triggered by weather changes or is associated with parasympathetic symptoms, such as nasal congestion, lacrimation, or rhinorrhea. When sinus inflammation is the source of headache, it is almost always accompanied by facial tenderness and pain, nasal congestion, or nasal discharge. Inflammation of the sinuses is called *sinusitis*, or *rhinosinusitis* when the nasal passages are also affected.

Patients perceive *maxillary sinus* pain in the cheek, gums, and upper teeth. *Frontal sinus* pain tends to involve the forehead. *Ethmoid sinusitis* causes pain behind or between the eyes. *Sphenoid sinusitis* is characterized by pain in variable locations, including the frontal, occipital, temporal, or vertex locations.

Symptoms lasting fewer than 7 days tend to be viral in origin. In contrast, acute bacterial rhinosinusitis presents with more than 7 days of purulent rhinorrhea, nasal congestion, facial or dental pain/pressure, cough, halitosis, and, if severe, fever (50% of adults). Fungal sinusitis may be acute or chronic (lasting >12 weeks) and is of particular concern in patients who are immunocompromised. Rhinosinusitis can usually be diagnosed on clinical suspicion. Diagnosing recurrent, chronic, or complicated disease depends on CT, MRI, or direct visualization with nasal endoscopy. Treatment involves the appropriate antibacterial or antifungal medications.

Sphenoid sinusitis is an uncommon infection that may manifest as acute or subacute headache associated with nausea and vomiting. It may accompany pansinusitis but, when isolated, may not have associated nasal symptoms. It can mimic many other causes of headache, including aseptic meningitis, migraine, and trigeminal neuralgia. Excessive tearing, photophobia, and paresthesias in the trigeminal nerve distribution may accompany sphenoid rhinosinusitis. This should be considered in patients with a severe, intractable new-onset headache that worsens with coughing, bending, or walking; interferes with sleep; is progressive in severity; and does not respond well to analgesics.

TEMPOROMANDIBULAR DISORDER

Pain from the *temporomandibular joint* (TMJ), with its associated musculature and ligaments, can be referred to the head. The manifesting symptom is usually pain in the preauricular area, TMJ, or muscles of mastication, aggravated by jaw motion. Associated ipsilateral ear pain is common. Patients may have TMJ noise (such as clicking or crepitus), locking on jaw opening, or limited or asymmetric jaw movement. Diagnosis is confirmed by CT of the maxilla and mandible, including open and closed position views of bilateral TMJs, and panoramic radiographs looking for bony pathology. Initial treatment is conservative, with an oral appliance or bite plate and physical therapy. Medication such as NSAIDs, muscle relaxants, and tricyclic antidepressants can also be used. Rarely, surgery is indicated for patients with medically refractory temporomandibular disorder.

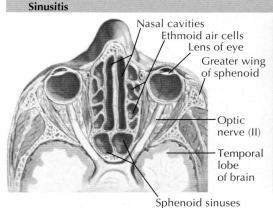

Sinusitis

Nasal cavities
Ethmoid air cells
Lens of eye
Greater wing of sphenoid
Optic nerve (II)
Temporal lobe of brain
Sphenoid sinuses

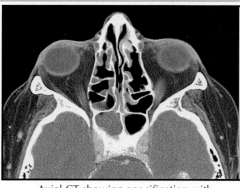

Axial CT showing opacification with fluid of the right sphenoid sinus

Temporomandibular disorder

Jaw closed
Articular tubercle
Mandibular fossa
Articular disk
Joint capsule

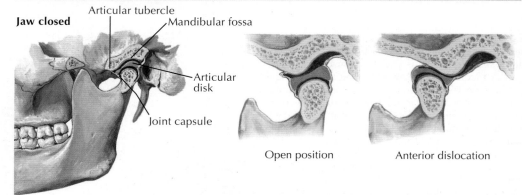

Open position

Anterior dislocation

Dental disease

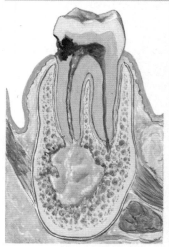

Dentoalveolar abscess

Glaucoma: primary closed angle

Consensual response preserved

Inflamed eye with nonreactive, mid-dilated pupil typical of acute attack

Pupillary block
Secondary block in angle
Primary block at pupil
Central anterior chamber shallow

Plateau iris
Primary block in angle
Central anterior chamber normal

Angle closure may result from primary pupillary block with bulging iris or from less common plateau iris (primary occlusion at periphery of iris).

DENTAL

Inflammatory dental disease may cause intense, throbbing, poorly localized unilateral pain that is generally provoked by stimulation of the offending tooth. This is often associated with increased sensitivity to hot and cold. Occasionally, infection of the dental pulp or apical root may cause neuralgic-type pain in the second and third trigeminal divisions, which is difficult to distinguish clinically from trigeminal neuralgia. For this reason, patients with trigeminal neuralgia may undergo one or more unnecessary dental procedures before the correct diagnosis is made. Conversely, it is important to exclude dental disease before making a diagnosis of trigeminal neuralgia.

GLAUCOMA

Acute angle-closure glaucoma occurs when the normal drainage of aqueous humor is blocked, leading to sudden increased intraocular pressure. This creates severe eye pain sometimes associated with a unilateral headache, nausea, vomiting, conjunctival injection, and a mid-dilated nonreactive pupil. Patients may describe intermittent visual blurring and seeing halos around objects. The severe unilateral headache may mimic migraine or CH. Dim light and certain medications (e.g., anticholinergics, sympathomimetics) that result in pupillary dilation may precipitate the pain. Chronic open-angle glaucoma, the more common form of glaucoma, is not a cause of headaches.

Plate 13.16

Headache

THUNDERCLAP HEADACHE AND OTHER HEADACHE PRESENTING IN THE EMERGENCY DEPARTMENT

Most patients who seek care in an emergency department have a primary headache disorder. Nevertheless, an emergency medicine physician must evaluate for the possibility of an underlying, secondary cause for the pain. New headaches beginning during vigorous exertion or after head or neck trauma require consideration of an intracranial hemorrhage or cervicocephalic arterial dissection. Most concerning are those patients presenting with an *explosive, debilitating,* or *"thunderclap" headache* often referred to as the "worst headache of my life" or "I felt like I was hit with a sledgehammer." Because of the urgency of diagnosis, every individual experiencing these symptoms must initially be investigated for a subarachnoid or intracranial hemorrhage. If hemorrhage is ruled out, other pathologic mechanisms for an acute severe headache require consideration (Plate 13.16).

Urgent evaluation is also needed for acute headache associated with neurologic symptoms, particularly focal motor or sensory loss, language dysfunction, or encephalopathic symptomatology such as confusion or seizures. Other features warranting further and immediate evaluation include older age, immunocompromised state, recent infection or fever, history of cancer, clotting or bleeding disorders (particularly including therapeutic anticoagulation), progressively worsening headache severity, or symptoms of systemic illness (weight loss, fatigue, myalgia, or unexplained anemia).

Any patient whose clinical presentation with headache includes fever, alteration in consciousness or mentation, or an overall toxic appearance requires an urgent evaluation for a possible underlying infection. Nuchal rigidity usually indicates meningeal irritation, which can be seen with either SAH or meningitis. Papilledema reflects increased intracranial pressure and warrants further investigation for disorders causing mass effect, such as tumor, infection, hemorrhage, or IIH.

SUBARACHNOID AND INTRAPARENCHYMAL HEMORRHAGE

Although the classic thunderclap presentation typically heralding the rupture of an intracerebral aneurysm with SAH is not easily overlooked, patients with SAH occasionally may present with more subtle symptoms. Any headache that is *unusual for the patient,* especially if there is associated neck pain or stiffness, raises the question of possible SAH. Intraparenchymal hemorrhage is more likely to cause relatively rapid evolution of focal neurologic symptoms as well as seizures and altered mentation, depending on the size and location of the hematoma. If the blood tracks into the CSF, intraparenchymal hemorrhage may also cause meningeal irritation and neck stiffness. A history of anticoagulation, especially in an older patient presenting with headache, is particularly concerning for hemorrhage. A CT scan is diagnostic. Information on evaluation and management of intracranial hemorrhage is detailed in Section 9.

REVERSIBLE CEREBRAL VASOCONSTRICTION SYNDROME

Reversible cerebral vasoconstriction syndrome is characterized by recurrent thunderclap headaches. Pain peaks within minutes, lasts minutes to hours, sometimes more than 1 day, and tends to recur over a few days to 2 weeks.

CAUSES OF THUNDERCLAP HEADACHE

	Headache	Typical Presentation	Diagnosis/Testing
Secondary	Subarachnoid hemorrhage	Sudden and severe HA ± N/V; may have ophthalmoplegia or altered mentation	CT without contrast; LP for xanthochromia
	Intracranial hemorrhage	Sudden and severe HA; focal neurologic signs; seizures; altered mentation	CT without contrast
	Cerebral venous sinus thrombosis	May mimic idiopathic intracranial hypertension	Examine for papilledema; MRV; CT with contrast for empty delta sign
	Arterial dissection	Sudden unilateral HA ± neck pain; may be posttraumatic; may mimic migraine	Examine for Horner sign; MRI/MRA head and neck (CTA or carotid ultrasound if MRI not available)
	Reversible cerebral vasoconstriction syndrome	Recurrent thunderclap HA; photophobia or nausea possible	Cerebral angiogram is the gold standard: however, can start with MRA or CTA
	Ischemic stroke	New neurologic deficits, in specific vascular distribution	MRI with DWI: large or subacute/chronic; may show on CT
	Pituitary apoplexy	HA; visual changes ± altered mentation	CT or MRI (MRI more sensitive)
	Third ventricular colloid cyst with hydrocephalus	Recurrent severe HA, sometimes relieved with recumbency	CT with contrast or MRI
	Spontaneous intracranial hypotension	Postural HA, worse upright ± symptoms of low CSF pressure	MRI with gadolinium; in some cases cisternogram, CT myelogram occasionally
	Posterior reversible leukoencephalopathy (PRES)	HA with vision changes, seizures, or altered mentation; marked hypertension on occasion	CT or MRI (MRI more sensitive)
	Intracranial infection (e.g., bacterial meningitis)	Fever, chills, meningismus, leukocytosis	Lumbar puncture for CSF, glucose, protein, and cells; MRI may show meningeal enhancement; CT before lumbar puncture if concern for mass effect
	Glaucoma	Ipsilateral HA with slowly responsive mid-dilated pupil	Ophthalmology consult
Primary	Primary sexual or exertional HA	Sudden onset before, during, or right after orgasm or peak of exertion	Diagnosis of exclusion especially if this is the first episode; consider MRI/MRA to rule out aneurysm with SAH
	Primary cough HA	Sudden onset with cough or strain, 1 second to 30 minutes in duration	Diagnosis of exclusion
	Primary thunderclap HA	Max intensity in <1 minute; lasts 1 hour to 10 days	Diagnosis of exclusion

CTA, Computed tomographic angiography; *DWI,* diffusion-weighted imaging; *HA,* headache; *LP,* lumbar puncture; *N/V,* nausea/vomiting; *SAH,* subarachnoid hemorrhage

Patients may have associated focal neurologic deficits, and one-third of patients experience seizures. Risk factors include hypertension, preeclampsia/eclampsia (i.e., postpartum angiopathy), sympathomimetic drugs or serotonergic agents (drug-induced cerebral vasculopathy), catecholamine-secreting tumors (i.e., pheochromocytoma), cannabis use, and binge alcohol drinking.

CSF is normal or near normal (mild elevations in protein or white blood cells). MRI and CT may be normal, may show features similar to PRES, or may show evidence of intracranial hemorrhage, especially cortical SAH. The diagnostic gold standard is conventional angiography demonstrating multifocal segmental vasoconstriction

subsequently reversible within 12 weeks after onset. However, MRA and CT angiography are less invasive and may provide supporting diagnostic evidence. Although there is no evidence-based study to support a specific therapy, nimodipine is the treatment most often recommended for the vasospasm.

ACUTE HYPERTENSIVE CRISIS/POSTERIOR REVERSIBLE ENCEPHALOPATHY SYNDROME

Patients with *hypertensive crisis* may present with acute or subacute posterior headaches sometimes accompanied by dyspnea, chest pain, lightheadedness, focal

Plate 13.17

Brain: PART I

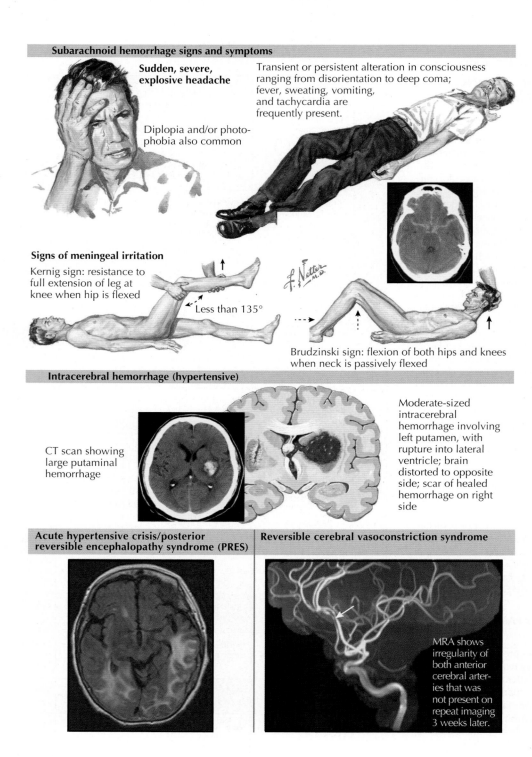

Subarachnoid hemorrhage signs and symptoms

Sudden, severe, explosive headache

Transient or persistent alteration in consciousness ranging from disorientation to deep coma; fever, sweating, vomiting, and tachycardia are frequently present.

Diplopia and/or photophobia also common

Signs of meningeal irritation

Kernig sign: resistance to full extension of leg at knee when hip is flexed

Less than 135°

Brudzinski sign: flexion of both hips and knees when neck is passively flexed

Intracerebral hemorrhage (hypertensive)

CT scan showing large putaminal hemorrhage

Moderate-sized intracerebral hemorrhage involving left putamen, with rupture into lateral ventricle; brain distorted to opposite side; scar of healed hemorrhage on right side

Acute hypertensive crisis/posterior reversible encephalopathy syndrome (PRES)

Reversible cerebral vasoconstriction syndrome

MRA shows irregularity of both anterior cerebral arteries that was not present on repeat imaging 3 weeks later.

THUNDERCLAP HEADACHE AND OTHER HEADACHE PRESENTING IN THE EMERGENCY DEPARTMENT (Continued)

neurologic deficits, and epistaxis. Markedly elevated blood pressure (generally >180/120 mm Hg) may be associated with hypertensive encephalopathy or malignant hypertension with retinal hemorrhages/exudates, papilledema, intracranial hemorrhage, or other organ damage, including pulmonary edema or malignant nephrosclerosis. The cause for the hypertension needs to be identified. Immediate commencement of rapidly acting antihypertensive therapies is the primary treatment;

general symptom management is also needed for dyspnea and chest pain, if present.

PRES is a syndrome involving vasogenic edema preferentially affecting the white matter of the posterior brain, including the occipital lobes and cerebellum. On MRI, the vasogenic edema appears as a relatively symmetric increased T2 signal not conforming to a particular vascular distribution. Patients present with headache that may be accompanied by seizures, visual changes, and altered mentation. This syndrome may be associated with hypertensive encephalopathy, preeclampsia/eclampsia, and certain cytotoxic and immunosuppressant drugs.

CEREBRAL VENOUS THROMBOSIS

Cerebral venous thrombosis most often has a subacute presentation; however, a minority of patients present

with thunderclap headache. Headaches are persistent and tend to be worse in the morning, in a recumbent position, and with Valsalva maneuvers, such as coughing or straining. Headaches may be accompanied by other signs of increased intracranial pressure, such as papilledema, seizures, and altered mentation. If venous infarction occurs, focal neurologic deficits may be present. If the venous thrombosis is in the superior sagittal sinus, a CT scan with contrast may show a filling defect around the thrombus, called the "empty delta" sign. However, CT and MRI may be unremarkable, requiring MR venography for diagnosis. When diagnosis is established, causative or predisposing conditions need to be identified, including thrombophilic states or occult malignancy. Patients are generally treated with anticoagulation.

Plate 13.18

Headache

Cerebral venous sinus thrombosis

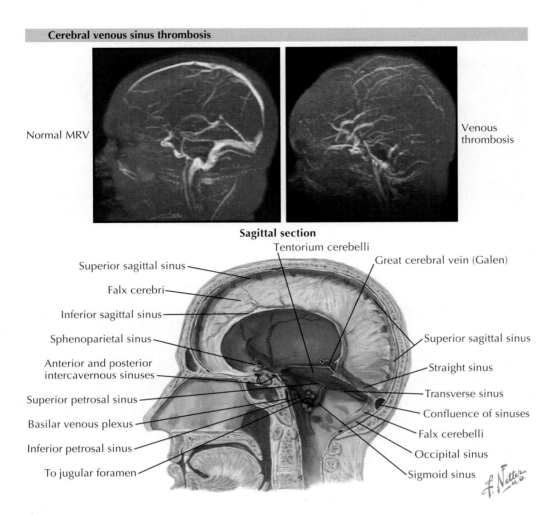

Normal MRV

Venous
thrombosis

Sagittal section

Tentorium cerebelli

Superior sagittal sinus

Great cerebral vein (Galen)

Falx cerebri

Inferior sagittal sinus

Sphenoparietal sinus

Anterior and posterior
intercavernous sinuses

Superior sagittal sinus

Superior petrosal sinus

Straight sinus

Basilar venous plexus

Transverse sinus

Inferior petrosal sinus

Confluence of sinuses

Falx cerebelli

To jugular foramen

Occipital sinus

Sigmoid sinus

Pituitary apoplexy

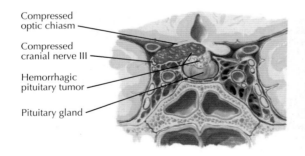

Compressed
optic chiasm

Compressed
cranial nerve III

Hemorrhagic
pituitary tumor

Pituitary gland

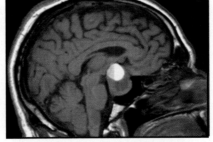

MRI showing pituitary tumor apoplexy. Sagittal
image shows fluid-fluid level within the area of
recent hemorrhage.

THUNDERCLAP HEADACHE AND OTHER HEADACHE PRESENTING IN THE EMERGENCY DEPARTMENT (Continued)

PITUITARY APOPLEXY

Acute pituitary apoplexy is an uncommon syndrome due to hemorrhage or infarction of the pituitary gland in the setting of a pituitary macroadenoma. Patients may present with a sudden and severe headache, ophthalmoplegia, visual disturbance, nausea/vomiting, altered mentation, meningismus, and sometimes fever. In the emergency department this may mimic a severe migraine or aseptic meningitis, and in severe cases it may cause adrenal crisis, coma, or death. Although pituitary pathology is usually noted on a noncontrast CT head scan, MRI is more sensitive.

COLLOID CYST

A colloid cyst is a benign cyst that arises in the anterior third ventricle just posterior to the foramen of Monro. Because of its location, it can act as a ball valve transiently obstructing the ventricular outflow and causing obstructive hydrocephalus. Patients may present with intermittent symptoms of increased intracranial pressure, including sudden and severe headache with nausea/vomiting; these symptoms often improve in a recumbent position. If obstructive hydrocephalus is prolonged, deterioration with altered mentation, seizures, coma, and death may occur. Diagnosis is made by CT or MRI, and early surgical intervention is necessary for symptomatic colloid cysts.

POSTTRAUMATIC HEADACHE

Most headaches after trauma mimic migraine or TTH. However, a history of trauma should alert the physician to the possibility of hemorrhage, especially in the setting of anticoagulation. This includes subarachnoid and intraparenchymal hemorrhage as mentioned above, as well as subdural or epidural hematoma (see Sections 9 and 14). Subdural hematomas may manifest

Plate 13.19

Brain: PART I

Colloid cyst

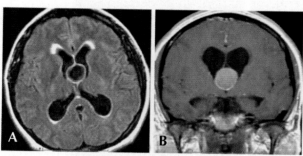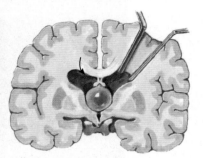

Colloid cyst. (**A**) Axial FLAIR and (**B**) coronal, T1-weighted gadolinium-enhanced images demonstrate a round cystic mass in the region of the foramina of Monro, with dilation of the lateral ventricles. The signal characteristics are variable. This cyst is hypointense on T2-weighted images and bright on T1-weighted imaging, with minimal peripheral enhancement.

Colloid cyst of 3rd ventricle and surgical approach via right prefrontal (silent) cerebral cortex

Bacterial meningitis

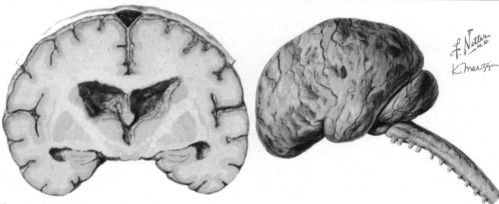

Thrombophlebitis of superior sagittal sinus and suppurative ependymitis, with beginning hydrocephalus

Inflammation and suppurative process on surface of leptomeninges of brain and spinal cord

Arterial dissection

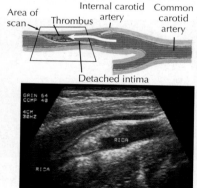

Area of scan   Thrombus   Internal carotid artery   Common carotid artery

Detached intima

Intimal tear allows blood flow to dissect beneath intimal layer, detaching it from arterial wall. Large dissection may occlude vessel lumen.

Carotid dissection. Ultrasound of the carotid artery with clot formed between layers of the artery (near the upper right internal carotid artery [RICA]).

THUNDERCLAP HEADACHE AND OTHER HEADACHE PRESENTING IN THE EMERGENCY DEPARTMENT (Continued)

insidiously with headache, decreased level of consciousness, balance or gait difficulty, cognitive impairment or memory loss, or focal neurologic deficits.

Carotid or vertebral arterial dissection may also occur after trauma. These often manifest as a unilateral headache, with or without neck pain, and may be associated with focal neurologic signs, such as Horner syndrome (ptosis and miosis unilaterally).

Local injury to neck structures, including cervical vertebra or disks, can create a referred headache with associated neck pain. Head trauma may be followed by the development of a postconcussive syndrome, and headaches may be accompanied by dizziness, fatigue, irritability, anxiety, insomnia, and decreased concentration.

INTRACRANIAL INFECTION

Meningitis or meningoencephalitis must be suspected in any patient with new headache accompanied by neck stiffness or fever, nausea/vomiting, and photophobia, sometimes mimicking a severe migraine. In addition to a lumbar puncture, blood cultures are drawn and antibiotics started empirically when bacterial meningitis is suspected. Patients with focal neurologic findings, papilledema, or altered mentation must have a CT or MRI before lumbar puncture to exclude a brain abscess with associated mass effect. In a patient with a new headache associated with altered mentation or seizure, rapid initiation of acyclovir is recommended to cover for herpes simplex virus while results of diagnostic testing are pending. Diagnosis and evaluation of intracranial infection are outlined in Section 11.

HEAD TRAUMA

Plate 14.1

Brain: PART I

SKULL: ANTERIOR VIEW

Frontal bone
Glabella
Supraorbital notch (foramen)
Orbital surface
Nasal bone
Lacrimal bone
Zygomatic bone
Frontal process
Orbital surface
Temporal process
Zygomaticofacial foramen
Maxilla
Zygomatic process
Orbital surface
Infraorbital foramen
Frontal process
Alveolar process
Anterior nasal spine

Coronal suture
Parietal bone
Nasion
Sphenoidal bone
Lesser wing
Greater wing
Temporal bone
Ethmoidal bone
Orbital plate
Perpendicular plate
Middle nasal concha
Inferior nasal concha
Vomer
Mandible
Ramus
Body
Mental foramen
Mental tubercle
Mental protuberance

SKULL: ANTERIOR AND LATERAL ASPECTS

The anterior, or facial, aspect of the skull is composed of the frontal part of the calvaria (skullcap) above and the facial bones below. The facial contours and proportions show considerable variations associated with age, sex, and ethnicity. The outer surface of the frontal bone underlies the brow. The facial skeleton is irregular, a feature accentuated by the presence of the orbital openings, the piriform aperture, and the superior and inferior dental arches of the oral cavity.

The convex anterior surface of the frontal bone is relatively smooth, but there are frontal tuberosities, or elevations, on each side. In early life, a median suture separates the two halves of the developing bone. This suture normally fuses between ages 6 and 10 years but occasionally persists as the metopic suture. The two *orbital openings* are roughly quadrangular and have supraorbital, infraorbital, medial, and lateral borders. The supraorbital notch, or fissure, carries the corresponding nerve and vessels. The infraorbital foramen, located about 1 cm below the infraorbital margin, transmits the nerve and vessels of the same name. The orbits are somewhat pyramidal in shape, with the quadrangular openings, or bases, directed forward and slightly outward, whereas the apexes correspond to the medial ends of the superior orbital fissures.

The *superior wall (roof)* separates the orbital contents from the brain and meninges in the anterior cranial fossa. Anteromedially, it is hollowed out by a variably sized frontal sinus, and anterolaterally, there is a shallow lacrimal fossa for the orbital part of the lacrimal gland. Posteriorly, the optic canal (foramen) lies between the two roots of the lesser wing of the sphenoid bone, just above the medial end of the superior orbital fissure; it transmits the optic (II) nerve and ophthalmic artery.

The *inferior wall (floor)* is formed mainly by the orbital surface of the maxilla, which separates the orbit from the maxillary sinus (antrum). A groove for the infraorbital nerve and vessels ends in the infraorbital foramen.

The thin *medial wall* separates the orbit from the ethmoidal air cells, the anterior part of the sphenoidal sinus, and the nasal cavity. At its anterior end, the lacrimal fossa is continuous below with the short nasolacrimal canal that opens into the inferior nasal meatus. The thicker *lateral wall* separates the orbit from the temporal fossa anteriorly and from the middle cranial fossa posteriorly. The orbital surface of the zygomatic bone shows a foramen for the zygomatic nerve, which bifurcates within the bone to emerge on the cheek and temporal

Right orbit: frontal and slightly lateral view

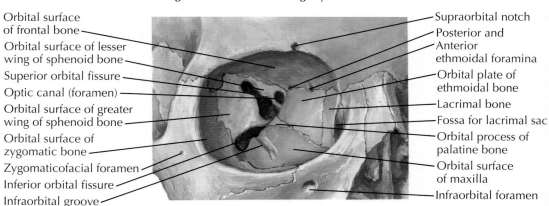

Orbital surface of frontal bone
Orbital surface of lesser wing of sphenoid bone
Superior orbital fissure
Optic canal (foramen)
Orbital surface of greater wing of sphenoid bone
Orbital surface of zygomatic bone
Zygomaticofacial foramen
Inferior orbital fissure
Infraorbital groove

Supraorbital notch
Posterior and Anterior ethmoidal foramina
Orbital plate of ethmoidal bone
Lacrimal bone
Fossa for lacrimal sac
Orbital process of palatine bone
Orbital surface of maxilla
Infraorbital foramen

fossa as the zygomaticofacial and zygomaticotemporal nerves, respectively.

The lateral wall and roof are continuous anteriorly but diverge posteriorly to bound the *superior orbital fissure,* which lies between the greater and lesser wings of the sphenoid bone and opens into the middle cranial fossa. The fissure transmits the oculomotor (III) and trochlear (IV) nerves; the lacrimal, frontal, and nasociliary branches of the ophthalmic nerve; the abducens

(VI) nerve; the ophthalmic veins; and small meningeal vessels.

The lateral wall and floor of the orbit are also continuous anteriorly but are separated posteriorly by the *inferior orbital fissure,* most of which is located between the greater wing of the sphenoid bone and the orbital surface of the maxilla. The inferior orbital fissure connects the orbit with the pterygopalatine and infratemporal fossae. The maxillary nerve passes from the pterygopalatine

Plate 14.2

Head Trauma

SKULL: ANTERIOR AND LATERAL ASPECTS (Continued)

fossa into the orbit through the inferior orbital fissure and continues forward as the infraorbital nerve. Anastomotic channels between the orbital and pterygoid venous plexuses, and orbital fascicles from the pterygopalatine ganglion, also traverse this fissure.

The *anterior nasal (piriform) aperture* is bounded by the nasal and maxillary bones. The nasal bones articulate with each other in the midline, with the frontal bone above and with the frontal processes of the maxillae behind. The irregular lower borders of the nasal bones give attachment to the lateral nasal cartilages.

The *lower face* is supported by both the maxillary alveolar processes and the mandible. The inferior margin of each *maxilla* projects downward as the curved alveolar process, which unites in front with its fellow to form the U-shaped alveolar arch containing the sockets for the upper teeth. The roots of the teeth produce slight surface elevations, the most obvious of which are produced by the canine teeth. The upper border of the body of the *mandible* is called the alveolar part and contains sockets for the lower teeth, whose roots also produce slight surface elevations.

Viewed from the side, the skull is divided into the larger ovoid braincase and the smaller facial skeleton. The two are connected by the zygomatic bone, which acts as a yoke (zygon) between the temporal, sphenoid (greater wing) and frontal bones, and the maxilla. Other features on the lateral aspect of the skull include parts of the sutures between the frontal, parietal, sphenoid, and temporal bones (which form most of the braincase), and the sutures between such facial bones as the nasal, lacrimal, ethmoid, and maxilla. Clearly seen are the parts of the mandible and the temporomandibular joint, the external acoustic meatus, and the various foramina that transmit nerves and vessels of the same name. Not readily visible are the foramen ovale (trigeminal nerve) and the foramen spinosum (middle meningeal artery).

Certain features deserve particular mention. The curved *superior* and *inferior temporal lines* arch upward and backward over the frontal bone from the vicinity of the frontozygomatic suture, pass over the coronal suture and the parietal bone, and then turn downward and forward across the temporal squama to end above the mastoid process. The superior and inferior temporal lines provide attachments, respectively, for the temporal fascia and the upper margin of the temporal muscle, which occupies most of the *temporal fossa*. This fossa is bounded above by the superior temporal line and below

by the infratemporal crest, separating the greater wing of the sphenoid bone from the pterygoid processes. The anteroinferior corner of the parietal bone usually fills the angle between the greater wing of the sphenoid and the frontal bone, although sometimes the squamous part of the temporal bone may extend forward to articulate directly with the frontal bone, thus excluding the sphenoid. This area is the *pterion,* and its internal surface is deeply grooved by the anterior branches of the middle meningeal vessels. It is situated about 3.5 cm behind the frontozygomatic suture (usually palpable as

a slight ridge) and 4 cm above the zygomatic arch. It is the most common site of damage to these vessels from a skull fracture.

The *infratemporal fossa* is an irregular space lying below the infratemporal crest. It is continuous above with the temporal fossa through the gap between the crest and the zygomatic arch. It is bounded medially by the lateral plate of the pterygoid process and the infratemporal surface of the maxilla and laterally by the ramus of the mandible. It communicates through the pterygomaxillary fissure with the pterygopalatine fossa.

SKULL: LATERAL VIEW

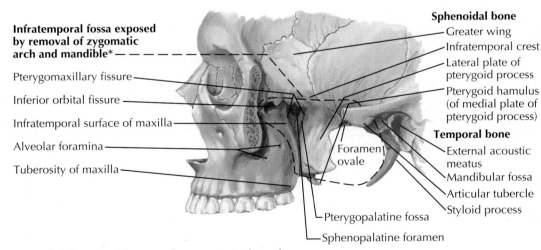

*Superficially, mastoid process forms posterior boundary.

Plate 14.3

Brain: PART I

SKULL: MIDSAGITTAL SECTION

The rigid braincase is formed by the bones of the calvaria (see Plate 14.4) and the base of the skull (see Plate 14.5), which is divided into anterior, middle, and posterior cranial fossae (see Plates 14.6 and 14.7). These divisions are less visible on a sagittal section of the skull.

The *occipital bone* bounds most of the posterior cranial fossa. It is pierced by the foramen magnum, through which the medulla oblongata and spinal cord, surrounded by their meninges, become continuous; it also transmits the vertebral arteries, a few small veins, the spinal roots of the accessory (XI) nerves, and the recurrent meningeal branches from the upper spinal nerves. The occipital condyle articulates with the homolateral superior atlanto-articular process. The hypoglossal (XII) nerve passes through the corresponding canal. The jugular foramen lodges the superior bulb of the internal jugular vein (in which the sigmoid and inferior petrosal sinuses end); the glossopharyngeal (IX), vagus (X), and accessory nerves pass through it anteromedial to the bulb, and it provides an entry for the recurrent meningeal branches of the vagus and small meningeal branches of the ascending pharyngeal and occipital arteries. The basilar part of the occipital bone unites with the body of the sphenoid to form a sloping platform anterior to the medulla oblongata.

The squamous part of the *temporal bone* is grooved by the posterior branches of the middle meningeal vessels, and the sulcus along the superior border of its petrous part is for the superior petrosal sinus. The inferior petrosal sinus lies in the sulcus between the petrous temporal and occipital bones. The internal acoustic meatus is a canal about 1 cm long, ending in a cribriform septum that separates it from the internal ear. It transmits the facial (VII) nerve and its nervus intermedius, the vestibulocochlear (VIII) nerve, and the internal auditory (labyrinthine) artery.

The *sphenoid bone* has a central body from which two greater and two lesser wings and two pterygoid processes arise. The body contains two air sinuses separated by a septum that is often incomplete. Its concave upper surface, the sella turcica, houses the pituitary gland. The optic canal transmits the optic (II) nerve and the ophthalmic artery.

The *nasal cavity* is roofed over mainly by the cribriform plate of the ethmoid bone, augmented anteriorly by small parts of the frontal and nasal bones, and posteriorly, by the anteroinferior surface of the sphenoidal body. Its floor is formed by the palatine processes of the maxillae and by the horizontal plates of the palatine bones. The *incisive canal* transmits the nasopalatine nerves and branches of the greater palatine arteries. Each lateral wall is formed above by the nasal surface of the ethmoid bone that covers the ethmoidal labyrinth and supports thin, shell-like projections, the *superior* and *middle nasal conchae*. These overhang the corresponding nasal meatuses. Below, each lateral wall is formed by the nasal surface of the maxilla, the perpendicular plate of the palatine bone, and the medial pterygoid plate. The maxillary and palatine bones articulate with a separate bone, the *inferior nasal concha*, overhanging the inferior nasal meatus. The sphenoidal air sinuses open into the nose through the *sphenoidal aperture* in the sphenoethmoidal recess posterosuperior to the superior concha. The frontal and maxillary air sinuses open into the middle meatus through a *semilunar hiatus*, and the multiple air cells forming the ethmoidal labyrinth open into the superior and middle meatuses. The lower opening of the *nasolacrimal duct* is near the anterior end of the inferior meatus. The *sphenopalatine foramen* behind the middle concha transmits the nasopalatine nerve.

The nasal cavity is subdivided by a more or less vertical *septum* formed by the perpendicular ethmoidal plate and the vomer. The triangular gap between them anteriorly is filled in by the nasal *septal cartilage* (not shown in the illustration).

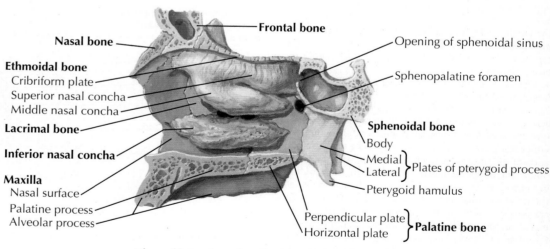

View of lateral nasal wall with nasal septum removed

Plate 14.4

Head Trauma

Superior view

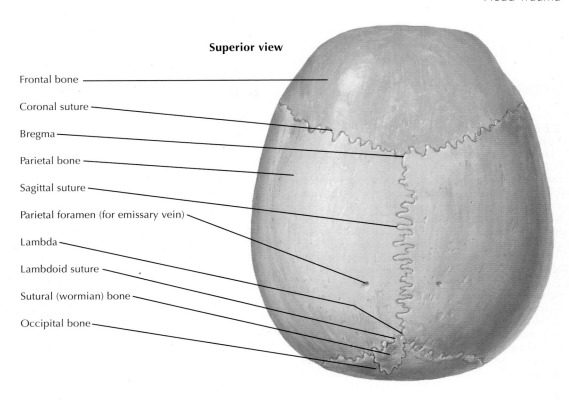

Frontal bone

Coronal suture

Bregma

Parietal bone

Sagittal suture

Parietal foramen (for emissary vein)

Lambda

Lambdoid suture

Sutural (wormian) bone

Occipital bone

Inferior view

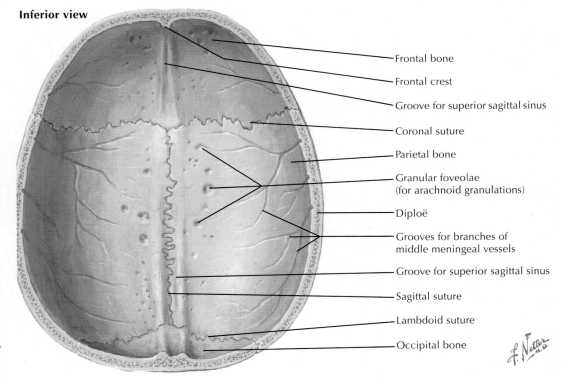

Frontal bone

Frontal crest

Groove for superior sagittal sinus

Coronal suture

Parietal bone

Granular foveolae
(for arachnoid granulations)

Diploë

Grooves for branches of
middle meningeal vessels

Groove for superior sagittal sinus

Sagittal suture

Lambdoid suture

Occipital bone

CALVARIA

The *calvaria,* or skullcap, is the roof of the cranium and is formed by the frontal, parietal, and occipital bones. It is ovoid in shape and widest toward the posterior parts of the parietal bones, but there are individual variations in size and shape associated with age, race, and sex; thus minor degrees of asymmetry are common.

The anterior part, or brow, is formed by the frontal bone, which extends backward to the *coronal suture* between the frontal bone and the parietal bones. The latter bones curve upward and inward to meet at the midline *sagittal suture.* Posteriorly, the parietal bones articulate with the triangular upper part of the occipital squama along the *lambdoid suture.* The meeting points of the sagittal suture with the coronal and lambdoid sutures are termed, respectively, *bregma* and *lambda.* In the fetal skull, they are the sites of the anterior and posterior fontanelles. The *vertex,* or highest point, of the skull lies near the middle of the sagittal suture. Parietal foramina are usually present; they transmit emissary veins passing between the superior sagittal sinus and the veins of the scalp.

The deeply concave internal, or endocranial, surface of the calvaria is made up of the inner aspects of the bones, sutures, and foramina mentioned above. The bones show indistinct impressions produced by related cerebral gyri, more evident grooves for dural venous sinuses and meningeal vessels, and small pits, or *foveolae,* for arachnoid granulations. Thus there is a median groove in the frontal, parietal, and occipital bones extending backward from the frontal crest to the internal occipital protuberance; it increases in width posteriorly

and lodges the *superior sagittal sinus.* The frontal crest seen in the midline is produced by the coalescence of the anterior ends of the lips of the groove for the superior sagittal sinus. There are other, narrower grooves for meningeal vessels. The largest of these, the *middle meningeal arteries and veins,* leave their imprints in particular on the parietal bones, and the channels containing them may become tunnels where the anteroinferior angles of the parietal bones meet the greater wings of the sphenoid bone. The skull varies in thickness, and

the area around the pterion is thin. It is relatively easily fractured by a blow to the side of the head, with possible tearing of the middle meningeal vessels. The resulting hemorrhage can be serious if it is not recognized and treated promptly.

The cut edge of the skullcap reveals that the constituent bones possess outer and inner laminae of compact bone separated by the *diploë,* a layer of cancellous bone. The outer lamina is thicker and tougher than the more brittle inner lamina.

Plate 14.5

Brain: PART I

EXTERNAL ASPECT OF SKULL BASE

The inferior surface of the base of the skull, the *norma basilaris*, is formed anteriorly by the arched hard palate, fringed by the maxillary alveolar processes and teeth; posteriorly by the wider occipital squama, pierced by the foramen magnum; and, in between, by an irregular area comprising several bony processes for muscular and tendinous attachments, articular and other fossae, and many foramina. The bones and fissures shown in Plate 14.5 need no added description, but the nerves and vessels traversing the foramina will be listed.

The *incisive foramen* transmits the terminal branches of the nasopalatine nerves and greater palatine vessels. The *major* and *minor palatine foramina* are traversed by the corresponding arteries and nerves. The *choanae* are the posterior nasal apertures.

The *foramen ovale* pierces the greater sphenoidal wing near the lateral pterygoid plate and the sulcus for the auditory tube; the mandibular nerve, the accessory meningeal artery, and communications between the cavernous sinuses and pterygoid venous plexus pass through it. The *foramen spinosum,* anteromedial to the sphenoidal spine, transmits the middle meningeal artery and the meningeal branch of the mandibular nerve.

The *foramen lacerum* is an irregular canal between the sphenoidal body, the apex of the petrous part of the temporal bone, and the basilar part of the occipital bone. The upper end of the carotid canal opens into it, and the internal carotid artery, with its nerves and veins, on emerging from the canal, turns upward to enter the cavernous sinus. Meningeal branches of the ascending pharyngeal artery and emissary veins from the cavernous sinus pass through the foramen lacerum, and the deep and greater petrosal nerves unite within it to form the nerve of the pterygoid canal.

The anterior part of the *mandibular fossa* articulates with the mandibular head and belongs to the temporal squama, but the posterior nonarticular part is derived from the tympanic plate. The *tympanosquamous fissure* between them is continued medially as the *petrotympanic fissure*, through which the chorda tympani nerve emerges. The *stylomastoid foramen* behind the root of the styloid process transmits the facial (VII) nerve and the stylomastoid branch of the posterior auricular artery.

The lower opening of the *carotid canal* is anterior to the *jugular fossa*, which lodges the superior bulb of the internal jugular vein. The canal bends at right angles within the petrous part of the temporal bone, and its upper end opens into the foramen lacerum. The *tympanic canaliculus* pierces the ridge between the carotid canal and the jugular fossa and conveys the tympanic branch of the glossopharyngeal (IX) nerve to the tympanic plexus. The *mastoid canaliculus* opens on the lateral wall of the fossa and transmits the auricular branch of the vagus (X) nerve. The *jugular foramen* in the depth of the fossa may be partly or completely divided into three parts by bony spicules. The anteromedial compartment transmits the inferior petrosal sinus and a meningeal branch of the ascending pharyngeal artery; the intermediate part transmits the glossopharyngeal, vagus, and accessory (XI) nerves; and the posterolateral part conveys the sigmoid sinus to the superior bulb of the internal jugular vein. Often seen near the posterior border of the mastoid process is a *mastoid foramen,* which is

Maxilla
Incisive fossa
Palatine process
Intermaxillary suture
Zygomatic process

Zygomatic bone

Frontal bone

Sphenoid bone
Pterygoid process
Hamulus
Medial plate
Pterygoid fossa
Lateral plate
Scaphoid fossa
Greater wing
Foramen ovale
Foramen spinosum
Spine

Temporal bone
Zygomatic process
Articular tubercle
Mandibular fossa
Styloid process
Petrotympanic fissure
Carotid canal
(external opening)
Tympanic canaliculus
External acoustic meatus
Mastoid process
Mastoid canaliculus
Stylomastoid foramen
Petrous part
Mastoid notch (for
digastric muscle)
Occipital groove
(for occipital artery)
Jugular fossa (jugular
foramen in its depth)
Mastoid foramen

Parietal bone

Occipital bone
Hypoglossal canal
Occipital condyle
Condylar canal and fossa
Basilar part
Pharyngeal tubercle
Foramen magnum
Inferior nuchal line
External occipital crest
Superior nuchal line
External occipital protuberance

Palatomaxillary suture

Palatine bone
Horizontal plate
Greater palatine
foramen
Pyramidal process
Lesser palatine
foramina
Posterior nasal spine

Choanae

Vomer
Ala

Groove for auditory
(pharyngotympanic,
eustachian) tube

Foramen lacerum

traversed by an emissary vein from the sigmoid sinus and a meningeal twig from the occipital artery. The anterior end of the *hypoglossal canal* (for the hypoglossal [XII] nerve and some small meningeal vessels) is above the anterior end of the occipital condyle. Behind the condyle is a shallow condylar fossa, usually pierced by a *condylar foramen* conveying an emissary vein between the sigmoid sinus and cervical veins.

The posterior part of the base of the skull is formed predominantly by the occipital squama; these are marked by nuchal lines, occipital crest, and so forth, which serve mainly for muscular and ligamentous attachments. However, the most notable feature is the *foramen magnum*, through which the medulla oblongata and spinal cord become continuous. The vertebral arteries, spinal roots of the accessory nerves, and recurrent meningeal branches from the upper cervical nerves ascend through the foramen magnum, whereas the anterior and posterior spinal arteries descend through it.

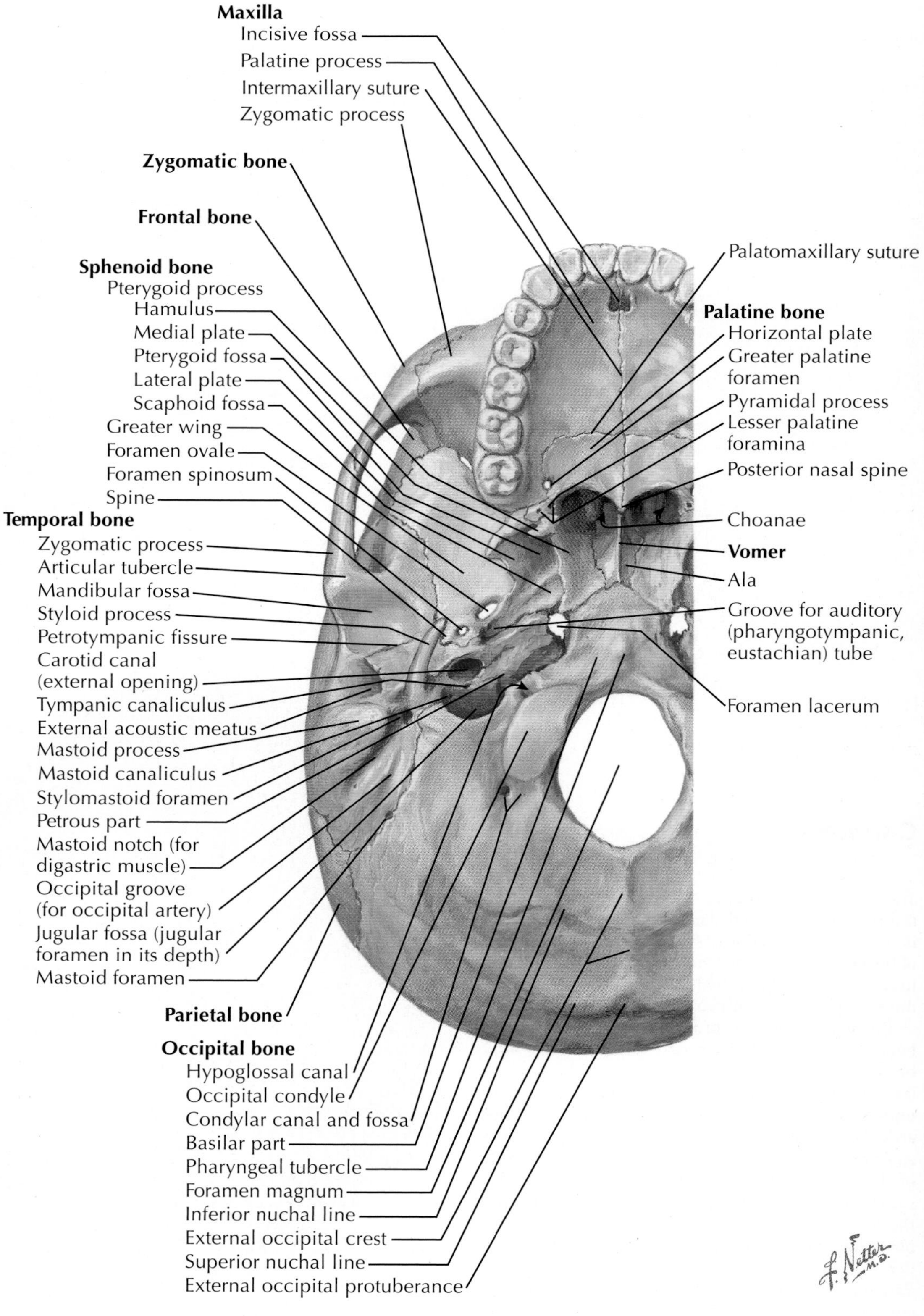

Plate 14.6

Head Trauma

BONES, MARKINGS, AND ORIFICES OF SKULL BASE

The internal surface of the base of the skull has adapted its shape to the configuration of the adjacent parts of the brain. It consists of three cranial fossae (the anterior, middle, and posterior), which are separated by conspicuous ridges and increase in size and depth from front to back.

The *anterior cranial fossa* is the shallowest of the three fossae and lodges the lower parts of the frontal lobes of the brain. The sulci and gyri of the lobes are mirrored in the irregularities of the bony surfaces. It is limited anteriorly and laterally by the frontal bone. On each side, the floor is formed by the slightly domed and ridged *orbital plate of the frontal bone*, which supports the orbital surface of the homolateral frontal lobe of the brain and its meninges and separates them from the orbit. Posterior extensions from the frontal air sinuses may expand the orbital plates for varying distances, and the medial parts of these plates overlie the ethmoidal labyrinths.

On each side of the midline *crista galli* are the grooved *ethmoidal cribriform plates* that help form the roof of the nasal cavity, lodge the olfactory bulbs, and provide numerous orifices for the delicate olfactory nerves. A small pit exists between the frontal crest and the crista galli, the *foramen cecum,* which occasionally transmits a tiny vein from the nose to the superior sagittal sinus. The crista galli and frontal crest give attachment to the anterior end of the falx cerebri.

Posterior to the ethmoid and frontal bones, the floor of the anterior cranial fossa is formed by the anterior part of the body of the sphenoid bone, the *jugum sphenoidale,* and on each side by the *lesser wings* of this bone. These lesser wings slightly overlap the anterior part of the middle cranial fossa and project into the stems of the lateral cerebral sulci, thus forming the upper boundaries of the superior orbital fissures.

The medial ends of the posterior borders of the lesser wings end in small, rounded projections, the *anterior clinoid processes,* which provide attachments for the anterior ends of the free border of the tentorium cerebelli. Each anterior process is grooved on its medial side by the internal carotid artery, and each may be joined to the inconstant middle clinoid process by a thin osseous bar, thus forming a narrow bony ring around the artery as it emerges from the cavernous sinus.

The *middle cranial fossa* is intermediate in depth between the anterior and posterior fossae. It is narrow and elevated medially but expands and becomes deeper at each side to lodge and protect the temporal lobes of the brain. It is bounded anteriorly by the posterior borders of the lesser wings of the sphenoid bone and the anterior margin of the prechiasmatic sulcus; posteriorly by the superior borders of the petrous parts of the temporal bones, which are grooved by the superior petrosal sinuses and by the dorsum sellae of the sphenoid; and laterally by the greater wings of the sphenoid, the frontal angles of the parietal bones, and the temporal squamae.

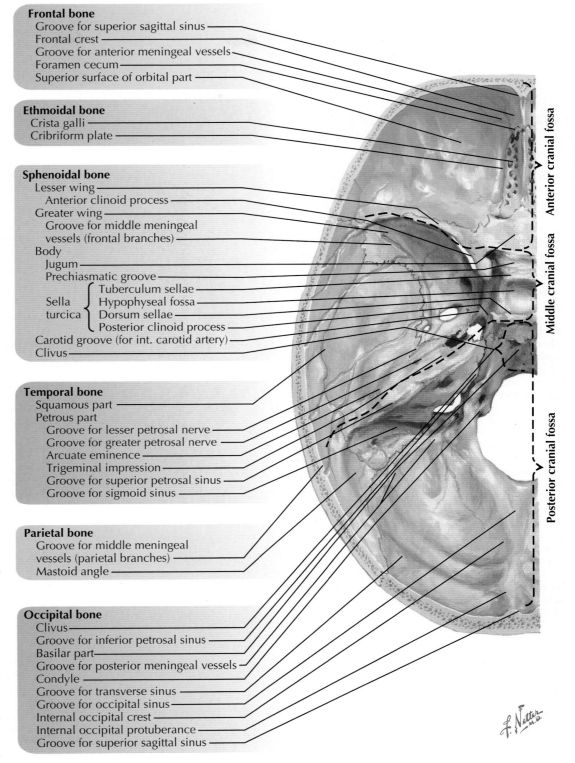

Frontal bone
Groove for superior sagittal sinus
Frontal crest
Groove for anterior meningeal vessels
Foramen cecum
Superior surface of orbital part

Ethmoidal bone
Crista galli
Cribriform plate

Sphenoidal bone
Lesser wing
Anterior clinoid process
Greater wing
Groove for middle meningeal vessels (frontal branches)
Body
Jugum
Prechiasmatic groove
Sella turcica { Tuberculum sellae
Hypophyseal fossa
Dorsum sellae
Posterior clinoid process
Carotid groove (for int. carotid artery)
Clivus

Temporal bone
Squamous part
Petrous part
Groove for lesser petrosal nerve
Groove for greater petrosal nerve
Arcuate eminence
Trigeminal impression
Groove for superior petrosal sinus
Groove for sigmoid sinus

Parietal bone
Groove for middle meningeal vessels (parietal branches)
Mastoid angle

Occipital bone
Clivus
Groove for inferior petrosal sinus
Basilar part
Groove for posterior meningeal vessels
Condyle
Groove for transverse sinus
Groove for occipital sinus
Internal occipital crest
Internal occipital protuberance
Groove for superior sagittal sinus

Anterior cranial fossa

Middle cranial fossa

Posterior cranial fossa

The floor in the median area is formed by the *body of the sphenoid bone,* containing the sphenoidal air sinuses. The lesser wings of the sphenoid are attached to its body by two roots, separated from each other by the *optic canals* that transmit the optic (II) nerves and ophthalmic arteries. Behind the prechiasmatic sulcus is a median elevation, the *tuberculum sellae,* and the *hypophyseal fossa* housing the pituitary gland. The fossa is limited behind by the *dorsum sellae,* an upward-projecting bony plate with a concave upper border expanding laterally into the *posterior clinoid processes.* Lateral to the sellae is a shallow, sinuous *groove for the internal carotid artery;* at its anterior end on the medial side may be a small tubercle, the *middle clinoid process.*

The lateral parts of the middle fossa are related in front to the orbits, on each side to the temporal fossae, and

Plate 14.7

Brain: PART I

INTERNAL ASPECTS OF BASE OF SKULL: ORIFICES

Foramen cecum ------- Emissary vein to superior sagittal sinus

Nasal slit / Anterior ethmoidal foramen } Anterior ethmoidal artery, vein, and nerve

Foramina of cribriform plate --------- Olfactory nerves

Posterior ethmoidal foramen ------ Posterior ethmoidal artery, vein, and nerve

Optic canal -------- { Optic nerve (II) / Ophthalmic artery

Superior orbital fissure -- { Oculomotor nerve (III) / Trochlear nerve (IV) / Lacrimal, frontal, and nasociliary branches of ophthalmic nerve (V₁) / Abducent nerve (VI) / Superior ophthalmic vein

Foramen rotundum ------ Maxillary nerve (V₂)

Foramen ovale -------- { Mandibular nerve (V₃) / Accessory meningeal artery / Lesser petrosal nerve

Foramen spinosum ----- { Middle meningeal artery and vein / Meningeal branch of mandibular nerve

Sphenoidal emissary foramen (of Vesalius) (inconstant)

Foramen lacerum------ Greater petrosal nerve

Carotid canal for ------ { Internal carotid artery / Internal carotid nerve plexus

Hiatus for ----------- Lesser petrosal nerve

Hiatus for ----------- Greater petrosal nerve

Internal acoustic meatus-- { Facial nerve (VII) / Vestibulocochlear nerve (VIII) / Labyrinthine artery

Opening of vestibular aqueduct------ Endolymphatic duct

Mastoid foramen------- (inconstant) Emissary vein (and occasional branch of occipital artery)

Jugular foramen ------ { Inferior petrosal sinus / Glossopharyngeal nerve (IX) / Vagus nerve (X) / Accessory nerve (XI) / Sigmoid sinus / Posterior meningeal artery

Condylar canal ------- (inconstant) { Emissary vein and meningeal branch of ascending pharyngeal artery

Hypoglossal canal --------- Hypoglossal nerve (XII)

Foramen magnum ------ { Medulla oblongata / Meninges / Vertebral arteries / Meningeal branches of vertebral arteries / Spinal roots of accessory nerves

F. Netter, M.D.

BONES, MARKINGS, AND ORIFICES OF SKULL BASE (Continued)

below to the infratemporal fossae. The middle fossa communicates with the orbits through the *superior orbital fissures*.

Various other, more or less symmetric openings exist on each side. The *foramen rotundum* pierces the greater wing of the sphenoid bone just below and behind the inner end of the superior orbital fissure, and then it opens anteriorly into the pterygopalatine fossa. The *foramen ovale* also penetrates the greater sphenoidal wing posterolateral to the foramen rotundum and leads downward into the infratemporal fossa. The smaller *foramen spinosum* lies posterolateral to the foramen ovale and opens below into the infratemporal fossa close to the sphenoidal spine; the sulcus for the middle meningeal vessels starts at this foramen. The *foramen lacerum* is an irregular aperture between the body and greater wing of the sphenoid bone and the apex of the petrous part of the temporal bone; it marks the point of entry of the internal carotid artery into the cavernous sinus. Behind the foramen lacerum is the shallow *depression for the trigeminal (semilunar) ganglion* on the anterior surface of the petrous temporal bone, and lateral to this are two narrow grooves leading to the hiatuses for the lesser (minor) and greater (major) petrosal nerves.

The *arcuate eminence* is produced by the superior semicircular canal of the internal ear. Anterolateral to this eminence is a thin plate of bone, the *tegmen tympani*, forming the roof of the tympanic cavity and mastoid antrum and extending forward and medially to cover the bony part of the auditory (pharyngotympanic) tube.

The *posterior cranial fossa* is the largest and deepest of the cranial fossae and lodges the cerebellum, pons, and medulla oblongata. It is bounded anteriorly by the dorsum sellae, the back of the body of the sphenoid bone, and the basilar part of the occipital bones; posteriorly by the squama of the occipital bone below the sulci for the transverse sinuses and the internal occipital protuberance; and laterally by the petrous and mastoid parts of the temporal bones, the mastoid angles of the parietal bones, and the lateral parts of the occipital bone.

The posterior fossa is pierced by several foramina and is grooved by various dural venous sinuses. A large median opening in the floor of the fossa, the *foramen magnum*, penetrates the occipital bone. The medulla oblongata and spinal cord and their surrounding meninges become directly continuous immediately below the foramen. The petrous part of the temporal bone and the occipital bone are separated by the *petro-occipital fissure* and the *sulcus for the inferior petrosal sinus*; the fissure ends behind, in the *jugular foramen*. The inferior petrosal and sigmoid sinuses pass through the anterior and posterior parts of this foramen, respectively, whereas the glossopharyngeal (IX), vagus (X), and accessory (XI) nerves occupy an intermediate position as they leave the skull.

Two canals are associated with the occipital condyles: the *hypoglossal canal*, for cranial nerve XII, and the *condylar canal*.

Above the jugular foramen, the *internal acoustic meatus* tunnels into the petrous part of the temporal bone. It is about 1 cm long and is separated laterally from the internal ear by a thin bony plate pierced by many apertures for fascicles of the facial (VII) and vestibulocochlear (VIII) nerves. Behind the orifice of this meatus is the slit-like opening of the *vestibular aqueduct*, which lodges the blind end of the endolymphatic duct.

The internal opening of the inconstant *mastoid foramen* is close to the *sulcus for the sigmoid sinus*, which winds downward from the transverse sinus to the jugular foramen, where it ends in the superior bulb of the internal jugular vein. The *internal occipital protuberance* is related to the confluence of the superior sagittal, straight, occipital, and transverse sinuses. The margins of the sulci for the transverse sinuses give attachment to the tentorium cerebelli.

Plate 14.8

Head Trauma

SKULL INJURIES

The mechanical forces resulting in traumatic brain injuries (TBIs) may produce a variety of different structural injuries, each of which requires different surgical or medical treatment.

Before the introduction of computed tomography (CT) scans, plain skull radiographs were of vital importance in evaluating patients with head injuries. The presence of a skull fracture strongly suggested the possibility of a significant, underlying intracranial injury. Fracture is present in 66% to 100% of patients with epidural hematoma, 18% to 60% with acute subdural hematoma (ASDH), and 40% to 80% with contusions or intracerebral hematoma. Such intracranial injuries are now immediately identified by CT, and an associated skull fracture is often noticed only in passing.

There are, however, several types of skull fracture that are of clinical significance. The most classic is the basilar skull fracture, which may be associated with cerebrospinal fluid (CSF) leak and cranial nerve injuries. Basilar skull fracture has been reported in up to 25% of patients sustaining a head injury. Even with CT, basilar skull fractures may not be identified because of their orientation to the plane of the scan. Special thin cuts or coronal views may be required. Most basilar skull fractures occur through the petrous bone or the anterior cranial fossa. Clival fractures are less common. Petrous bone fractures occur either transversely or longitudinally, and their orientation predisposes to various complications.

The classic clinical presentation of a petrous bone fracture is with the Battle sign, a retromastoid hematoma. Raccoon eyes, or periorbital hematomas, may be seen with anterior skull base fractures. CSF leaks, otorrhea, and rhinorrhea have been reported in approximately 10% of patients with basal skull fractures. Otorrhea is typically associated with petrous fractures, whereas rhinorrhea may emanate from either frontal fossa fractures through the cribriform plate or the petrous bone through the eustachian canal. In either case, with bed rest and head elevation, the CSF leak ceases spontaneously in more than 85% of patients. The administration of antibiotics is not advised because this may predispose to antibiotic-resistant infection. Persisting leaks may be treated with a lumbar drain; only a small number require direct or endoscopic surgical repair.

If there is any question as to whether drainage from the nose or ear represents CSF, the fluid can be checked for glucose, which typically is greater than 30 mg/mL in CSF, or β2-transferrin, which is found only in the CSF.

Cranial nerve injuries may complicate up to 5% of basal skull fractures, the most common of which is facial nerve injury in association with petrous fractures. Such an injury may occur in up to 50% of patients with transverse and 20% with longitudinal fractures. The facial nerve is especially prone to injury in the narrow fallopian canal as swelling occurs or by compression from fracture fragments. If facial paralysis is immediate and complete, the chances of recovery are small. More minor injuries tend to recover well, and steroids are often used for treatment. Some advocate early surgical exploration and decompression of the nerve.

Two other types of skull fractures require specific clinical management: open depressed and frontal sinus fractures.

Open, or compound, depressed skull fractures have been said to be associated with infection and posttraumatic epilepsy. They definitely are associated with

Open fracture

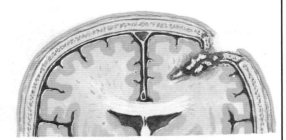

In-driven fragments of bone

Depressed fracture

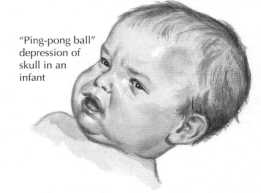

"Ping-pong ball" depression of skull in an infant

Basilar skull fractures

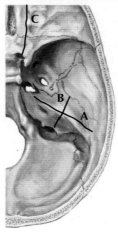

Longitudinal (*A*) and transverse (*B*) fractures of petrous pyramid of temporal bone, and anterior basal skull fracture (*C*)

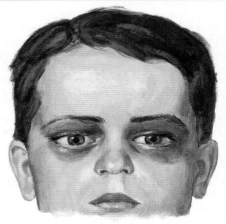

"Panda bear" or "raccoon" sign due to leakage of blood from anterior fossa into periorbital tissues. Absence of conjunctival injection differentiates fracture from direct eye trauma.

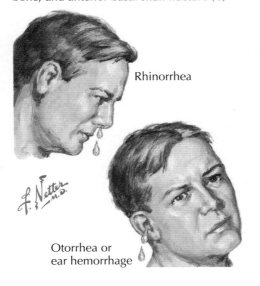

Rhinorrhea

Otorrhea or ear hemorrhage

Battle sign: postauricular hematoma

potentially significant underlying brain injury. Common practice until recently was to operate on all such fractures. Contemporary literature, however, has shown that the risk of posttraumatic epilepsy is not significantly increased, and the risk of infection may be greater in patients treated operatively than those treated nonoperatively. It thus appears possible to manage conservatively all but the most contaminated and comminuted fractures with reasonable safety.

The primary concern over frontal sinus fractures is the status of the posterior wall of the sinus, with the possibility of dural violation and the risk of CSF leak, pneumocephalus, and infection. In general, unless there is overt evidence of CSF leak or pneumocephalus with posterior wall fragments in-driven more than 3 to 4 mm, nonoperative management is usually successful. Some, however, advocate surgery on most frontal sinus fractures to prevent the development of a mucocele.

Plate 14.9

Brain: PART I

CONCUSSION

A concussion is a type of TBI that changes the way the brain normally works and is caused by traumatic forces to the head or body. Most concussions occur without loss of consciousness. The Centers for Disease Control and Prevention (CDC) estimates that between 1.6 and 3.8 million concussions occur in sports and recreational activities each year. Concussions or mild TBIs can result in short- and long-term health risks. In athletes, there is an association between repetitive concussions and a neurodegenerative disease called *chronic traumatic encephalopathy*. There is also an entity known as *second impact syndrome*. The potential public health problem of concussion is such that most states in the United States have either laws or pending bills addressing the problem of concussions in youth sports.

At the level of the neuron, linear and rotational forces can lead to structural and metabolic changes that transiently impair function and contribute to physical, cognitive, and emotional symptoms. The molecular substrate for these acute clinical changes is the subject of much current research on cellular ionic transients in sodium and calcium, axonal integrity, bioenergetics, neurovascular coupling, and genetics. What is apparent in those who have experienced a concussion is that symptoms may persist for days, weeks, or months after a concussive event.

CLINICAL SYMPTOMATOLOGY

The signs and symptoms of concussions are diverse. Typically, individuals have difficulty with thinking and memory skills, and their emotions may be affected. The physical problems include headache, nausea, and visual disturbances. The CDC advocates that any athlete suspected of having a concussion should be immediately removed from play, evaluated by a healthcare professional, and only allowed to return when cleared by a healthcare professional. At present, there are no "neuroprotective" drugs that can be used for this condition, and it is recommended that, for safety, physical and mental activities that excessively stimulate the injured brain should be discontinued. Furthermore, a graded return-to-play system is recommended as the safest way to bring an athlete back to full-contact activities.

SECOND IMPACT SYNDROME

Second impact syndrome is the most devastating, yet rare, consequence of repeat concussion in the postinjury phase. This condition occurs when an individual experiences a second traumatic episode to the brain before the brain has fully recovered from the initial traumatic injury. These subjects rapidly develop global cerebral edema, coma, severe neurologic impairment, and the potential for death. This rare condition has been observed mainly in youths younger than 21 years. At present, there are no methods for determining the recovery period after a concussion or even the duration of a "window of vulnerability" after a concussion. Hence much of the current emphasis in the management of concussion and return to playing of sports in young athletes is on reducing any potential for second impact syndrome.

REPEAT CONCUSSIONS AND CHRONIC TRAUMATIC ENCEPHALOPATHY

Individuals who experience an isolated concussive event should recover completely if they allow an appropriate time for recovery, with rest and cessation of sports.

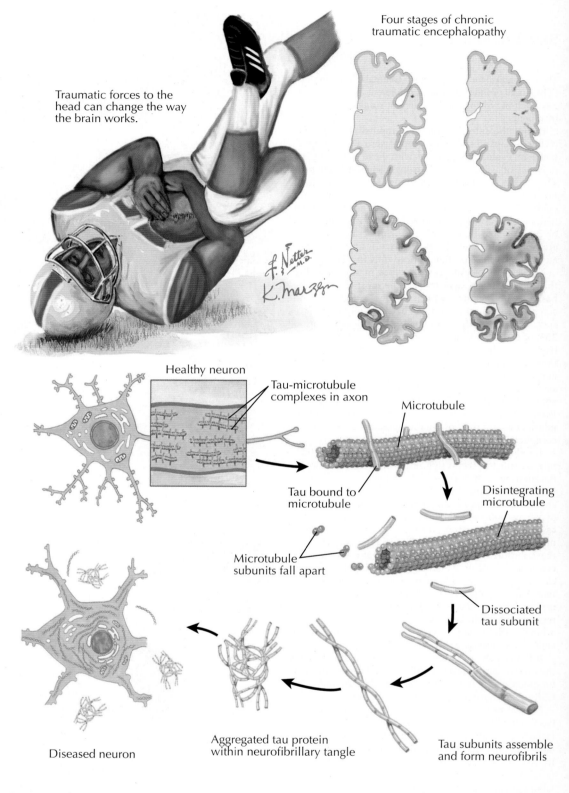

Traumatic forces to the head can change the way the brain works.

Four stages of chronic traumatic encephalopathy

Healthy neuron

Tau-microtubule complexes in axon

Microtubule

Tau bound to microtubule

Disintegrating microtubule

Microtubule subunits fall apart

Dissociated tau subunit

Diseased neuron

Aggregated tau protein within neurofibrillary tangle

Tau subunits assemble and form neurofibrils

In contrast, brain autopsy studies of former professional athletes in contact sports, such as boxing, football, and hockey, have revealed a chronic, neurodegenerative disease termed *chronic traumatic encephalopathy* (see Plate 14.9). This disease was first described in 1928 as *dementia pugilistica* in deceased boxers. The clinical syndrome associated with this pathology, the so-called punch drunk condition, was believed to be limited to boxers who displayed progressive cognitive, emotional, and behavioral symptoms, such as depression, agitation, and dementia, years after repeated TBIs. However, many other cases of chronic traumatic encephalopathy have been described in deceased players from other sports, including football, hockey, and wrestling.

The US National Institutes of Neurological Disorders and Stroke consensus group has provided a description of required criteria for the pathologic diagnosis of chronic traumatic encephalopathy. The feature that differentiates the condition from other tauopathies is an "abnormal perivascular accumulation of tau in neurons, astrocytes, and cell processes in an irregular pattern at the depths of the cortical sulci."

Plate 14.10

Head Trauma

Temporal fossa hematoma

Skull fracture crossing middle meningeal artery

Shift of normal midline structures

Compression of posterior cerebral artery

Shift of brainstem to opposite side may reverse lateralization of signs by tentorial pressure on contralateral pathways

Herniation of temporal lobe under tentorium cerebelli

Compression of oculomotor (III) nerve leading to ipsilateral pupil dilation and third cranial nerve palsy

Herniation of cerebellar tonsil

Compression of corticospinal and associated pathways, resulting in contralateral hemiparesis, deep tendon hyperreflexia, and Babinski sign

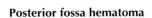

Subfrontal hematoma

Frontal trauma: headache, poor cerebration, intermittent disorientation, anisocoria

Posterior fossa hematoma

Occipital trauma and/or fracture: headache, meningismus, cerebellar and cranial nerve signs, Cushing triad

Bone flap turned down from cracking uncut segment of margin, exposing epidural hematoma, which is removed by suction, spoon, or Penfield dissector

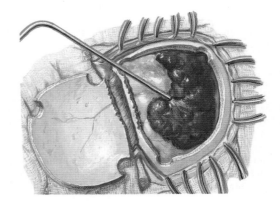

ACUTE EPIDURAL HEMATOMA

The overall incidence of acute epidural hematoma (EDH) after head injury is approximately 5%, but it approaches 10% in patients presenting in coma. EDHs are almost always traumatic in nature. There are rare reports of spontaneous occurrence in association with anticoagulation or thrombocytopenia. The classic clinical presentation is with a loss of consciousness that is followed by a lucid interval and then by progressively severe headache and decreasing level of consciousness. However, most EDHs result from motor vehicle collisions, and greater than 60% of patients are unconscious at the scene or on hospital arrival.

CT scan shows a variably sized oval or lens-shaped hyperdensity between the bone and the dura.

The most common clinical location for an EDH is the temporal fossa, typically associated with a temporal bone fracture that lacerates the middle meningeal artery and leads to arterial bleeding. This can result in the well-known transtentorial herniation syndrome. As the ipsilateral temporal lobe is forced medially, the third nerve is trapped against the brainstem, resulting in ipsilateral pupillary dilation. As more pressure develops, the ipsilateral posterior cerebral artery may be so severely compressed as to result in an occipital lobe stroke that is typically seen on CT scan a day or two after the event. With increasing shift of the brain to the opposite side, the brainstem is compressed, and the cerebral peduncle is forced into the edge of the tentorium, creating a so-called Kernohan notch and resulting in hemiparesis ipsilateral to the dilated pupil. If the compression remains severe for too long, Duret hemorrhages occur in the brainstem from compression or tearing of the small perforating arteries coming off the basilar artery. Such hemorrhages can be seen on magnetic resonance imaging (MRI) and portend a poor prognosis.

Venous epidural hematomas may also occur and are most common in the posterior fossa in children.

The following are recently published guidelines by the Brain Trauma Foundation (New York) for the treatment of EDH:

- An EDH greater than 30 cm³ should be surgically evacuated regardless of the patient's score on the Glasgow Coma Scale (GCS).
- An EDH less than 30 cm³ and with less than 15-mm thickness and with less than a 5-mm midline shift in patients with a GCS score greater than 8 without focal neurologic deficit can be managed conservatively with serial CT scanning and close neurologic observation in a neurosurgical center.
- It is strongly recommended that patients with an acute EDH in coma (GCS < 9) with anisocoria undergo surgical evacuation as soon as possible.

In a truly urgent situation when, for example, weather or distance precludes getting the patient to a center with neurosurgical capabilities, a burr hole may release sufficient blood to be lifesaving. Definitive treatment is evacuation through a large "trauma" bone flap. An active bleeding point is virtually always found on the dura. Occasionally, bleeding may be seen to be coming from underneath the temporal lobe, and the middle meningeal artery will be found lacerated at or within the foramen spinosum. With rapid, aggressive treatment, mortality across all age groups and all GCS scores is less than 10%.

Plate 14.11

Brain: PART I

ACUTE SUBDURAL HEMATOMA

Acute subdural hematoma (ASDH) is the primary structural abnormality in up to 30% of patients after severe TBI and, in most instances, is associated with other significant structural injuries such as contusions.

The injury occurs typically after a high-speed motor vehicle collision. ASDH, however, is being increasingly seen in elderly patients after same-height falls, and especially in patients on anticoagulant or antiplatelet medication. Bleeding is typically venous in nature, resulting from shearing of cortical veins, bridging veins, or veins from one of the cerebral venous sinuses.

A CT scan typically shows a hyperdense crescent of blood between the dura and the brain. Despite a relatively small amount of blood, there is typically significant underlying hemispheric cerebral edema with associated midline shift. An entity known as *hyperacute ASDH* has been described on CT: the presence of mixed hyperdensity indicates ongoing active bleeding. Contusions are also frequent and typically will worsen after surgical evacuation of the ASDH.

The decision to operate is based on several factors, but increased age is an extremely strong independent factor indicating a poor prognosis.

The following recommendations by the Brain Trauma Foundation have been proposed for surgical management:

- An ASDH with a thickness greater than 10 mm or a midline shift greater than 5 mm should be surgically evacuated regardless of the patient's GCS score.
- All patients with ASDH with a GCS score less than 9 should undergo intracranial pressure (ICP) monitoring.
- A patient with a GCS score less than 9 and with an ASDH less than 10 mm thick and a midline shift less than 5 mm should undergo surgical evacuation of the lesion if the GCS score decreases by 2 or more points between injury and hospital admission and/or the patient presents with asymmetric or fixed and dilated pupils and/or the ICP exceeds 20 mm Hg.
- Patients with ASDH and indications for surgery should have evacuation performed as soon as possible.

The issue of "as soon as possible" for surgical intervention has been widely studied. In a landmark paper in 1981, it was found that patients undergoing surgery within 4 hours of injury had a lower mortality rate (30%) than those undergoing surgery after more than 4 hours (90%). A subsequent paper in 1991 did not find any significant difference in mortality for patients undergoing surgery within or after 4 hours. It has been suggested that the degree and extent of underlying brain injury are probably the more important determinants of recovery than is the absolute timing of surgery.

The goal of surgery is the most complete evacuation of the ASDH as is possible through a large "trauma craniotomy" flap. Attention should be directed to coagulating any bleeding cortical veins or bridging veins. If there appears to have been avulsion of a vein from one of the venous sinuses, unless there has been adequate exposure of the area, it is best controlled by packing with hemostatic agents. If there is significant brain swelling, it is often best not to replace the craniotomy flap.

"Question mark" skin incision (black); outline of free bone flap and burr holes (red)

Catheter to monitor intracranial pressure, emerging through burr hole and stab wound

Skin flap reflected (Raney clips control bleeding); free bone flap removed and dura opened; clot evacuated by irrigation, suction, and forceps

Bone and skin flaps replaced and sutured

Jackson-Pratt drain, emerging from subdural space via burr hole and stab wound

Section showing acute subdural hematoma on right side and subdural hematoma associated with temporal lobe intracerebral hematoma ("burst" temporal lobe) on left

Unfortunately, despite the most aggressive neurocritical care, the mortality rate from ASDH remains high, ranging from 40% to 60% across all GCS categories and greater than 70% in patients presenting in coma.

CONTUSIONS

Contusions are parenchymal mass lesions that occur in up to 35% of patients with severe TBI. Approximately 30% will enlarge progressively or become associated with significant surrounding edema. Although most can be managed medically, it has been recommended that surgery be considered in the following settings: patients with GCS scores of 6 to 8 with frontal or temporal contusions greater than 20 cm³ in volume, patients with midline shift of at least 5 mm and/or cisternal compression on CT scan, and patients with any lesion greater than 50 cm³ in volume.

DIFFUSE AXONAL INJURY

Diffuse axonal injury (DAI) or shear injury, as the name implies, results from stretching and tearing of axons throughout the brain. Although the injury is diffuse, two of the most common areas of involvement are the corpus callosum and the posterolateral quadrants of the upper brainstem. CT scans may show discrete punctate hemorrhages in these and other white matter tracts. MRI is very sensitive to DAI lesions, which appear hyperintense on T2-weighted images. Severe DAI is associated with a poor outcome.

Plate 14.12

Head Trauma

CT Scans and Magnetic Resonance Images of Intracranial Hematomas

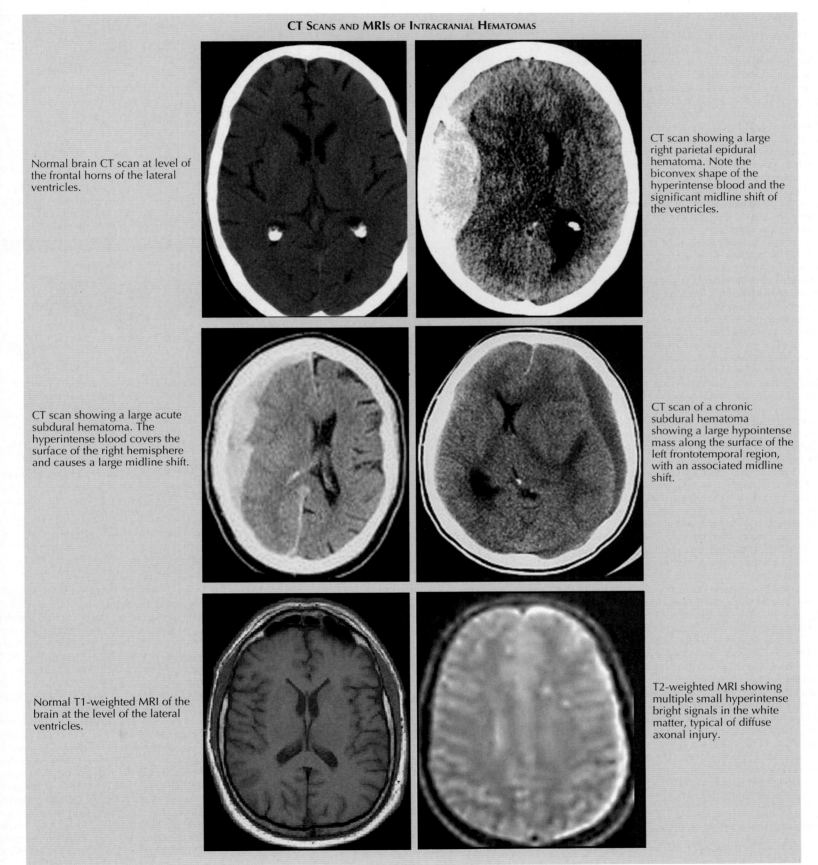

CT Scans and MRIs of Intracranial Hematomas

Normal brain CT scan at level of the frontal horns of the lateral ventricles.

CT scan showing a large right parietal epidural hematoma. Note the biconvex shape of the hyperintense blood and the significant midline shift of the ventricles.

CT scan showing a large acute subdural hematoma. The hyperintense blood covers the surface of the right hemisphere and causes a large midline shift.

CT scan of a chronic subdural hematoma showing a large hypointense mass along the surface of the left frontotemporal region, with an associated midline shift.

Normal T1-weighted MRI of the brain at the level of the lateral ventricles.

T2-weighted MRI showing multiple small hyperintense bright signals in the white matter, typical of diffuse axonal injury.

Plate 14.13

Brain: PART I

VASCULAR INJURY

CAROTID-CAVERNOUS FISTULA

Carotid-cavernous fistula (CCF), occurring in less than 3% of patients with head injuries, is the most well-characterized sequela of intracranial vascular injury, having first been described in 1757. Although CCF may arise from other causes such as ruptured intracavernous aneurysm or infection, trauma is the most common cause. CCF occurs when there has been an injury to the cavernous sinus segment of the carotid artery, resulting in redirection, overfilling, and pressurization of the venous inflow and outflow of the cavernous sinus. The resulting clinical syndrome is characterized by pulsating exophthalmos and a bruit.

The carotid artery enters the cavernous sinus as it exits the foramen lacerum at the base of the skull. It then rises toward the posterior clinoid process before acutely turning anteriorly for approximately 2 cm (the horizontal segment), leaving the cavernous sinus just below the anterior clinoid. There are several small branches of the carotid artery inside the cavernous sinus, including the meningohypophyseal trunk and the artery of the inferior cavernous sinus. The cavernous sinus itself is an intricate plexus of venous channels surrounding the carotid artery. It lies lateral to the pituitary gland and sphenoid sinus, extending from the superior orbital fissure to the apex of the petrous bone. Among many other venous and sinus connections, the superior and inferior ophthalmic veins and the central retinal artery drain into the cavernous sinus, the former accounting for the exophthalmos and the latter for the possibility of intracranial hemorrhage. The third, fourth, and all three branches of the fifth cranial nerve run within the lateral wall of the cavernous sinus; the sixth nerve passes directly through the sinus alongside the carotid artery, whereas ocular sympathetic fibers form a plexus on the wall of the carotid artery.

The classic signs and symptoms of the syndrome resulting from CCF include pulsating exophthalmos, a bruit that patients often appreciate, chemosis (conjunctival injection), diplopia, visual loss, and headache. These may evolve over the course of several weeks or months. Their pathophysiologic basis can be deduced readily from the previously described anatomy.

Although a CCF can typically be seen on CT or MRI, angiography is necessary to define the anatomy of the fistula and to identify the associated abnormal venous drainage to allow for planning of optimal treatment. Because traumatic CCFs rarely resolve spontaneously, surgical intervention is usually indicated. The timing of intervention depends on the degree and extent of visual loss. Visual deterioration is due to ischemia secondary to increased intraocular pressure and subsequent hypoxia as a result of reduced arterial flow and venous hypertension.

The current treatment of choice is selective endovascular balloon occlusion of the fistulous connection itself, preserving the carotid artery and its branches. The fistula may be accessed by a variety of routes, including the superior ophthalmic vein, the carotid artery, and the superior petrosal sinus. Large series of patients with CCFs treated endovascularly have demonstrated a 99% occlusion rate with less than 5% complications.

SUBARACHNOID HEMORRHAGE

Subarachnoid hemorrhage (SAH) occurs in approximately 10% of cases of severe TBI from injury to small

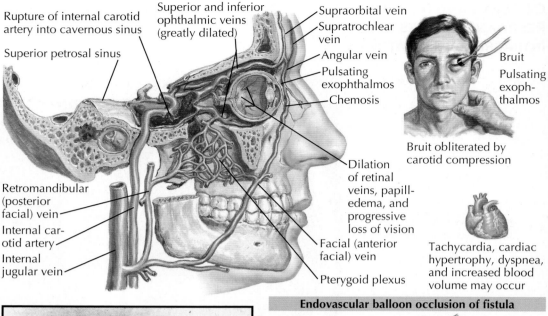

Rupture of internal carotid artery into cavernous sinus

Superior petrosal sinus

Superior and inferior ophthalmic veins (greatly dilated)

Supraorbital vein

Supratrochlear vein

Angular vein

Pulsating exophthalmos

Chemosis

Bruit
Pulsating exophthalmos

Bruit obliterated by carotid compression

Retromandibular (posterior facial) vein

Internal carotid artery

Internal jugular vein

Dilation of retinal veins, papilledema, and progressive loss of vision

Facial (anterior facial) vein

Pterygoid plexus

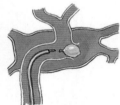

Tachycardia, cardiac hypertrophy, dyspnea, and increased blood volume may occur

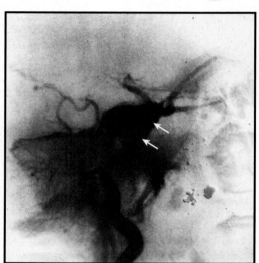

Carotid arteriography, early phase, reveals prominent opacificaton of cavernous sinus *(arrows)* via carotid-cavernous fistula.

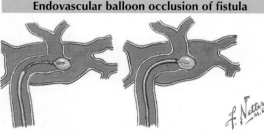

Endovascular balloon occlusion of fistula

Balloon inflated with radiopaque fluid occluding fistula

Outer catheter advanced over inner catheter to engage balloon cuff

Balloon liberated by slight pull on inner catheter. Balloon neck spontaneously constricted by tense latex tie. All catheters then withdrawn.

intracranial vessels, and severe vasospasm may develop. If a patient with traumatic SAH is not improving despite intensive treatment, vasospasm should be considered and appropriate studies undertaken to confirm this. Because of the possibility of injury to the intracranial vasculature, some are advocating routine CT angiography in all patients with severe TBI.

SECONDARY COMPLICATIONS OF TRAUMATIC BRAIN INJURY

A significant number of patients die or are left severely disabled after TBI, not by the primary injury itself but by the secondary insults that follow. The most common of these are hypotension and hypoxia.

Hypoxia (oxygen saturation <90%) and/or hypotension (systolic blood pressure [BP] <90 mm Hg) was found to occur in greater than one-third of patients with severe TBI in the National Coma Data Bank. A single episode of hypotension at any point is associated with a doubling of mortality, a single episode of hypoxia is associated with a 33% increase, and the combination

with a 75% increase. Thus every effort should be made to prevent or minimize the occurrence of these events.

Another serious secondary insult is intracranial hypertension. It is reasonably well established that maintaining ICP below 20 mm Hg at all times is associated with greater than 90% survival, controlling ICP below this level for greater than 50% of the time is associated with greater than 50% survival, and an inability to bring ICP below 20 mm Hg at any time is accompanied by a greater than 90% mortality.

An important but still uncontrolled problem is the damaging biochemical cascade that is initiated shortly after injury. The final common pathway to energy failure, and ultimately to cell death, relates to loss of calcium homeostasis and to mitochondrial damage. Opening the cellular membranes to calcium influx is triggered by a variety of mechanisms, including oxygen free-radical production, excitatory neurotoxicity, caspases, and cytokines. The resulting damage may exceed that created by the primary injury. Randomized controlled clinical trials of pharmacologic agents to block this biochemical cascade have not yielded benefit.

Plate 14.14

Head Trauma

Glasgow Coma Scale Score

Teasdale and Jennett introduced the Glasgow Coma Scale (GCS) in 1974 as an objective measure of level of consciousness after TBI. The GCS quickly became universally accepted as the best clinical measure of the severity of TBI, allowing for a reliable, standardized method of assessing and reporting sequential evaluation across all healthcare providers. The GCS measures level of consciousness, not neurologic deficits. An appropriate neurologic examination should accompany the GCS.

The GCS evaluates three independent neurologic responses: eye opening, motor response, and verbal response. All parameters may be significantly affected by systemic factors such as severe hypotension or significant drug/alcohol intoxication or by local factors, including ocular trauma, intubation, extremity fractures, and spinal cord injury. Iatrogenic paralysis and sedation affect the score and may render the GCS inapplicable.

The eye opening and verbal responses are simple to record. The motor response has traditionally been recorded as the best reaction in response to deep pressure or pain. Thus a patient who is hemiplegic may still receive a motor score of 6. In their original paper, Teasdale and Jennett specifically prescribed the manner in which the evaluation of all three parameters was to be undertaken. Noxious stimuli to the nail bed were to be applied to elicit decorticate or decerebrate responses, whereas painful stimuli to the head, neck, or trunk were used to test for localization. Eye opening in response to pain was to be tested distant to the face to prevent a grimacing reflex from keeping the eye shut.

It is generally accepted that a GCS score of 13 to 15 is associated with minor TBI, a score of 9 to 12 reflects moderately severe TBI, and a score of 3 to 8 indicates severe TBI. It is common practice to attach a modifier ("t") after the score if a verbal response cannot be recorded due to intubation.

The GCS cannot be used in preverbal children, and a separate children's coma scale has been developed. The eye and motor responses mirror those of the GCS. For the verbal response, a score of 5 is given if the child smiles, orients to sounds, follows objects, and interacts. Scores of 4 to 1 include both a component related to crying and one to interaction. Thus a score of 4 indicates that the child cries consolably and interacts inappropriately; 3, that crying is inconsistently consolable and there is moaning; 2, that the child cries inconsolably and is restless; and 1, that there is an absence of crying or interaction.

Several studies have shown an association between both a prehospital and in-hospital GCS score and outcome. As an example, patients having a score of 6 to 15 in the field were 30 times more likely to have a good outcome than those with a score less than 6. A prospective study of emergency medical service and in-hospital GCS determination found a positive predictive value of 77% for a poor outcome (dead, vegetative, or severely disabled) in patients with a score of 3 to 5 and 26% with a score of 6 to 8.

From a clinical perspective, the GCS is routinely recorded at regular intervals during the neurocritical care phase of TBI management. Various clinical decisions have come to be based on GCS thresholds, such as the need for intubation and consideration of ICP monitoring when the score is less than 8. Similarly, during ongoing evaluation, a decline of 2 or more points is generally considered clinically significant.

Efforts in developing the GCS have been extended to outcome assessment. The Glasgow Outcome Scale (GOS) was introduced in 1975 and is the cornerstone in outcome assessment, with high intrarater reliability. There are five potential outcomes: death, persistent vegetative state, severe disability, moderate disability, and a good outcome.

A good recovery is defined as a resumption of a normal life despite minor ongoing disability. With moderate disability, a patient is disabled but independent, able to perform all activities of daily living, and work in a sheltered setting. With severe disability, a patient is conscious but totally dependent on others for care. In the persistent vegetative state, the patient is unresponsive and speechless but may open the eyes and appear to be able to track.

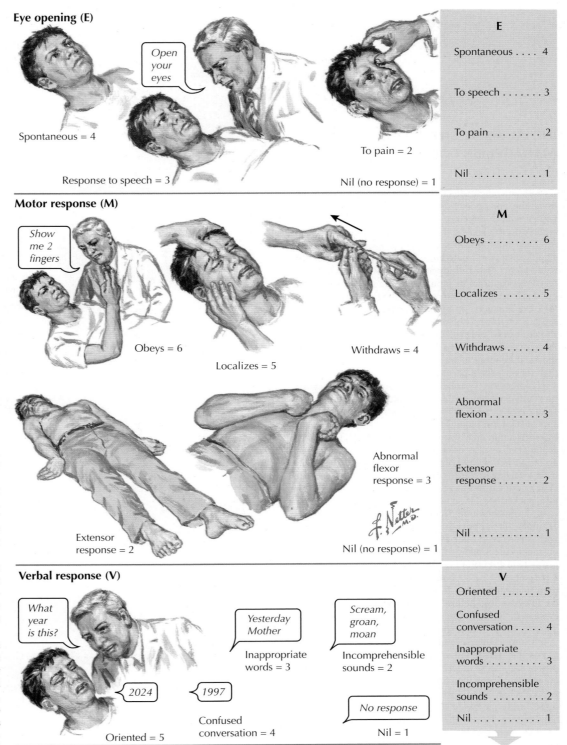

Eye opening (E)

Spontaneous = 4

Open your eyes

Response to speech = 3

To pain = 2

Nil (no response) = 1

E	
Spontaneous	4
To speech	3
To pain	2
Nil	1

Motor response (M)

Show me 2 fingers

Obeys = 6

Localizes = 5

Withdraws = 4

Abnormal flexor response = 3

Extensor response = 2

Nil (no response) = 1

f. Netter, M.D.

M	
Obeys	6
Localizes	5
Withdraws	4
Abnormal flexion	3
Extensor response	2
Nil	1

Verbal response (V)

What year is this?

2024   1997

Oriented = 5

Confused conversation = 4

Yesterday Mother

Inappropriate words = 3

Scream, groan, moan

Incomprehensible sounds = 2

No response

Nil = 1

V	
Oriented	5
Confused conversation	4
Inappropriate words	3
Incomprehensible sounds	2
Nil	1

Coma score (E + M + V) = 3 to 15

Plate 14.15

Brain: PART I

INITIAL ASSESSMENT AND MANAGEMENT OF HEAD INJURY

As with any potentially life-threatening injury, the airway, breathing, and circulation protocol takes precedence. In a patient who is comatose and whose airway has not been secured in the prehospital phase, intubation takes priority. Even brief episodes of hypoxia are associated with significantly worse outcomes. Rapid-sequence intubation using agents such as thiopental or propofol with a muscle relaxant is optimal in minimizing the risk of aspiration, but it also renders uninterpretable the findings on neurologic examination. Thus it is preferable that a reliable GCS score is established before intubation. Initial ventilation should aim to normalize PaO_2 at greater than 90% and PCO_2 at 35 to 40 mm Hg. Hyperventilation is not advised unless attempting to treat suspected increased ICP, and then for only short periods.

Hypotension (systolic BP < 90 mm Hg) may increase mortality markedly after head injury. Lactated Ringer solution or normal saline are the resuscitation fluids of choice. Glucose solutions should be avoided because hyperglycemia may worsen the outcome. Hypertonic saline (HS) is also used. Effective resuscitation can be accomplished with as little as 1 to 2 mL/kg, and HS may have a variety of neuroprotective effects. If an adequate systolic BP cannot be restored with 2 to 3 L of crystalloid, packed red blood cells should be given.

It is important to rigorously follow the Advanced Trauma Life Support guidelines. Up to 70% of patients with severe head injuries will have thoracic, abdominal, or major orthopedic injuries that may require more immediate attention than the head injury. On occasion, a patient may be so hemodynamically unstable as to require urgent thoracotomy, laparotomy, or endovascular intervention before the head injury can be fully evaluated. Simultaneous ICP monitoring during the ongoing intervention should be considered.

It is important to obtain a CT scan of the head as soon as possible during initial management to determine the degree and extent of structural damage to the brain and prepare for immediate operative intervention, if appropriate. When a large mass lesion or early evidence of significantly increased ICP (such as obliteration of the basal cisterns) is present, mannitol 0.5 to 1.0 mg/kg may be given to reduce ICP. However, mannitol may initiate diuresis that causes or exacerbates hypotension.

Additional problems are posed by patients taking anticoagulants or antiplatelet medications. If such a history cannot be elicited, an important component to the initial laboratory studies is determination of the international normalized ratio (INR) and clotting time. If the patient is on warfarin and has any evidence of traumatic intracranial bleeding, the INR must be corrected with vitamin K and fresh frozen plasma or prothrombin concentrate complex (PCC). Recombinant factor VIIa is often used for this purpose. Andexanet can be used for apixaban and rivaroxaban reversal. Dabigatran can be reversed with idarucizumab or PCC. Dealing with current antiplatelet agents is particularly problematic because platelet function may be impaired for up to 7 days. Platelet

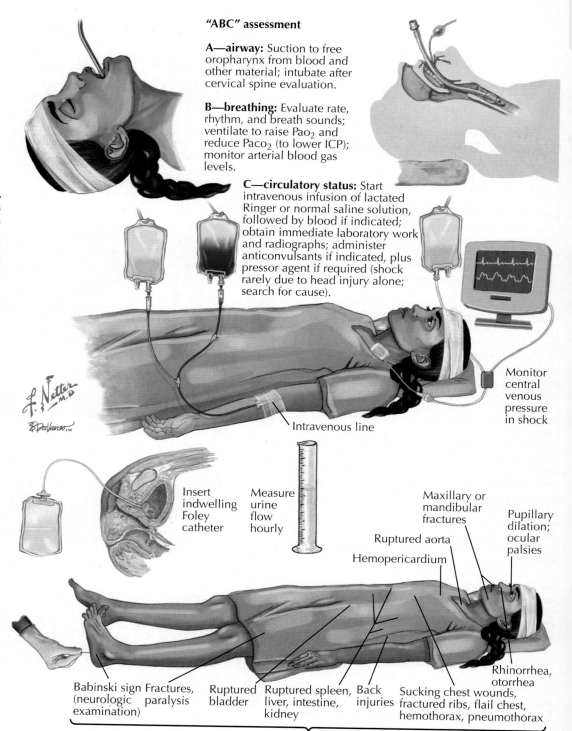

"ABC" assessment

A—airway: Suction to free oropharynx from blood and other material; intubate after cervical spine evaluation.

B—breathing: Evaluate rate, rhythm, and breath sounds; ventilate to raise PaO_2 and reduce $PaCO_2$ (to lower ICP); monitor arterial blood gas levels.

C—circulatory status: Start intravenous infusion of lactated Ringer or normal saline solution, followed by blood if indicated; obtain immediate laboratory work and radiographs; administer anticonvulsants if indicated, plus pressor agent if required (shock rarely due to head injury alone; search for cause).

Monitor central venous pressure in shock

Intravenous line

Insert indwelling Foley catheter

Measure urine flow hourly

Maxillary or mandibular fractures

Pupillary dilation; ocular palsies

Ruptured aorta

Hemopericardium

Rhinorrhea, otorrhea

Babinski sign (neurologic examination)

Fractures, paralysis

Ruptured bladder

Ruptured spleen, liver, intestine, kidney

Back injuries

Sucking chest wounds, fractured ribs, flail chest, hemothorax, pneumothorax

Conduct complete physical examination and repeat periodically

transfusions may be helpful. Desamino-D-arginine vasopressin (DDAVP) can be administered as well.

Unless a patient is on chronic steroid therapy, steroids are contraindicated as a treatment for head injury. Anticonvulsant prophylaxis should be initiated as soon as possible after severe head injury and maintained for 7 days unless the patient seizes. Phenytoin and levetiracetam are the most frequently used drugs for this purpose.

At some early point, the spine must be evaluated, as spinal injury occurs in more than 5% of patients with severe head injuries. Cervical immobilization must be maintained with a collar until structural injury to the

cervical spine is definitively excluded. It is important to remove a hard backboard as soon as possible, while maintaining the patient flat, to immobilize the thoracolumbar spine. Skin ischemia, potentially leading to decubiti, can begin after 30 minutes on a backboard, especially in patients who are hypotensive.

A plain radiograph of the spine, supplemented with CT scan, will rule out most bony injuries, but the possibility of a significant ligamentous injury remains. MRI within the first 24 to 48 hours of injury has been advocated as a reliable method of assessing for ligamentous damage, but many physicians prefer to leave a cervical collar in place until clinical assessment is complete.

Plate 14.16

Head Trauma

NEUROCRITICAL CARE AND MANAGEMENT AFTER TRAUMATIC BRAIN INJURY

Care of the patient with severe injuries is challenging and requires a team approach. Systemic and intracranial physiology may vary at different times. In 1996 the Brain Trauma Foundation, in conjunction with the American Association of Neurologic Surgeons, published the first evidence-based guidelines for the medical management of severe TBI, which are updated regularly.

The first priority in severe TBI is to establish complete and rapid physiologic resuscitation, which includes a secure airway and maintenance of O_2 saturation of greater than 90% and arterial systolic pressure greater than 90 mm Hg. If not already performed, endotracheal intubation should be undertaken in any patient with a GCS score less than 9 or one who remains hypoxic despite supplemental oxygen. It is routine to place an arterial line for continuous BP recording. Central or Swan Ganz lines may be helpful in guiding fluid resuscitation. The optimal resuscitation and maintenance intravenous fluids have been discussed earlier.

Once the patient is medically and surgically stabilized, the next priority is to establish ICP monitoring in those with a GCS score less than 9 who have abnormal CT scans. ICP monitoring is also important in patients who are comatose with normal CT scans if two of the following are present: age greater than 40 years, systolic BP less than 90 mm Hg, or presence of unilateral or bilateral motor posturing.

There are various devices for ICP monitoring. The intraventricular catheter is considered the gold standard and allows for the drainage of CSF when ICP is elevated. However, placement of a ventricular catheter may be difficult in the swollen and/or shifted brain, and a variety of parenchymal monitors may serve as reasonable substitutes.

Brain oxygen saturation (PBO_2) level is being increasingly monitored in severe TBI; however, its true usefulness is unclear. Early information suggests that a PBO_2 less than 20 mm Hg may be associated with worse outcomes, but it is unclear whether this represents the severity of the underlying brain injury or a potentially treatable secondary injury.

Less commonly used is cerebral microdialysis, which can measure a variety of neurotransmitters and metabolites, such as glutamate, aspartate, and lactate. It is likewise unclear how information obtained in this way will play a role in the institution of a specific therapy.

The central tenet of severe TBI management is control of ICP and, by extension, cerebral perfusion pressure (CPP). CPP is the mean arterial pressure minus the ICP and is the driver of cerebral blood flow. As has been noted, persistently elevated ICP (>20 mm Hg) is associated with significant mortality. An optimal CPP is generally in the range of 60 to 70 mm Hg.

DEVICES FOR MONITORING INTRACRANIAL PRESSURE

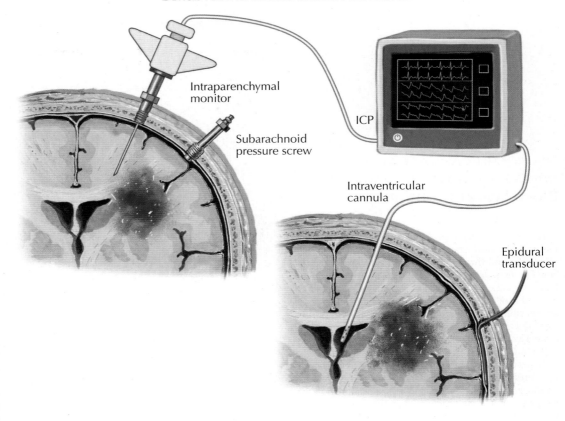

Intraparenchymal monitor

Subarachnoid pressure screw

ICP

Intraventricular cannula

Epidural transducer

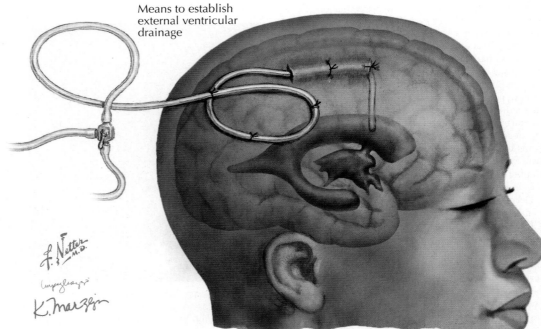

Means to establish external ventricular drainage

First-line therapies for ICP control include sedation, paralysis, head-of-bed elevation to 20 to 30 degrees, and avoidance of hyperthermia (>38.5°C).

Mannitol is the most commonly used pharmacologic agent to lower ICP. The primary action of mannitol is in inducing an osmotic gradient between plasma and cells, thus drawing edema fluid from the brain into the circulation. This causes an expansion of blood volume and a potential elevation in BP but ultimately results in a diuresis that may lower BP. Secondary effects of mannitol include a reduction in blood viscosity, which increases cerebral blood and cerebral oxygen delivery. Effective doses of mannitol range from 0.25 to 1 g/kg and lead to ICP reduction within 15 to 30 minutes.

Because mannitol is an osmotic diuretic, it is excreted entirely by the kidneys and thus should be used with caution in patients with renal failure. It is important to monitor serum sodium and osmolality and limit use if serum sodium is elevated to greater than 155 mEq/L or osmolality is greater than 320 mOsm/L.

Plate 14.17

Brain: PART I

DECOMPRESSIVE CRANIECTOMY

Increased intracranial pressure refractory to medical management

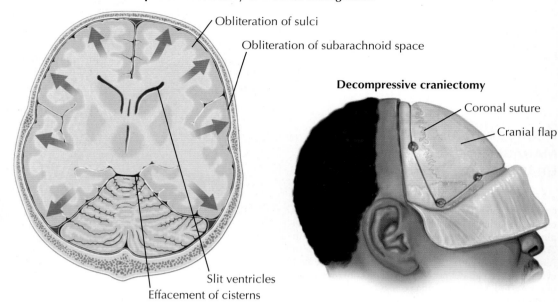

- Obliteration of sulci
- Obliteration of subarachnoid space
- Slit ventricles
- Effacement of cisterns

Decompressive craniectomy

- Coronal suture
- Cranial flap

NEUROCRITICAL CARE AND MANAGEMENT AFTER TRAUMATIC BRAIN INJURY (Continued)

HS (3%) is increasingly being used to treat intracranial hypertension. Its mechanism of action is clearance of edema fluid through bulk flow. Additional potential benefits include immunomodulation—prevention of leukocyte adherence and release of prostaglandins—and inhibition of excitotoxity. Typically, administered doses are intermittent boluses of 250 mL or a continuous infusion of 1 mL/kg/hr. As with mannitol, use should be limited if serum sodium exceeds 155 mEq/L or osmolality of 320 mOsm/L.

Hyperventilation can rapidly decrease ICP by causing vasoconstriction and reducing intracranial blood volume. Prolonged prophylactic hyperventilation was previously a mainstay of ICP management but has been found to worsen outcome, probably by inducing ischemia. Currently, it is recommended that hyperventilation should only be used for short periods and that P_{CO_2} be kept above 30 mm Hg.

If the ICP is uncontrollable despite these measures, high-dose barbiturate therapy may be necessary. This suppresses metabolism and lessens cerebral blood-flow requirements. The patient must, however, be hemodynamically stable because barbiturates can have a direct cardiac depressant effect. Pentobarbital is the barbiturate most commonly used. A typical loading dose is 10 mg/kg over 30 minutes, followed by 5 mg/kg hourly for three doses, with a maintenance dose of 1 mg/kg/hr. Continuous electroencephalographic monitoring is necessary, as the goal of therapy is to induce burst suppression.

Decompressive craniectomy (DC) has come to supplant barbiturates as the "final" treatment for intractable ICP elevations. Originally introduced in the 1960s, the procedure fell out of favor because, although mortality was lowered after severe TBI, the quality of survival was unchanged. The procedure involves removal of large portions of the skull in an attempt to control ICP. Over the past decade, numerous published articles on DC have used different ICP-based criteria for undergoing the procedure, such as ICP greater than 20 mm Hg for more than 30 minutes or ICP greater than 30 mm Hg for more than 20 minutes. However, DC is also performed frequently as part of the treatment of ASDH. Regardless of the criteria used, there is a direct correlation between the amount of bone removed and the ability to control ICP. There is a less than 40% reduction in ICP if bone removal is less than 8000 mm³ and greater than 80% reduction with removal of more than 12,000 mm³.

The DC may be unilateral or bilateral. When unilateral, bone is removed from the supraorbital ridge anteriorly to the inion posteriorly, superiorly to within 1 cm of the superior sagittal sinus, and inferiorly to the floor of the temporal fossa. Bilateral DC is typically bifrontal

After bifrontal craniectomy

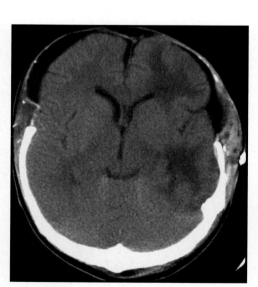

CT appearance after extensive bifrontal craniectomy for ICP control. Note that all of the cranial bone from the coronal suture forward has been removed.

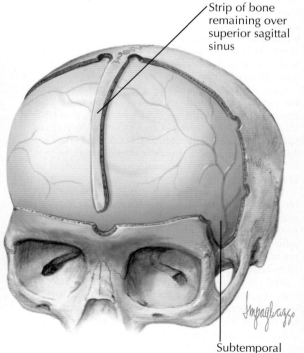

- Strip of bone remaining over superior sagittal sinus
- Subtemporal decompression

from the supraorbital ridge to behind the coronal suture (including a generous subtemporal decompression), leaving a 1-cm strip of bone over the superior sagittal sinus. The bone is saved for later replacement either by implantation into an abdominal subcutaneous pocket or by freezing. It is typically replaced within 1 to 3 months. Some advocate replacement of the bone before hospital discharge to minimize the risk of infection, especially if the bone has been implanted, and other complications associated with DC. More than 20% of patients will

develop symptomatic hydrocephalus or subdural hygromas after DC. This is related in part to the brain being exposed to atmospheric pressure once the ICP has normalized.

A recent metaanalysis of all published trials to date concluded that secondary DC, performed as a treatment for either early or late refractory ICP elevation, is suggested to reduce ICP and duration of intensive care, although the relationship between these effects and favorable outcome is uncertain.

Section 1: Normal and Abnormal Development

American Psychiatric Association. *Diagnostic and Statistical Manual of Mental Disorders (DSM-4-TR). Text Revision*. 4th ed. American Psychiatric Association; 2000.
Lord C, Bishop SL. Autism spectrum disorders: diagnosis, prevalence and services for children and families. *Soc Policy Rep*. 2010;24:1-21.
Park TS, Ghatan S, Scott RM. Pediatrics. In: Winn HR, ed. *Youmans Neurological Surgery*. vol 2. 6th ed. Elsevier; 2011:1861-2358.
Scarpinato N, Bradley J, Kurbjun K, Bateman X, Holtzer B, Ely B. Caring for the child with an autism spectrum disorder in the acute care setting. *J Spec Pediatr Nurs*. 2010;15:244-254.
Strock M. *Autism Spectrum Disorders (Pervasive Developmental Disorders)*. NIH publication no. NIH-04-5511. Bethesda, MD: National Institute of Mental Health, National Institutes of Health, U.S. Department of Health and Human Services; 2004. Available at: https://www.nimh.nih.gov/health/publications/autism-spectrum-disorder

Section 2: Cerebral Cortex and Neurocognitive Disorders

Bonelli RM, Cummings JL. Frontal-subcortical dementias. *Neurologist*. 2008;14:100-107.
Burns JM, Morris JC, eds. *Early Diagnosis and Treatment of Mild Cognitive Impairment*. Wiley Press; 2008.
Burns JM, Swerdlow RH. Right orbitofrontal tumor presenting as pedophilia symptom and constructional apraxia sign. *Arch Neurol*. 2003;60:437-440.
Gorno-Tempini ML, Hillis AE, Weintraub S. Classification of primary progressive aphasia and its variants. *Neurology*. 2011;76:1006-1014.
Kandel ER. The biology of memory: a forty-year retrospective. *J Neurosci*. 2009;294:12748-12756.
McKeel DW, Burns JM, Meuser TM, Morris JC, eds. *Dementia, An Atlas of Investigation and Diagnosis*. Clinical Publishing; 2007.
McKeith IG, Boeve BF, Dickson DW, et al. Diagnosis and management of dementia with Lewy bodies: Fourth consensus report of the DLB Consortium. *Neurology*. 2017;89(1):88-100.
Mesulam MM, edr. *Principles of Behavioral and Cognitive Neurology*. Oxford University Press; 2000.
Swerdlow RH, Anderson H, Burns JM. Alzheimer's disease. In: Kreutzer JS, DeLuca J, Caplan B, editors. *Encyclopedia of clinical neuropsychology*. Springer; 2011:105-110.

Section 3: Epilepsy

Berg AT, Berkovic SF, Brodie MJ, et al. Revised terminology and concepts for organization of seizures and epilepsies: report of the ILAE Commission on Classification and Terminology, 2005–2009. *Epilepsia*. 2010;51:676-685.
Berkovic SF. Epilepsy: insights into causes and treatment dilemmas. *Lancet Neurol*. 2010;9:9-11.
Engel Jr J. A practical guide for routine EEG studies in epilepsy. *J Clin Neurophysiol*. 1984;1:109-142.
Gorji A, Speckmann EJ. Epileptiform EEG spikes and their functional significance. *Clin EEG Neurosci*. 2009;40:230-233.
Kossoff EH, Zupec-Kania BA, Amark PE, et al. Optimal c linical management of children receiving the ketogenic diet: recommendations of the International Ketogenic Diet Study Group. *Epilepsia*. 2009;50:304-317.
McNamara JO. Cellular and molecular basis of epilepsy. *J Neurosci*. 1994;14:3413-3425.
Neville BG, Chin RF, Scott RC. Childhood convulsive status epilepticus: epidemiology, management and outcome. *Acta Neurol Scand Suppl*. 2007;186:21-24.
Obeid M, Wyllie E, Rahi AC, Mikati MA. Approach to pediatric epilepsy surgery: state of the art, part I: general principles and presurgical workup. *Eur J Paediatr Neurol*. 2009;13:102-114.
Obeid M, Wyllie E, Rahi AC, Mikati MA. Approach to pediatric epilepsy surgery: state of the art, part II: approach to specific epilepsy syndromes and etiologies. *Eur J Paediatr Neurol*. 2009;13:115-127.
Pitkanen A, Lukasiuk K. Mechanisms of epileptogenesis and potential treatment targets. *Lancet Neurol*. 2011;10:173-186.
Rogawski MA, Loscher W. The neurobiology of antiepileptic drugs. *Nat Rev Neurosci*. 2004;5:553-564.
Scharfman HE. The neurobiology of epilepsy. *Curr Neurol Neurosci Rep*. 2007;7:348-354.
Shewmon DA. What is a neonatal seizure? Problems in definition and quantification for investigative and clinical purposes. *J Clin Neurophysiol*. 1990;7:315-368.
Shields WD. Catastrophic epilepsy in childhood. *Epilepsia*. 2000;41(suppl 2):S2-S6.
Shorvon S, ed. *Status Epilepticus: Its Clinical Features and Treatment in Children and Adults*. Cambridge University Press; 2006.
Spencer S, Huh L. Outcomes of epilepsy surgery in adults and children. *Lancet Neurol*. 2008;7:525-537.
Spreafico R, Blumcke I. Focal cortical dysplasias: clinical implication of neuropathological classification systems. *Acta Neuropathol*. 2010;120:359-367.
Stockler-Ipsiroglu S, Plecko B. Metabolic epilepsies: approaches to a diagnostic challenge. *Can J Neurol Sci*. 2009;36(suppl 2):S67-S72.
Wiebe S, Blume WT, Girvin JP, Eliasziw M. A randomized, controlled trial of surgery for temporal-lobe epilepsy. *N Engl J Med*. 2001;345: 311-318.
Wyllie E, Cascino GD, Gidal BE, Goodkin HP, eds. *Wyllie's Treatment of Epilepsy: Principles and Practice*. Lippincott Williams & Wilkins; 2010.

Section 4: Psychiatry

Limbic System

Catani M, Dell'acqua F, Thiebaut de Schotten M. A revised limbic system model for memory, emotion and behaviour. *Neurosci Biobehav Rev*. 2013;37(8):1724-1737.
Rolls ET. Limbic systems for emotion and for memory, but no single limbic system. *Cortex*. 2015;62:119-157.
Vogt BA. Cingulate cortex in the three limbic subsystems. *Handb Clin Neurol*. 2019;166:39-51.

Major Depressive Disorder

American Psychiatric Association. *Diagnostic and Statistical Manual of Mental Disorders (DSM-5)*. 5th ed. American Psychiatric Association; 2013.
Hasin DS, Sarvet AL, Meyers JL, et al. Epidemiology of adult DSM-5 major depressive disorder and its specifiers in the United States. *JAMA Psychiatry*. 2018;75(4):336-346.

Depression/Bipolar Disorder

Bergink V, Rasgon N, Wisner KL. Postpartum psychosis: madness, mania, and melancholia in motherhood. *Am J Psychiatry*. 2016; 173(12):1179-1188.
Di Florio A, Mei Kay Yang J, Crawford K, et al. Post-partum psychosis and its association with bipolar disorder in the UK: a case-control study using polygenic risk scores. *Lancet Psychiatry*. 2021;8(12): 1045-1052.
Zorumski CF, Paul SM, Covey DF, Mennerick S. Neurosteroids as novel antidepressants and anxiolytics: GABA-A receptors and beyond. *Neurobiol Stress*. 2019;11:100196.

Bipolar Disorder

McIntyre RS, Berk M, Brietzke E, et al. Bipolar disorders. *Lancet*. 2020;396:1841-1856.
Merikangas KR, Jin R, He JP, et al. Prevalence and correlates of bipolar spectrum disorder in the world mental health survey initiative. *Arch Gen Psychiatry*. 2011;68:241-251.
Philips ML, Swartz HA. A critical appraisal of neuroimaging studies of bipolar disorder: toward a new conceptualization of underlying neural circuitry and a road map for future research. *Am J Psychiatry*. 2014;171:821-843.
Stahl EA, Breen G, Forstner AJ, et al. Genome-wide association study identifies 30 loci associated with bipolar disorder. *Nat Genet*. 2019;51:793-803.

Generalized Anxiety Disorder

American Psychiatric Association. *Diagnostic and Statistical Manual of Mental Disorders (DSM-5)*. 5th ed. American Psychiatric Association; 2013.
Ruscio AM, Hallion LS, Lim CCW, et al. Cross-sectional comparison of the epidemiology of DSM-5 generalized anxiety disorder across the globe. *JAMA Psychiatry*. 2017;74(5):465-475.

Posttraumatic Stress

American Psychiatric Association. *Diagnostic and Statistical Manual of Mental Disorders (DSM-5)*. 5th ed. American Psychiatric Association; 2013.
Pai A, Suris AM, North, CS. Posttraumatic stress disorder in the DSM-5: Controversy, change, and conceptual considerations. *Behav Sci (Basel)*. 2017;7(1):7.
U.S. Department of Health and Human Services, National Institutes of Health, National Institute of Mental Health. *Post-traumatic Stress Disorder*. 2019. Available at: https://www.nimh.nih.gov/health/topics/post-traumatic-stress-disorder-ptsd.

Obsessive-Compulsive Disorder

Dantzer R, O'Connor JC, Freund GG, Johnson RW, Kelley KW. From inflammation to sickness and depression: when the immune system subjugates the brain. *Nat Rev Neurosci*. 2008;9:46-56.
Dougherty DD, Brennan BP, Stewart SE, Wilhelm S, Widge AS, Rauch SL. Neuroscientifically informed formulation and treatment planning for patients with obsessive-compulsive disorder: a review. *JAMA Psychiatry*. 2018;75(10):1081-1087.
Jenike MA. Clinical practice. Obsessive-compulsive disorder. *N Engl J Med*. 2004;350:259-265.
Ruscio AM, Stein DJ, Chiu WT, Kessler RC. The epidemiology of obsessive-compulsive disorder in the National Comorbidity Survey Replication. *Mol Psychiatry*. 2010;15:53-63.

Schizophrenia

Brown AS, Derkits EJ. Prenatal infection and schizophrenia: a review of epidemiologic and translational studies. *Am J Psychiatry*. 2010;167:261-280.
Fusar-Poli P, Salazar de Pablo G, Correll CU, et al. Prevention of psychosis: advances in detection, prognosis, and intervention. *JAMA Psychiatry*. 2020;77(7):755-765.
Howes OD, Kapur S. The dopamine hypothesis of schizophrenia: version III—the final common pathway. *Schizophrenia Bull*. 2009;35:549-562.

Addiction

Amato L, Minozzi S, Davoli M. Efficacy and safety of pharmacological interventions for the treatment of the alcohol withdrawal syndrome. *Cochrane Database Syst Rev*. 2011;(6):CD008537.
Global Status Report on Alcohol and Health 2018. World Health Organization; 2018. https://www.who.int/publications/i/item/9789241565639
Knox J, Scodes J, Witkiewitz K, et al; Alcohol Clinical Trials (ACTIVE) Workgroup. Reduction in world health organization risk drinking levels and cardiovascular disease. *Alcohol Clin Exp Res*. 2020;44(8):1625-1635.
Rockett IRH, Caine ED, Banerjee A, et al. Fatal self-injury in the United States, 1999-2018: unmasking a national mental health crisis. *EClinicalMedicine*. 2021;32:100741.
Substance Abuse and Mental Health Services Administration. Key substance use and mental health indicators in the United States: Results from the 2020 National Survey on Drug Use and Health (HHS Publication No. PEP21-07-01-003, NSDUH Series H-56). Center for Behavioral Health Statistics and Quality, Substance Abuse and Mental Health Services Administration; 2021. Available at: https://www.samhsa.gov/data/.
Weiss RD, Rao V. The Prescription Opioid Addiction Treatment Study: what have we learned. *Drug Alcohol Depend*. 2017;173 (suppl 1):S48-S54.

Somatoform/Conversion Disorders

Beutel ME, Wiltink J, Ghaemi Kerahrodi J, et al. Somatic symptom load in men and women from middle to high age in the Gutenberg Health Study—association with psychosocial and somatic factors. *Sci Rep*. 2019;9(1):4610.
Donnachie E, Schneider A, Enck P. Comorbidities of patients with functional somatic syndromes before, during and after first diagnosis: a population-based study using bavarian routine data. *Sci Rep*. 2020;10(1):9810.
Harvey AG, Tang NKY. (Mis)perception of sleep in insomnia: a puzzle and a resolution. *Psychol Bull*. 2012;138(1):77-101.
Henningsen P. Management of somatic symptom disorder. *Dialogues Clin Neurosci*. 2018;20(1):23-31.
Leaviss J, Davis S, Ren S, et al. Behavioural modification interventions for medically unexplained symptoms in primary care: systematic reviews and economic evaluation. *Health Technol Assess*. 2020;24(46):1-490.
Okur Güney ZE, Sattel H, Witthöft M, Henningsen P. Emotion regulation in patients with somatic symptom and related disorders: a systematic review. *PLoS One*. 2019;14(6):e0217277.

Conversion Disorder

Ali S, Jabeen S, Pate RJ, et al. Conversion disorder: mind versus body: a review. *Innov Clin Neurosci*. 2015;12(5-6):27-33.
Canna M, Seligman R. Dealing with the unknown. Functional neurological disorder (FND) and the conversion of cultural meaning. *Soc Sci Med*. 2020;246:112725.
Ejareh Dar M, Kanaan RA. Uncovering the etiology of conversion disorder: insights from functional neuroimaging. *Neuropsychiatr Dis Treat*. 2016;12:143-153.

Intimate Partner Violence

Domestic Violence National Statistics. NCADV: National Coalition Against Domestic Violence; 2015. Available at: https://www.ncadv.org/statistics.
Messing JT, Campbell JC, Snider C. Validation and adaptation of the Danger Assessment-5: A brief intimate partner violence risk assessment. *J Adv Nurs*. 2017;73(12):3220-3230.

Abuse in Later Life

Acierno R, Hernandez MA, Amstadter AB, et al. Prevalence and correlates of emotional, physical, sexual, and financial abuse and potential neglect in the United States: the National Elder Mistreatment Study. *Am J Public Health*. 2010;100(2):292-297.
Domestic Violence National Statistics. NCADV: National Coalition Against Domestic Violence; 2015. Available at: https://www.ncadv.org/statistics.
McGarry J, Ali P, Hinchliff S. Older women, intimate partner violence and mental health: a consideration of the particular issues for health and healthcare practice. *J Clin Nurs*. 2017;26(15-16):2177-2191.

Yon Y, Mikton CR, Gassoumis ZD, Wilber KH. Elder abuse prevalence in community settings: a systematic review and meta-analysis. *Lancet Glob Health.* 2017;5(2):e147-e156.

Yon Y, Ramiro-Gonzalez M, Mikton CR, Huber M, Sethi D. The prevalence of elder abuse in institutional settings: a systematic review and meta-analysis. *Eur J Public Health.* 2019;29(1):58-67.

Child Psychiatry

American Academy of Child and Adolescent Psychiatry. Practice parameter for the assessment and treatment of children and adolescents with attention-deficit/hyperactivity disorder. *J Am Acad Child Adolesc Psychiatry.* 2007;46:894-921.

American Academy of Child and Adolescent Psychiatry. Practice parameter for the assessment and treatment of children and adolescents with depressive disorders. *J Am Acad Child Adolesc Psychiatry.* 2007;46:1503-1526.

American Academy of Child and Adolescent Psychiatry. Practice parameter for the assessment and treatment of children and adolescents with oppositional defiant disorder. *J Am Acad of Child Adolesc Psychiatry.* 2007;46:126-141.

Posner J, Polanczyk GV, Sonuga-Barke E. Attention-deficit hyperactivity disorder. *Lancet.* 2020;395(10222):450-462.

Borg KB, Hodes DH. G71(P) beyond risk management in child sexual abuse: Understanding a resilience-based approach. *Arch Dis Child.* 2017;102:A29-A30.

Bruno A, Celebre L, Torre G, et al. Focus on Disruptive Mood Dysregulation Disorder: A review of the literature. *Psychiatry Res.* 2019;279:323-330.

CAPTA Reauthorization Act of 2010 (P.L. 111-320), 42 U.S.C. § 5101, Note (§ 3). Available at: http://www.congress.gov/111/crpt/srpt378/CRPT-111srpt378.pdf.

Cash RE, Valley-Gray S, Worton S, Newman A. Evidence-based interventions for persistent depressive disorder in children and adolescents. In: Theodore LA, ed. *Handbook of Evidence-Based Interventions for Children and Adolescents.* Springer; 2017:301-311.

Kimber M, MacMillan HL. Child Psychological Abuse. *Pediatr Rev.* 2017;38(10):496-498.

Marques L, Alegria M, Becker AE, et al. Comparative prevalence, correlates of impairment, and service utilization for eating disorders across U.S. ethnic groups: Implications for reducing ethnic disparities in health care access for eating disorders. *Int J Eat Disord.* 2011;44:412-420.

Merikangas KR, He JP, Burstein M, et al. Lifetime prevalence of mental disorders in US adolescents: results from the National Comorbidity Survey Replication-Adolescent Supplement (NCS-A). *J Am Acad Child Adolesc Psychiatry.* 2010;49(10):980-989.

Merry SN, Hetrick SE, Cox GR, et al. Cochrane review: psychological and educational interventions for preventing depression in children and adolescents. *Evid Based Child Health.* 2012;7(5):1409-1685.

Mondale WF, Sargent J, Hanson RF, Reece RM. *Treatment of Child Abuse: Common Ground for Mental Health, Medical, and Legal Practitioners.* 2nd ed. Baltimore: Johns Hopkins University Press; 2014.

Rosen DS. American Academy of Pediatrics Committee on Adolescence. Identification and management of eating disorders in children and adolescents. *Pediatrics.* 2010;126:1240-1253.

Stice E, Gau JM, Rohde P, Shaw H. Risk factors that predict future onset of each DSM-5 eating disorder: Predictive specificity in high-risk adolescent females. *J Abnorm Psychol.* 2016;126:38-51.

Strawn JR, Lu L, Peris TS, Levine A, Walkup JT. Research review: pediatric anxiety disorders—what have we learnt in the last 10 years? *J Child Psychol Psychiatry.* 2021;62(2):114-139.

Sukhodolsky DG, Smith SD, McCauley SA, Ibrahim K, Piasecka JB. Behavioral interventions for anger, irritability, and aggression in children and adolescents. *J Child Adolesc Psychopharmacol.* 2016;26(1):58-64.

Wilens TE, Spencer TJ. Understanding Attention-Deficit/Hyperactivity Disorder from Childhood to Adulthood. *Postgrad Med.* 2010;122(5):97-109.

Vasa, Roma A, Krain Roy A. *Pediatric Anxiety Disorders: A Clinical Guide.* Springer; 2013.

Walter HJ, Bukstein OG, Abright AR, et al. Clinical practice guideline for the assessment and treatment of children and adolescents with anxiety disorders. *J Am Acad Child Adolesc Psychiatry.* 2020;59;10:1107-1124.

Section 5: Hypothalamus, Pituitary, Sleep, and Thalamus

Abbott SB, Machado NL, Geerling JC, Saper CB. Reciprocal control of drinking behavior by median preoptic neurons in mice. *J Neurosci.* 2016;36:8228-8237.

Adamantidis AR, Schmidt MH, Carter ME, Burdakov D, Peyron, Scammell TE. A circuit perspective on narcolepsy. *Sleep.* 2020;43:1-9.

Barion A, Zee PC. A clinical approach to circadian rhythm sleep disorders. *Sleep Med.* 2007;8:566-577.

Burstein R. Somatosensory and visceral input to the hypothalamus and limbic system. *Prog Brain Res.* 1996;107:257-267.

Fontes MA, Xavier CH, de Menezes RC, Dimicco JA. The dorsomedial hypothalamus and the central pathways involved in the cardiovascular response to emotional stress. *Neuroscience.* 2011;184:64-74.

Gautron L, Elmquist JK, Williams KW. Neural control of energy balance: translating circuits to therapies. *Cell.* 2015;161:133-145.

Machado NLS, Bandaru SS, Abbott SBG, Saper CB. EP3R-Expressing glutamatergic neurons mediate inflammatory fever. *J Neurosci.* 2020;40:2573-2588.

Nunn N, Womack M, Dart C, Barrett-Jolley R. Function and pharmacology of spinally-projecting sympathetic pre-autonomic neurones in the paraventricular nucleus of the hypothalamus. *Curr Neuropharmacol.* 2011;9:262-277.

Saper CB. The hypothalamus. In: Mai JK, Paxinos G, eds. *The Human Nervous System.* 3rd ed. Academic Press; 2012.

Saper CB, Chou TC, Elmquist JK. The need to feed: homeostatic and hedonic control of eating. *Neuron.* 2002;36:199-211.

Saper CB, Machado NLS. Flipping the switch on the body's thermoregulatory system. *Nature.* 2020;583:34-36.

Saper CB, Scammell TE, Lu J. Hypothalamic regulation of sleep and circadian rhythms. *Nature.* 2005;437:1257-1263.

Scammell TE. The neurobiology, diagnosis, and treatment of narcolepsy. *Ann Neurol.* 2003;53:154-166.

Scammell TE, Arrigoni E. Lipton JO. Neural circuitry of wakefulness and sleep. *Neuron.* 2017;93:747-765.

Todd WD, Fenselau H, Wang JL, et al. A hypothalamic circuit for the circadian control of aggression. *Nat Neurosci.* 2018;21:717-724.

Section 6: Disorders of Consciousness (Coma)

Booth CM, Boone RH, Tomlinson G, Detsky AS. Is this patient dead, vegetative, or severely neurologically impaired? Assessing outcome for comatose survivors of cardiac arrest. *JAMA.* 2004;291:870-879.

Giacino JT, Katz DI, Schiff ND, et al. Practice guideline update recommendations summary: Disorders of consciousness: Report of the guideline development, dissemination, and implementation subcommittee of the American Academy of Neurology; the American Congress of Rehabilitation Medicine; and the National Institute on Disability, Independent Living, and Rehabilitation Research. *Neurology.* 2018;91:450-460.

Greer DM. Determination of brain death. *N Engl J Med.* 2021;385:2554-2561.

Greer DM, Shemie SD, Lewis A, et al. Determination of brain death/death by neurologic criteria: the World Brain Death Project. *JAMA.* 2020;324:1078-1097.

Jennett B. *The Vegetative State: Medical Facts, Ethical and Legal Dilemmas.* Cambridge University Press; 2002.

Medical aspects of the persistent vegetative state. The Multi-Society Task Force on PVS. *N Engl J Med.* 1994;330:1499-1508.

Nakagawa TA, Ashwal S, Mathur M, Mysore M. Clinical report: guidelines for the determination of brain death in infants and children: an update of the 1987 task force recommendations. *Pediatrics.* 2011;128:e720-e740.

Posner JB, Saper CB, Schiff ND, Claassen J. *Plum and Posner's Diagnosis and Treatment of Stupor and Coma.* 5th ed. Oxford University Press; 2019.

Teasdale G, Jennett B. Assessment of coma and impaired consciousness: a practical scale. *Lancet.* 1974;2:81-84.

Teasdale G, Maas A, Lecky F, Manley G, Stocchetti N, Murray G. The Glasgow Coma Scale at 40 years: standing the test of time. *Lancet Neurol.* 2014;13:844-854.

Thibaut A, Bodien YG, Laureys S, Giacino JT. Minimally conscious state "plus": diagnostic criteria and relation to functional recovery. *J Neurol.* 2020;267:1245-1254.

Topjian AA, de Caen A, Wainwright MS, et al. Pediatric post-cardiac arrest care: a scientific statement from the American Heart Association. *Circulation.* 2019;140:e194-e233.

Van Erp WS, Lavrijsen JCM, Vos PE, Laureys S, Koopmans RTCM. Unresponsive wakefulness syndrome: outcomes from a vicious circle. *Ann Neurol.* 2020;87:12-18.

Wijdicks EFM. *Brain Death.* 3rd ed. Oxford University Press; 2017.

Wijdicks EFM. *The Comatose Patient.* 2nd ed. Oxford University Press; 2014.

Wijdicks EFM, Bamlet WR, Maramattom BV, Manno EM, McClelland RL. Validation of a new coma scale: the four score. *Ann Neurol.* 2005;58:585-593.

Section 7: Basal Ganglia and Movement Disorders

Parkinsonism

Galvez-Jimenez N, ed. *Scientific Basis for the Treatment of Parkinson's Disease.* 2nd ed. Taylor & Francis; 2005.

Galvez-Jimenez N, Tuite P, eds. *Unusual Causes of Movement Disorders.* Cambridge University Press; 2011.

Jankovic J, Tolosa E, eds. *Parkinson's Disease and Movement Disorders.* 5th ed. Lippincott Williams & Wilkins; 2007.

Tarsy D, Vitek J, Lozano LM, eds. *Surgical Treatment of Parkinson's Disease and Other Movement Disorders.* Humana Press; 2003.

Dystonia

Bressman SB, de Leon D, Kramer PL, et al. Dystonia in Ashkenazi Jews: clinical characterization of a founder mutation. *Ann Neurol.* 1994;36:771-777. Erratum *Ann Neurol.* 1995;37:140.

Brin MF, Comella C, Jankovic J, eds. *Dystonia: Etiology, Clinical Features, and Treatment.* Lippincott Williams & Wilkins; 2004.

Epidemiological Study of Dystonia in Europe (ESDE) Collaborative Group. A prevalence study of primary dystonia in eight European countries. *J Neurol Neurosurg Psychiatry.* 2000;247:787-792.

Tarsy D, Simon DK. Dystonia. *N Engl J Med.* 2006;355:818-829.

Chorea/Ballism

Walker FO. Huntington's disease. *Lancet.* 2007;369:218-228.

Walker R, ed. *The Differential Diagnosis of Chorea.* Oxford University Press; 2011.

Zomorrodi A, Wald ER. Sydenham's chorea in western Pennsylvania. *Pediatrics.* 2006;117:e675-e679.

Tremor

Fahn S, Jankovic J, Hallett M, eds. *Principles and Practice of Movement Disorders.* 2nd ed. Saunders; 2011.

Koller WC, Busenbark K, Miner K. The relationship of essential tremor to other movement disorders: report on 678 patients. Essential Tremor Study Group. *Ann Neurol.* 1994;35:717-723.

Lemon RN, Edgley SA. Life without a cerebellum. *Brain.* 2010;133 (Pt 3):652-654.

Tics and Tourette Syndrome

Cohen DJ, Jankovik J, Goetz CG, eds. *Tourette Syndrome. Advances in Neurology.* vol 85. Lippincott Williams & Wilkins; 2001.

Lees AJ, ed. *Tics and Related Disorders.* Churchill Livingstone; 1985.

Singer H, Mink JW, Gilbert DL, Jankovik J, eds. *Movement Disorders in Childhood.* Saunders; 2010.

Myoclonus

Fahn S, Jankovic J, Hallett M, eds. *Principles and Practice of Movement Disorders.* 2nd ed. Saunders; 2011.

Galvez-Jimenez N, Tuite P, eds. *Unusual Causes of Movement Disorders.* Cambridge University Press; 2011.

Koenig MA, Geocadin R. Global hypoxia-ischemia and critical care seizures. In: Varelas P, ed. *Seizures in Critical Care: A Guide to Diagnosis and Therapeutics: Current Clinical Neurology.* 2nd ed. Humana Press; 2010:157-178.

Lance JW, Adams RD. The syndrome of intention or action myoclonus as a sequel to hypoxic encephalopathy. *Brain.* 1963;86:111-136.

Wilson Disease

El-Youssef M. Wilson disease. *Mayo Clin Proc.* 2003;78:1126-1136.

Liebeskind DS, Wong S, Hamilton RH. Faces of the giant panda and her cub: MRI correlates of Wilson's disease. *J Neurol Neurosurg Psychiatry.* 2003;74:682.

Cerebral Palsy

Ashwal S, Russman BS, Blasco PA, et al. Practice parameter: diagnostic assessment of the child with cerebral palsy: report of the Quality Standards Subcommittee of the American Academy of Neurology and the Practice Committee of the Child Neurology Society. *Neurology.* 2004;62:851-863.

Mutch L, Alberman E, Hagberg B, Kodama K, Perat MV. Cerebral palsy epidemiology: where are we now and where are we going? *Dev Med Child Neurol.* 1992;34:547-551.

Section 8: Cerebellum and Ataxia

Anheim M, Tranchant C, Koenig M. The autosomal recessive cerebellar ataxias. *N Engl J Med.* 2012;366(7):636-646.

Boltshauser E, Schmahmann JD, eds. *Cerebellar Disorders in Children. Clinics in Developmental Medicine No. 191–2.* MacKeith Press; 2012.

Brice A, Pulst SM, eds. *Spinocerebellar Degenerations: The Ataxias and Spastic Paraplegias: Blue Books of Neurology Series, vol 31.* Butterworth-Heinemann; 2007.

Buckner RL, Krienen FM, Castellanos A, Diaz JC, Yeo BT. The organization of the human cerebellum estimated by intrinsic functional connectivity. *J Neurophysiol.* 2011;106(5):2322-2345.

De Zeeuw CI, Cicirata F, eds. Creating coordination in the cerebellum. *Prog Brain Res.* 2005;148:X-XIII, 1-411.

Durr A. Autosomal dominant cerebellar ataxias: polyglutamine expansions and beyond. *Lancet Neurol.* 2010;9(9):885-894.

Highsteen SM, Thach WT, eds. The cerebellum: recent developments in cerebellar research. *Ann NY Acad Sci.* 2002;978:1-551.

Ito M. *The Cerebellum and Neural Control.* Raven Press; 1984.

Leiner HC, Leiner AL, Dow RS. Does the cerebellum contribute to mental skills? *Behav Neurosci.* 1986;100(4):443-454.

Manto MU. *Cerebellar Disorders: A Practical Approach to Diagnosis and Management.* Cambridge University Press; 2010.

Manto MU, Gruol D, Schmahmann JD, Koibuchi N, Rossi F, eds. *Handbook of the Cerebellum and Cerebellar Disorders.* Springer; 2012.

Schmahmann JD. An emerging concept: the cerebellar contribution to higher function. *Arch Neurol.* 1991;48:1178-1187.

Schmahmann JD, ed. The cerebellum and cognition. *Neurosci Lett.* 2019;688:62-75.

Schmahmann JD. Disorders of the cerebellum. Ataxia, dysmetria of thought, and the cerebellar cognitive affective syndrome. *J Neuropsychiatry Clin Neurosci.* 2004;16(3):367-378.

Schmahmann JD. The role of the cerebellum in cognition and emotion: personal reflections since 1982 on the dysmetria of thought hypothesis, and its historical evolution from theory to therapy. *Neuropsychol Rev.* 2010;20(3):236-260.

Schmahmann JD, Doyon J, Toga A, Petrides M, Evans A. *MRI Atlas of the Human Cerebellum.* Academic Press; 2000.

Schmahmann JD, Pandya DN. Anatomic organization of the basilar pontine projections from prefrontal cortices in rhesus monkey. *J Neurosci.* 1997;17:438-458.

Schmahmann JD, Pandya DN. The cerebrocerebellar system. In: Schmahmann JD, ed. *The Cerebellum and Cognition.* Academic Press; 1997.

Schmahmann JD, Sherman JC. The cerebellar cognitive affective syndrome. *Brain.* 1998;121:561-579.

Stoodley CJ, Valera EM, Schmahmann JD. Functional topography of the cerebellum for motor and cognitive tasks: an fMRI study. *NeuroImage.* 2012;59(2):1560-1570.

Strick PL, Dum RP, Fiez JA. Cerebellum and nonmotor function. *Annu Rev Neurosci.* 2009;32:413-434.

Voogd J. Cerebellar zones: a personal history. *Cerebellum.* 2011;10(3):334-350.

Voogd J, Glickstein M. The anatomy of the cerebellum. *Trends Neurosci.* 1998;21(9):370-375.

Section 9: Cerebrovascular Circulation and Stroke

Albers GW, Marks, MP, Kemp S, et al. Thrombectomy for Stroke at 6 to 16 hours with selection by perfusion imaging. *N Engl J Med.* 2018;378:708-718.

Berkefeld J, Chaturvedi S. The International Carotid Stenting Study and the North American Carotid Revascularization Endarterectomy versus Stenting Trial: fueling the debate about carotid artery stenting. *Stroke.* 2010;41:2714-2715.

Brott TG, Halperin JL, Abbara S, et al. 2011 ASA/ACCF/AHA/AANN/AANS/ACR/ASNR/CNS/SAIP/SCAI/SIR/SNIS/SVM/SVS guideline on the management of patients with extracranial carotid and vertebral artery disease. *J Am Coll Cardiol.* 2011;57(8):e16-e94.

Capecchi M, Abbattista M, Martinelli I. Cerebral venous sinus thrombosis. *J Thromb Haemost.* 2018;16(10):1918-1931.

Caplan LR, ed. *Caplan's Stroke: A Clinical Approach.* 4th ed. Saunders; 2009.

Caplan LR, Biller J. *Uncommon Causes of Stroke.* Cambridge University Press; 2018.

Caplan LR, Van Gyn J, eds. *Stroke Syndromes.* 3rd ed. Cambridge University Press; 2012.

Christensen AF, Christensen H. Editorial: Imaging in acute stroke—New options and state of art. *Front Neurol.* 2017;8:736.

Claiborne Johnston S, Amarenco P, Denison H, et al. Ticagrelor and aspirin or aspirin alone in acute ischemic stroke or TIA. *N Engl J Med.* 2020;383:207-217.

Connolly Jr ES, Rabinstein AA, Carhuapoma JR, et al. Guidelines for the management of aneurysmal subarachnoid hemorrhage: a guideline for healthcare professionals from the American Heart Association/American Stroke Association. *Stroke.* 2012;43(6):1711-1737.

Edlow JA, Caplan LR. Avoiding pitfalls in the diagnosis of subarachnoid hemorrhage. *N Engl J Med.* 2000;342(1):29-36.

Ellenbogen RG, Sekhar LN, Kitchen N. *Principles of Neurological Surgery,* 4th ed. Elsevier; 2018.

Frieden IJ, Reese V, Cohen D. PHACE syndrome. The association of posterior fossa brain malformations, hemangiomas, arterial anomalies, coarctation of the aorta and cardiac defects, and eye abnormalities. *Arch Dermatol.* 1996;132:307-311.

Goldstein LB, Bushnell CD, Adams RJ, et al. Guidelines for the primary prevention of stroke: a guideline for Healthcare Professionals from the American Heart Association/American Stroke Association. *Stroke.* 2011;42:517-584.

Grotta, JC, Albers GW, Broderick JP. *Stroke: Pathophysiology, Diagnosis, and Management.* 7th ed. Elsevier; 2021.

Halan T, Ortiz JF, Reddy D, Altamimi A, Ajibowo AO, Fabara SP. Locked-in syndrome: a systematic review of long-term management and prognosis. *Cureus.* 2021;13(7):e16727.

Harrigan MR, Deveikis JP. *Handbook of Cerebrovascular Disease and Neurointerventional Technique.* 3rd ed. Springer; 2018.

Kilburg C, McNally JS, Havernon A, et al. Advanced imaging in acute ischemic stroke. *Neurosurgical Focus.* 2017;42(4):E10.

Kleindorfer DO, Towfighi A, Chaturvedi S, et al. 2021 Guideline for the prevention of stroke in patients with stroke and transient ischemic attack: a guideline from the American Heart Association/American Stroke Association. *Stroke.* 2021;52:e364-e467.

Komatsubara I, Kondo J, Akiyama M, et al. Subclavian steal syndrome: a case report and review of advances in diagnostic and treatment approaches. *Cardiovasc Revasc Med.* 2016;17(1):54-58.

Nogueira RG, Jadhav AP, Haussen DC, et al. Thrombectomy 6 to 24 Hours after Stroke with a Mismatch between Deficit and Infarct. *N Engl J Med.* 2018;378:11-21.

Potter BJ, Pinto DS. Subclavian steal syndrome. *Circulation.* 2014;129(22):2320-2323.

Powers WJ, Rabinstein AA, Ackerson T, et al. Guidelines for the early management of patients with acute ischemic stroke: 2019 update to the 2018 guidelines for the early management of acute ischemic stroke: a guideline for healthcare professionals from the American Heart Association/American Stroke Association. *Stroke.* 2019;50(12):e344-e418.

Rantner B, Kollerits B, Roubin GS, et al. Early endarterectomy carries a lower procedural risk than early stenting in patients with symptomatic stenosis of the internal carotid artery: results from 4 randomized controlled trials. *Stroke.* 2017;48(6):1580-1587.

Salvarani, C, Brown Jr RD, Christianson TJ, et al. Adult primary central nervous system vasculitis treatment and course: analysis of one hundred sixty-three patients. *Arthritis Rheumatol.* 2015;67(6):1637-1645.

Saposnik G, Barinagarrementeria F, Brown Jr RD, et al. Diagnosis and management of cerebral venous thrombosis: a statement for healthcare professionals from the American Heart Association/American Stroke Association. *Stroke.* 2011;42(4):1158-1192.

Scott RM, Smith JL, Robertson RL, Madsen JR, Soriano SG, Rockoff MA. Long-term outcome in children with moyamoya syndrome after cranial revascularization by pial synangiosis. *J Neurosurg.* 2004;100(Suppl 2 Pediatrics):142-149.

Spence, DJ, de Freitas GR, Pettigrew LC, et al. Mechanisms of stroke in COVID-19. *Cerebrovasc Dis.* 2020;49(4):451-458.

Vagal A, Wintermark M, Nael K, et al. Automated CT perfusion imaging for acute ischemic stroke. Pearls and pitfalls for real-world use. *Neurology.* 2019;93(20):888-898.

Wardlaw JM, Brazzelli M, Chappell FM, et al. ABCD2 score and secondary stroke prevention. Meta-analysis and effect per 1,000 patients triaged. *Neurology.* 2015;85(4):373-380.

Woranush W, Moskopp ML, Sedghi A, et al. Preventive approaches for post-stroke depression: where do we stand? A systematic review. *Neuropsychiatr Dis Treat.* 2021;17:3359-3377.

Section 10: Multiple Sclerosis and Other Central Nervous System Autoimmune Disorders

Multiple Sclerosis

Batista FD, Harwood NE. The who, how and where of antigen presentation to B cells. *Nat Rev Immunol.* 2009;9:15-27.

Brinkman V. FTY720 (fingolimod) in multiple sclerosis: therapeutic effects in the immune and the central nervous system. *Br J Pharmacol.* 2009;158:1173-1182.

Crotty S. Follicular helper CD4 T cells (TFH). *Annu Rev Immunol.* 2011;29:621-663.

Dalla Libera D, Di Mitri D, Bergami A, et al. T regulatory cells are markers of disease activity in multiple sclerosis patients. *PLoS One.* 2011;6:e21386.

Davis MD, Kehrl JH. The influence of sphingosine-1-phophate receptor signaling on lymphocyte trafficking: how a bioactive lipid mediator grew up from an "immature" vascular maturation factor to a "mature" mediator of lymphocyte behavior and function. *Immunol Res.* 2009;43:187-197.

Dhib-Jalbut S, Marks S. Interferon-b mechanisms of action in multiple sclerosis. *Neurology.* 2010;74(suppl 1):S17-S24.

Fabriek BO, Zwemmer JNP, Teunissen CE, et al. In vivo detection of myelin proteins in cervical lymph nodes of MS patients using ultrasound guided fine-needle aspiration cytology. *J Neuroimmunol.* 2005;161:190-194.

Fainardi E, Rizzo R, Melchiorri L, et al. CSF levels of soluble HLA-G and Fas molecules are inversely associated to MRI evidence of disease activity in patients with relapsing remitting multiple sclerosis. *Mult Scler.* 2008;14:446-454.

Feng X, Reder NP, Yanamandala M, et al. Type I interferon is high in lupus and neuromyelitis optica but low in multiple sclerosis. *J Neurol Sci.* 2012;313:48-53.

Frischer JM, Bramow S, Dal-Bianco A, et al. The relation between inflammation and neurodegeneration in multiple sclerosis brains. *Brain.* 2009;13:1175-1189.

Gay D, Esiri M. Blood-brain barrier damage in acute multiple sclerosis plaques. *Brain.* 1991;114:557-572.

Gold R, Kappos L, Arnold D, et al. Placebo-controlled phase 3 study of oral BG-12 for relapsing-remitting multiple sclerosis. *N Engl J Med.* 2012;367(12):1098-1107.

Goodin DS, Arnason BG, Coyle PK, Frohman EM, Paty DW. The use of mitoxantrone (Novantrone) for the treatment of multiple sclerosis. *Neurology.* 2003;61:1332-1338.

Hartung HP, Freedman MS, Polman CH, et al. Interferon beta-1b-neutralizing antibodies 5 years after clinically isolated syndrome. *Neurology.* 2011;77:835-843.

Hauser SL, Waubant E, Arnold DL, et al. B-cell depletion with rituximab in relapsing-remitting multiple sclerosis. *N Engl J Med.* 2008;358:676-688.

Howell OW, Rundle JL, Garg A, et al. Activated microglia mediate axoglial disruption that contributes to axonal injury in multiple sclerosis. *J Neuropathol Exp Neurol.* 2010;69:1017-1033.

International Multiple Sclerosis Genetics Consortium, Wellcome Trust Case Control Consortium 2, Sawcer S, et al. Genetic risk and a primary role for cell-mediated immune mechanisms in multiple sclerosis. *Nature.* 2011;476:214-219.

Kappos L, Li D, Calabresi PA, et al. Ocrelizumab in relapsing-remitting multiple sclerosis: a phase 2, randomized, placebo-controlled, multicenter trial. *Lancet.* 2011;378:1779-1787.

Katakai T, Hara T, Lee JH, Gonda H, Sugai M, Shimizu A. A novel reticular stromal structure in lymph node cortex: an immuno-platform for interactions among dendritic cells, T cells and B cells. *Int Immunol.* 2004;16:1133-1142.

Kim HJ, Miron VE, Dukala D, et al. Neurobiological effects of sphingosine 1-phosphate receptor modulation in the cuprizone model. *FASEB J.* 2011;25:1509-1518.

Kitano M, Moriyama S, Ando Y, et al. Bcl6 protein expression shapes pre-germinal center B cell dynamics and follicular helper T cell heterogeneity. *Immunity.* 2011;34:961-972.

Kivisakk P, Imitola J, Rasmussen S, et al. Localizing central nervous system immune surveillance: meningeal antigen-presenting cells activate T cells during experimental autoimmune encephalomyelitis. *Ann Neurol.* 2008;65:457-469.

Kooi EJ, van Horssen J, Witte ME, et al. Abundant extracellular myelin in the meninges of patients with multiple sclerosis. *Neuropathol Appl Neurobiol.* 2009;35:283-295.

Linker RA, Lee DH, Demir S, et al. Functional role of brain-derived neurotrophic factor in neuroprotective autoimmunity: therapeutic implications in a model of multiple sclerosis. *Brain.* 2010;133:2248-2263.

Magliozzi R, Howell O, Vora A, et al. Meningeal B-cell follicles in secondary progressive multiple sclerosis associate with early onset of disease and severe cortical pathology. *Brain.* 2007;130:1089-1104.

Moore GRW, Esiri MM. The pathology of multiple sclerosis and related disorders. *Diagnostic Histopathol.* 2011;17:225-231.

Munger KL, Levin LI, O'Reilly EJ, Falk KI, Ascherio A. Anti-Epstein-Barr virus antibodies as serological markers of multiple sclerosis: a prospective study among United States military personnel. *Mult Scler.* 2011;17:1185-1193.

Murphy KM, Stockinger B. Effector T cell plasticity: flexibility in the face of changing circumstances. *Nat Immunol.* 2010;11:674-680.

Polman CH, Reingold SC, Banwell B, et al. Diagnostic criteria for multiple sclerosis: 2010 revisions to the McDonald criteria. *Ann Neurol.* 2011;69:292-302.

Prodinger C, Bunse J, Kruger M, et al. CD11c-expressing cells reside in the juxtavascular parenchyma and extend processes into the glia limitans of the mouse nervous system. *Acta Neuropathol.* 2011;121:445-458.

Racke MK, Lovett-Racke AE, Karandikar NJ. The mechanism of action of glatiramer acetate in multiple sclerosis. *Neurology.* 2010;74(suppl 1):S25-S30.

Reich DS, Lucchinetti CF, Calabresi PA. Multiple sclerosis. *N Engl J Med.* 2018;378(2):169-180.

Schreiber RD, Old LJ, Smyth MJ. Cancer immunoediting: integrating immunity's roles in cancer suppression and promotion. *Science.* 2011;331:1565-1570.

Smolders J, Damoiseaux J, Menheere P, Hupperts R. Vitamin D as an immune modulator in multiple sclerosis: a review. *J Neuroimmunol.* 2008;194:7-17.

Tennakoon DK, Mehta RS, Ortega SB, et al. Therapeutic induction of regulatory, cytotoxic, CD8^{1} T cells in multiple sclerosis. *J Immunol.* 2006;176:7119-7129.

Verhey LH, Branson HM, Shroff MM, et al. CNS: MRI parameters for prediction of multiple sclerosis diagnosis in children with acute demyelination: a prospective national cohort study. *Lancet Neurol.* 2011;10:1065-1073.

Weller RO, Galea I, Carare RO, Minagar A. Pathophysiology of the lymphatic drainage of the central nervous system: implications for pathogenesis and therapy of multiple sclerosis. *Pathophysiology.* 2010;17:295-306.

Wheeler D, Venkata V, Bandaru R, et al. A defect of sphingolipid metabolism modifies the properties of normal appearing white matter in multiple sclerosis. *Brain.* 2008;131:3092-3102.

Zhou L, Chong MMW, Littman DR. Plasticity of CD4^{1} T cell lineage differentiation. *Immunity.* 2011;30:646-655.

ADEM, Tumescent MS

Gutrecht JA, Berger JR, Jones HR, Mancall AC. Monofocal acute inflammatory demyelination (MAID): a unique disorder simulating brain neoplasm. *South Med J.* 2002;95:1180-1186.

Hurst EW. Acute haemorrhagic leucoencephalitis: a previously undefined entity. *Med J Aust.* 1941;2:1-6.

Leake JA, Billman GF, Nespeca MP, et al. Pediatric acute hemorrhagic leukoencephalitis: report of a surviving patient and review. *Clin Infect Dis.* 2002;34:699-703.

Neuromyelitis Optica

Matà S, Lolli F. Neuromyelitis optica: an update. *J Neurol Sci.* 2011;303:13-21.

Other Neuroimmunology

Darnell RB, Posner JB. *Paraneoplastic Syndromes.* Oxford University Press; 2011.

Lachance DH, Lennon VA. Paraneoplastic neurological autoimmunity. In: Kalman B, Brannagan T III, eds. *Neuroimmunology in Clinical Practice.* Blackwell Publishing Ltd; 2008:210-217.

Lachance DH, Lennon VA, Pittock SJ, et al. An outbreak of neurological autoimmunity with polyradiculoneuropathy in

workers exposed to aerosolised porcine neural tissue: a descriptive study. *Lancet Neurol*. 2010;9:55-66.
McKeon A, Pittock SJ. Paraneoplastic encephalomyelopathies: pathology and mechanisms. *Acta Neuropathol*. 2011;122:381-400.
Pittock SJ, Kryzer TJ, Lennon VA. Paraneoplastic antibodies coexist and predict cancer, not neurological syndrome. *Ann Neurol*. 2004;56(5):715-719.
Vincent A, Bien CG, Irani SR, Waters P. Autoantibodies associated with diseases of the CNS: new developments and future challenges. *Lancet Neurol*. 2011;10(8):759-772.

Stiff-Person Syndrome

Burns TM, Jones Jr HR, Phillips LH II, Bugawan TL, Erlich HA, Lennon VA. Two generations of clinically disparate stiff man syndrome confirmed by significant elevations of GAD65 autoantibodies. *Neurology*. 2003;61:1291-1293.
Mas N, Saiz A, Leite MI, et al. Antiglycine-receptor encephalomyelitis with rigidity. *J Neurol Neurosurg Psychiatry*. 2011;82:1399-1401.
McKeon A, Robinson MT, McEvoy K, et al. Stiff-man syndrome and variants. *Arch Neurol*. 2012;69:230-239.
Moersch FP, Woltman HW. Progressive fluctuating muscular rigidity and spasm ("stiff-man" syndrome): report of a case and some observations in 13 other cases. *Mayo Clin Proc*. 1956;31:421-427.

Section 11: Infections of the Nervous System

Halperin JJ. Nervous system Lyme disease: is there still a controversy? *Semin Neurol*. 2011;31:317-324.
Major EO, Yousry TA, Clifford DB. Pathogenesis of progressive multifocal leukoencephalopathy and risks associated with treatment for multiple sclerosis: a decade of lessons learned. *Lancet Neurol*. 2018;17(5):467-480.
Moore P, Esmail F, Qin S, et al. Hypercoagulability of COVID-19 and neurological complications: a review. *J Stroke Cerebrovasc Dis*. 2022:31(1):106163.
Portegies P, Berger JR, eds. *HIV/AIDS and the Nervous System. Handbook of Clinical Neurology. Vol 85*. Elsevier; 2007.
Roos KL. Neurologic complications of Lyme disease. *Continuum (Minneap Minn)*. 2021;27(4);1040-1050.
Roos KL. *Principles of Neurologic Infectious Diseases*. McGraw-Hill; 2005.
Roos KL, Tunkel AR, eds. *Bacterial Infections of the Central Nervous System. Handbook of clinical neurology. Vol 96*. Elsevier; 2010.
Thwaites GE, Fisher M, Hemingway C, British Infection Society. British Society guidelines for the diagnosis and treatment of tuberculosis of the central nervous system in adults and children. *J Infect*. 2009;59:167-187.
Tunkel AR, Glaser CA, Bloch KC, et al. The management of encephalitis: clinical practice guidelines by the Infectious Diseases Society of America. *Clin Infect Dis*. 2008;47:303-327.
Trevelyan B, Smallman-Raynor M, Cliff AD. The spatial dynamics of poliomyelitis in the United States: from epidemic emergence to vaccine-induced retreat, 1910–1971. *Ann Assoc Am Geogr*. 2005;95:269-293.
White AC, Coyle CM, Rajshekhar V, et al. Diagnosis and treatment of neurocysticercosis: 2017 clinical practice guidelines by the Infectious Diseases Society of America (IDSA) and the American Society of Tropical Medicine and Hygiene (ASTMH). *Clin Infect Dis*. 2018;66:e49-e75.

Section 12: Neuro-oncology

Amirian ES, Armstrong TS, Aldape KD, et al. Predictors of survival among pediatric and adult ependymoma cases: a study using Surveillance, Epidemiology, and End Results data from 1973 to 2007. *Neuroepidemiology*. 2012;39:116-124.
Aoyama H, Shirato H, Tago M, et al. Stereotactic radiosurgery plus whole-brain radiation therapy vs stereotactic radiosurgery alone for treatment of brain metastases: a randomized controlled trial. *JAMA*. 2006;295:2483-2491.
Brandsma D, Stalpers L, Taal W, et al. Clinical features, mechanisms, and management of pseudoprogression in malignant gliomas. *Lancet Oncol*. 2008;9:453-461.
Brat DJ, Aldape K, Colman H, et al. cIMPACT-NOW update 3: recommended diagnostic criteria for "Diffuse astrocytic glioma, IDH-wildtype, with molecular features of glioblastoma, WHO grade IV." *Acta Neuropathol*. 2018;136:805-810.
Brown PD, Gondi V, Pugh S, et al. Hippocampal avoidance during whole-brain radiotherapy plus memantine for patients with brain metastases: phase III trial NRG oncology CC001. *J Clin Oncol*. 2020;38:1019-1029.
Brown PD, Pugh S, Laack NN, et al. Memantine for the prevention of cognitive dysfunction in patients receiving whole-brain radiotherapy: a randomized, double-blind, placebo-controlled trial. *Neuro Oncol*. 2013;15:1429-1437.
Cho YJ, Tsherniak A, Tamayo P, et al. Integrative genomic analysis of medulloblastoma identifies a molecular subgroup that drives poor clinical outcome. *J Clin Oncol*. 2011;29:1424-1430.
Ellison DW, Aldape KD, Capper D, et al. cIMPACT-NOW update 7: advancing the molecular classification of ependymal tumors. *Brain Pathol*. 2020;30:863-866.
Hegi ME, Diserens AC, Gorlia T, et al. MGMT gene silencing and benefit from temozolomide in glioblastoma. *N Engl J Med*. 2005;352:997-1003.
Kalkanis SN, Kondziolka D, Gaspar LE, et al. The role of surgical resection in the management of newly diagnosed brain metastases: a systematic review and evidence-based clinical practice guideline. *J Neurooncol*. 2010;96:33-43.
Khuong-Quang DA, Buczkowicz P, Rakopoulos P, et al. K27M mutation in histone H3.3 defines clinically and biologically distinct subgroups of pediatric diffuse intrinsic pontine gliomas. *Acta Neuropathol*. 2012;124:439-447.
Louis DN, Perry A, Reifenberger G, et al. The 2016 World Health Organization classification of tumors of the central nervous system: a summary. *Acta Neuropathol*. 2016;131:803-820.
Louis DN, Perry A, Wesseling P, et al. The 2021 WHO classification of tumors of the central nervous system: a summary. *Neuro Oncol*. 2021;23:1231-1251.
Lu-Emerson C, Duda DG, Emblem KE, et al. Lessons from anti-vascular endothelial growth factor and anti-vascular endothelial growth factor receptor trials in patients with glioblastoma. *J Clin Oncol*. 2015;33:1197-1213.
Michael AP, Watson VL, Ryan D, et al. Effects of 5-ALA dose on resection of glioblastoma. *J Neurooncol*. 2019;141:523-531.
Nassiri F, Liu J, Patil V, et al. A clinically applicable integrative molecular classification of meningiomas. *Nature*. 2021;597:119-125.
Northcott PA, Korshunov A, Witt H, et al. Medulloblastoma comprises four distinct molecular variants. *J Clin Oncol* 2011;29:1408-1414.
Parsons DW, Jones S, Zhang X, et al. An integrated genomic analysis of human glioblastoma multiforme. *Science*. 2008;321:1807-1812.
Plotkin SR, Stemmer-Rachamimov AO, Barker FG II, et al. Hearing improvement after bevacizumab in patients with neurofibromatosis type 2. *N Engl J Med*. 2009;361:358-367.
Preusser M, Brastianos PK, Mawrin C. Advances in meningioma genetics: novel therapeutic opportunities. *Nat Rev Neurol*. 2018;14:106-115.
Roder C, Bisdas S, Ebner FH, et al. Maximizing the extent of resection and survival benefit of patients in glioblastoma surgery: high-field iMRI versus conventional and 5-ALA-assisted surgery. *Eur J Surg Oncol*. 2014;40:297-304.
Ruda R, Reifenberger G, Frappaz D, et al. EANO guidelines for the diagnosis and treatment of ependymal tumors. *Neuro Oncol*. 2018;20:445-456.
Stieber VW, Mehta MP. Advances in radiation therapy for brain tumors. *Neurol Clin*. 2007;25:1005-1033.
Stupp R, Hegi ME, Mason WP, et al. Effects of radiotherapy with concomitant and adjuvant temozolomide versus radiotherapy alone on survival in glioblastoma in a randomised phase III study: 5-year analysis of the EORTC-NCIC trial. *Lancet Oncol*. 2009;10:459-466.
Stupp R, Mason WP, van den Bent MJ, et al. Radiotherapy plus concomitant and adjuvant temozolomide for glioblastoma. *N Engl J Med*. 2005;352:987-996.
Stupp R, Taillibert S, Kanner A, et al. Effect of tumor-treating fields plus maintenance temozolomide vs maintenance temozolomide alone on survival in patients with glioblastoma: a randomized clinical trial. *JAMA*. 2017;318:2306-2316.
Stupp R, Wong ET, Kanner AA, et al. NovoTTF-100A versus physician's choice chemotherapy in recurrent glioblastoma: a randomised phase III trial of a novel treatment modality. *Eur J Cancer*. 2012;48:2192-2202.
Tawbi HA, Forsyth PA, Algazi A, et al. Combined Nivolumab and Ipilimumab in melanoma metastatic to the brain. *N Engl J Med*. 2018;379:722-730.
Verhaak RG, Hoadley KA, Purdom E, et al. Integrated genomic analysis identifies clinically relevant subtypes of glioblastoma characterized by abnormalities in PDGFRA, IDH1, EGFR, and NF1. *Cancer Cell*. 2010;17:98-110.
Wen PY, Weller M, Lee EQ, et al. Glioblastoma in adults: a Society for Neuro-Oncology (SNO) and European Society of Neuro-Oncology (EANO) consensus review on current management and future directions. *Neuro Oncol*. 2020;22:1073-1113.

Section 13: Headache

Burch RC, Buse DC, Lipton RB. Migraine: epidemiology, burden, and comorbidity. *Neurol Clin*. 2019;37(4):631-649.
Goadsby PJ, Holland PR. An update: pathophysiology of migraine. *Neurol Clin*. 2019;37(4):651-671.
Hadjikhani N, Sanchez Del Rio M, Wu O, et al. Mechanisms of migraine aura revealed by functional MRI in human visual cortex. *Proc Natl Acad Sci U S A*. 2001;98:4687-4692.
Headache Classification Committee of the International Headache Society (IHS). The International Classification of Headache Disorders, 3rd edition. *Cephalalgia*. 2018;38:1-211.
Lagman-Bartolome AM, Lay C. Pediatric migraine variants: a review of epidemiology, diagnosis, treatment, and outcome. *Curr Neurol Neurosci Rep*. 2015;15(6):34.
Loder E, Rizzoli P. Tension-type headache. *BMJ*. 2008;336:88-92.
Pascual J, Gonzalez-Mandly A, Oterino A, Martin R. Primary cough headache, primary exertional headache, and primary headache associated with sexual activity. *Handb Clin Neurol*. 2010;97:459-468.
Robbins MS. Diagnosis and management of headache: a review. *JAMA*. 2021;325(18):1874-1885.
Robertson C. Cranial Neuralgias. *Continuum (Minneap Minn)*. 2021;27(3):665-685.
Schwedt TJ. Thunderclap headaches: a focus on etiology and diagnostic evaluation. *Headache*. 2013;53(3):563-569.
Schievink WI. Spontaneous intracranial hypotension. *N Engl J Med*. 2021;385:2173-2178.
Silberstein SD, Lipton RB, Dodick DW, eds. *Wolff's Headache and Other Head Pain*. 8th ed. Oxford University Press; 2007.
Tfelt-Hansen PC. History of migraine with aura and cortical spreading depression from 1941 and onwards. *Cephalalgia*. 2010;30:780-792.
Wei DY, Khalil M, Goadsby PJ. Managing cluster headache. *Pract Neurol*. 2019;19:521-528.

Section 14: Head Trauma

Badjatia N, Carney N, Crocco TJ, et al. Brain Trauma Foundation; BTF Center for Guidelines Management. Guidelines for prehospital management of traumatic brain injury 2nd ed. *Prehosp Emerg Care*. 2008;12(suppl 1):S1-S52.
Brain Trauma Foundation. *Guidelines for the Management of Severe Traumatic Brain Injury*. 4th ed. 2016. Available at: https://braintrauma.org/coma/guidelines/guidelines-for-the-management-of-severe-tbi-4th-ed.
Brain Trauma Foundation; American Association of Neurological Surgeons; Congress of Neurological Surgeons; Joint Section on Neurotrauma and Critical Care, AANS/CNS, Bratton SL, Chesnut RM, Ghajar J, et al. Guidelines for the management of severe traumatic brain injury. XV. Steroids. *J Neurotrauma*. 2007;24(suppl 1):S91-S95.
Brain Trauma Foundation; American Association of Neurological Surgeons; Congress of Neurological Surgeons; Joint Section on Neurotrauma and Critical Care, AANS/CNS, Bratton SL, Chestnut RM, Ghajar J, et al. Guidelines for the management of severe traumatic brain injury. XIV. Hyperventilation. *J Neurotrauma*. 2007;24(suppl 1):S87-S90.
Bullock MR, Chesnut R, Ghajar J, et al. Surgical management of acute epidural hematomas. *Neurosurgery*. 2006;58(suppl 3):S7-S15.
Bullock MR, Chesnut R, Ghajar J, et al. Surgical management of acute subdural hematomas. *Neurosurgery*. 2006;58(suppl 3):S16-S24.
Bullock MR, Chesnut R, Ghajar J, et al. Surgical management of depressed cranial fractures. *Neurosurgery*. 2006;58(suppl 3):S56-S60.
Bullock MR, Chesnut R, Ghajar J, et al. Surgical management of traumatic parenchymal lesions. *Neurosurgery*. 2006;58(suppl 3):S25-S46.
Gabriel EJ, Ghajar J, Jagoda A, et al. Guidelines for prehospital management of traumatic brain injury. *J Neurotrauma*. 2002;19:111-174.
Godoy DA, Rabinstein AA. How to manage traumatic brain injury without invasive monitoring? *Curr Opin Crit Care*. 2022;28(2):111-122.
Hawryluk GWJ, Rubiano AM, Totten AM, et al. Guidelines for the management of severe tbi: 2020 update of the decompressive craniectomy recommendations. *Neurosurgery*. 2020;87:427-434.
Isokuortti H, Iverson GL, Silverberg ND, et al. Characterizing the type and location of intracranial abnormalities in mild traumatic brain injury. *Neurosurgery*. 2022;90:170-179.
Jha RM, Kochanek PM, Simard JM. Pathophysiology and treatment of cerebral edema in traumatic brain injury. *Neuropharmacology*. 2019;145:230-246.
Mangat HS. Severe traumatic brain injury. *Continuum (Minneap Minn)*. 2012;18:532-546.
Marion DW. Evidenced-based guidelines for traumatic brain injuries. *Prog Neurol Surg*. 2006;19:171-196.
van Essen TA, den Boogert HF, Cnossen MC, et al. Variation in neurosurgical management of traumatic brain injury: a survey in 68 centers participating in the CENTER-TBI study. *Acta Neurochir (Wien)*. 2019;161(3):435-449.
Whitehouse DP, Vile AR, Adatia K, et al. Blood biomarkers and structural imaging correlations post-traumatic brain injury: a systematic review. *Neurosurgery*. 2022;90:170-179.